W9-AZG-214

MEDICAID SOURCE BOOK: BACKGROUND DATA AND ANALYSIS
(A 1993 Update)

A REPORT

PREPARED BY THE

CONGRESSIONAL RESEARCH SERVICE

FOR THE USE OF THE

SUBCOMMITTEE ON HEALTH AND THE ENVIRONMENT

OF THE

COMMITTEE ON ENERGY AND COMMERCE
U.S. HOUSE OF REPRESENTATIVES

JANUARY 1993

U.S. GOVERNMENT PRINTING OFFICE
WASHINGTON : 1993

61-899

For sale by the U.S. Government Printing Office
Superintendent of Documents, Mail Stop: SSOP, Washington, DC 20402-9328
ISBN 0-16-039943-2

LETTER OF TRANSMITTAL

ONE HUNDRED SECOND CONGRESS

HENRY A. WAXMAN, CALIFORNIA, CHAIRMAN

GERRY SIKORSKI, MINNESOTA
TERRY L. BRUCE, ILLINOIS
J. ROY ROWLAND, GEORGIA
EDOLPHUS TOWNS, NEW YORK
GERRY E. STUDDS, MASSACHUSETTS
PETER H. KOSTMAYER, PENNSYLVANIA
JAMES H. SCHEUER, NEW YORK
MIKE SYNAR, OKLAHOMA
RON WYDEN, OREGON
RALPH M. HALL, TEXAS
BILL RICHARDSON, NEW MEXICO
JOHN BRYANT, TEXAS
JOHN D. DINGELL, MICHIGAN
(EX OFFICIO)

WILLIAM E. DANNEMEYER, CALIFORNIA
THOMAS J. BLILEY, JR., VIRGINIA
JACK FIELDS, TEXAS
MICHAEL BILIRAKIS, FLORIDA
ALEX McMILLAN, NORTH CAROLINA
J. DENNIS HASTERT, ILLINOIS
CLYDE C. HOLLOWAY, LOUISIANA
NORMAN F. LENT, NEW YORK
(EX OFFICIO)

KAREN NELSON, STAFF DIRECTOR

U.S. HOUSE OF REPRESENTATIVES

COMMITTEE ON ENERGY AND COMMERCE

SUBCOMMITTEE ON HEALTH AND THE ENVIRONMENT

2415 RAYBURN HOUSE OFFICE BUILDING
WASHINGTON, DC 20515
PHONE (202) 225-4952

December 23, 1992

Honorable John D. Dingell
Chairman
Committee on Energy and Commerce
U.S. House of Representatives
Washington, D.C.   20515

Dear Mr. Chairman:

I am enclosing for your review a report entitled The Medicaid Source Book: Background Data and Analysis, which was prepared at the request of the Subcommittee on Health and the Environment by the Education and Public Welfare Division of the Congressional Research Service.

As you know, the Subcommittee has jurisdiction over Medicaid, our nation's largest source of health care financing for the poor. In FY 1993, according to the Congressional Budget Office, the Federal and State governments will spend an estimated $140.9 billion to purchase basic health care services on behalf of some 34.4 million low-income people. How Medicaid and the populations it serves are to be treated is an issue central to the design of any health care reform plan.

This report is a revision of a similar report issued by the Subcommittee in November, 1988, which has come to be known as the "Yellow Book." I am confident that this updated version will be of great value not only to Members, but also to program administrators, policy analysts, and others. This document merits widespread distribution, and I therefore request that it be published as a Committee Print.

Sincerely,

HENRY A. WAXMAN, Chairman

Congressional Research Service • The Library of Congress • Washington, D.C. 20540

December 23, 1992

Honorable Henry A. Waxman,
Chairman, Subcommittee on
  Health and the Environment
Committee on Energy and Commerce
House of Representatives
Washington D.C. 20515

Dear Mr. Chairman:

     I am pleased to submit to you this report, *Medicaid Source Book: Background Data and Analysis*, in response to your request for a comprehensive study on Medicaid. As you know, the Congressional Research Service prepared a similar study in 1988 for the Subcommittee. However, Medicaid has changed significantly over the last 4 years. Eligibility rules have changed and the program has experienced historical increases in the number of beneficiaries and spending. Financing and reimbursement policies have been examined, and questioned. The program has been changed by the Congress, the executive branch, State legislatures and administrators. All of these differences called for another examination of the program.

     Like the earlier version of this report, the research team assigned to this project attempted to produce a comprehensive, easy to understand document, one that would help the requesting Subcommittee and the Congress discern the many intricacies of Medicaid and potential sources of future program issues.

     We hope this report will be useful to Members of your Subcommittee and to the Congress in their deliberations and consideration of legislation affecting the program.

Sincerely,

Joseph E. Ross
Director

(v)

PREFACE

Medicaid, the means-tested entitlement program that finances medical assistance to persons with low income, has been controversial in recent years. For some, the program is viewed as an important source of health insurance for people with limited means to acquire coverage, and a potential source for the 35 million Americans currently estimated to be without health insurance. For others, the program is viewed as a drain on State and Federal budgets because of its recent 20 to 30 percent annual spending increases.

Medicaid is financed by Federal and State funds. Federal contributions to each State are based in part on a State's willingness to finance covered medical services and a matching formula. Each State designs and administers its own program under the general oversight of the Health Care Financing Administration (HCFA), Department of Health and Human Services (HHS). In FY 1992, it is estimated that total Federal and State spending on Medicaid will be about $119 billion. No other means-tested cash or noncash program comes close to approaching this spending level. In fact, of all federally supported social welfare programs, only Social Security and Medicare spend more.

To many the program is an enigma. The program's complexity surrounding who is eligible, what services will be paid for, and how those services can be paid for is one source of confusion. State Medicaid plan variability is the rule rather than the exception. For example, income eligibility levels vary, the services covered vary, and the amount of reimbursement for the services vary from State to State. The program acts as a form of health insurance providing access to health services traditionally covered by private health insurance. However, it also provides payment for services such as nursing homes and community-based long-term care, services that have traditionally been outside the umbrella of private insurance. Furthermore, Medicaid is a program that is targeted at individuals with low incomes; but not all the poor are covered, and not all who are covered are poor.

Over the 4 years since the original *Medicaid Source Book* was published, the program has undergone significant change. For example, eligibility criteria for the program have changed. Partly as a result of the changes, the number of beneficiaries has increased from 22.5 million in 1986 to 28.3 million in 1991. More States are offering optional Medicaid services. Furthermore, innovations in the types of services provided under the program have continued and become more widespread. For example, spending on home and community-based waiver programs, which provide services to those with chronic ailments in noninstitutional settings, has increased from $406 million in 1986 to $1.2 billion in 1991. The adequacy of State reimbursement rates for hospitals and nursing homes has been questioned. Numerous lawsuits have been filed calling for increased reimbursement rates.

PURPOSE AND SCOPE OF STUDY

Like the previous *Medicaid Source Book*, the main purpose of this report is to help answer some of the more frequently asked questions about the Medicaid program. The complexity of Medicaid presents an enormous challenge to anyone attempting to make generalizations about the program. Perhaps because of this complexity, there has not been one single source that explains the program's major components. This report attempts to provide answers to some of the more basic questions about the program:

- Who is eligible for Medicaid?

- What services are covered?

- How is the program administered? How is the program financed?

- What does the program's recent spending trend look like? What might it look like in the future?

- What is the controversy surrounding States' use of provider donations and provider specific taxes as program revenue sources?

- How have recent legislative actors changed Medicaid?

- How does the program address the needs of special populations like the mentally ill, the mentally retarded, individuals with AIDS, and individuals with substance abuse problems?

- What is a Medicaid "waiver"? Who receives these "waiver" services and how has "waiver" spending changed over time?

In order to answer these and other questions, this report is organized into three parts. The first part (chapters I through XI) describes how the Medicaid program works. This section of the report begins with an overview that provides a primer on the program. The overview is followed by a discussion on trends in spending, eligibility, services, reimbursement, alternate delivery options and waivers, administration, and financing. The first section ends with a compendium on legislative changes since 1980, a chapter dealing with current (fiscal year 1991) program beneficiary and payment statistics, and a selected bibliography.

The second part of the report (appendices A through F) describes Medicaid's effect on specific groups. Appendix A provides estimates of the Medicaid coverage rate of the poor and adds a discussion on the uninsured. Appendix B describes Medicaid's recent emphasis on prenatal care and how the program affects young children. Appendix C explores Medicaid's important role as a primary source of payment for long-term care and its use by the aged. Appendix D underlines the increasing role of community-based care for those who are developmentally disabled and the continued substantial spending on institutional services. Appendix E describes the rules associated with institutions for mental disease and how they affect the program's support of services for those with mental illness. Appendix F endeavors to explore Medicaid's role in providing substance abuse treatment services.

The third part of the report (appendices G through I) provides insight into a number of timely topics. Appendix G discusses the topic of managed care, a method used in some States to provide access to the health care system as well as to control costs. Appendix H describes Medicaid as a form of health insurance. This appendix explores Medicaid's role in allowing access to health care services. Finally, appendix I examines the effect of the HIV epidemic on Medicaid.

In order to help the readers find their way through the labyrinth of information in this report, we have made some changes from the 1988 version. First, the overview chapter has been restructured. The primary purpose of this chapter is to provide a complete and easy to understand description of Medicaid without forcing the reader to understand all the program's details. Second, the eligibility chapter has been rewritten to reflect how specific groups of persons (children, women, the disabled, and the aged) qualify for Medicaid. In the previous edition, the discussion paralleled the eligibility classifications in Medicaid law. This new approach highlights the many different ways particular individuals can meet the program's eligibility criteria. Finally, we have added a chapter discussing Medicaid and substance abuse treatment.

DATA SOURCES

There is no single primary source to turn to in describing the Medicaid program. Program statistics are collected by the States on a number of different HCFA forms. Often, the accounting methods and categories used on each of these forms differ. In some instances HCFA needs to estimate information because State provided information is unavailable or incomplete. In order to provide a comprehensive description of the program this report relies on a number of different HCFA data sources. Beneficiary and payment information for fiscal years 1975 through 1991 is based on data provided to HCFA using the *Statistical Report on Medical Care: Eligibles, Recipients, Payments and Services*. This report is commonly referred to by its form number, HCFA Form 2082. Information from this data source was augmented by spending information contained in *State Quarterly Statements of Medicaid Expenditures for the Medical Assistance Program*, HCFA Form 64. Projected and estimated spending trends were provided to us by the Congressional Budget Office (CBO). Additional historical outlay information was obtained from the Office of Management and Budget.

Estimates on Medicaid coverage of the poor and the number of people without health insurance are based on an analysis of the March Current Population Survey annual supplement of income. This supplement provides information on an individual's income and selected program participation for the previous calendar year. Information contained in this report relies on these March supplements from 1980 through 1992. Questionnaire and other technical changes took place over the course of the 12 years covered by the data series and are noted in appendix A.

It should be noted that there is no single and comprehensive source on Medicaid program characteristics in each of the States. Information contained in this report relies on data collected by HCFA and a special survey of eligibility and service characteristics commissioned by the Congressional Research Service (CRS) and performed by the National Governors' Association.

Each of these data sources has its own strengths and weaknesses. Using these rather distinct sources the study confirms previous findings about the program, and questions "common folklore" about how the program currently works.

ACKNOWLEDGMENTS

A team of CRS analysts worked together and agreed on the scope and methods employed in describing the Medicaid program in this report. The authors of the report are noted at the beginning of each chapter. The project was directed by Richard Rimkunas. The principal authors include: Mark Merlis, Jennifer O'Sullivan, Richard Price, Richard Rimkunas, Edward Klebe, Melvina Ford, Mary Smith, Dawn Nuschler, and Madeleine Smith. Research assistance was provided by Dawn Nuschler. Mike O'Grady helped in the analysis of Current Population Survey data. Gene Falk helped in exploring how Medicaid fits into the Federal budget process. Mark Merlis needs to be singled out as a continual source of expertise and encouragement in helping us all understand the inner workings of this complicated program. Dawn Nuschler provided a quiet strength, helping with every research task she could: from data gathering, to questioning analytic points and helping support staff with the monumental effort of putting this report together.

The authors make up only one component of a skilled research and production team. At CRS, production of the report was enhanced by the reliable and patient team of Phillip Brogsdale, Waymond Elliott, Flora Dean, and Brenda Freeman. Janet Kline, Ken Cahill, and Earl Canfield of the Education and Public Welfare Division helped throughout many stages of this report: encouraging staff to explore new approaches, providing necessary support to accomplish our task, and providing insightful review comments. The CRS team was further supported by the work of Mike Flanigan, printing editor of the House Energy and Commerce Committee, and his colleagues.

The authors would like to acknowledge the help, encouragement (and patience!) of majority and minority staff of the House Subcommittee on Health and the Environment, and the Senate Finance Committee. Many of the innovations in this version of the report were hatched after discussions with this group.

This report could not be completed without the help and insight of a number of individuals outside CRS. The list of analysts who provided information to individual authors is long. Officials at HCFA cooperated with this research effort by providing program data and some important insights into the program. Analysts at CBO, notably Jean Hearne and Pat Purcell, provided cost estimates and budget projections. The State Medicaid Information Center, National Governors' Association provided the research team with information on eligibility and service characteristics. Information on county contributions to State Medicaid financing was graciously provided by Kathy Gramp, National Association of Counties.

Time and space force this list of acknowledgments to be short. The authors benefitted from informal discussions and insightful writings of many Medicaid experts. Their assistance is greatly appreciated.

CONTENTS

CHAPTER II. TRENDS IN MEDICAID PAYMENTS
AND BENEFICIARIES

CHAPTER III. ELIGIBILITY

CHAPTER IV. SERVICES

CHAPTER V. REIMBURSEMENT

CHAPTER VIII. FINANCING

CHAPTER IX. RECENT LEGISLATIVE HISTORY

APPENDIX B. MEDICAID AND MATERNAL
AND CHILD HEALTH

APPENDIX E. MEDICAID SERVICES FOR
THE MENTALLY ILL

APPENDIX F. MEDICAID SERVICES FOR SUBSTANCE ABUSE TREATMENT

APPENDIX I. MEDICAID AND HIV DISEASE

LIST OF TABLES

LIST OF FIGURES

CHAPTER I. OVERVIEW[1]

Medicaid is a joint Federal-State entitlement program that pays for medical services on behalf of certain groups of low-income persons. The program was enacted in 1965, in the same legislation that created the Federal Medicare program for the aged and disabled. Medicaid is estimated to have served 31.4 million persons in FY 1992, at a combined cost to the Federal, State, and local governments of $118.8 billion, about 15 percent of total national health spending. (Figure I-1 shows the relative size of Medicaid and other public and private sources of health spending in calendar year 1990.)

The Federal share of Medicaid spending in FY 1992 is estimated to have been $67.8 billion, about 57 percent of the total, with State and local governments paying the remainder. Medicaid is the third largest social program in the Federal budget, exceeded only by Social Security and Medicare. It is also one of the fastest growing components of Federal and State budgets.

This overview begins with a basic explanation of how Medicaid works: who is covered, what services they may receive, and how the program operates and is financed. This is followed by a history of the program and a more detailed look at the program's performance in serving its targeted populations. The last section summarizes trends that may affect the program in the near future.

I. BASIC PROGRAM DESCRIPTION

Medicaid is administered by the States with partial Federal funding. Each State designs its own program within Federal guidelines.[2] States must provide Medicaid to certain population groups and have the option of covering others. Similarly, a State must cover certain basic services and may cover additional services if it chooses. States set their own payment rates for services, with some limitations. There is thus considerable variation in Medicaid programs; some are relatively limited, others very generous. Over the last decade, Congress has gradually expanded the minimum standards that all States must meet. Still, the program is by no means uniform across States.

---

[1]This chapter was written by Mark Merlis.

[2]Arizona is the only State without a Medicaid program. Since 1982, it has received Federal funds under a demonstration waiver for an alternative medical assistance program for low-income persons, the Arizona Health Care Cost Containment System, or AHCCCS.

FIGURE I-1. National Health Expenditures by Payer, CY 1990

Total spending = $666.2 billion

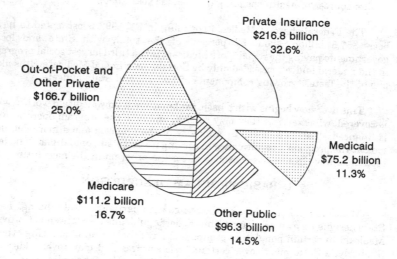

Private Insurance
$216.8 billion
32.6%

Out-of-Pocket and
Other Private
$166.7 billion
25.0%

Medicaid
$75.2 billion
11.3%

Medicare
$111.2 billion
16.7%

Other Public
$96.3 billion
14.5%

Source: Figure prepared by Congressional Research Service based on data from HCFA.

The following discussion provides basic information about program eligibility, covered services, payment for services, and alternative delivery and payment systems. It also provides an overview of Medicaid administration and financing.

A. Eligibility for Medicaid Benefits

Medicaid is a means-tested program. Applicants' income and other resources must be within program financial standards.[3] These standards vary among States, and different standards apply to different population groups within a State. With some exceptions, Medicaid is available only to persons with very low incomes. However, Medicaid does not cover everyone who is poor. Only 47 percent of persons in poverty received Medicaid benefits at any time during 1990. There are two basic reasons for this. First, many types of applicants must meet income limits that are based on cash welfare standards and are usually well below the poverty level. Second, Medicaid eligibility is subject to *categorical restrictions*.

Medicaid is available only to members of families with children and pregnant women, and to persons who are aged, blind, or disabled. Persons not falling into those categories--such as single adults and childless couples--cannot qualify, no matter how low their income is. Even within the covered groups there are categorical distinctions that are based on those traditionally used in cash assistance (welfare) programs. For example, all the members of a single-parent family may receive Medicaid. In a two-parent family with one parent working full time, only the children may receive continuous coverage; the mother is eligible only during pregnancy, and the father is never eligible.

The Medicaid statute defines over 50 distinct population groups as potentially eligible, including those for which coverage is mandatory in all States and those that may be covered at a State's option. The various eligibility groups have traditionally been divided into two basic classes, the "categorically needy" and the "medically needy." The two terms once distinguished between welfare-related beneficiaries and those qualifying only under special Medicaid rules. However, nonwelfare groups have been added to the "categorically needy" list over the years. As a result, the terms are no longer especially helpful in sorting out the various populations for whom mandatory or optional Medicaid coverage has been made available, and some analysts believe they should be abandoned. However, the distinction between the categorically and medically needy is still an important one, because the scope of covered services that States must provide to the categorically needy is much broader than the minimum scope of services for the medically needy (see the discussion of service requirements in the next section).

Despite the complexity of Medicaid eligibility, most of the coverage categories fall into six basic groups:

---

[3]"Resources" include bank accounts and similar liquid assets, as well as real estate, automobiles, and other personal property whose value exceeds specified limits.

- *Current and some former recipients of cash assistance*, either Aid to Families with Dependent Children (AFDC), which covers single-parent families and two-parent families with an unemployed principal earner, or Supplemental Security Income (SSI), which covers low-income persons who are aged, blind, or disabled. All recipients of AFDC receive Medicaid automatically, as do SSI recipients in all but a few States. AFDC and SSI recipients account for 61 percent of Medicaid beneficiaries. Medicaid is also available to some persons whose cash assistance has been terminated or who fail to receive cash assistance for technical reasons.

- *Low-income pregnant women and children* who do not qualify for AFDC, either because their income is too high or because they fail to meet the program's categorical restrictions. Coverage of some children in this category (the "Ribicoff children") was made optional when Medicaid was first enacted in 1965. As will be discussed below, expansion of mandatory and optional coverage for non-AFDC pregnant women and children was a major theme of Medicaid legislation in the 1980s.

- *The medically needy*, persons who do not meet the financial standards for cash assistance programs but meet the categorical standards and have income and resources within special medically needy limits established by the States. Persons whose incomes or resources are above those standards may qualify by "spending down," incurring medical bills that reduce their income and/or resources to the necessary levels. Coverage of the medically needy is optional; as of October 1991, 41 States and other jurisdictions covered at least some groups of the medically needy.

- *Persons requiring institutional care*. Special eligibility rules apply to persons receiving care in nursing facilities (NFs) or intermediate care facilities for the mentally retarded (ICFs/MR) or who are participating in alternative community care programs for the aged and disabled. Many of these persons may have incomes well above the poverty level but qualify for Medicaid because of the very high cost of their care.

- *Low-income Medicare beneficiaries*. Medicaid pays required Medicare premiums, deductibles, and coinsurance on behalf of low-income aged and disabled Medicare beneficiaries. (Coverage is restricted to Medicare cost-sharing unless the beneficiary also qualifies for Medicaid in some other way.)

- *Low-income persons losing employer coverage* and entitled to purchase continuation coverage through the employer's group health plan under the provisions of the Consolidated Omnibus Budget Reconciliation Act of 1985 (COBRA, Public Law 99-272). At the State's option, Medicaid may pay the premiums for continued private coverage on behalf of certain individuals.

Figures I-2 and I-3 show two different ways of grouping the 28.3 million persons receiving Medicaid benefits in FY 1991. Because of limitations in the data reported by States, neither corresponds to the groupings listed above (or to those in Medicaid law). Figure I-2 classes beneficiaries into those receiving AFDC or SSI, the medically needy, and non-AFDC or SSI groups. The latter would include low-income pregnant women and children and low-income Medicare beneficiaries qualifying under recent Medicaid expansions, as well as persons eligible under the special rules for institutional care. Figure I-3 classes beneficiaries by demographic group.[4]

The following discussion provides a more detailed look at the various populations eligible for Medicaid. It describes the mandatory and optional coverage groups under four broad headings (families, pregnant women, and children; aged and disabled; the medically needy; and persons receiving institutional or other long-term care), along with the COBRA premium payment option.

1. Families, Pregnant Women and Children

Medicaid-eligible families, pregnant women, and children fall into two basic groups: those receiving AFDC or meeting AFDC standards, and those qualifying under the series of targeted Medicaid expansions that began in the 1980s.

a. AFDC-Related Groups

States must provide Medicaid to families receiving AFDC benefits, and eligibility for some other groups is tied to AFDC standards. Each State sets its own income limits for AFDC. As of January 1992, limits on countable income for a family of three ranged from $1,440 per year in Alabama to $11,088 per year in Alaska. The median State's limit was $4,464, or 38 percent of the Federal poverty level for a family of three.[5]

Mandatory. States must provide Medicaid to all persons receiving cash assistance under AFDC, as well as to additional AFDC-related groups who are not actually receiving cash payments. (Examples include persons who do not receive a payment because the amount would be less than $10 and persons whose payments are reduced to zero because of recovery of previous overpayments.)

---

[4]The large number of beneficiaries shown as "other/unknown" in both figures is the result of inconsistencies in State reporting practices. Many of the beneficiaries in this group are Ribicoff children.

[5]U.S. Congress. House. Committee on Ways and Means. *Overview of Entitlement Programs (1992 Green Book).* Committee Print 102-44, 102d Cong., 2d Sess. Washington, GPO, May 1992. p. 636-637. (House Ways and Means Committee, *1992 Green Book*)

FIGURE I-2. Medicaid Beneficiaries by Assistance Status, FY 1991

Total beneficiaries = 28.3 million

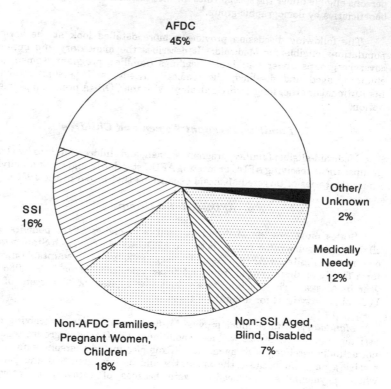

AFDC
45%

SSI
16%

Other/
Unknown
2%

Medically
Needy
12%

Non-AFDC Families,
Pregnant Women,
Children
18%

Non-SSI Aged,
Blind, Disabled
7%

NOTE: The total number of beneficiaries shown is an unduplicated total.
Source: Figure prepared by Congressional Research Service based on data from HCFA.

FIGURE I-3. Medicaid Beneficiaries
by Basis of Eligibility, FY 1991

Total beneficiaries = 28.3 million

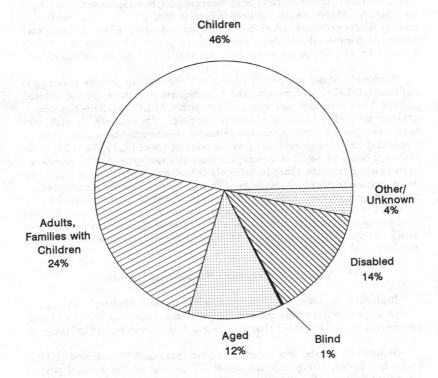

NOTE: The total number of beneficiaries shown is an unduplicated total.
Source: Figure prepared by Congressional Research Service based on data from HCFA.

States are required to continue Medicaid for specified periods for certain families losing AFDC benefits after receiving them in at least 3 of the preceding 6 months. If the family loses AFDC benefits because of increased earnings or hours of employment, Medicaid coverage must be extended for 12 months. (During the second 6 months a premium may be imposed, the scope of benefits may be limited, or alternate delivery systems may be used.) If the family loses AFDC because of increased child or spousal support, coverage must be extended for 4 months. States are also required to furnish Medicaid to certain two-parent families whose principal earner is unemployed and who are not receiving cash assistance because the State is one of those permitted (under the Family Support Act of 1988) to set a time limit on AFDC coverage for such families.

Optional. States are permitted, but not required, to provide coverage to additional AFDC-related groups. The most important of these are the "Ribicoff children," whose income and resources are within AFDC standards but who do not meet the AFDC definition of "dependent child." For example, the child may be in a two-parent family where the principal breadwinner is not unemployed. States may cover these children up to a maximum age of 18, 19, 20, or 21, at the State's option, and may limit coverage to reasonable subgroups, such as children in two-parent families, those in privately subsidized foster care, or those who live in certain institutional settings. (This group will become largely obsolete as States are required to phase in coverage of children under age 19 with incomes below poverty. However, some States may still choose to cover Ribicoff children aged 19 and 20.) States may also furnish Medicaid to persons who would receive AFDC if the State's AFDC program were as broad as permitted under Federal law.

b. Non-AFDC Pregnant Women and Children

Beginning in 1984, Congress gradually extended Medicaid coverage to groups of pregnant women and children who are defined in terms of family income and resources, rather than in terms of their ties to the AFDC program.

Mandatory. States are required to cover pregnant women and children under age 6 with family incomes below 133 percent of the Federal poverty income guidelines. (The State may impose a resource standard that is no more restrictive than that for SSI, in the case of pregnant women, or AFDC, in the case of children.) Coverage for pregnant women is limited to services related to the pregnancy or complications of the pregnancy; children receive full Medicaid coverage.

Effective July 1, 1991, States are also required to cover all children who are under age 19, who were born after September 30, 1983, and whose family income is below 100 percent of the Federal poverty level. (Coverage of such children through age 7 has been optional since Omnibus Budget Reconciliation Act of 1987 (OBRA 87).) The 1983 start date means that coverage of 18 year olds will take effect during FY 2002.

Optional. States are permitted, but not required, to cover pregnant women and infants under 1 year old with incomes below a State-established maximum that is above 133 percent of the poverty level but no more than 185 percent. As of January 1992, 30 States had made use of this option; 23 had set their income limits at the maximum of 185 percent.[6]

Figure I-4 shows the maximum income eligibility thresholds for children through age 19.

2. Aged and Disabled Persons

a. SSI-Related Groups

SSI was established in 1972, replacing previous federally funded cash assistance programs for the aged, blind, and disabled. Income and resource standards are defined by Federal law. For 1992 the maximum income is $442 per month for an individual and $653 for a couple (higher limits apply to persons with wage income). However, States have the option of supplementing SSI payments for aged persons living independently, resulting in income maximums above the Federal limits. All but nine States or jurisdictions do so. In the States with supplements, the median resulting increase in 1992 income limits was $32 per month for an individual.[7]

Mandatory. States are generally required to cover recipients of SSI. However, States may use more restrictive eligibility standards for Medicaid than those for SSI if they were using those standards on January 1, 1972 (before the implementation of SSI). States that have chosen to apply more restrictive standards are known as "section 209(b)" States, after the section of the Social Security Amendments of 1972 (Public Law 92-603) that established the option. There are 12 section 209(b) States:

Connecticut	Minnesota	North Dakota
Hawaii	Missouri	Ohio
Illinois	New Hampshire	Oklahoma
Indiana	North Carolina	Virginia

These States may use different definitions of disability, more restrictive income and resource limits, or methodologies for determining income and resources different from those used under SSI. States using more restrictive income standards must allow applicants to "spend down": deduct incurred medical expenses from income before determining eligibility. For example, if an applicant has a monthly income of $600 (not including any SSI or State supplement payment (SSP)) and the State's maximum allowable income is $500, the applicant would be required to incur $100 in medical expenses before qualifying for Medicaid. As will be discussed below, the spend-down process is also used in establishing medically needy eligibility.

---

[6]National Governors' Association.

[7]House Ways and Means Committee, *1992 Green Book*, p. 791.

FIGURE I-4. Income Eligibility Thresholds for Medicaid Coverage of Non-AFDC Children, July 1992

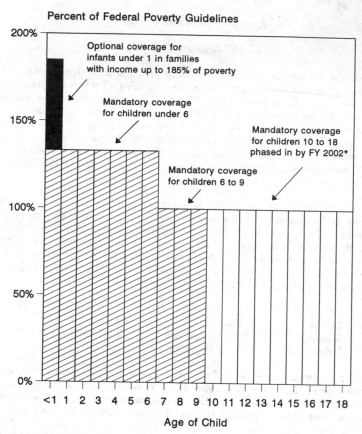

*Phased in coverage for children born after September 30, 1983.

Source: Figure prepared by Congressional Research Service.

States must continue Medicaid coverage for several defined groups of individuals who have lost SSI or SSP eligibility. The "qualified severely impaired" are disabled persons who have returned to work and have lost eligibility as a result of employment earnings, but still have the condition that originally rendered them disabled and meet all nondisability criteria for SSI except income. Medicaid must be continued if such an individual needs continued medical assistance to continue employment and the individual's earnings are not sufficient to provide the equivalent of SSI, Medicaid, and attendant care benefits the individual would qualify for in the absence of earnings. States must also continue Medicaid coverage for persons who were once eligible for both SSI and Social Security payments and who lose SSI because of a cost of living adjustment (COLA) in their Social Security benefits. Similar Medicaid continuations have been provided for certain other persons who lose SSI as a result of eligibility for or increases in Social Security or veterans' benefits. Finally, States must continue Medicaid for certain SSI-related groups who received benefits in 1973, including "essential persons" (persons who care for a disabled individual).

Optional. States are permitted to provide Medicaid to individuals who are not receiving SSI but are receiving State-only supplementary cash payments.

b. *Qualified Medicare Beneficiaries*

States must provide limited Medicaid coverage for "qualified Medicare beneficiaries" (QMBs). These are aged and disabled persons who are receiving Medicare, whose income is below 100 percent of the Federal poverty level, and whose resources do not exceed twice the allowable amount under SSI.

Mandatory. States must pay Medicare Part B premiums (and, if applicable, Part A premiums) for QMBs, along with required Medicare coinsurance and deductible amounts. Coverage is restricted to Medicare cost-sharing unless the beneficiary also qualifies for Medicaid in some other way.

Effective January 1, 1993, all States must pay Part B premiums (but not Part A premiums or Part A or B coinsurance and deductibles) for beneficiaries who would be QMBs except that their incomes are between 100 percent and 110 percent of the poverty level; the upper limit rises to 120 percent on January 1, 1995.

States are also required to pay Part A premiums, but no other expenses, for "qualified disabled and working individuals." These are persons who formerly received Social Security disability benefits and hence Medicare, have lost eligibility for both programs, but are permitted under Medicare law to continue to receive Medicare in return for payment of the Part A premium. Medicaid must pay this premium on behalf of such individuals who have incomes below 200 percent of poverty and resources no greater than twice the SSI standard.

Optional. States are permitted to provide full Medicaid benefits, rather than just Medicare premiums and cost-sharing, to QMBs who meet a State-established income standard that is no higher than 100 percent of the Federal poverty level.

3. The Medically Needy

As of October 1991, 41 States and other jurisdictions provided Medicaid to at least some groups of "medically needy" persons. These are persons who meet the nonfinancial standards for inclusion in one of the groups covered under Medicaid, but who do not meet the applicable income or resource requirements for categorically needy eligibility. The State may establish higher income or resource standards for the medically needy. In addition, individuals may spend down to the medically needy standard by incurring medical expenses, in the same way that SSI recipients in section 209(b) States may spend down to Medicaid eligibility.

The State may set its separate medically needy income standard for a family of a given size at any level up to 133 1/3 percent of the maximum payment for a similar family under the State's AFDC program. States may limit the groups of individuals who may receive medically needy coverage. If the State provides any medically needy coverage, however, it must include all children under 18 who would qualify under one of the mandatory categorically needy groups, and all pregnant women who would qualify under either a mandatory or optional group, if their income or resources were lower.

4. Persons Receiving Institutional or Other Long-Term Care

States may provide Medicaid to certain otherwise ineligible groups of persons who are in Nfs or other institutions, or who would require institutional care if they were not receiving alternative services at home or in the community.

States may establish a special income standard for institutionalized persons, not to exceed 300 percent of the basic SSI benefit that would be payable to a person who was living at home and had no other income ($1,266 per month in 1992). In States without a medically needy program, this "300 percent rule" is an alternative way of providing NF coverage to persons with incomes above SSI or SSP levels. (Unlike the medically needy, however, persons with incomes above the 300 percent limit cannot spend down to Medicaid eligibility, even if their income is insufficient to cover the costs of their care.)

Both the medically needy and those becoming eligible under the 300 percent rule must contribute their available income to the costs of their care, retaining only a small personal needs allowance ($30 to $75 per month in 1991, depending on the State) for clothing and other incidental expenses. Medicaid has distinct post-eligibility rules to determine how much of a beneficiary's income must be applied to the cost of care before Medicaid makes its payment. Special rules exist for the treatment of income and resources of married couples when one of the spouses requires nursing home care and the other remains in the community. These rules are referred to as the "spousal impoverishment" protections of Medicaid law, because they are intended to prevent the impoverishment of the spouse remaining in the community.

A State may obtain a waiver under section 1915(c) of the Act to provide home and community-based services to a defined group of individuals who would otherwise require institutional care.[8] Persons served under such a waiver may include persons who would be eligible under the 300 percent rule if they were in an institution. Such individuals may also be covered in a State that terminates its waiver program in order to take advantage of a new, no-waiver home and community-based services option created by OBRA 90.

A State may also provide Medicaid to several other classes of persons who need the level of care provided by an institution and would be eligible if they were in an institution. These include children who are being cared for at home, persons of any age who are ventilator-dependent, and persons receiving hospice benefits in lieu of institutional services.

5. Medicaid Purchase of COBRA Coverage

The COBRA 85 (COBRA, provides that employees or dependents leaving an employee health insurance group in a firm with 20 or more employees must be offered an opportunity to continue buying insurance through the group for 18 to 36 months (depending on the reason for leaving the group). The employer may charge a premium of no more than 102 percent of the average plan cost (150 percent for months 19 to 29 for certain disabled persons).

The OBRA 90 permits State Medicaid programs to pay the premiums for COBRA continuation coverage when it is cost-effective to do so. States may pay premiums for individuals with incomes below 100 percent of poverty and resources less than twice the SSI limit who are eligible for continuation coverage under a group health plan offered by an employer with 75 or more employees. As of March 1992, only two States, Montana and Washington, were reported by Health Care Financing Administration (HCFA) to be making use of this option.

B. Covered Services

1. Mandatory and Optional Services

Each State defines its own package of covered medical services within broad Federal guidelines. Thus, there is considerable variation among the States in types of services covered and the amount of care provided under specific service categories.

Federal Medicaid law draws a distinction between mandatory services (those States are required to cover) and optional services (those they may elect to cover). The mandatory services for the categorically needy are as follows:

---

[8]These waivers, also known as section 2176 waivers after the section of OBRA 81 that established them, are discussed below in the section on alternative delivery and payment systems.

- inpatient and outpatient hospital services,

- NF services[9] for individuals 21 or older,

- physicians' services,

- laboratory and X-ray services,

- early and periodic screening, diagnostic and treatment (EPSDT) services for individuals under age 21,

- family planning services,

- home health services for any individual entitled to NF care,

- rural health clinic and federally qualified health center (FQHC) services, and

- services of nurse-midwives, certified pediatric nurse practitioners, and certified family nurse practitioners (to the extent these individuals are authorized to practice under State law).

(As will be discussed below, EPSDT services for beneficiaries under age 21 include both screening examinations and follow-up services required to treat problems uncovered during a screening. As a result, States may be required to cover services for children that would be optional for adults.)

States may also offer any of a broad range of optional services. Among the most important, in terms of program expenditure, are prescribed drugs, dental and optical services, clinic services, and care in ICFs/MR and in institutions for mental diseases (IMDs). Many of the optional services are listed in law or regulations; coverage of any other medical service may be approved at the request of a State.

States that have chosen to cover the medically needy may offer more restricted benefits to these beneficiaries than to the categorically needy (the reverse is not true). States having medically needy programs are required, at a minimum, to offer the following:

- prenatal and delivery services for pregnant women;

- ambulatory services for individuals under 18 and individuals entitled to institutional services; and

- home health services for individuals entitled to NF services.

---

[9]The former distinction between skilled nursing facilities (SNFs) and ICFs has been eliminated. ICFs/MR remain a distinct service type.

Broader requirements apply if a State has chosen to provide coverage for medically needy persons in ICFs/MR or in IMDs. In this case the State is required to cover either the same services as those which are mandatory for the categorically needy or alternatively the care and services listed in 7 of the 21 paragraphs in the law defining covered mandatory and optional services.

Table I-1 lists the mandatory and optional services currently defined in Medicaid law and regulations. It should be noted that the Secretary has approved coverage of additional services at the request of individual States. Among those not listed in table I-1 but covered in one or more States are adult day care, blood and blood products, durable medical equipment, ambulatory surgical centers, and various types of mental health and substance abuse clinics.

Figure I-5 shows FY 1991 Medicaid spending by major service category. Four mandatory services (inpatient and outpatient hospital, NF, and physician) accounted for 52 percent of total program spending. Two optional services, prescription drugs and ICF/MR, accounted for another 17 percent.

States may place certain limits on the coverage of all services. For example, they may place limits on the number of covered hospital days [10] or the number of covered physician visits. States are also permitted to impose nominal cost-sharing charges, with certain major exceptions, in connection with the use of covered services.

2. Other Coverage Rules

In addition to covering the mandatory services specified in law, States must meet four basic requirements in designing their benefit packages:

Amount, duration, and scope. Each covered service must be sufficient in amount, duration, and scope to reasonably achieve its purpose. The State may not arbitrarily deny or reduce the amount, duration, or scope of services solely because of the type of illness or condition. The State may place appropriate limits on a service based on such criteria as medical necessity.

Comparability. The services available to any categorically needy beneficiary in a State must generally be equal in amount, duration, and scope to those available to any other categorically needy beneficiary in the State. Similarly, services available to an individual in a covered medically needy group must be equal in amount, duration, and scope to those available to all persons in the covered medically needy group.

---

[10]Public Law 100-360 prohibits States (effective July 1, 1989) from imposing limits on the number of covered hospital days with respect to infants receiving services in hospitals serving a disproportionate number of low-income patients.

TABLE 1–1. Mandatory and Optional Medicaid Services for Categorically and Medically Needy Populations

	CATEGORICALLY NEEDY	MEDICALLY NEEDY
MANDATORY SERVICES	◆ Inpatient hospital services ◆ Outpatient hospital services ◆ Rural health clinic services ◆ Federally qualified health center services ◆ Other laboratory and x–ray services ◆ Nursing facility (NF) services (age 21 or over) ◆ Home health services for individuals entitled to NF care ◆ Early and Periodic Screening, Diagnostic, and Treatment (EPSDT) services (under age 21) ◆ Family planning services ◆ Physicians' services ◆ Nurse–midwife services ◆ Certified pediatric and family nurse practitioners' services	◆ Prenatal and delivery services ◆ Ambulatory services (individuals under age 18 and individuals entitled to institutional services) ◆ Home health services (individuals entitled to NF services) ◆ In States choosing to cover the medically needy in ICFs/MR or institutions for mental disease (IMDs), broader requirements apply.
	CATEGORICALLY AND MEDICALLY NEEDY	
OPTIONAL SERVICES	◆ Podiatrists' services ◆ Optometrists' services ◆ Chiropractors' services ◆ Other practitioners' services ◆ Private duty nursing ◆ Clinic services ◆ Dental services ◆ Physical therapy ◆ Occupational therapy ◆ Speech, hearing, and language disorder ◆ Prescribed drugs ◆ Prosthetic devices ◆ Dentures ◆ Eyeglasses ◆ Other diagnostic, screening, preventive, and rehabilitative services	◆ Inpatient hospital services (age 65 or over in mental institution) ◆ Nursing facility services (age 65 or over in mental institution) ◆ IMD (over age 65 or under age 21) and ICF/MR services ** ◆ Inpatient psychiatric hospital services (under age 21) ◆ Christian Science nurses ◆ Christian Science sanitoria ◆ Nursing facility services (under age 21) ◆ Emergency hospital services ◆ Personal care services ◆ Transportation services ◆ Case management services ◆ Hospice services ◆ Respiratory care services ◆ Other services approved by the Secretary

NOTE: States may offer optional services to the categorically needy only, or to both the categorically and medically needy.

**If a State covers these services, it is required to cover in their medically needy program either the same services as those which are mandatory for the categorically needy (except certified nurse practitioners' and certified family nurse practitioners' services), or the care and services listed in 7 of the 21 paragraphs in the law defining covered mandatory and optional services.

Source: Table prepared by the Congressional Research Service.

FIGURE I-5. Medicaid Payments by Type of Service, FY 1991

Total payments = $77.0 billion

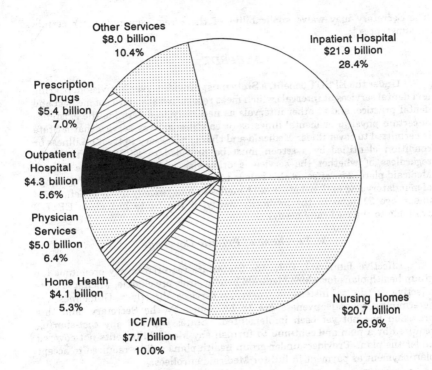

Other Services
$8.0 billion
10.4%

Inpatient Hospital
$21.9 billion
28.4%

Prescription
Drugs
$5.4 billion
7.0%

Outpatient
Hospital
$4.3 billion
5.6%

Physician
Services
$5.0 billion
6.4%

Home Health
$4.1 billion
5.3%

ICF/MR
$7.7 billion
10.0%

Nursing Homes
$20.7 billion
26.9%

NOTE: "Other Services" category includes dental, clinic, and lab and x-ray services among others.
Source: Figure prepared by Congressional Research Service based on data from HCFA Form 2082.

Statewideness. Generally, a State plan must be in effect throughout an entire State; that is the amount, duration, and scope of coverage must be the same statewide.

Freedom-of-Choice. Beneficiaries must be free to obtain services from any institution, agency, pharmacy, person, or organization that undertakes to provide the services and is qualified to perform the services.

The Secretary may waive applicability of these requirements under certain circumstances.[11]

3. EPSDT

Under the EPSDT benefit, a State must provide screening, vision, hearing and dental services at intervals which meet recognized standards of medical and dental practice, and at other intervals as necessary to determine the existence of certain physical or mental illnesses or conditions. Any service that a State is permitted to cover under Medicaid and that is necessary to treat an illness or condition identified by a screen must be provided to EPSDT participants, regardless of whether the service is otherwise included under the State's Medicaid plan. The effect of this rule is to require States to offer the full range of mandatory and optional Medicaid benefits to categorically needy beneficiaries under age 21 (and to the medically needy, if the State has made EPSDT available to the medically needy).

4. Purchase of Private Coverage

Effective January 1, 1991, the States are required to pay premiums for group health plans for which Medicaid beneficiaries are eligible, when it is cost-effective to do so instead of covering services directly. Guidelines for determining cost-effectiveness are to be issued by the Secretary, and this provision has not yet been implemented. States will pay any cost-sharing required by a plan and continue to furnish any Medicaid benefits not covered under the plan. Providers under group health plans will be required to accept plan payment as payment in full for Medicaid enrollees.

C. Payment for Services

Under Medicaid law, States now have considerable freedom to develop their own methods and standards for reimbursement of Medicaid services. This section reviews States' methods for determining provider payment and for collecting amounts due from other potential sources of payment for Medicaid beneficiaries.

---

[11]See the discussion of waivers below.

1. Institutional Services

Before 1980, Medicaid programs were required to use the same methods as Medicare in paying for hospital and NF services. Facilities were paid on the basis of the actual costs they incurred in providing care. Legislative changes in 1980 and 1981 (the Boren amendment) permitted States to develop their own reimbursement methodologies for these services. Most States have now moved to "prospective" payment systems, under which the amount of payment for a defined unit of service (such as a day of care in a NF or full treatment of an inpatient hospital case) is established in advance. Some of these systems are comparable to Medicare's prospective payment system (PPS) for hospital services, under which reimbursement varies according to the classification of each case into a diagnosis related group, or DRG. In other States, hospitals are paid a flat rate, for each day of care or for total care for each patient, without regard to diagnosis. Finally, States may develop rates through negotiation with hospitals. In a number of States, the Medicaid program participates in an "all-payer" system, under which most insurers in the State agree to a single method for paying hospitals. States are required to make additional payment to "disproportionate share" hospitals, those that serve a higher than average number of Medicaid and other low-income patients.[12]

Data collected by the American Hospital Association (AHA) indicate that, at least until recently, most States have been paying less than the full cost incurred by hospitals in serving Medicaid beneficiaries. In the median State in 1989, Medicaid covered 81.6 percent of estimated costs; in the aggregate, AHA estimates that Medicaid nationally covered 78.3 percent of hospital costs. Courts have found Medicaid reimbursement inadequate in several States, and hospitals have filed suit for higher reimbursement in several more. Data for more recent years show dramatic growth in Medicaid inpatient spending, a matter that will be discussed further below.

For NF services, Medicaid law formerly distinguished between two types of facilities: SNFs and ICFs. The distinction between the two types of care was eliminated effective October 1, 1990. Nearly all States have adopted prospective payment systems for NF services, although they may pay on a retrospective basis for certain cost components. Rates may be set for individual facilities or for peer groups (based on such factors as size and location). As of 1989, twelve States had adopted "case mix" reimbursement systems, under which higher payments are made to facilities that accept more severely ill patients.

2. Physician and Outpatient Services

For services of physicians or other individual practitioners, payment amounts are usually the lesser of the provider's actual charge for the service or a maximum allowable charge established by the State. Payments may be determined through "prevailing charge" screens, under which the maximum is

---

[12]Legislation in 1991 limited national aggregate spending for these payment adjustments to 12 percent of total program spending. The reason for this change is discussed in the section on program history, below.

set at a fixed percentile of the customary charges of area providers for comparable services. Or the State may use a fee schedule, specifying a flat maximum payment amount for each service. In 1989, 41 States and the District of Columbia used fixed fee schedules. The Physician Payment Review Commission has estimated that State payment rates for physician services in that year averaged 73.7 percent of what would have been allowed under Medicare for the same services.

States use a wide variety of methods for reimbursing hospital outpatient services. Hospitals may be paid their actual costs for providing outpatient care, or the State may pay fixed rates. These may be based on a hospital's historic costs or may involve a fee schedule comparable to those used for physician services. As of 1989, only 10 States were still paying on the basis of actual costs; the rest had adopted some form of prospective rates or a fee schedule.

3. Prescription Drugs

For prescription drugs, States are required to establish a system that pays a pharmacy's cost for acquiring a drug plus a fixed dispensing fee. Payment for drugs that exist in both brand-name and generic versions is generally limited to the price of the least expensive readily available generic equivalent. The pharmacy thus has an incentive to substitute the generic drug unless the physician specifically requests that the brand-name version be furnished. OBRA 90 requires pharmaceutical manufacturers to grant rebates to Medicaid programs for the drugs they purchase, thus giving Medicaid discounts comparable to those offered to other high-volume purchasers.

4. Other Services

Although Medicaid programs cover numerous other kinds of services, the law establishes specific payment rules for only a few of them. Payment to rural health clinics, hospices, and clinical laboratories must generally follow Medicare rules. For some services, including laboratory services, durable medical equipment, and eyeglasses, States are permitted to establish "volume purchasing" programs, selecting a sole source for the service through competitive bidding or other means.

5. Medicaid and Other Payers

With minor exceptions, Medicaid is the "payer of last resort," secondary to any other insurance coverage a beneficiary may have or to any other third party who may be liable for medical payments or medical support on the beneficiary's behalf.

Some Medicaid beneficiaries may also have private health insurance, or may be eligible for payments through automobile or liability insurance or workers' compensation. Finally, an absent parent may be responsible for medical support payments. Applicants for Medicaid benefits are required to disclose any potential payment sources, and Medicaid programs must have a system for pursuing third party claims. For most services, States have adopted a "cost avoidance" system, denying payment of claims for which third party liability is known to exist. For a few types of services, Medicaid programs pay the claims and then seek to collect from the responsible party.

Most aged Medicaid beneficiaries and many of the disabled are also eligible for Medicare benefits. States enter into "buy-in" agreements with the Department of Health and Human Services (DHHS) for these dual eligibles. The State pays Medicare premiums on the beneficiaries' behalf. Medicare pays its allowed amounts for the services it covers, with Medicaid paying beneficiary cost-sharing, the deductibles and coinsurance required under Medicare.[13] For beneficiaries fully eligible under both programs, Medicaid also pays for services that Medicare does not cover but that are included in the State's Medicaid plan, such as prescription drugs and most NF care. For QMBs (see above), Medicaid pays only the Medicare cost-sharing amounts.

D. Alternative Delivery and Payment Systems

Medicaid law provides a number of options for States wishing to use innovative methods for delivering or paying for Medicaid services. Since the earliest years of the Medicaid program, States have arranged for the voluntary enrollment of Medicaid beneficiaries under contracts with health maintenance organizations (HMOs) or comparable organizations. OBRA 81 established two new options, the section 1915(b) (freedom-of-choice) and section 1915(c) (home and community-based services) waiver programs.[14] Under these provisions, the Secretary may waive certain statutory requirements, on application by a State, in order to allow the State to develop cost-effective alternative methods of service delivery or reimbursement. The purpose of these provisions was to give States greater flexibility in managing their Medicaid programs.

In the case of the 1915(b) waiver option, the greater flexibility was intended to offset the temporary reductions in Federal Medicaid funding imposed by the same Act. The waivers allow States to require beneficiaries to enroll in HMOs or other managed care programs, or to select cost-effective providers from whom beneficiaries must obtain all nonemergency care. The 1915(c) option was intended to correct a perceived "institutional bias" in Medicaid services for the chronically ill by providing States an alternative of offering a broad range of home and community-based care to persons at risk of institutionalization. Two other home and community-based care waiver programs were subsequently established in Medicaid--one to allow States to serve elderly persons at risk of needing nursing home care and a second to allow them to provide services to certain children infected with the acquired immune deficiency syndrome (AIDS) virus or who are drug dependent at birth.

---

[13]Some States pay less than the full cost-sharing amounts if the sum of Medicare and Medicaid payment would be greater than the maximum payable by Medicaid alone.

[14]These are also known as section 2175 and 2176 waivers, respectively, after the sections of OBRA 81 that created them.

Most recently, OBRA 90 established two new optional Medicaid benefits, home and community-based care for functionally disabled elderly persons and community supported living arrangements for the developmentally disabled. These benefits may be provided at a State's option, without waivers. However, total Federal contributions are subject to national caps ($70 million for the elderly and $10 million for the developmentally disabled in 1992). In addition, no more than 8 States may furnish community supported living arrangements.

Finally, States have periodically been granted waivers of Medicaid requirements in order to conduct demonstration projects. Some of these projects have been authorized by the Secretary under general statutory provisions allowing for tests of possible program improvements. Others have been specifically authorized by Federal legislation.

Arizona's medical assistance program, under which beneficiaries receive all services through HMO-like contractors, has been operated under demonstration waivers since 1982.

E. Administration

At the Federal level, Medicaid is administered by the HCFA in DHHS, the same agency that administers the Medicare program. In 1990, a separate Medicaid bureau was established within HCFA, and most Medicaid functions were shifted to the new bureau.

Each State operates its Medicaid program through a single state agency, usually the department responsible for welfare and social services programs, the health department, or a combination of the two. (Eligibility determination must be performed by the agency that manages the State's AFDC and SSI programs.) The program in each State is operated in accordance with a *State plan* for medical assistance, which describes the State's basic eligibility, coverage, reimbursement, and administrative policies. The State plan must be approved by HCFA and is periodically updated to reflect changes in State policy or to conform to new Federal requirements. HCFA may use several mechanisms to insure State compliance with Federal requirements. The method generally chosen is the disallowance action, under which HCFA retrospectively disallows and recovers Federal matching payments for State expenditures made in violation of Federal requirements. An alternative process is the compliance action, under which HCFA could prospectively withhold Federal funds if it makes a determination that the State plan no longer complies with Federal requirements or that the administration of the plan is noncompliant; this process has never yet been carried to the point of actual withholding of funds.

A Medicaid program pays claims for medically necessary covered services rendered by qualified providers to eligible beneficiaries. This basic program description defines the chief functions performed by the single State agency.

1. *Eligibility Determination*

Many Medicaid beneficiaries qualify automatically as a result of their eligibility for cash assistance. Determination of Medicaid eligibility for persons receiving AFDC must be performed by the same agency that determines AFDC eligibility. In States where recipients of SSI are automatically eligible, the State may contract with the Social Security Administration to determine eligibility for these beneficiaries, as well as for other aged, blind, or disabled applicants, or it may perform its own determinations. A State that uses more restrictive standards for Medicaid eligibility than for SSI (so-called "209(b) States"; see *Chapter III, Eligibility*) must conduct its own Medicaid determinations. States generally conduct their own determinations for the medically needy. The State must verify the information furnished on applications, largely through data exchange with other agencies.

Establishment of eligibility for Medicaid is not permanent. The State must conduct periodic redetermination of eligibility and must also take action between redeterminations if it learns of changes in a beneficiary's circumstances. The Secretary has established by regulation that redetermination must occur at least every 12 months; longer intervals are permissible for blind or disabled beneficiaries. Redetermination intervals for recipients of AFDC and SSI are set by the regulations for those programs; the interval is 6 months for AFDC and varies for different groups of SSI beneficiaries. Applicants who are denied eligibility must be given notice and an opportunity for a fair hearing.

States have the option to establish "presumptive eligibility" for low-income pregnant women, in order to ensure that prenatal care is not delayed by the process of establishing Medicaid eligibility. Certain providers of care may make a preliminary determination that a pregnant woman may be financially eligible for Medicaid benefits. The woman may then receive ambulatory prenatal care while the State is reviewing her Medicaid application. States are also now required to "outstation" eligibility workers, to give individuals the opportunity to apply for Medicaid at the sites where they receive health care.

2. *Claims Processing*

Most Medicaid payments must be issued directly to the provider furnishing the service, not to the beneficiary. Many States use outside fiscal agents to process claims. Three States have entered into arrangements under which the fiscal agent assumes direct financial responsibility for payment of some services. The State issues a fixed monthly payment to the agent, known as a "health insuring organization" or HIO, for each eligible beneficiary. The HIO uses the funds to reimburse providers, and may retain some of the savings--or suffer a loss--if amounts paid to providers differ from the total payment received from the State.

3. *Provider Certification*

States must determine which providers of services are eligible to participate in the program. Federal law is specific about the standards and certification procedures for institutional providers, such as hospitals and NFs. For certain other kinds of providers, such as physicians and pharmacies, States generally follow their own laws on licensure and monitoring. (OBRA 1990 established minimum Federal standards for physicians furnishing Medicaid-covered pediatric or obstetric services.)

Both Medicare and Medicaid use State certification agencies to determine compliance by institutional providers with program standards. (The Secretary also conducts direct reviews of some facilities.) For hospital certification, both Medicare and Medicaid may rely on the findings of one of two organizations (the Joint Commission on the Accreditation of Health Care Organizations or the American Osteopathic Association, whichever is appropriate) for determining whether an institution meets the majority of program requirements. A State may terminate the certification of a facility that no longer meets the requirements for participation. If the deficiencies do not immediately jeopardize the health and safety of patients, the provider may be granted a reasonable period of time to achieve compliance and may be subject to other sanctions.

States generally follow their own procedures for certifying physicians and other health care practitioners and certain other noninstitutional providers such as pharmacies. The Medicare and Medicaid Patient and Program Protection Act of 1987 (Public Law 100-93) established a data exchange system to disseminate information on adverse licensing actions among the States, Federal agencies, and other parties.[15]

4. Program Controls

A Medicaid agency must engage in a variety of activities to ensure that the program is properly administered:

- Medicaid, like other federally funded, State administered programs, has quality control systems, under which each State identifies eligibility errors that may result in improper Federal payments. States with high error rates may be subject to financial penalties.

- Most States are required to operate a computerized Medicaid Management Information System (MMIS), which maintains information on beneficiaries and providers, processes claims, and produces program reports. As of January 1991, only one State-- Rhode Island--was exempt from the requirement to have an operational MMIS.

- Medicaid law and regulations include detailed provisions relating to the quality and appropriateness of care rendered to Medicaid beneficiaries. Required State activities include development of a utilization review plan and provision for external reviews of

---

[15]This system is coordinated with the National Practitioner Data Bank, established by the Health Care Quality Improvement Act of 1986 (P.L. 99-660), which collects data on malpractice awards.

certain facilities. Activities conducted by the facilities themselves include initial and periodic recertification of each patient's need for care, development of plans for the care of each patient, and operation of an approved utilization review (UR) program.

- The "nursing home reform" provisions of OBRA 87 established new minimum standards for nursing homes participating in Medicaid, restructured the survey and certification process, and included new sanctions and enforcement actions for noncompliant facilities. The new standards address such issues as levels of staffing in the facility, the qualifications of staff, and residents' rights. NFs must also now conduct periodic assessments of residents' functional capacity.

- Each State is required to establish methods for identifying and investigating cases of potential fraud and abuse. Special Federal funding is available for State Medicaid fraud control units (MFCUs), which investigate State law fraud violations. Federal agencies may also act on their own to pursue Medicaid fraud or abuse cases.

F. Program Financing

Medicaid services and associated administrative costs are jointly financed by the Federal Government and the States. The Federal share of a State's payments for services is known as the Federal medical assistance percentage (FMAP). FMAPs are calculated annually based on a formula designed to provide a higher Federal matching rate to States with lower per capita incomes. No State may have an FMAP lower than 50 percent or higher than 83 percent. In FY 1992, 11 States and the District of Columbia received the minimum 50 percent FMAP, while Mississippi received the highest FMAP, 79.99 percent. (FMAPs for the territories are fixed at 50 percent; there are also overall caps on Federal funding for the territories' Medicaid programs.) The Federal share of administrative costs is 50 percent for all States, though higher rates are applicable for specific items. Overall, the Federal share of Medicaid payments is an estimated 57 percent in FY 1992.

Participating States are responsible for the nonfederal share of Medicaid payments. (Some States require local governments to share a part of the cost.) Like the Federal Government, States usually rely on general funds for Medicaid spending. In recent years, however, many States have developed special revenue sources for Medicaid, some of them controversial. In the face of rising Medicaid costs, States have used funds donated by health care providers or taxes paid by those providers to draw greater Federal matching payments. For example, hospitals might donate funds to the State. The State would use these funds as the State share of Medicaid spending, receive Federal matching funds, then repay the hospitals their donations plus the Federal funds. Similar increases in Federal funds could be generated through taxes or mandatory assessments on providers. The Medicaid Voluntary Contribution and Provider-Specific Tax

Amendments of 1991 (P.L. 102-234) prohibit the use of provider donations after 1992 (or mid-1993, in certain States) and limit the use of provider-specific taxes.

G. Medicaid and the Federal Budget

From a Federal budget perspective, Medicaid is viewed as an entitlement program. Entitlement programs provide benefits to all people or jurisdictions who are eligible and receive benefits. Spending levels for entitlements are determined, not by the annual appropriation process, but by the number of persons who participate in the program and program benefit levels. However, Medicaid spending is still drawn from Federal general funds. There is no trust fund like that established for some other entitlement programs (such as Social Security and Part A of Medicare).

Under the Budget Enforcement Act of 1990 (Title XIII of OBRA 90, P.L. 101-508), Medicaid spending falls into the "pay-as-you-go" category with other entitlement programs. The budget law requires that for fiscal years 1991 through 1995 any legislation affecting these programs should be deficit neutral for the whole class of entitlement programs. That is, any legislative change in one of these programs that would increase spending over current law levels must by offset by changes in the same program or other "pay-as-you-go" programs, in order to avoid increasing the size of the Federal deficit.

II. MEDICAID PROGRAM HISTORY

A. Predecessor Programs and Enactment of Medicaid

Medicaid was enacted in 1965, in the same legislation that created the Medicare program, the Social Security Amendments of 1965 (P.L. 89-97). It grew out of and replaced two earlier programs of Federal grants to States to provide medical care to low-income persons. The first was the vendor payment program for welfare recipients, enacted in 1950. The second was the Kerr-Mills medical assistance program for the aged, enacted in 1960.

TABLE I-2. Major Medicaid Legislation, 1965 to 1991

1965 ◆ **Social Security Amendments of 1965 (P.L. 89−97)**
Established the Medicaid program

1967 ◆ **Social Security Amendments of 1967 (P.L. 90−248)**
Limited financial standards for the medically needy
Established the Early and Periodic Screening, Diagnostic and Treatment (EPSDT) program to improve child health
Permitted Medicaid beneficiaries to use providers of their choice

1971 ◆ **Act of December 14, 1971 (P.L. 92−223)**
Allowed States to cover services in intermediate care facilities (ICFs) and ICFs for the mentally retarded (ICFs/MR)

1972 ◆ **Social Security Amendments of 1972 (P.L. 92−603)**
Repealed 1965 provision requiring States to move toward comprehensive Medicaid coverage
Allowed States to cover care for beneficiaries under age 22 in psychiatric hospitals

1977 ◆ **Medicare−Medicaid Anti−Fraud and Abuse Amendments of 1977 (P.L. 95−142)**
Established Medicaid Fraud Control Units

1980 ◆ **Mental Health Systems Act (P.L. 96−398)**
Required most States to develop a computerized Medicaid Management Information System (MMIS)

◆ **Omnibus Reconciliation Act of 1980 (P.L. 96−499)**
Boren amendment permitted States to establish payment systems for nursing home care in lieu of Medicare's rules

1981 ◆ **Omnibus Budget Reconciliation Act of 1981 (OBRA 81, P.L. 97−35)**
Enacted 3−year reductions in Federal matching percentages for States whose spending exceeded growth targets
Established section 1915(b) and 1915(c) waiver programs (freedom−of−choice and home and community−based services)
Extended the Boren amendment to inpatient hospital services
Eliminated special penalties for noncompliance with EPSDT requirements and gave States with medically needy programs broader authority to limit coverage

1984 ◆ **Deficit Reduction Act of 1984 (DEFRA, P.L. 98−369)**
Eliminated categorical tests for certain pregnant women and young children

Continued on next page.

TABLE I–2. Major Medicaid Legislation, 1965 to 1991––Continued

1986
- **Consolidated Omnibus Budget Reconciliation Act of 1985 (COBRA, P.L. 99–272)**
  Extended coverage to all pregnant women meeting AFDC financial standards

- **Omnibus Budget Reconciliation Act of 1986 (OBRA 86, P.L. 99–509)**
  Allowed coverage of pregnant women and young children to 100 percent of poverty
  Established a new optional category of "qualified Medicare beneficiaries" (QMBs)

1987
- **Medicare and Medicaid Patient and Program Protection Act of 1987 (P.L. 100–93)**
  Strengthened authorities to sanction and exclude providers

- **Omnibus Budget Reconciliation Act of 1987 (OBRA 87, P.L. 100–203)**
  Allowed coverage of pregnant women and infants to 185 percent of poverty
  Strengthened quality of care standards and monitoring of nursing homes
  Strengthened OBRA 81 requirement that States provide additional payment to hospitals treating a disproportionate share of low–income patients

1988
- **Medicare Catastrophic Coverage Act of 1988 (MCCA, P.L. 100–360)**
  Mandated coverage of pregnant women and infants to 100 percent of poverty
  Expanded coverage of low–income Medicare beneficiaries
  Established special eligibility rules for institutionalized persons whose spouse remained in the community to prevent "spousal impoverishment"

- **Family Support Act of 1988 (P.L. 100–485)**
  Extended work transition coverage for families losing AFDC because of increased earnings and expanded coverage for two–parent families whose principal earner was unemployed

1989
- **Omnibus Budget Reconciliation Act of 1989 (OBRA 89, P.L. 101–239)**
  Mandated coverage of pregnant women and children under age 6 to 133 percent of poverty
  Expanded EPSDT program requirements
  Mandated coverage and full–cost reimbursement of federally qualified health centers (FQHCs)

1990
- **Omnibus Budget Reconciliation Act of 1990 (OBRA 90, P.L. 101–508)**
  Phased in coverage of children ages 6 through 18 to 100 percent of poverty
  Expanded coverage of low–income Medicare beneficiaries
  Established Medicaid prescription drug rebate program

1991
- **Medicaid Voluntary Contribution and Provider–Specific Tax Amendments of 1991 (P.L. 102–234)**
  Restricted use of provider donations and taxes as State share of Medicaid spending; limited disproportionate share hospital payments

Source: Table prepared by the Congressional Research Service.

Before 1950, welfare payments might include a small amount nominally earmarked for medical expenses, but the payments were made to the recipient and could be used for any purpose the recipient chose. The Social Security Amendments of 1950 provided Federal matching funds for direct State payments to medical care providers (or "vendors") on behalf of recipients of public assistance. Total spending under these programs reached $0.5 billion by 1960. In that year, the Kerr-Mills Act created a new program, Medical Assistance for the Aged. This program provided Federal matching funds to States that chose to cover the "medically needy" aged, persons whose incomes were above cash assistance levels but who needed help with medical bills. As of 1965, 40 States and the District of Columbia, along with Puerto Rico, the Virgin Islands, and Guam, had implemented Kerr-Mills programs. Combined spending under the vendor payment and Kerr-Mills programs had reached $1.3 billion.[16]

By 1965, improving medical coverage for the elderly had become a major congressional priority. Congress considered a number of approaches, including a universal system based on Social Security, a voluntary program supported in part by beneficiary premiums, and an expansion of the means-tested Kerr-Mills program for the low-income elderly only. What was adopted in the Social Security Amendments of 1965 represented a combination of all three approaches. Medicare hospital insurance (Part A) was a social insurance program covering nearly all of the elderly, while Medicare's supplementary medical insurance program (Part B) was a voluntary program. However, both programs could leave some elderly beneficiaries exposed to substantial costs for premiums, deductibles, and coinsurance payments, as well as costs for uncovered services. A third component, an expansion of Kerr-Mills to be called Medicaid, was included in order to help the low-income elderly meet these costs. At the same time the new program would consolidate and simplify the other existing Federal efforts to provide medical assistance to the poor, the vendor payment programs for cash assistance recipients. It would also extend the Kerr-Mills concept of medical need to other populations, including families with children, the blind, and the disabled.

The new Medicaid program carried over two key features of its predecessors. First, States were given substantial latitude to design their own programs, so long as they met minimum Federal standards. (States were required, as a condition of continued funding, to make steady progress towards development of a "comprehensive" program by raising eligibility levels and expanding services; this requirement was repealed in 1972.) Second, coverage was largely confined to the populations traditionally eligible for welfare--certain families with children (chiefly single-parent families) and the aged, blind, and disabled. One exception was created by the Ribicoff amendment--States could choose to cover children who met the financial standards for welfare eligibility but not the categorical standards (because, for example, they were in two-parent families with a working parent). As passed by the Senate, the Ribicoff amendment would also have allowed coverage of the children's caretakers, in

---

[16]U.S. Congress. Senate. Committee on Finance. *Medicare and Medicaid: Problems, Issues, and Alternatives.* Unnumbered Committee Print, 91st Cong., 2d Sess., Feb. 9, 1970. Washington, GPO, 1970.

effect opening the program to all types of low-income families. This provision was dropped in conference, and two-parent families with a working parent are excluded from the program to this day, as are single adults and childless couples who are not aged or disabled.[17]

On the other hand, the law specified no upper income limits for program eligibility, and States were free to provide medically needy coverage for higher income persons in the traditional welfare categories. Despite this flexibility, Medicaid was not expected to result in a dramatic expansion of coverage. Maximum new Federal expenditures, even if all States took full advantage of the new program, were projected to be $238 million per year above those under the vendor payment/Kerr-Mills programs.[18] In fact this level was reached in the first year, although only six States had implemented programs.

B. Medicaid in the 1960s and 1970s

Twenty-six States implemented Medicaid programs in 1966, and another 11 in 1967. Program spending grew much more rapidly than had been anticipated. Combined Federal and State spending under Medicaid and its predecessors (which were not fully phased out until 1970) was $1.7 billion in FY 1966, but rose 43 percent, to $2.4 billion in FY 1967. Spending grew even faster in FY 1968, rising 57 percent, to $3.7 billion.

One factor in the unexpected early growth in the program was liberal eligibility standards for the medically needy. New York in particular established a very high protected income level, $6,000 per year for a family of four in 1966. (By July 1991, 25 years later, 13 States with medically needy programs had not reached this level.) It was projected that up to 45 percent of the State's population in 1966 could have potentially qualified for Medicaid coverage.[19]

Congress responded in 1967 by limiting medically needy eligibility. States that chose to cover the medically needy were required to set upper income limits no greater than 133 1/3 percent of the maximum payment for a family of the same size under AFDC. This meant that States could not expand Medicaid eligibility without expanding their cash assistance programs as well.

---

[17]The OBRA 89 established a demonstration project under which up to four States are permitted to extend Medicaid to low-income individuals and families not meeting categorical requirements.

[18]U.S. Congress. Senate. Committee on Finance. *Social Security Amendments of 1965*. (Report to accompany H.R. 6675.) Senate Report No. 404, 89th Cong., 1st Sess., June 30, 1965. Washington, GPO, 1965. p. 85.

[19]Stevens, Robert, and Rosemary Stevens. *Welfare Medicine in America*. New York, Free Press, 1974. p. 86, 92. The protected income level is the amount of countable income a medically needy family may retain after spending any excess on medical bills.

The Social Security Amendments of 1967 (P.L. 90-248) included two other key changes in Medicaid. First, the law established the EPSDT program in conjunction with other, non-Medicaid initiatives to improve child health. Second, the law provided that Medicaid beneficiaries had to be permitted to obtain covered services from any qualified provider "who undertakes to provide [the beneficiary] such services." Under the pre-Medicaid vendor payment programs, a State could contract with specific providers, such as clinics or hospitals, to serve as the sources of care for public assistance recipients. As enacted in 1965, Medicaid continued to allow States the option of making direct arrangements for beneficiaries' care. The new "freedom-of-choice" requirement meant that States could no longer establish separate systems of care for Medicaid beneficiaries. Instead, Medicaid would allow low-income citizens to use providers of their choice, to enter the mainstream of American health care. (Whether they could actually do so depended on whether providers were prepared to participate in the program, an issue to be discussed further below.)

Even in the earliest years of the program, some States were already finding Medicaid a strain on State budgets and began to consider restrictions in eligibility or benefits. They were briefly prevented from doing so by a Secretarial ruling that States could not reduce coverage under an already approved State plan. This ruling was reversed by Congress in 1969. Congress also delayed, and in 1972 repealed, the provision of the original 1965 legislation requiring States to progress steadily towards comprehensive Medicaid coverage. Early expectations for the program had been lowered, and States undertook a variety of cost containment efforts, including benefit limitations, requirements for prior authorization of services, and reductions in payment levels. Some States also began contracting with HMOs or similar entities to provide coverage on a prepaid basis to beneficiaries who agreed to obtain all services through the organization.

Congress also took steps in the early 1970s to control spending under both Medicare and Medicaid; many of these measures were joint initiatives affecting both programs. Professional Standards Review Organizations (PSROs, the predecessors of today's peer review organizations, or PROs) were established to monitor inpatient utilization, and States were required to develop their own systems for monitoring nursing home care. In response to the view that growth in the supply of medical facilities was fueling health care demand, States were required to develop health planning programs, which were supposed to limit unnecessary expansion of hospitals and NFs. Start-up funds were authorized for new HMOs, in the hope of achieving savings for both private purchasers and public programs. These early cost control efforts had mixed results. PSROs had little impact on utilization, while State health planning programs had some success in controlling the growth in nursing home beds. Federal funding promoted rapid growth in the HMO industry, but few of the new entities were prepared to accept Medicaid beneficiaries.

Even as it undertook these early cost containment initiatives, Congress added new optional Medicaid services that were to have a significant impact on program spending in the years ahead. Amendments in 1971 and 1972 allowed States to cover care in ICFs, ICFs/MR and, for beneficiaries under age 22, in psychiatric hospitals (care in mental hospitals for beneficiaries aged 65 and over was included in the original Medicaid package). Federal funding for ICFs was already available through the cash assistance programs; the transfer of this service to Medicaid made it available to the medically needy (some of whom were instead being treated in more costly SNFs).

The two new services, ICF/MR and care in psychiatric hospitals, had long been a State responsibility. ICF/MR services were added to Medicaid partly in response to growing concern about inadequate care in some State facilities, with the expectation that States would have to improve those facilities to qualify for Federal payment. Inpatient psychiatric care was added in the view that helping mentally ill children become functional members of society was in keeping with Medicaid's objectives.

Addition of these services had the effect of federalizing a significant component of State health spending. States that chose to shift these services to Medicaid had to meet "maintenance of effort" requirements; that is, Federal matching was available only for expenditures in excess of what the State had been spending before adding the services to Medicaid. These thresholds were passed rapidly, and ICF/MR soon became a major factor in Medicaid spending. Figure I-6 illustrates the impact. While it is sometimes alleged that long-term care for the aged crowded out spending for families and children during the 1970s, the data do not support this view. Spending for NFs (other than ICFs/MR) accounted for roughly the same share of program spending in 1970 as they did in 1990.[20] On the other hand, spending for ICF/MR services grew from nothing in 1967 to over 8 percent of program spending by 1980 and 11 percent in 1990.

Overall program spending grew an average of 17.3 percent a year in the decade 1970-1980, despite a decline in the number of beneficiaries in the latter part of the decade. Much of this growth was attributable to general inflation and the even higher price increases in the medical sector. After correction for medical price inflation, spending per beneficiary rose at an average rate of 3.3 percent per year in the 1970s.

Congress continued to explore ways of controlling Medicaid spending growth. Two approaches that received considerable attention during this period were reduction in fraud and abuse and changes in provider reimbursement methods.

---

[20]The 1970 figures include ICF spending under the cash assistance programs before ICF was transferred to Medicaid.

FIGURE I-6. Share of Medicaid Spending
by Type of Service, Selected Years

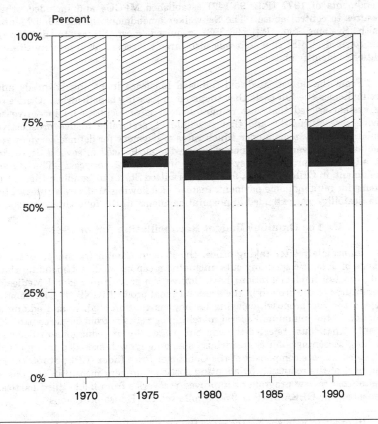

Source: Figure prepared by Congressional Research Service based on data from HCFA.

Fraud and abuse had been a concern since the earliest years of the program. There were continuing concerns about "Medicaid mills," clinics that treated large numbers of beneficiaries in brief and perfunctory visits, about fraudulent billing by individual practitioners and inflated cost reports from institutional providers. The Medicare-Medicaid Anti-Fraud and Abuse Amendments of 1977 (P.L. 95-142) established MFCUs and included other measures to control abuse. The Schweiker amendment (in the 1980 Mental Health Systems Act, P.L. 96-398) required most States to develop a computerized MMIS; this step was also largely directed at improving States' abilities to identify abuse.

From the outset, Medicaid followed Medicare in paying hospitals and nursing homes the full costs they incurred in treating beneficiaries. Critics of this system argued that cost reimbursement gave facilities no incentive to provide care efficiently, and that it would be preferable to use prospective reimbursement systems, under which rates of payment for defined services are established in advance. Demonstrations were authorized in several States to test alternative prospective systems for institutional services. The Boren amendment, in OBRA 80 (P.L. 96-499), permitted States to establish their own systems for nursing home payment, instead of following Medicare's rules. The same flexibility was extended to hospital payments in the following year.

C. The Omnibus Budget Reconciliation Act of 1981

Immediately after taking office, the Reagan Administration proposed a package of domestic spending cuts, including a cap on Medicaid spending that would (on full implementation) have limited the growth in Federal Medicaid expenditures to the growth in the gross national product (GNP).[21] The Senate accepted the cap proposal, delaying its implementation slightly and adding a reduction in the minimum Federal matching percentage from 50 percent to 40 percent. The House rejected the cap but passed 3-year reductions in Federal matching percentages for States whose spending growth exceeded targets tied to the medical care component of the Consumer Price Index (CPI); States could avoid part of the reduction by adopting cost-containment measures, such as a hospital cost review program or improved recoveries from liable third parties. As enacted, the OBRA 81 (P.L. 97-35) followed the House provisions.

In order to help the States meet the spending limits, OBRA 81 included a variety of provisions to increase State flexibility, perhaps the most important of which were the establishment of the section 1915(b) and 1915(c) waiver programs (freedom-of-choice and home and community-based services) and the extension to inpatient hospital services of the Boren amendment, which allowed States to develop reimbursement systems different from Medicare's. (Among other changes, the bill also eliminated special penalties for noncompliance with

---

[21]Federal Medicaid spending grew from $17.1 billion in FY 1981 to $52.5 billion in FY 1991, an increase of 214 percent. The Reagan proposal would have permitted 10-year growth of just 47 percent, reducing FY 1991 Federal spending to $25.1 billion.

EPSDT requirements and gave States with medically needy programs broader authority to limit coverage.)

While many States moved to take advantage of the new waiver options,[22] they also responded to the Federal spending limits by cutting services and reimbursement or limiting eligibility. Among the most common measures during this period were imposition of day limits for inpatient hospital services, reductions in prescription drug coverage, and limits or decreases in hospital and physician reimbursement.[23] Other domestic spending cuts in 1981 also affected Medicaid indirectly. In particular, changes in AFDC rules made it more difficult for working mothers to qualify for cash assistance and hence for Medicaid. Partly as a result of this change, the number of persons receiving AFDC declined even as the number of persons in poverty was rising during the recession that began in 1981. Overall, the number of Medicaid beneficiaries, relative to the population in poverty, reached its low point in 1983.

Growth in Medicaid spending dropped sharply, from an average of 17 percent a year in FY 1979 through 1981 to just 7 percent per year in FY 1982 through 1984. Only part of this drop was attributable to program changes; much of it reflected the decline in general inflation, which also helped to slow increases in medical spending by other payers. Still, the moderation in Medicaid spending helped to shift the policy focus from cost containment to possible program expansion. While the Administration's FY 1985 budget proposal would have made permanent the OBRA 81 limits in Federal matching payments for States exceeding growth targets, Congress let them lapse and has rejected subsequent proposals to cap Medicaid spending growth.

D. Program Expansion: 1984-1990

Beginning with the Deficit Reduction Act of 1984 (P.L. 98-369), Congress moved to expand Medicaid eligibility to increasing numbers of pregnant women and children, in order to reduce infant mortality and improve access to child health services. To some extent these expansions, which continued almost annually for the remainder of the decade, worked in a stepwise fashion--States would be given the option to extend coverage in one year's legislation, while subsequent legislation would make the extensions mandatory. These changes allowed higher-income persons to qualify for Medicaid and also partially severed the link between Medicaid and the cash assistance programs, by extending coverage to families that did not fit into traditional welfare categories. The sequence of expansions was as follows:

---

[22]See *Chapter VI, Alternate Delivery Options and Waiver Programs* for a year-by-year summary of State waiver applications.

[23]Intergovernmental Health Policy Project, as cited in U.S. General Accounting Office. *Medicare and Medicaid: Effects of Recent Legislation on Program and Beneficiary Costs.* Report to the Chairman, House Select Committee on Aging. GAO/HRD-87-53, Apr. 1987. Washington, 1987. p. 32-33.

Deficit Reduction Act of 1984 (DEFRA, P.L. 98-369). Required States to provide Medicaid to first-time pregnant women and those in two-parent families whose principal earner was unemployed, as well as to children up to age 5 born after September 30, 1983, who met AFDC financial standards but not the categorical tests for eligibility.

Consolidated Omnibus Budget Reconciliation Act of 1985 (COBRA, P.L. 99-272). Required States to cover all remaining pregnant women meeting AFDC financial standards (that is, those in two-parent families with an employed principal earner).

Omnibus Budget Reconciliation Act of 1986 (OBRA 86, P.L. 99-509). Permitted States to cover pregnant women and infants under age 1 (and, on a phased basis, children up to age 5) meeting a State-established income standard as high as 100 percent of the Federal poverty level. Permitted States to establish presumptive eligibility for pregnant women (allowing payment for prenatal care while their Medicaid applications were pending).

Omnibus Budget Reconciliation Act of 1987 (OBRA 87, P.L. 100-203). Permitted States to cover pregnant women and infants with family incomes up to 185 percent of the poverty level and allowed more rapid phase-in of coverage of children aged 1 through 5 with incomes below 100 percent of poverty. Extended to age 7 (or at the State's option, to age 8) the required coverage of children born after September 30, 1983, who met financial but not categorical eligibility standards.

Medicare Catastrophic Coverage Act of 1988 (MCCA, P.L. 100-360). Required States to phase in coverage of pregnant women and infants under age 1 with incomes under 100 percent of poverty. (Note that this and other Medicaid-related provisions of MCCA were not affected by the 1989 repeal of MCCA's Medicare expansions.)

Omnibus Budget Reconciliation Act of 1989 (OBRA 89, P.L. 101-239). Required States to cover pregnant women and children up to age 6 born after September 30, 1983, with incomes under 133 percent of the poverty level.

Omnibus Budget Reconciliation Act of 1990 (OBRA 90, P.L. 101-508). Required States to cover all children under age 19 born after September 30, 1983, with family incomes under 100 percent of the poverty level. (The effect is to phase in coverage of all children in poverty by 2002).

Figures I-7, I-8, and I-9 show, for 1983 through 1992, the highest mandatory and optional income level in effect at any time during the year for a non-AFDC child whose age was under 1, 4, or 6 at any time during the year. For example, figure I-7 shows that in 1983 a State had the option of covering a non-AFDC infant with family income up to that State's medically needy level (shown here as 133 1/3 percent of the median State's AFDC level); no coverage of non-AFDC children was mandatory in that year. In 1984, coverage of infants up to the AFDC level was mandated, while coverage up to the higher medically needy level remained optional. In 1987 and 1988, optional income levels rose to 100 percent of poverty and then to 185 percent, while the mandatory level remained the same. Since then, the maximum optional level has gone unchanged, while the mandatory level rose to 75 percent of poverty in 1989 and to 133 percent in 1990.[24]

The shift from AFDC-based eligibility standards to standards based on the poverty guidelines is significant, not only because the poverty guidelines are much higher than most States' AFDC payment levels, but also because the poverty guidelines keep pace with inflation while AFDC payments may not. The median State's maximum AFDC payment dropped from 45.5 percent of poverty in 1984 (when the first mandatory coverage of children up to AFDC levels took effect) to 38.6 percent of poverty in 1992. Continued use of AFDC standards to establish Medicaid eligibility could thus have led to a gradual erosion of coverage of poor children in recent years, instead of the expansion that has actually occurred (see below).

Through a similar process, Congress gradually extended limited benefits to low-income Medicare beneficiaries not otherwise eligible. Most States had always paid Medicare premiums, deductibles, and coinsurance amounts for aged and disabled beneficiaries qualifying under both programs. These "dual eligibles," who had to meet ordinary Medicaid financial eligibility standards, were also entitled to any Medicaid benefits not available under Medicare, such as prescription drugs or long-term care beyond Medicare's limited coverage. OBRA 86 established a new optional eligibility category (now known as "QMBs"), who met a State-established income standard no higher than 100 percent of the poverty level and whose resources were no more than twice the SSI limit. States could extend full Medicaid coverage to QMBs or could limit coverage to payment of Medicare cost-sharing amounts. MCCA required States to cover at least premiums and Medicare cost-sharing for all Medicare beneficiaries with incomes below 100 percent of poverty. OBRA 90 required payment of Medicare premiums (but not deductibles or coinsurance) for beneficiaries up to 110 of poverty by FY 1993, and up to 120 percent by FY 1995.

---

[24]All income levels are for a child in a family of three. AFDC levels are the median maximum payment amount. Optional medically needy levels are 133 1/3 of the AFDC levels. All levels for a year are expressed as a percent of the Federal poverty guideline for that year.

FIGURE I-7. Medicaid Income Limit, Non-AFDC Child Under 1 Year Old

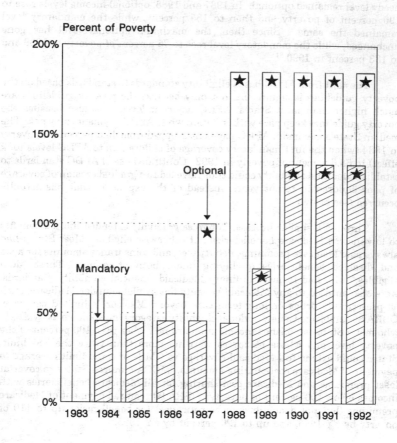

Percent of Poverty

★ = Eligibility levels based on Federal poverty guidelines.
All others based on median maximum AFDC payment levels.
Source: Figure prepared by Congressional Research Service.

FIGURE I-8. Medicaid Income Limit, Non-AFDC Child 4 Years Old

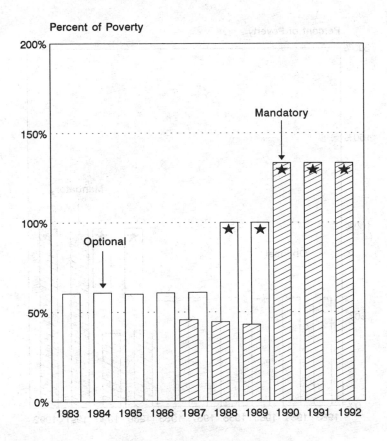

★ = Eligibility levels based on Federal poverty guidelines.
All others based on median maximum AFDC payment levels.
Source: Figure prepared by Congressional Research Service.

FIGURE I-9. Medicaid Income Limit, Non-AFDC Child 6 Years Old

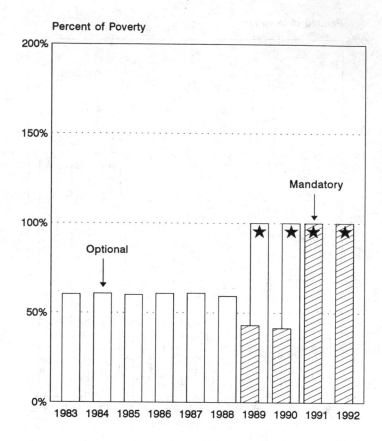

★ = Eligibility levels based on Federal poverty guidelines.
All others based on median maximum AFDC payment levels.
Source: Figure prepared by Congressional Research Service.

While most eligibility expansions in this period focused on these two target populations, women and children and low-income Medicare beneficiaries, Congress also expanded coverage for other groups as well. The Family Support Act of 1988 (P.L. 100-485) extended work transition coverage for families losing AFDC because of increased earnings, and also expanded coverage for two-parent families whose principal earner was unemployed. OBRA 87 established special eligibility rules for institutionalized persons whose spouse remained in the community, in order to prevent "spousal impoverishment," the reduction of the community spouse to poverty before the institutionalized spouse could receive Medicaid. Finally, there were measures to provide coverage for certain chronically ill or disabled persons who would have qualified for Medicaid if they had been in an institution but could not meet Medicaid standards if they were cared for in the community.

In addition to the eligibility expansions, Congress has required States to improve certain aspects of service coverage and raise reimbursement levels. In the area of services, new standards of quality for NF care were established by OBRA 87; States were required to raise payments to NFs to reflect the costs of meeting the new standards. EPSDT program requirements were expanded by OBRA 89; States must now provide the services needed to treat any problem or condition uncovered during a screening, even if the services are optional benefits that the State has chosen not to make available to other beneficiaries. New services have been added to the list of mandatory benefits that all States must provide, chiefly in order to expand access to care in underserved areas. States must now cover services of nurse practitioners (if the State licenses such providers) and services in FQHCs, facilities such as community and migrant health centers that are receiving or meet the requirements for grants under several Public Health Service programs.

Both Congress and the courts have taken steps to improve Medicaid provider reimbursement. Congress added to the statute a long-standing regulatory requirement that Medicaid payment rates had to be sufficient to attract enough providers to provide reasonable access. OBRA 89 spelled out detailed procedures for enforcing this requirement with respect to payment for services of pediatricians and obstetricians. Steps were also taken to strengthen an OBRA 81 requirement that States provide additional payment to hospitals treating a disproportionate share of low-income patients. In response to reports that few States had complied with the rule, OBRA 87 included minimum standards for the payment adjustments. For reasons to be discussed below, disproportionate share payments have been an important component of recent growth in Medicaid spending.

More recently, courts have begun more vigorous enforcement of the Boren amendment, the 1980 (1981 for hospitals) change that allowed States to depart from Medicare's cost reimbursement system for hospitals and nursing homes. Many States responded to the new flexibility by reducing payments to levels below the cost of treating Medicaid beneficiaries. However, the amendment included a requirement that States' payments to hospitals and nursing homes be sufficient to meet the cost of "efficiently and economically operated" facilities. A 1990 Supreme Court decision affirmed that facilities could seek review in

Federal courts of States' compliance with this requirement.[25] As of mid-1991, Boren amendment lawsuits had been filed by hospitals, nursing homes, or both in 29 States. Many of these suits have resulted in changes in reimbursement systems, either through court orders or through settlements.

Most of the legislative changes in Medicaid in the 1984-1990 period represented increases in spending above "current law" levels (the amount spending would have grown in the absence of legislation). While Medicare spending was repeatedly cut in an effort to meet deficit reduction targets, Medicaid was allowed to grow. In addition, the 1985 Gramm-Rudman-Hollings Act (P.L. 99-177), which provided for automatic spending reductions (sequestration) if necessary to meet deficit reduction targets, exempted Medicaid and other low-income entitlement programs.

The most recent Medicaid expansions, in OBRA 90, represent an exception to the pattern of legislated spending increases. Measures intended to produce program savings were included along with program expansions.[26]

The OBRA 90 required manufacturers of prescription drugs to provide rebates to State Medicaid programs, to give Medicaid the benefit of discounts accorded to other major payers. In return, States were required to cover all the drugs manufactured by a firm entering into a rebate agreement. A second savings measure in OBRA 90 requires States to pay premiums for group health plans for which Medicaid beneficiaries are eligible, when it is cost-effective to do so. This requirement was scheduled to take effect January 1, 1991, but had not been implemented as of June 1992.

E. The Cost Explosion

Growth in spending by Medicaid and other health care purchasers, which had been in double digits every year since the enactment of Medicare and Medicaid, slowed down in the early 1980s. As figure I-10 shows, rates of increase in the middle of the decade were at the lowest level in the program's history.

These relatively moderate cost increases paralleled the experience of Medicare and private insurers. In part the change reflected a drop in the rate of general inflation. However, many analysts believed the slowdown in medical care spending growth could be attributed to the success of cost containment efforts. In particular, they pointed to declining hospital admissions, which stemmed from changes in medical practice and in part from the widespread adoption of preadmission certification programs.

---

[25]*Wilder vs. Virginia Hospital Association*, 110 Sup.Ct. 2510.

[26]The Medicaid expansions included in the Medicare Catastrophic Coverage Act were originally projected to be partially offset by savings for dual Medicare/Medicaid beneficiaries resulting from the Medicare expansions in the Act. These savings were eliminated when the Medicare changes were repealed in 1989.

FIGURE I-10. Annual Rate of Growth in Medicaid Spending, FY 1966 to FY 1991

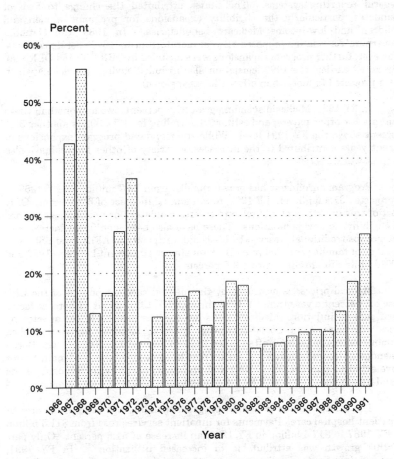

Source: Figure prepared by Congressional Research Service based on data contained in the Budget of the United States Government, Fiscal Years 1969 to 1993.

The slowdown in medical spending growth was shortlived. Spending by all payers resumed double digit growth in 1988, and Medicaid cost increases soon outpaced those for other health care purchasers. Many States were aware of the turnaround in Medicaid spending in 1989, before it was fully apparent in Federal reporting systems. The States attributed the change to Federal mandates, particularly the eligibility expansions for pregnant women and children and low-income Medicare beneficiaries. In 1989, the National Governors' Association proposed a 2-year moratorium on new Federal mandates. However, further program expansions were included in OBRA 89 and OBRA 90. (As noted earlier, the 1990 legislation also included savings provisions which were projected to more than offset the expansions.)

In FY 1991, Medicaid spending grew 27.8 percent, two and one-half times the rate for other payers, and estimated spending for FY 1992 is another 30.1 percent above the FY 1991 level. While the mandated program expansions of recent years contributed to the increases, a variety of other factors have also been at work.

Program enrollment has grown rapidly, from 24.7 million in FY 1989 to a projected 31.4 million in FY 1992, for an annual increase of 8.3 percent. Only part of this growth is attributable to recent mandatory or optional expansions of eligibility to new populations. There have also been significant increases in the groups traditionally served by Medicaid, recipients of AFDC and SSI. The number of families enrolled in AFDC rose almost 19 percent between 1989 and 1991, while SSI enrollment rose 9.5 percent.

Medical prices, as measured by the medical care component of the CPI, rose 8.4 percent a year from FY 1988 through FY 1991, about 71 percent faster than general inflation. Medicaid costs have in the past been less affected by price increases than costs for other payers, because State-established reimbursement rates have often failed to keep pace with inflation. The Boren amendment lawsuits mentioned earlier may have changed this, and many States have acted to improve physician reimbursement, partially in response to the standards imposed by OBRA 89 for obstetric and pediatric care payments.

The most dramatic growth in program spending has been in the area of inpatient hospital care. Payments for inpatient services rose from $11.5 billion in FY 1987 to $17.4 billion in FY 1990, an increase of 51.8 percent. Only part of this growth was attributable to increased utilization.[27] In FY 1991, Medicaid inpatient spending grew another 44.7 percent. In a few States, inpatient spending increases may have been related to Boren amendment suits. However, much of the growth appears to be related to two factors that emerged as a central issue in Medicaid policy in 1991--State reliance on provider donations and provider-specific taxes as revenue sources, and the rapid growth in State payments to hospitals serving a disproportionate share of Medicaid and uninsured patients.

---

[27]The AHA data indicate that total Medicaid inpatient days rose 13.1 percent in calendar years 1987-1990, or slightly more than the growth in Medicaid enrollment in the same period.

Beginning in 1986, States developed programs to use funds donated by health care providers or taxes paid by those providers to draw greater Federal matching payments. Table I-3 illustrates how a typical provider donation program might work in a State whose Federal matching percentage was 60 percent. A hospital gives the State $40; the State pays the hospital $100 and receives $60 in Federal matching funds. The State's share is $40, or zero after crediting the hospital donation. Some State provider tax programs worked in a similar way. A State might pay a hospital $100 and claim from HCFA the $60 Federal matching payment, then tax the hospital $40, leaving no net State expenditure from general funds.

TABLE I-3. Effect of Typical State Provider Donation Program
(Federal matching rate = 60 percent)

Hospital donation	$ 40
State payment to hospital	100
Amount allowed by HCFA	100
Computed Federal share	60
State share	40
Net cost to State	$ 0
(State share less donation)	

The Administration first proposed to outlaw these financing mechanisms in 1988, contending that they allowed States to receive Federal funds without having incurred any real costs. The States responded that the Federal Government had no authority to scrutinize State revenue sources and argued that donation and tax programs were essential to maintaining Medicaid services. Congress repeatedly delayed the Secretary's authority to regulate in this area. By late 1991, 34 States had or were planning some form of donation program or provider-specific tax. The Administration estimated that revenues from such sources would total $4.5 billion in FY 1992, or 9.2 percent of the States' share of Medicaid spending.

States used the additional Federal funds for a variety of purposes, including financing program expansions or simply maintaining current services in the face of State budget shortfalls. However, one use that was of particular concern to the Administration was increasing payments to disproportionate share hospitals (DSHs). As was discussed earlier, these payments were first required in 1981, and minimum standards for DSH adjustments were enacted in 1987. By 1989, 41 States responding to a survey by the National Association of Public Hospitals reported DSH payments of $569 million. Late in 1991, however, HCFA projected on the basis of State estimates that DSH payments would total $14.3 billion in FY 1992, or over 12 percent of total Medicaid spending.

In 1986, Congress had prohibited the Secretary from limiting DSH payments, making these payments the only area of Medicaid reimbursement not subject to Federal regulation. The Administration contended that the growth in DSH payments was tied to the use of donations and taxes and that States were designating hospitals as DSHs inappropriately. A State could increase DSH payments by any amount it chose, tax away the increase, and draw unlimited Federal funds.

In 1991, the Administration again proposed to regulate donations and taxes and also proposed to limit the hospitals that could be designated as DSHs. While there were questions about the Secretary's authority to impose the new rules, the Administration and the States negotiated a compromise that was enacted by Congress in the Medicaid Voluntary Contribution and Provider-Specific Tax Amendments of 1991 (P.L. 102-234). The Act prohibits the use of most provider donations and phases out the use of provider taxes that are not "broad based" (such as taxes imposed solely on Medicaid revenues), although States currently using such revenues are permitted to phase them out in 1992 and 1993. Total revenues from donations and taxes (whether or not broad-based) are limited to 25 percent of the State's share of Medicaid, again with exceptions for States that were relying more heavily on these revenues.

The Act also limits national aggregate spending for DSH payment adjustments to 12 percent of total Medicaid program spending, roughly the level initially projected for FY 1992. States with DSH payments already exceeding 12 percent may not increase those payments; other States may do so, subject to the national cap. (Actual FY 1992 DSH payments are estimated to have reached 16.1 percent of program spending, well above the level anticipated when the Act was considered.)

III. THE THREE MEDICAID PROGRAMS

While Medicaid is structured at the Federal level as a program of grants to States, at the State level it operates essentially as an insurance plan--it pays claims from qualified medical providers for covered services furnished to enrolled beneficiaries. One key difference between Medicaid and other public and private insurance plans is in the scope of benefits it covers. While most health plans are limited to coverage of costs for acute medical care, Medicaid also covers long-term care in NFs, ICFs/MR, facilities for the chronically mentally ill, and community settings. As the largest single source of financing for long-term care, Medicaid has taken on a more active role in shaping and regulating the delivery of these services than is customary for a health insurer. In addition, the persons receiving these services often become eligible for Medicaid in different ways from other beneficiaries and form distinct populations. As a result, many people speak of Medicaid as constituting three separate programs:

- It is a basic medical plan for most of its beneficiaries.

- It is a financing program for long-term medical and social services for the frail elderly and the disabled.

- It is a funding stream for programs (largely State-operated) for the developmentally disabled and the mentally ill.

These "programs" overlap to a considerable extent. For example, persons eligible in the community may later enter long-term care, while those in long-term care may also receive Medicaid-funded acute care services. In addition, while the three basic functions account for the bulk of Medicaid spending, Medicaid performs other roles as well, such as providing supplemental coverage to low-income Medicare beneficiaries. Nevertheless, the division of Medicaid into three key functions is a useful way of examining the program. The following provides an overview of each of the three major components of Medicaid.

A. Health Insurance

Medicaid serves as the nearest equivalent to conventional health insurance for most of its beneficiaries. Recent congressional steps to expand eligibility, along with proposals for further expansions to reach more of the uninsured, have focused increasing attention on questions of how well Medicaid functions as an insurance program. How well does it reach low-income population groups targeted for coverage, and what effect have recent eligibility expansions had? For those the program does insure, does Medicaid provide access to care of adequate quality? Has it helped its beneficiaries enter the "mainstream" of medical care?

1. Medicaid as a Source of Insurance

Medicaid is the third most important source of health insurance coverage in the United States (after employment-based coverage and Medicare). As figure I-11 indicates, 10.6 percent of the noninstitutionalized population was covered by Medicaid at some time during 1991.[28] For persons in poverty, as shown in figure I-12, Medicaid is by far the largest source of coverage, reaching 47.3 percent of persons with family incomes below the Federal poverty level.

Medicaid enrollment has grown significantly in recent years, as a result of the congressionally mandated eligibility expansions and a rising AFDC caseload. Its performance in providing coverage to the poor population has improved accordingly. The percentage of the poor receiving Medicaid has grown from 39.1 percent in 1979 to 47.3 percent in 1991.[29] As would be expected, given the congressional focus in recent expansion efforts, the greatest gains have occurred among children. The Medicaid coverage rate for poor children under age 7 has risen from 49.8 percent in 1979 to 73.7 percent in 1992; coverage of poor children aged 7 to 17 has grown from 47.2 percent to 58.5 percent.

---

[28]This and other estimates in this section are based on Congressional Research Service analysis of the March 1992 Current Population Survey (CPS) conducted by the Census Bureau, which asked questions about insurance coverage during 1991.

[29]Because of changes in the CPS questionnaire, estimates for years before 1987 are not strictly comparable to those for more recent years.

FIGURE I-11. Health Insurance Coverage by Type of Insurance, CY 1991

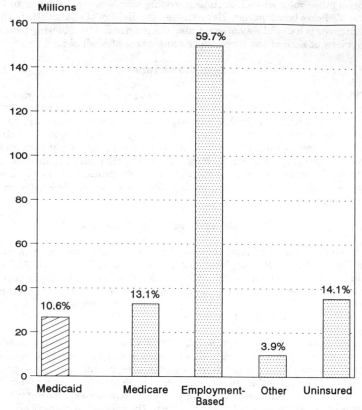

Total population = 251.2 million

Millions

NOTE: "Other" includes CHAMPUS, VA, or military health care.
Percentages represent share of total population covered by each type of health insurance. They sum to more than 100% because an individual may have more than one type of coverage.

Source: Figure prepared by Congressional Research Service based on data from the Census Bureau.

FIGURE I-12. Health Insurance Coverage of Persons Below the Poverty Level by Type of Insurance, CY 1991

Total population = 35.7 million

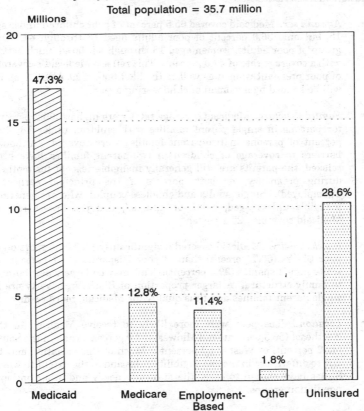

NOTE: "Other" includes CHAMPUS, VA, or military health care.
Percentages represent share of total population covered by each type of health insurance. They sum to more than 100% because an individual may have more than one type of coverage.

Source: Figure prepared by Congressional Research Service based on data from the Census Bureau.

Coverage rates for different subgroups of the poor vary widely. Medicaid is available only to certain populations specified in law, and financial eligibility standards differ by State and by the defined population into which an individual falls. The following is a summary of differences in coverage rates for specified population characteristics.

- *Age and sex.* Medicaid covered 65.5 percent of poor children under age 18, but only 36.0 percent of poor adults aged 18 through 64. One group of poor adults, women aged 18 through 44, fared much better, with a coverage rate of 47.9 percent. This reflects Medicaid's coverage of poor pregnant women as well as the likelihood that AFDC families will be headed by a woman of childbearing age.

- *Family structure.* Medicaid coverage rates were highest, 69.2 percent, for persons in single parent families with children under 18; 40.3 percent of persons in two-parent families were covered. Although barriers to coverage of children in two-parent families have been relaxed, the parents are still generally ineligible (except for mothers during pregnancy, or both parents if the principal earner is unemployed). Single adults and childless couples, who are generally ineligible unless aged, blind, or disabled, had the lowest rate of Medicaid coverage, 25.1 percent.

- *Race/ethnicity.* Medicaid covered a significantly higher proportion of poor Blacks (60.7 percent) than of poor Hispanics (47.7 percent) or white non-Hispanics (39.4 percent). This may be largely attributable to family structure. A larger proportion of Blacks in poverty are in single parent families and thus qualify for Medicaid more readily.

- *Location.* The poor were more likely to receive Medicaid in the Northeast (56.3 percent) and Midwest (52.0 percent) than in the South (42.2 percent) or West (44.3 percent). Much of this variation may be due to differences in income eligibility rules and in the extent to which States have chosen to cover the medically needy and other optional population groups.

- *Degree of poverty.* Within the poor population, those with the lowest incomes had a greater likelihood of coverage. Of persons with family incomes below 50 percent of poverty, 54.2 percent received Medicaid; of those with incomes between 75 and 100 percent of poverty, 35.6 percent received Medicaid. This reflects the fact that in most States financial eligibility standards (except for the newly covered groups of pregnant women and children) are well below the poverty level.

Variation in Medicaid coverage rates for different subgroups of the population in poverty may reflect, not only the effects of Medicaid policies, but also the extent to which different groups have access to alternative sources of insurance. Because of the complexity of the application process and the "welfare stigma" attached to the program, Medicaid may function as the insurer of last resort, attracting chiefly persons who have not obtained coverage elsewhere. It may, then, be useful to ask how well Medicaid fills in the gaps left by other public and private sources of coverage.

Table I-4 answers the question, of poor persons with no other form of insurance, how many receive Medicaid and how many remain uninsured? The patterns are essentially the same as those observed in the preceding discussion: Medicaid is most successful in reaching children, members of single parent families, and the very poor. Single individuals and childless couples are most likely to be left uninsured.

All of the figures cited so far represent people who received Medicaid at any time during the year. However, eligibility for Medicaid can be affected both by fluctuations in earnings and other income and by other events that can affect categorical eligibility (such as a change in family structure or disability status). As a result, many people gain or lose Medicaid over the course of a year. One Census Bureau study found that, of persons receiving Medicaid at any time in 1987, only 57 percent were covered for the entire year; 18 percent were covered for 4 months or less.[30]

TABLE I-4. Medicaid Coverage of the Poor Without Other Public or Private Coverage, 1991
(numbers in thousands)

	Covered by Medicaid only	Uninsured	Total without non-Medicaid coverage[a]	Percent covered by Medicaid
Age:				
Under 18	8,421	2,935	11,356	74.2%
18-44	4,436	5,562	9,998	44.4%
45-64	973	1,618	2,591	37.6%
Family structure:				
Single parent family	9,118	2,814	11,932	76.4%
Two parent family	3,345	3,576	6,921	48.3%
Husband/wife	234	795	1,029	22.7%
Single person	1,142	3,036	4,178	27.3%
Race:				
White (non-Hispanic)	5,456	4,912	10,368	52.6%
Black (non-Hispanic)	5,142	2,282	7,424	69.3%
Hispanic	2,595	2,566	5,161	50.3%
Other (non-Hispanic)	646	459	1,105	58.5%

See notes at end of table.

[30]U.S. Dept. of Commerce. Bureau of the Census. *Health Insurance Coverage: 1987-90.* Prepared by Kathleen Short. Current Population Reports, Household Economic Studies, Series P-70, no. 29, May 1992. Washington, 1992.

TABLE I-4. Medicaid Coverage of the Poor Without Other
Public or Private Coverage, 1991--Continued
(numbers in thousands)

	Covered by Medicaid only	Uninsured	Total without non-Medicaid coverage[a]	Percent covered by Medicaid
Region:				
Midwest	3,480	1,808	5,288	65.8%
Northeast	2,772	1,141	3,913	70.8%
South	4,693	4,561	9,254	50.7%
West	2,895	2,710	5,605	51.7%
Family income relative to poverty ratio:				
Under 50 percent	6,924	4,059	10,983	63.0%
50 to 74 percent	4,400	2,884	7,284	60.4%
75 to under 100 percent	2,516	3,277	5,793	43.4%
Total	13,840	10,220	24,060	57.5%

[a]Sum of persons without insurance and persons receiving Medicaid only.

NOTE: All figures are estimates of the noninstitutionalized poverty populations. Medicaid totals omit persons reporting both Medicaid and another form of coverage during the year.

Source: Table prepared by the Congressional Research Service based on data contained in the Mar. 1992 Current Population Survey.

Changes in employment are the most important single reason for the loss of Medicaid benefits. Another study found that 45 percent of persons losing Medicaid had an employment change (a new job, increased hours of work, or increased hourly wages).[31] This does not mean, however, that individuals leaving Medicaid necessarily shift to employment-based health insurance or other coverage. On the contrary, most persons losing Medicaid became uninsured.

One consequence is a concern that Medicaid may serve as a "work disincentive"--some families may remain on welfare instead of seeking employment because they are afraid of losing health coverage. The extended work transition coverage provisions of the Family Support Act of 1988 (see above) were designed to address this problem by continuing Medicaid for up to a year after a family loses AFDC benefits. The effects of this provision are not yet known.

[31]Short, Pamela, J. Cantor, and A. Monheit. The Dynamics of Medicaid Enrollment. *Inquiry*, v. 25, no. 1, winter 1988. p. 504-516.

2. Medicaid and Access to Care

a. Basic Access

The simplest way to measure Medicaid's relative success in facilitating access to care is to count services. Beneficiaries' use of services can be compared, on the one hand, to that of comparable persons with no insurance coverage at all and, on the other, to that of persons with private insurance coverage. (However, it must be emphasized that health insurance coverage is just one of many factors that help to determine whether and to what an extent an individual will receive medical care, including the physical availability of health services, individual propensity to seek medical treatment, and basic need for care.)

In terms of simple quantity of services used, Medicaid beneficiaries appear to have significantly better access to care than comparable uninsured individuals. Medicaid enrollees are about as likely as persons with private insurance to have at least one ambulatory physician contact during a year, and much more likely than the uninsured. Those who do see a physician have (after correction for health status) about the same number of visits as the privately insured. For some types of care, however, the pattern may be different. Women covered by Medicaid are only slightly more likely to obtain prenatal care in the first trimester of pregnancy than are uninsured women, and much less likely than the insured. Only about a third of Medicaid-covered children are known to receive preventive care; comparable figures for privately insured children are not available.

Persons with Medicaid receive more inpatient hospital care than either the privately insured or the uninsured, again after correction for health status. Their hospital stays for any particular diagnosis tend to be longer. This may reflect greater severity within diagnoses or social factors, such as delays in discharge because of difficulties arranging for nursing home placement or home care.

An alternative measure of basic access is the extent to which patients are able to establish an ongoing relationship with a regular source of care. Medicaid beneficiaries do relatively well on this measure; they are less likely than the privately insured, and much less likely than the uninsured, to report that they have no usual source of care. However, they are also more likely than the privately insured to report that their usual source of care is a hospital outpatient department or emergency room, rather than an office-based physician. This does not mean that many beneficiaries rely exclusively on hospital-based care. Instead, they are more likely than the privately insured to see a mix of hospital and office-based physicians.

b. Mainstreaming

For a variety of reasons, many medical care providers refuse to accept Medicaid patients or limit the number of such patients they will treat. As a result, some people argue that Medicaid has failed to achieve the goal of mainstreaming and has led to the development of a two-tier system of medical care.

The willingness of physicians to accept Medicaid patients varies by specialty. Surgical specialists and primary care physicians are most likely to accept Medicaid, while obstetricians and psychiatrists are the least likely. Studies in the mid-1980s indicated that Medicaid patients accounted for a declining share of caseloads in most specialties. More recent studies have shown a drop in participation in two key specialties--obstetrics/gynecology and pediatrics. A 1987 survey found that only 63 percent of obstetricians were accepting Medicaid, while the percentage of pediatricians accepting Medicaid patients dropped from 85 percent to 77 percent between 1978 and 1989. Low Medicaid fee schedules, relative to the physicians' usual charges to other payers, are the major deterrent to participation. Physicians may also be influenced by what they perceive as cumbersome bureaucratic requirements, delays in claim payment, or characteristics of Medicaid beneficiaries themselves (including a view, refuted by several recent studies, that beneficiaries are more likely to sue for malpractice).

Virtually all hospitals participate in Medicaid. However, the extent of participation varies widely. For inpatient services, Medicaid beneficiaries are much more likely to be treated in public nonfederal hospitals than are other patients, and are less likely to be admitted to private facilities, including both for-profit and nonprofit hospitals. Teaching hospitals, those with medical residency programs, also have a higher Medicaid patient load than others. Factors other than hospital admission policies, such as location or the nature of the hospital's services, may affect a hospital's Medicaid caseload. At least in some States, however, private hospitals may be reluctant to admit Medicaid patients because of low Medicaid reimbursement rates or restrictive coverage policies.

Concern over the failure to mainstream Medicaid beneficiaries does not stem simply from the fact that providers used by Medicaid beneficiaries may not be identical to those used by other patients. Simple geography might often dictate that the providers most accessible to low-income persons would be different from those most convenient to higher-income persons. However, there is some evidence that Medicaid beneficiaries must travel longer than other patients to their usual source of care and must wait longer to be seen. There are also quality issues, raised by continuing reports of "Medicaid mills" (clinics that treat large numbers of beneficiaries in brief and perfunctory visits) and by concerns about the lack of continuity in care furnished by hospital outpatient departments.

Finally, there is limited evidence that, even when Medicaid beneficiaries receive care from the same sources used by other patients, they may be treated differently. Some providers may spend less time with lower-paying patients, and Medicaid patients may be less likely to receive costly procedures (such as coronary artery bypass grafts) than comparable privately insured patients. So far, however, there is little information on whether the actual outcomes of care differ for Medicaid and privately insured patients.

3. Medicaid and Maternal and Child Health

While availability of Medicaid coverage and access to care for Medicaid beneficiaries are important issues for all the populations served by the program, the greatest attention in recent years has been devoted to improving coverage and access for pregnant women and children. A number of factors have contributed to this focus. The United States performs poorly in comparison to other industrialized countries on such standard measures as infant mortality rates, incidence of low birthweight babies, and immunization of young children. Inadequate access to prenatal and early childhood care may have long-term social costs, in terms of lifetime disability and lost productivity. They may also have immediate financial consequences: for example, the cost of providing comprehensive prenatal care has been shown to be considerably less than that of providing the medical care associated with poor birth outcomes. In response to these concerns, Congress and the States have taken a variety of steps to remove barriers to Medicaid eligibility for pregnant women and children and to overcome other, nonfinancial barriers to access.

a. Eligibility

During the 1980s, Congress repeatedly raised both mandatory and optional Medicaid income limits for pregnant women and children, and eliminated the categorical rules that had tied Medicaid eligibility to eligibility for cash assistance (such as limitations on coverage of members of two-parent families). These expansions were traced earlier in this chapter. However, income standards are not the only key to Medicaid eligibility. Applicants must also meet resource standards (limitations on cash and other assets) and must complete an eligibility determination process that can be cumbersome and time-consuming. A number of recent measures have addressed these other barriers to eligibility:

- The OBRA 86 allowed States to use different asset tests, or none at all, for pregnant women and children potentially qualifying under the new poverty-related income standards. As of January 1992, 48 States had made use of this option.

- States have the option to establish "presumptive eligibility" for low-income pregnant women; certain providers of care may make a preliminary determination that a pregnant woman may be financially eligible for Medicaid benefits. The woman may then receive ambulatory prenatal care while the State is reviewing her Medicaid application. Presumptive eligibility was used in 26 States in January 1992.

- The OBRA 90 required States to "outstation" eligibility workers, so that pregnant women and children can apply for Medicaid at the places where they receive care (such as hospitals and community health centers) instead of at welfare offices. Some States are also accepting mail-in or telephone applications.

- Finally, 33 States have developed a shorter Medicaid application form for pregnant women and children, and some have taken steps to expedite the review of completed applications.

b. Access

Because Medicaid eligibility alone may not ensure access to medical services, Congress and the States have also sought to address barriers to care not directly related to insurance status. Perhaps the most important of these has been a shortage of providers willing to accept Medicaid payment. As was noted earlier, participation by obstetricians has always been low, while the willingness of pediatricians to accept Medicaid has been dropping. OBRA 89 provided for closer Federal monitoring of Medicaid payment rates for obstetric and pediatric services. In addition, States are now required to cover alternate providers of these services, such as nurse midwives and certified pediatric or family nurse practitioners. States are also required to cover (and reimburse at reasonable cost) services of FQHCs, such as community health centers and similar entities. These centers are a major source of perinatal and child health care in medically underserved areas. Finally, some States have explored the possibility of Medicaid payment for services in school health clinics, although Medicaid participation in these clinics has been limited so far.

Even when services are accessible, not all beneficiaries are aware of what services are available or of the benefits of prenatal and early childhood care. Some States have developed outreach programs (using non-Medicaid funding sources) to encourage high-risk clients to obtain appropriate care. Outreach to EPSDT-eligible children has long been a Medicaid requirement, although Federal standards in this area were relaxed in the early 1980s.[32]

Finally, there have been measures to improve the coordination between Medicaid and other Federal and State programs that provide services to pregnant women and children, including the Special Supplemental Food Program for Women, Infants, and Children (WIC) and programs funded under the Maternal and Child Health (MCH) block grant. Beneficiaries using one program must be notified of the availability of others, and DHHS and the Department of Agriculture have developed a combined application form for federally assisted maternal and child programs.

B. Long-Term Care

Long-term care refers to a broad range of medical, social, personal care, and supportive services needed by individuals who have lost some capacity for self-care because of a chronic illness or condition. Chronic illnesses or conditions often result in both functional impairment and physical dependence on others for an extended period of time. These conditions include heart disease, strokes, arthritis, and Alzheimer's and related dementias. Long-term care services can be provided either in institutions, such as nursing homes, or in home and

---

[32]A lawsuit is now pending in Pennsylvania over whether the State, among other things, has failed to conduct adequate EPSDT outreach.

community-based care settings. Although chronic conditions occur in individuals of all ages, the elderly are the largest group in need of long-term care. It is estimated that the elderly account for two-thirds of the 10.6 million persons of all ages needing long-term care and living in institutions and the community. The following discussion will therefore focus on Medicaid services for the elderly. Services for the other major population receiving Medicaid long-term care coverage, the developmentally disabled, are discussed in the next section.

1. *Medicaid Coverage of Long-Term Care Services for the Elderly*

Medicaid funds a broad range of long-term care services for the elderly, including:

- *Nursing facility services.* States are required to cover under their Medicaid plans NF services for individuals 21 years of age and older.

In determining whether persons should be covered for Medicaid's NF benefit, many States use preadmission screening programs that go beyond the State's income and assets standards used for eligibility. Preadmission screening programs include an on-site assessment of a person's functional impairments and need for nursing home care.

The OBRA 87 comprehensively revised the statutory authority that applies to nursing homes participating in Medicaid. The so-called nursing home reform law eliminated the Medicaid program's previous distinction between SNFs and ICFs and established a single category called "NF". It strengthened the requirements that must be met by NFs in order to participate in Medicaid, modified the survey and certification process that States must use for determining whether nursing homes comply with these requirements; and established new sanctions and enforcement actions that the States and HCFA may impose against noncompliant nursing homes.

The new standards for participation address such issues as the scope of services a NF must provide, levels of staffing in the facility and the qualifications of staff, residents' rights, and the physical environment of the facility. OBRA 87 requires States to take into account in their payments to NFs the costs of complying with these and other new requirements. Some States may also have to increase nursing home reimbursement as a result of Boren amendment lawsuits, comparable to the suits by hospitals discussed earlier.

- *Home health care.* States are required to cover home health for any person who is entitled to NF services under the State's Medicaid plan.

Medicaid's home health benefit has a skilled medical care orientation and is not intended to provide personal care and other nonmedical supportive assistance that many elderly persons with chronic conditions require in order to remain in the community.

- *Personal care.* Personal care includes services provided in an individual's home by a qualified person who is supervised by a registered nurse and who is not a member of the individual's family.

Personal care services include bathing, dressing, ambulation, feeding, and grooming. Household services offered by most programs include meal preparation and clean-up, light cleaning, laundry, and shopping. As of October 1, 1991, 28 States covered personal care under their Medicaid plans. Beginning October 1, 1994, Medicaid law will require States to cover personal care for any person entitled to NF services under the State's Medicaid plan.

- *Home and community-based care waiver services.* States have an option of covering persons needing home and community-based care services, if these persons would otherwise require institutional care that would be covered by Medicaid. These services are provided under waiver programs authorized in section 1915(c) and 1915(d) of Medicaid law.

With HCFA approval, States may provide a wide variety of nonmedical, social, and supportive services that have been shown to be critical in allowing chronically ill and disabled persons to remain in their homes. These include case management, homemaker/home health aide services, personal care, adult day health, and respite care, among others. States are using waiver programs to provide services to a diverse long-term care population, including the elderly, and others who are disabled or who have chronic mental illness, mental retardation and developmental disabilities, and AIDS. As of December 1991, 40 States operated 49 1915(c) waiver programs serving the aged/disabled. The aged/disabled represented 73 percent of all persons served in FY 1991, but accounted for only 31 percent of total waiver spending. The mentally retarded/developmentally disabled accounted for 21 percent of total waiver participants, but 65 percent of total spending.

- *Optional home and community-based care services.* States may also provide home and community-based care to elderly persons under a new optional Medicaid benefit called home and community-based care for functionally disabled elderly persons (the "frail elderly").

This new benefit, established by OBRA 90, allows States to cover a variety of home and community-based services without going through the process of applying for a 1915(c) waiver. (A similar nonwaiver benefit was created for the developmentally disabled; see below.) This optional benefit is different from others, in that Federal matching payments are capped. Federal matching payments cannot exceed $40 million for FY 1991; $70 million for FY 1992; $130 million for FY 1993; $160 million for FY 1994; and $180 million for FY 1995. (No cap applies after FY 1995.) As of July 1992, only two States, Texas and Rhode Island, had made use of the new option.

2. Medicaid Long-Term Care Spending

Long-term care spending, and especially nursing home spending, accounts for the great bulk of Medicaid's spending for the elderly. Two-thirds of total Medicaid spending for the elderly, or $14.5 billion of $21.5 billion, was for nursing home care in FY 1990. Much smaller amounts were spent for various home care services--$1.7 billion, or 8.1 percent of total spending for the elderly, in FY 1990. Together these two categories of long-term care spending amounted to three-quarters of total Medicaid spending for the elderly.

There is considerable variation among States in the proportion of beneficiaries who are elderly, the proportion of program payments made on their behalf, and the magnitude of difference between these two ratios. The percentage of elderly Medicaid beneficiaries in a State's Medicaid program ranged from 7.0 percent in Alaska to 22.6 percent in New Hampshire. The proportion of total program payments for the elderly ranged from 18.2 percent in Utah to 50.4 percent in Connecticut. Average payments per elderly beneficiary ranged from $2,814 in Mississippi to $14,824 in New York, with Kansas representing the median value of $6,037. Variation in these ratios can be explained by differences in the scope of benefits covered, reimbursement rates for benefits, and eligibility policies for coverage.

After relatively modest rates of growth of 6 to 9 percent in the mid-1980s, nursing home spending increased by 14 percent in 1990 and 17 percent in 1991. These increases may be the result of higher reimbursement rates required as the result of OBRA 87 nursing home reform revisions as well as court cases that have required States to increase payments to facilities. While payments for noninstitutional long-term care services are growing even more rapidly, they represent a much smaller share of Medicaid spending, just 2.7 percent of the total in FY 1991.

3. Medicaid Long-Term Care and the Non-Poor

As figure I-13 shows, Medicaid is the largest source of third-party funding for long-term care. Medicare has very limited long-term care benefits, restricted to short-term nursing home and home health care following hospitalization. Employer and other private health insurance plans commonly have similar restrictions. Private insurance specifically for long-term care is growing rapidly but is still comparatively rare. Medicaid is therefore left to fill the gaps left by other insurance. It serves, not only the low-income elderly and disabled, but higher income persons who must turn to Medicaid after exhausting their own resources to pay for their care.

At an average cost of $30,000 a year, nursing home costs can quickly deplete the resources of most elderly individuals, especially after long stays. A number of different State studies have looked at the percentage of Medicaid residents of nursing homes who were not eligible for Medicaid when they were originally admitted. They found that somewhere between 27 and 45 percent of residents "spent down" while in nursing homes; that is, they used up their savings and became eligible for Medicaid.

FIGURE I-13. Sources of Funding for Nursing Home Care, CY 1990

Total spending = $53.1 billion

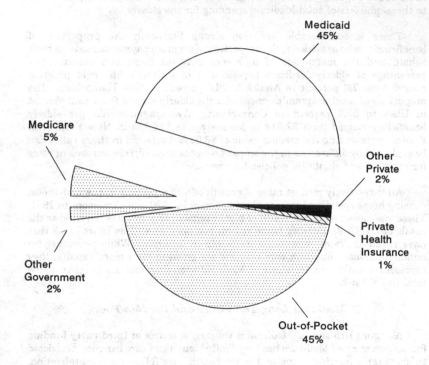

Medicaid
45%

Medicare
5%

Other
Private
2%

Private
Health
Insurance
1%

Other
Government
2%

Out-of-Pocket
45%

Source: Figure prepared by Congressional Research Service based on data from Office of the Actuary, Division of National Cost Estimates.

Medicaid's spending for long-term care for the elderly is thus largely driven by its coverage of persons who need nursing home care and who are not poor by cash welfare standards. States cover these persons either under a medically needy program or a special income rule, referred to as the "300 percent rule." As was discussed earlier, medically needy programs allow States to cover persons who have incurred medical expenses that deplete their resources and incomes to levels that make them needy according to State-determined standards. Under the 300 percent rule, States are allowed to cover persons needing nursing home care so long as their income does not exceed 300 percent of the basic SSI cash welfare payment (in 1992, 300 percent of $422, or $1,266 a month).

Figure I-14 shows the shares of Medicaid NF spending and spending for other services that go to the medically needy, the categorically needy without cash assistance (such as persons covered under the 300 percent rule), the categorically needy with cash assistance (SSI recipients), and other beneficiaries. The medically needy and categorical noncash groups accounted for 88 percent of NF spending and 75 percent of total spending for aged beneficiaries in FY 1990. It is nursing home spending for the non-poor that largely explains the fact that elderly Medicaid beneficiaries over the years have accounted for a disproportionately large portion of Medicaid payments for services. In FY 1990, elderly beneficiaries represented 13 percent of total Medicaid beneficiaries, while their share of program payments amounted to 33 percent of total program payments.

While Medicaid allows States to extend coverage to people with incomes in excess of cash welfare program standards, it also requires these persons first to deplete their assets before they can become eligible. In an effort to assure that these persons actually apply their assets to the cost of their care and do not give them away (for example, to their children) in order to gain Medicaid eligibility sooner than they otherwise would, Medicaid law contains provisions prohibiting most transfer of assets for less than fair market value during the 30-month period prior to an application for coverage. If a transfer has occurred, States must establish a period of ineligibility beginning with the month the resources were transferred.

Despite these requirements, anecdotal reports and a recent survey of Medicaid officials in six States suggest that increasing numbers of non-poor elderly persons finding ways to avoid applying their wealth to the costs of long-term care services. They may shelter assets in certain types of trusts or convert them into noncountable resources (for example, using cash, which is countable, to buy down the mortgage on their home, which is not countable). How extensively these and other strategies are being used to protect assets, so that Medicaid ends up paying sooner than it otherwise would, is unknown. Some argue that the scope of the problem is overstated, since few elderly persons are wealthy enough to be motivated to protect assets.

FIGURE I-14. Medicaid Payments for Aged Beneficiaries by Service Category and Eligibility Status, FY 1990

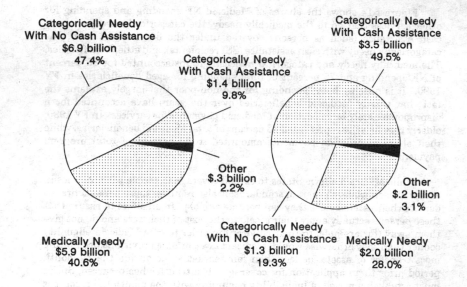

Nursing Facility Care
Spending = $14.5 billion

All Other Services
Spending = $7.0 billion

Categorically Needy
With No Cash Assistance
$6.9 billion
47.4%

Categorically Needy
With Cash Assistance
$1.4 billion
9.8%

Categorically Needy
With Cash Assistance
$3.5 billion
49.5%

Other
$.3 billion
2.2%

Other
$.2 billion
3.1%

Medically Needy
$5.9 billion
40.6%

Categorically Needy
With No Cash Assistance
$1.3 billion
19.3%

Medically Needy
$2.0 billion
28.0%

Total spending = $21.5 billion

Source: Figure prepared by Congressional Research Service based on data from HCFA Form 2082.

Some States have been exploring ways to link private long-term care insurance and Medicaid. Recently, HCFA approved proposals from four States that would allow them to establish more liberal asset standards for persons with private long-term care insurance coverage. If a person with such coverage exhausted the policy's maximum benefits during a nursing home stay and needed to turn to Medicaid for assistance, assets equal to the amount paid out by the private policy would be "protected"--could be retained by the beneficiary instead of being spent down. The goal is to encourage higher-income persons to make advance provisions for their own long-term care needs. Because a long period can elapse between the purchase of insurance and actual need for long-term care, it will be many years before it can be determined whether this approach can help control Medicaid spending. In addition, some people contend that this approach amounts to using a means-tested program to help higher-income persons protect their estates.

C. Developmentally Disabled and Mentally Ill

Medicaid is a major source of Federal support for State and private programs to serve the mentally retarded and other developmentally disabled individuals. Institutional and community-based services for the developmentally disabled account for more than 10 percent of Medicaid spending. To a limited extent, Medicaid also supports treatment for the mentally ill. However, the mentally ill population has never emerged, as has the mentally retarded population, as a distinct population served by the Medicaid program. Medicaid provides some services to some segments of the mentally ill population under certain conditions.

1. Medicaid Services for the Developmentally Disabled

Persons with developmental disabilities (including mental retardation and other related conditions) require special care and services to achieve their potential. Most are able to live at home with their families or in community-based facilities. These persons can generally participate in daytime activities, including programs that offer training ranging from self-help habilitation programs to prevocational or supported employment programs. However, some persons require more intensive services, and many of these most severely impaired persons are served in residential facilities that offer comprehensive, continual care.

Medicaid is a major source of funding for services to the developmentally disabled, chiefly through coverage of services in ICFs/MR and more limited support for community-based services. Of an estimated $20.2 billion in Federal and State spending for benefits and services for developmental disabilities in FY 1988, Medicaid accounted for $7.0 billion, or over one third. ICF/MR services made up 87 percent of this amount, with the rest going to programs operated under section 1915(c) home and community-based services waivers and to day treatment programs covered as optional Medicaid clinic or rehabilitation services.

Most persons with developmental disabilities who qualify for Medicaid do so by meeting the disability criteria and financial standards for SSI. Of 1.3 million disabled SSI beneficiaries aged 18 to 64 in 1991, an estimated 28 percent qualified on the basis of mental retardation. In addition, mental retardation was the primary diagnosis for 45 percent of the 382,000 children receiving SSI disability payments.[33] Thus a total of about 550,000 disabled SSI recipients qualified on the basis of mental retardation in 1991. In addition, an unknown number of persons with developmental disabilities may qualify for Medicaid on some other basis (for example, AFDC or SSI for the aged or blind) or have a primary disability under SSI other than mental retardation.

Whatever the total number of beneficiaries with developmental disabilities, they account for a disproportionate share of Medicaid spending. The $7.0 billion in FY 1988 spending for services specifically designed for the developmentally disabled (ICFs/MR and the waiver and day habilitation programs) represented 14 percent of Medicaid service spending in that year. By FY 1991, spending for ICFs/MR and waiver services alone is estimated to have reached $9.1 billion. This amount is a lower share of total spending than earlier, about 10 percent, because spending for these services has been growing less rapidly in the last several years than spending for acute care, such as inpatient hospital services.

a. ICFs/MR and Other Institutional Services

Care for the mentally retarded was for many years a State responsibility, with most persons receiving essentially custodial care in large State facilities. Concerns about the quality of care in these facilities prompted Congress to add ICF/MR as an optional Medicaid service in 1971 (P.L. 92-223). To qualify for Medicaid funding, States would have to improve their facilities to meet new Federal standards that would ensure that ICF/MR residents received active treatment. As the Senate Finance Committee noted, "The purpose here is to improve medical care and treatment of the mentally retarded rather than to simply substitute Federal dollars for State dollars."[34] The Act included a "maintenance of effort" requirement; Federal matching was available only for expenditures in excess of what the State had been spending before adding the services to Medicaid.

Most States acted promptly to take advantage of the new option; 43 States covered ICF/MR services by 1977. Between 1975 and 1980, Medicaid spending for ICF/MR services rose at an average rate of 37 percent a year, nearly 3 times the rate of overall Medicaid spending. Growth in ICF/MR spending was more moderate in the 1980s, but still faster than general Medicaid growth, 14 percent per year compared to 10.7 percent. By 1990 the share of spending attributable to ICF/MR services had reached 11.3 percent, one in nine Medicaid dollars.

---

[33]House Ways and Means Committee, *1992 Green Book*, p. 800-801.

[34]Report language on a previous version of the ICF/MR amendment inserted in Senator Long's floor statement on H.R. 10604. *Congressional Record*, v. 117, Dec. 4, 1971. p. 44721.

Growth in the first years of ICF/MR coverage was partially attributable to increasing numbers of persons served, as more States added ICF/MR coverage and more facilities were certified. The number of beneficiaries receiving ICF/MR services rose from 69,000 in 1975 to a peak of 151,000 in 1981. Since then, the Medicaid ICF/MR population has been stable; the figure for 1990 was 147,000. However, per capita spending has grown significantly, from about $16,000 per beneficiary in 1980 to about $50,000 in 1990.

Most ICF/MR beneficiaries continue to be served in large State and non-State facilities (defined as those with 15 or more beds). However, a growing number--16 percent in 1988--are now cared for in small State and private facilities. This is one reflection of a general movement away from institutionalization and towards community-based treatment of the developmentally disabled. In recent years, large public institutions have served a declining population of older and more profoundly disabled residents, while the moderately disabled have gradually been shifted to smaller facilities or group homes or are remaining with their families.

Medicaid spending patterns do not fully reflect this trend, in part because many smaller facilities do not qualify for Medicaid reimbursement. In 1989, 9 out of 10 residents of larger facilities were in facilities that were certified as ICFs/MR. Only 23 percent of residents in small facilities (those with fewer than 15 beds) were in certified facilities. Although States could gain Federal funding by bringing more facilities into compliance with ICF/MR standards, States may not have chosen to incur the additional staffing and other costs involved in certification for smaller facilities that serve less severely disabled residents.

Some Medicaid beneficiaries with developmental disabilities are cared for, not in ICFs/MR, but in ordinary NFs. Estimates from the 1987 National Medical Expenditure Survey indicate that 57,849 NF residents in that year had mental retardation or a related condition as a primary diagnosis, while another 32,538 with a different primary diagnosis were also reported as developmentally disabled. (The number whose stays were covered by Medicaid was not reported.)[35]

In response to reports that many of these NF residents were inappropriately placed and were not receiving active treatment, Congress included in the nursing home reform provisions of OBRA 87 (see above) a requirement for screening of NF residents who were mentally retarded or mentally ill. States must determine whether the placement of any new mentally ill or mentally retarded patient in an NF is appropriate, or whether the patient would be more appropriately cared for in some other setting, and must also review current residents to determine whether continued care at the current level is appropriate. However, there have been delays in implementing the requirements, and there are concerns about whether persons diverted from or discharged from NFs will be directed to other appropriate sources of care.

---

[35]Lakin, K. Charlie et al. *Intermediate Care Facilities for Persons with Mental Retardation (ICFs-MR): Program Utilization and Resident Characteristics*. Minneapolis, Mar. 1990. p. 68-69.

b. Community-Based Services

Most States have developed home and community-based services programs for the developmentally disabled under the section 1915(c) authority discussed earlier. In FY 1988, 36 States had 1915(c) programs for the developmentally disabled, and it is projected that nearly all will by the end of FY 1992. The population served under these waiver programs is also growing rapidly, from just over 29,000 in FY 1988 to an estimated 69,000 in FY 1992. Spending under waivers for the developmentally disabled has increased from $447 million in FY 1988 to an estimated $1.1 billion in FY 1991.

The waiver programs may be functioning chiefly as a way of avoiding the expansion of institutional services, rather than promoting the discharge of persons already resident in ICFs/MR. As was noted earlier, the number of Medicaid beneficiaries receiving ICF/MR services has been virtually stable since 1981, before the waiver programs began. Waiver services have thus added to, not replaced, previous Medicaid spending for the developmentally disabled. Further growth in these services is potentially constrained by the requirement that section 1915(c) programs be budget neutral; that is, result in Medicaid spending no greater than would have been incurred in the absence of the waiver. A State would ordinarily have to show that it was reducing its ICF/MR population and that waiver expenditures were thus replacing ICF/MR spending. However, some States appear to be meeting the cost-effectiveness requirement by showing instead that they would have to expand ICFs/MR if waiver services were not available.

The OBRA 90, P.L. 101-508, authorized a new limited option under the Medicaid program to permit from two to eight States to provide "community supported living arrangements services," comparable to services under waiver programs, for individuals with developmental disabilities who live at home or in very small group residences.[36] Unlike section 1915(c) waiver services, services under this option are available without regard to whether participants are at risk of institutionalization. In addition, the States are not required to demonstrate budget neutrality. Federal Medicaid expenditures for this program are limited to $10 million for FY 1992 and increase annually to $35 million for FY 1995, with such sums as may be provided by Congress for fiscal years thereafter.

2. Medicaid Services for the Mentally Ill

Medicaid is an important source of funding for the treatment of mental illness, including long-term serious mental illness and short-term acute problems. In fiscal year 1990, over $1.7 billion in Medicaid funds went to mental institutions, while additional funds were spent on services for mental

---

[36]Effective Oct. 1991, the following States are participating in this program: California, Colorado, Florida, Illinois, Maryland, Michigan, Rhode Island, Wisconsin.

illness in ordinary hospitals and nursing homes and in the community.[37] However, Medicaid's role in covering the mentally ill has always been restricted, in part by certain policy decisions made in the early years of the program and in part by the nature of the mentally ill population, which is heterogeneous and ill-defined, with widely differing problems and needs.

Medicaid has no special eligibility rules or conditions for mentally ill persons. Those in the community may qualify by receiving SSI disability benefits, while those in institutions may qualify under the special eligibility rules for institutional coverage discussed earlier. As in the case of the mentally retarded, then, the number of mentally ill Medicaid beneficiaries cannot be firmly established. However, approximately 380,000 persons receiving SSI disability payments in December 1990 had a primary disability of mental disorder (other than mental retardation). The number of persons receiving Medicaid-covered services in mental institutions during fiscal year 1990 was 92,386. In addition, data from the 1985 National Nursing Home Survey indicated that 149,811 mentally ill persons were receiving Medicaid nursing home services during that year. (Note that the latter two figures would include some SSI recipients.)

a. Institutional Services

State Medicaid programs may, at their option, cover services in two types of institutional mental health providers: "IMDs," and inpatient psychiatric hospitals. Services in IMDs, which are facilities with more than 16 beds that primarily serve patients with mental diseases, may be covered only for beneficiaries aged 65 and older. Services in inpatient psychiatric hospitals may be covered only for beneficiaries age 21 and under.[38] The effect of these rules is to exclude Medicaid coverage of services for persons between 21 and 65 years old in mental institutions.[39] (States are required to cover short-term acute care for mental illness in general hospitals for all beneficiaries, just as they must cover inpatient hospital care for physical problems. Stays with a diagnosis related to mental illness account for a large of Medicaid inpatient spending in some States.)

The mentally ill aged between 21 and 65 may receive Medicaid services in facilities that do not specialize in mental health care, such as ordinary NFs. One consequence of this policy is that a significant number of mentally ill patients reside in nonpsychiatric institutions. In 1985, for example, 29 percent

---

[37]Medicaid data do not distinguish expenditures for treatment of mental as opposed to physical problems by providers other than mental institutions.

[38]Beneficiaries who are under 21 at the time they enter such a facility may continue receiving care until they reach 22.

[39]Persons between 21 and 65 in group homes and other small residential facilities with fewer than 16 beds may receive Medicaid benefits for physician, clinic, or other services they may require, but Medicaid will not pay the costs of room and board in the facility.

of nursing home residents under age 65, and 17 percent of those over 65, had a primary diagnosis of mental illness. The presence of large numbers of mentally ill Medicaid beneficiaries in facilities classified as ordinary nursing homes has raised two major issues. The first is whether some facilities that are actually IMDs have been classified as NFs, possibly in order to circumvent the exclusion of Medicaid coverage for persons aged 21 to 65 in IMDs. OBRA 89 required the Secretary to report to Congress by October 1990 on appropriate changes in IMD classification and coverage; the report had not been submitted as of July 1992. The second, complementary question--discussed above in the context of developmental disability--is whether mentally ill persons in facilities that do not specialize in the treatment of mental illness are appropriately placed and are receiving the active treatment they need. The OBRA 87 screening and evaluation requirements thus apply to the mentally ill as well as to the mentally retarded.

b. Noninstitutional Services

Medicaid programs furnish mental health care outside institutional settings as part of the general coverage of services rendered by physicians, clinics, hospitals, and other providers. In most States, Medicaid beneficiaries may obtain services from psychiatrists under the same rules that apply to other physician services; however, psychiatrists have been less willing than any other group of physicians to accept Medicaid patients. Only a minority of States cover the services of other types of mental health professionals in independent practice, such as clinical psychologists or social workers.

States may also cover mental health care services in clinics or similar settings. According to a 1989 survey, 38 States cover mental health clinic services provided in community mental health centers. These clinic providers may include State or county facilities, often funded through the Federal Alcohol, Drug Abuse, and Mental Health Services Block Grant.[40] The survey also showed that 24 States also covered services provided in private mental health clinics.[41] Forty-one States cover mental health services furnished in general hospital outpatient departments; 18 States cover outpatient mental health services in a psychiatric hospital.[42] In a number of States, outpatient mental health services may include "partial hospitalization" or "psychiatric day care" programs.

Some States have imposed coverage limits for mental health care services that are more restrictive than those applied to other services furnished by the same providers. A State may, for example, distinguish between an ordinary

---

[40]Fox, Wicks, McManus, and Kelly, p. 49-50.

[41]The OBRA 87 provided that States could cover as clinic services, services provided by clinic personnel outside the actual clinic facility. This provision permits clinics to furnish offsite care to homeless chronically mentally ill patients in shelters or other locations.

[42]Fox, Wicks, McManus, and Kelly, p. 42-44.

physician office visit and a "psychotherapy visit," and limit coverage of the latter. Despite these limitations, it has been found that Medicaid beneficiaries are more likely to obtain mental health care than other low-income persons without Medicaid or even than higher-income persons.[43]

A number of observers have suggested that Medicaid and other public mental health policies have resulted in discontinuous and uncoordinated care for the seriously mentally ill. States have experimented with a variety of systems meant to improve the management of Medicaid mental health services. As of December 1990, 20 States had approved targeted case management services for chronically mentally ill persons: A few States have used other options, such as 1915(b) freedom-of-choice waivers or 1915(c) home and community-based services waivers to structure care systems for the mentally ill. Finally, OBRA 87 authorized special waivers of Medicaid rules to facilitate a set of demonstrations of coordinated service systems emphasizing continuity of care, a full range of services, a housing plan, and new sources of financing.

IV. THE FUTURE OF MEDICAID

Medicaid has become one of the fastest-growing components of both Federal and State budgets. Program spending doubled between FY 1989 and FY 1992 and is projected to grow another 86 percent by FY 1997. By that year, combined Federal and State Medicaid spending is projected to be $221 billion, nearly equal to the $224 billion projected for Medicare.

A. Spending Trends

Table I-5 shows the growth in combined Federal and State Medicaid spending from FY 1980 through FY 1992, along with Congressional Budget Office (CBO) projections through FY 1997. As the table shows, CBO projects sharp increases in Medicaid spending through FY 1993 and slightly more moderate growth, about 12 percent per year, through FY 1997. A variety of factors could influence Medicaid spending trends in the years ahead:

- The number of Medicaid beneficiaries is expected to continue growing, from an estimated 31.4 million in FY 1992 to 35.8 million in FY 1997, partly because of the continued phase-in of mandatory coverage of older children below the poverty level. However, this rate of projected population growth, 2.7 percent a year, is well below the annual growth rate of 8.3 percent in FY 1989 through FY 1992.

- Medicaid programs may be increasingly burdened by the costs of health problems that are associated with lower socioeconomic status, such as drugs and drug-related violence and--to an increasing extent-- human immunodeficiency virus (HIV) disease. As many as 40 percent of persons with AIDS become eligible for Medicaid at some point in the

---

[43]Taube, Carl A., and Agnes Rupp. The Effect of Medicaid on Access to Ambulatory Mental Health for the Poor and Near-Poor Under 65. *Medical Care*, v. 24, no. 8, Aug. 1986. p. 677-686.

course of their illness. Medicaid spending for AIDS treatment is projected to total $2.1 billion in FY 1992 and $3.9 billion by FY 1997. Newly emergent problems, such as the recent outbreak of tuberculosis, could also have a disproportionate effect on Medicaid.

• To the extent that States' use of provider donations and taxes helped to contribute to spending increases, the restrictions enacted in 1991 are expected to slow program growth.

TABLE I-5. Medicaid Spending, Fiscal Years 1980 to 1997
(payment amounts are in millions)

Fiscal year	Federal spending	Percent change	State spending	Percent change	Total spending	Percent change
1980	14,550	18.6	11,231	18.4	25,781	18.5
1981	17,074	17.3	13,303	18.4	30,377	17.8
1982	17,514	2.6	14,931	12.2	32,446	6.8
1983	18,985	8.0	15,971	7.0	34,956	7.5
1984	20,065	6.1	17,508	9.6	37,569	7.7
1985	22,655	12.9	18,262	4.3	40,917	8.9
1986	24,995	10.3	19,856	8.7	44,851	9.6
1987	27,435	9.8	21,909	10.3	49,344	10.0
1988	30,462	11.0	23,654	8.0	54,116	9.7
1989	34,604	13.6	26,642	12.6	61,246	13.2
1990	41,103	18.8	31,389	17.8	72,492	18.4
1991[a]	52,533	27.8	39,856	26.9	92,389	27.4
1992[a]	67,827	29.1	50,959	27.9	118,786	28.6

CBO Projections of Federal Medicaid Spending, FY 1993 to 1997

1993	79,590	17.3	59,797[b]	16.4[b]	139,387[b]	16.4[b]
1994	89,048	11.9	66,903[b]	11.9[b]	155,951[b]	11.9[b]
1995	100,184	12.5	75,270[b]	12.5[b]	175,454[b]	12.5[b]
1996	112,573	12.4	84,578[b]	12.4[b]	197,151[b]	12.4[b]
1997	126,339	12.2	94,920[b]	12.2[b]	221,259[b]	12.2[b]

[a]Preliminary estimate.

[b]State spending amounts and total amounts are not prepared by the Congressional Budget Office. Totals shown are estimates prepared by the Congressional Research Service based on the assumption that Federal spending will represent 57.1 percent of total Medicaid funds. These State and total amounts provide a very rough estimate of overall program spending. Federal spending has represented a growing share of total program outlays over the last few years.

NOTE: All spending amounts are in millions. Spending amounts represent payments for benefits, administration, fraud and control, and survey and certification. All projected numbers are subject to revision.

Source: Based on data contained in the Budget of the United States Government, fiscal years 1969 to 1993; and data from the Health Care Financing Administration, Division of the Budget. Federal spending estimates for fiscal years 1993 to 1997 prepared by the Congressional Budget Office in Aug. 1992. Total spending estimates for fiscal years 1993 to 1997 prepared by the Congressional Research Service.

- Some States are reportedly "federalizing" existing State programs, by restructuring services in such as a way as to qualify for Medicaid reimbursement. For example, some social services provided to foster children or other distinct group of beneficiaries may be coverable under Medicaid as optional targeted case management services. Federal funding is then available at the matching rate for Medicaid services, instead of the (usually lower) matching rate for foster care administration.

- Over the very long term, aging of the population is expected to increase demand for long-term care, although the full effect will not be felt until the first baby boomers reach the age of higher risk for nursing home care, in the 2020s. The impact on Medicaid might be reduced if current efforts to develop workable private long-term care insurance systems were to succeed.

At least some of these factors operate independently of any State or Federal policy decisions. Because Medicaid is an entitlement program, much of its spending is driven by demographic changes, fluctuations in the performance of the United States economy, emerging health problems, and changes in the pattern of medical practice. However, States are taking some measures to bring spending under control. In addition, there are proposals at both the State and Federal levels for a more sweeping restructuring of the Medicaid program. The remainder of this section provides a brief summary of recent State action and broader Medicaid reform proposals.

B. State Action

States have responded to the growing burden of Medicaid spending in two major ways. Some have limited program eligibility or reduced benefits, while others have developed or expanded managed care initiatives in the hope of improving program efficiency.

1. Program Cutbacks

Since every State covers some optional population groups and/or optional services, one way States have often responded to Medicaid budget overruns is by eliminating optional coverages or limiting coverage of mandatory services (for example, by reducing the number of allowed inpatient days per beneficiary). In the past, many States have also controlled costs by freezing or reducing provider reimbursement rates. Such changes have become less feasible since the recent wave of Boren amendment lawsuits; courts have specifically overruled reimbursement changes found to be driven by budgetary considerations.

Despite the budget problems experienced by many States in the last several years, relatively few appear to have resorted to direct cuts in their Medicaid programs. A survey of 1991 changes in State programs affecting low-income persons found that 4 States reduced their coverage of the medically needy, and

15 States eliminated or reduced coverage of certain services.[44] In the same year, 10 States expanded eligibility, while 20 expanded service coverage. Many more States, however, made changes that affected Medicaid indirectly. For example, 40 States cut or froze AFDC benefits, potentially reducing Medicaid rolls as well. (Some persons losing AFDC eligibility might have been able to continue receiving Medicaid on some other basis.)

The Medicaid eligibility cuts that did occur were relatively minor. The reductions in medically needy coverage in 4 States were estimated to have affected fewer than 10,000 people. Most of the service changes involved imposition of copayments, chiefly for pharmacy services. Some were more significant, involving new quantitative limits on coverage of physician visits, home health visits, or inpatient days.

The most severe cuts in 1991 involved non-Medicaid State-funded medical assistance programs. Many States provide cash assistance and related medical benefits to persons who are categorically ineligible for Federal benefits, such as single adults; these programs are usually known as "general assistance." In 1991, 12 States limited general assistance eligibility and one, Michigan, eliminated the entire program. In addition, 8 States reduced the medical coverage available under general assistance or other wholly State-funded medical assistance programs.

Full information on Medicaid changes in 1992 is not available at this writing. A March 1992 survey by the National Association of State Budget Officers indicated that 15 States were considering Medicaid budget cuts. Organizations that monitor State legislative activity report that few States had enacted significant Medicaid reductions by mid-year. However, some large States were still in the middle of budget debates, and some States may have reduced Medicaid spending through regulatory (rather than legislative) action. Other States, while not actually cutting benefits, may have eliminated or postponed planned Medicaid expansions. For example, one State that was planning to offer medically needy coverage for the first time in 1992 has now delayed that initiative. Another has abandoned plans to raise the eligibility standard for pregnant women to 185 percent of poverty and increase payments for pediatric and obstetrical services.[45]

2. Managed Care

In recent years Medicaid programs, like other health care purchasers, have shown increasing interest in managed care programs--systems in which the overall care of a patient is overseen by a single provider or organization. The basic model for managed care is the HMO, which receives a fixed periodic payment (known as a capitation payment or premium) for each individual served

---

[44]Shapiro, Isaac, et al. *The States and the Poor: How Budget Decisions in 1991 Affected Low Income People.* Washington, Center on Budget and Policy Priorities, 1991.

[45]Personal communication, Intergovernmental Health Policy Project.

and accepts financial responsibility for all the medical care required by that individual. The risk arrangement is intended to give the HMO a financial incentive to furnish services more efficiently.

The managed care concept has been of interest to Medicaid programs, as well as to other purchasers of health care, because it appears to offer a way of changing provider and beneficiary behaviors which may have contributed to rising costs in the traditional fee-for-service system. In at least some areas, many Medicaid beneficiaries receive routine health services in hospital outpatient departments and emergency rooms, at greater cost than if they had used office-based physician services. In other areas, some beneficiaries engage in "doctor shopping," visiting multiple providers for a single complaint. The providers themselves, paid for each service they perform, may have an incentive to maximize their own services and may have no reason to control the referral services they order. Managed care, it is argued, can provide control over the beneficiaries' behavior and change the incentives for providers.

States have contracted with HMOs for voluntary enrollment of Medicaid beneficiaries since the earliest years of the program. Since 1981, many States have used the section 1915(b) freedom-of-choice waiver option to require specified groups of beneficiaries to enroll in HMOs or similar organizations.[46] Others have developed systems that retain some of the managed care features of HMOs but that do not involve the substantial risks (and hence the need for capital and experienced management) presented by HMOs. Some States have used fee-for-service case management. Individual physicians or groups are paid a fee to manage the care of assigned patients but are not at direct financial risk for the services the patients use. Other States have developed "partial capitation systems." The providers are paid a premium for each enrollee and accept financial risk for a limited group of services, such as all physician and diagnostic services, but are not at risk for the most expensive services, such as hospital inpatient. Overall, 31 States were operating some form of managed care program by 1991, with 2.3 million beneficiaries enrolled.

Critics of managed care programs say that providers may respond to the new incentives, not just by providing care more efficiently, but also by denying needed services. Reports of quality problems and other abuses in some Medicaid managed care experiments have led Congress to place restrictions on the types of organizations that may participate and on the terms under which the programs may operate. Advocates of further managed care expansion contend that these restrictions are excessive and that the 1915(b) waiver process is burdensome. The Administration and others have proposed giving the States greater flexibility to develop managed care programs. Opponents of these proposals argue that Medicaid beneficiaries might be forced into substandard plans serving Medicaid-only populations. They also question whether managed

---

[46]Some States operate such programs under the Secretary's general demonstration waiver authority or under specific waivers enacted by Congress, instead of under the 1915(b) authority. Arizona's program, under which all beneficiaries are enrolled in HMO-like entities, has operated under a demonstration waiver since 1982.

care can achieve additional savings in States where Medicaid is already paying considerably less than providers' costs or usual charges.

C. Proposals for Program Restructuring

Broader proposals for changes in the Medicaid program have been characterized, like the general debate over options for health care reform, by two conflicting goals--improving access and coverage and controlling costs. Some people argue that recent spending trends reflect a program that is out of control; they would enact strict limits on further spending growth. Others contend that Medicaid has not succeeded in ensuring access to care and that it should be redefined or replaced. One approach would be to increase the Federal role in the program, to promote greater uniformity or make up for insufficient State resources. Another option would be to allow each State to redefine the program, possibly in the context of a system to provide universal health care coverage for the State's residents.

1. Capping Medicaid Spending

Because Medicaid and other social welfare programs represent the largest single component of Federal spending, some people believe that controlling growth in these programs must be a key part of any plan to reduce the Federal deficit. In 1992, a number of proposals have been advanced for "entitlement caps"--fixed limits, tied to growth in the GNP or other factors, on annual increases in spending for entitlement programs. Narrower proposals to cap Medicaid growth have been advanced in the past. The Reagan administration repeatedly proposed some form of spending limit. Congress never acted on these proposals, although it did approve, in OBRA 81, short-term reductions in Federal matching funds for States whose Medicaid spending growth exceeded targets tied to the medical care component of the CPI.

The Bush Administration included a Medicaid cap in the Comprehensive Health Care Reform package put forward in February 1992. Instead of receiving Federal matching payments based on actual expenditures for Medicaid services, States would have received a fixed per capita amount for acute services to nonelderly beneficiaries. The per capita amount would have been indexed for inflation but not for overall growth in health spending. The Administration contended that States would be able to hold down spending growth by adopting managed care systems; use of such systems generally would have been made mandatory.

2. Redefining Federal and State Responsibilities

Variation among States in Medicaid eligibility and coverage, as well as disparities in States' ability to finance the program, have led to proposals that some or all of Medicaid should be converted to a uniform Federal program. The U.S. Bipartisan Commission on Comprehensive Health Care (the Pepper Commission) proposed in 1990 that the acute care component of Medicaid be replaced by a Federal program to cover all persons lacking employer-based or Medicare coverage. (The current joint Federal-State Medicaid program would continue to offer some long-term care services.) A federalized Medicaid program, or a new public program for low-income persons, was part of a number of universal coverage proposals introduced in the 102nd Congress, while others would leave low-income coverage with the States, possibly with enhanced Federal funding.[47]

There have also been proposals to split Medicaid into a fully Federal program for acute care and a fully State program for long-term care. This option was proposed in 1982, as part of President Reagan's "New Federalism" program, and has begun to receive some discussion again in the last several years. If FY 1991 spending patterns continued, the effect of the trade-off would be a slight gain for the States as a whole; individual States with different acute/long-term care spending breakdowns might have larger gains or losses.[48] Proponents of this proposal believe that States are in a better position to control long-term care spending, through such means as controlling nursing home bed supply and developing new community-based programs. As was suggested earlier, however, aging of the population could place a much heavier burden on States over the very long term.

Finally, there are suggestions for a redesign of the Federal Medicaid matching formula to better target assistance to States, without necessarily shifting the overall balance of Federal/State responsibilities. The current formula, under which the Federal percentage is inversely proportional to a State's per capita income has been criticized on the grounds that it provides insufficient help to the neediest States. The General Accounting Office (GAO) and others have proposed systems under which the percentage would be based on the proportion of a State's population in poverty and some measure of the State's revenue-raising capacity.[49] One alternative studied by GAO would have reduced some States' Federal funding by as much as 36 percent in FY 1989, while raising funding for other States by as much as 21 percent. Precisely because these proposals shift money among States, they face formidable barriers to enactment. However, redesigned funding formulas are included in some proposals for new joint Federal/State universal coverage plans.

---

[47]Still others would eliminate any separation between coverage of the poor and coverage of the rest of the population. Some would assist the poor in buying private coverage, while others would create a single public program for all U.S. residents.

[48]In FY 1991, Medicaid spending totalled $51.8 billion for acute care services and $35.8 for long-term care, with the Federal Government paying 57 percent of the cost. Under a split program, the States would pay an additional $20.4 billion for long-term care and save $22.3 billion on acute care, for a net gain of $1.9 billion.

[49]U.S. General Accounting Office. *Medicaid: Alternatives for Improving the Distribution of Funds.* GAO/HRD-91-66FS, May 1991. Washington, 1991.

3. Unified State Systems

Although health care reform emerged as one of the central domestic policy issues in the 102nd Congress and is a high priority for the new Administration, many people argue that a Federal solution may still be some years away and that States should be given greater freedom to develop their own approaches. There are a number of proposals to waive Federal Medicaid (and perhaps Medicare) requirements, so that States could use Federal funds to help establish a system that would cover all their residents.

Hawaii is the first State actually to implement a comprehensive system. Employers are required to provide health coverage to full-time workers. Low-income residents who do not meet Medicaid eligibility criteria may enroll in the State Health Insurance Program (SHIP). SHIP is entirely State-funded, and the Medicaid program conforms to Federal rules. As a result, Hawaii has not needed Medicaid waivers. However, the mandatory employee coverage component of its program did require a congressionally authorized exemption from the Employee Retirement Income Security Act of 1974 (ERISA), which ordinarily prohibits States from regulating employee benefit plans.

Other States, including Florida and Vermont, are also considering seeking Medicaid waivers to develop a unified system. (Whether ERISA waivers would also be required would depend on whether the States opt for an employer-based system like Hawaii's.) Colorado's legislature passed a bill instructing the State to seek Federal waivers for the development of an alternative to Medicaid (not necessarily in the context of a universal coverage program); in the absence of waivers, the State would have developed its own replacement for Medicaid without Federal funding. The bill was vetoed by the Governor in June 1992.

Widespread attention has been given to a universal coverage proposal enacted by Oregon in 1989 but not yet implemented. The Oregon plan has three basic components--a high-risk pool for "uninsurable" individuals (those with costly preexisting conditions), a requirement that all employers provide coverage to their workers, and an expansion and restructuring of Medicaid. Only the first component, the high-risk pool, was operational as of July 1991; the employer component has been postponed and might require ERISA waivers. As a result, most discussion has centered on the proposed restructuring of Medicaid.

The Medicaid proposal would extend eligibility to all persons with family incomes below 100 percent of the Federal poverty level, including groups currently excluded by Medicaid's categorical limits, such as single adults and childless couples who are not aged or disabled. In order to limit the cost of this expansion, the State also proposes to establish a minimum benefit package that is less comprehensive than the basic Medicaid benefits required by Federal law. (Certain classes of beneficiaries, such as the aged and disabled, would continue to receive current Medicaid benefits, at least initially.) The standard benefit package developed for Medicaid would also constitute the minimum package to be offered to workers under the employer mandate. In addition, the State would require participants to enroll in managed care programs.

Oregon's process for developing its standard benefit package has been the source of considerable controversy and was the ultimate basis for denial of its Medicaid waiver request. Instead of including or excluding entire categories of services (such as outpatient physician care or prescription drugs), the State developed a system for prioritizing specific treatments for specific conditions. A Health Care Commission defined 709 condition/treatment pairs--some relatively specific, such as "appendicitis/appendectomy," others broader, such as "imminent death regardless of diagnosis/comfort care." After a process that included provider consultation and public surveys, the Commission ranked the condition/treatment pairs in descending order, from "essential services," such as appendectomies and obstetrical care, to the least useful services, such as heroic measures for patients in the final stages of terminal illness. Cost estimates were obtained for providing each service on the list to the expanded Medicaid population. In 1991, the Oregon legislature authorized funding sufficient to cover the first 587 services on the list; the rest would be excluded from coverage in the first 2 years of the plan. In future years, the list of covered services might be shorter or longer, depending on the amount of money Oregon chose to devote to the plan.

The proposed Oregon system, dubbed "prioritization" by the State and "rationing" by some of its critics, was evaluated by the Office of Technology Assessment (OTA) at congressional request. OTA found that, while the prioritization process was relatively subjective, the final list of 587 covered services was not clearly better or worse than the Federal minimum Medicaid package. The list excluded some services that are currently mandatory, but included others that are now optional, such as adult preventive care, prescription drugs, and dental care. However, OTA expressed concern that Oregon might have underestimated program costs and that the list could be cut further, with adverse consequences for beneficiaries, in the event of budget shortfalls.[50] Opponents of the plan have also argued that it is inequitable to finance services for the low-income uninsured by reducing Medicaid benefits for other low-income persons.

Oregon's proposal would require Federal Medicaid demonstration waivers, in order to allow the State to cover persons otherwise ineligible; depart from the minimum Medicaid benefit package; and require enrollment in managed care arrangements that do not meet all current statutory requirements. Oregon applied for the waiver in August 1991. The application was rejected by the Secretary in August 1992, chiefly on the basis that the program would have violated the Americans with Disabilities Act. One factor considered in the process of prioritizing services was the expected quality of life of persons receiving those services. DHHS argued that the use of this factor was improper, because stereotyped perceptions about the quality of life of the disabled had contributed to the assignment of low priority to certain services benefiting the disabled. Oregon submitted a revised application in November 1992.

---

[50]U.S. Congress. Office of Technology Assessment. *Evaluation of the Oregon Medicaid Proposal*, May 1992. Washington, GPO, 1992.

CHAPTER II. TRENDS IN MEDICAID PAYMENTS AND BENEFICIARIES[1]

SUMMARY

In 1991, Medicaid financed health services to more people than in any year over its entire history. Twenty eight million people had health services paid for by this program, an increase of 1.7 million beneficiaries from fiscal year (FY) 1990. For the first time since the mid-1970s, increases in the number of Medicaid beneficiaries coincided with increases in the number of the poor. Along with this large increase in beneficiaries has come substantial increases in program spending. Since 1986, total Medicaid spending (spending by Federal, State and local governments) has more than doubled. This rapid spending growth is projected to continue. In FY 1991 total Medicaid spending equalled $92 billion. By 1993, assuming recent Federal and State spending patterns, total program spending could exceed $139 billion.

The trend in Medicaid spending can be divided into four distinct periods: an early period, 1966-1974, dominated by large increases in the number of beneficiaries; a second period from the mid-1970s to early 1980s, where spending growth occurred without increases in beneficiaries but with increased service utilization; a period of more moderate growth from 1982 through 1988; and the recent period of rapid spending increases.

Comparing Medicaid spending to overall national health spending suggests that after the program's initial start up period and through 1989, overall Medicaid spending grew at a rate that is comparable to national health spending. However, the recent Medicaid spending increase has outpaced overall national health spending.

Medicaid spending represents an increasing share of both Federal and State and local budgets. In 1981 Medicaid spending equalled about 21 percent of all Federal health spending. After declining during the early 1980s, its share increased to 22 percent in 1990. Growth also has occurred at the State and local level. In 1980, about 35 percent of State and local health spending was for Medicaid; a share that increased to 37 percent by 1990. Perhaps more indicative of the program's rapid growth is the share of all State and local expenditures spent on the program. In 1980, about 4.7 percent of all State and local expenditures went to Medicaid; in 1990 the program consumed 5.7 percent of all State and local spending.

---

[1] This chapter was written by Richard Rimkunas with the assistance of Dawn Nuschler.

One factor associated with the recent spending increase is an increase in the number of beneficiaries. Between 1975 and 1985 the total number of Medicaid beneficiaries hovered around 22 million. However, between 1985 and 1991 the number of beneficiaries increased to 28.0 million. Projected beneficiary trends suggest this increase will continue over the next few years.

Undoubtedly, some of this beneficiary growth is the result of Congress broadening access to Medicaid. For example, beginning in the mid-1980s Congress enacted measures that: expanded Medicaid eligibility to poor pregnant women and children; and extended limited benefits to poor and near-poor Medicare beneficiaries. These expansions are reflected in the beneficiary trend when looking at whether a beneficiary receives cash assistance payments. The traditional road to Medicaid eligibility was through the receipt of cash assistance payments. In 1975, more than 75 percent of all Medicaid beneficiaries also received Aid to Families with Dependent Children (AFDC) or Supplemental Security Income (SSI) payments. By expanding access to poor and near-poor persons, eligibility criteria ignore these cash assistance programs. By 1991 the share of beneficiaries receiving cash assistance payments was reduced to 61 percent.

In 1991, inpatient hospital spending represented the largest single program payment category (representing 28 percent of the total). In 1990 hospital spending increased rather sharply, registering the largest single year rate of increase over the previous 14 years. Prior to 1990, the largest single service spending category was nursing homes. In 1991, nursing home spending was the second largest category representing more than 27 percent of total service payments. Over the last 5 years, Medicaid's service categories experiencing the most rapid growth include: home health services, laboratory and radiological services, and outpatient hospital services.

I. INTRODUCTION

Since FY 1989 total Medicaid spending has been growing rapidly. Between FY 1989 and 1990, total Medicaid spending increased by 18.4 percent, the largest single year increase since the early 1970s. State and Federal spending exceeded $72 billion. Between FY 1990 and 1991, the annual increase is estimated to be even larger, 26.9 percent. Federal Medicaid funding increased by 27.8 percent. Currently, projected spending trends have the program's expenditures more than doubling in 5 years. Of the more than 70 benefit programs that provide cash or noncash aid directed primarily toward persons with limited income, Medicaid spends the most by far.[2]

---

[2]This comparison is based on programs that rely on some income-tested or need-based benefits and excludes social insurance programs such as Social Security or Medicare that may provide benefits to those with low income, but those with low income are not the primary focus of the program. See U.S. Library of Congress. Congressional Research Service. *Cash and Noncash Benefits for Persons with Limited Income: Eligibility Rules, Recipients, and Expenditure Data, FY 1988-90.* CRS Report for Congress No. 91-741 EPW, compiled by Vee Burke, Sept. 30, 1991. Washington, 1991.

The Medicaid program helps States to finance health care for low-income and medically needy persons. It is an avenue of support for services for families with children. It also provides payments for some of the chronically disabled, the developmentally disabled and the aged. While the program runs under Federal guidelines there is substantial State discretion in determining who is eligible, what is the scope of the services provided, and how health care providers should be reimbursed for those services. The multifaceted nature of this in-kind entitlement program is reflected in describing Medicaid, not as a single program, but rather as 150 separate programs (i.e., 50 different State programs for children; the aged; and the disabled). Any discussion of Medicaid trends needs to take this complexity into account.

This chapter concentrates on Medicaid spending and beneficiary trends in order to answer some of the more basic questions about the program:

- How rapid has growth in Medicaid spending been? Is it more rapid than in other public health programs? Has spending kept up with inflation? What is program spending likely to be in the near future?

- What factors account for program growth? An increase in beneficiaries? The effect of inflation? Changes in the volume and type of services used by beneficiaries?

- What service categories seem to spur program growth? Are there particular service categories that have grown more rapidly than others?

- What beneficiary categories have experienced the most rapid growth, and why?

- What State programs have experienced the most rapid growth? How are these programs different from other State Medicaid programs that have experienced more moderate rates of growth?

II. OVERALL SPENDING TREND, 1966-1991

In July 1965, the Social Security Amendments of 1965 (P.L. 89-97) established *Title XIX, Grants to States for Medical Assistance Programs*--the Medicaid program. Six States implemented Medicaid programs in January 1966, the earliest possible date for the program's implementation: Hawaii, Illinois, Minnesota, North Dakota, Oklahoma, and Pennsylvania. California began its program in March 1966, while New York established its program in May. All told, by the end of 1966, 26 States had Medicaid programs in place. An additional 11 States implemented plans in 1967. By July 1970 only Alaska and Arizona did not have Medicaid programs.[3]

---

[3]An important aspect of the early Medicaid program was that it acted to replace Federal matching payments for medical assistance in the cash assistance programs and the Kerr-Mills program. Federal matching payments for these

(continued...)

A. Describing Overall Beneficiary and Payment Trends

1. The Early Years, 1966-1974

Table II-1 provides information on total (Federal and State/local) Medicaid spending from 1966 to 1992. Total spending represents all payments to physicians, hospitals, long-term care facilities and other health providers, as well as payments for other covered services and supplies such as prescription drugs in each fiscal year. The payments also include payments for Medicare deductibles and coinsurance, as well as the administrative costs of the program.[4]

---

[3](...continued)
other programs ended in Dec. 1969. Alaska established a Medicaid program in 1972. In 1982, Arizona initiated a Medicaid-like program through a Medicaid demonstration waiver (see *Appendix G, Managed Care*).

[4]Later in this chapter detailed spending trends will focus on medical vendor payments only. The information contained in table II-1 and figure II-1 is based on budget data and differs somewhat from the vendor payment information. Total program spending portrayed in these tables is comparable to projected budget trends presented in the next section of this chapter.

83

TABLE II-1. Medicaid Spending, Fiscal Years 1966 to 1992
($ in millions)

Fiscal year	Federal spending	Percent change	State spending	Percent change	Total spending	Percent change
1966[a]	$ 789	--	$ 869	--	$ 1,658	
1967[a]	1,209	53.2%	1,159	33.4%	2,368	42.8%
1968[a]	1,837	51.9	1,849	59.5	3,686	55.7
1969[a]	2,276	23.9	1,890	2.2	4,166	13.0
1970[a]	2,617	15.0	2,235	18.3	4,852	16.5
1971	3,374	28.9	2,802	25.4	6,176	27.3
1972	4,361	29.3	4,074	45.4	8,434	36.6
1973	4,998	14.6	4,113	1.0	9,111	8.0
1974	5,833	16.7	4,396	6.9	10,229	12.3
1975	7,060	21.0	5,578	26.9	12,637	23.6
1976	8,312	17.7	6,332	13.5	14,644	15.9
1977	9,713	16.9	7,389	16.7	17,103	16.8
1978	10,680	10.0	8,269	11.9	18,949	10.8
1979	12,267	14.9	9,489	14.8	21,755	14.8
1980	14,550	18.6	11,231	18.4	25,781	18.5
1981	17,074	17.3	13,303	18.4	30,377	17.8
1982	17,514	2.6	14,931	12.2	32,446	6.8
1983	18,985	8.0	15,971	7.0	34,956	7.5
1984	20,065	6.1	17,508	9.6	37,569	7.7
1985	22,655	12.9	18,262	4.3	40,917	8.9
1986	24,995	10.3	19,856	8.7	44,851	9.6
1987	27,435	9.8	21,909	10.3	49,344	10.0
1988	30,462	11.0	23,654	8.0	54,116	9.7
1989	34,604	13.6	26,642	12.6	61,246	13.2
1990	41,103	18.8	31,389	17.8	72,492	18.4
1991[b]	52,533	27.8	39,856	26.9	92,389	27.4
1992[b]	67,827	29.1	50,959	27.9	118,786	28.6

Average annual rate of change:

1966-1970		35.0%		26.6%		30.8%
1970-1975		22.0		20.1		21.1
1975-1980		14.8		14.3		14.5
1980-1985		9.3		10.2		9.7
1985-1992		17.0		15.8		16.4

See notes on following page.

TABLE II-1. Medicaid Spending, Fiscal Years 1966 to 1992--Continued

ᵃSpending amounts for these years represent spending for Medicaid and its predecessor programs, such as Kerr-Mills. Federal matching payments were made for these programs through Dec. 1969.

ᵇPreliminary estimate.

NOTE: All spending amounts are in millions. The Federal fiscal year began on July 1 until FY 1976 when the beginning of the fiscal year was moved to Oct. 1. Percentage change reported for FY 1976 represents change in spending over 5 quarters. Spending amounts represent payments for benefits, administration, fraud and control, and survey and certification.

Source: Table prepared by the Congressional Research Service based on data contained in the *Budget of the United States Government, Fiscal Years 1969-1993*, and Health Care Financing Administration, Division of the Budget.

FIGURE Ii-1.
Total Medicaid Spending and Beneficiaries, FY 1966-1991

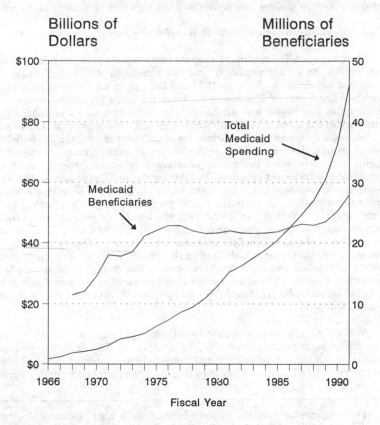

NOTE: Spending between 1966 and 1972 includes spending on related programs such as the Kerr-Mills and other programs.

Source: Figure prepared by Congressional Research Service based on data from HCFA.

The program's early period, from 1966 through 1974, was marked by rapid growth in both payments and beneficiaries. Between 1966 and 1974, spending grew by 500 percent, while beneficiaries grew from less than 11 million to over 21 million.[5] Analyses of this early period have focused on three factors contributing to the brisk growth: the dramatic increase in the number of persons on AFDC rolls and the concomitant increase in Medicaid beneficiaries; rapid increases in medical care prices; and the high cost of nursing home care.[6]

2. Spending Growth Without Beneficiary Increases, 1975-1981

Program spending continued to grow fairly rapidly over the next 6 years. But, unlike the earlier period, it was not associated with increases in the number of beneficiaries. Between 1975 and 1981, program spending grew at an average annual rate of 15.8 percent. Over the same period the number of beneficiaries essentially was unchanged, hovering around 22 million. This constancy in the number of beneficiaries highlights two important dimensions of Medicaid's spending and beneficiary trends. First, the program's beneficiary trends do not directly coincide with changes in overall program spending. During the early years increasing beneficiary rolls and program start up contributed to increased spending, but during the mid-1970s and early 1980s beneficiary growth was not a dominant factor. Second, the beneficiary trends do not coincide with changes in the size of the poverty population (see figure II-2 and table II-2). Between 1975 and 1981 the number of poor increased by 23 percent. Much of this increase occurred between 1979 and 1981. In contrast, the number of Medicaid beneficiaries remained about the same, declining by 27 thousand over the 6-year period. During this period, much of the growth in the poverty population was a result of increases in the number of poor people in two-parent families. These are families that historically were excluded from Medicaid (see Chapter III, Eligibility and Appendix A, Medicaid, the Poor, and Health Insurance).[7]

While Medicaid is a means-tested entitlement program, this does not mean that every poor person is eligible for coverage. For example, nonaged nondisabled childless couples and single individuals are generally not eligible for the program. In addition to a limited category of the poor being eligible during

---

[5]These figures compare the combined spending for Kerr-Mills and Medicaid in 1966 with Medicaid in 1974.

[6]See, Davis, Karen and Cathy Schoen. Health and the War on Poverty: A Ten Year Appraisal. Washington, Brookings Institution, 1978. p. 59-62.

[7]Poverty statistics and Medicaid beneficiary statistics are not strictly comparable. Many individuals who are poor do not meet the categorical eligibility criteria for Medicaid. It should also be noted that individuals in medical need (i.e., high medical expenses relative to their income) are also eligible for Medicaid. These individuals can have gross incomes in excess of the poverty threshold. Finally, as figure II-2 displays, the reduction in the ratio of Medicaid beneficiaries to the poor during the 1980s is the result of a decline in the number of poor, not an increase in Medicaid beneficiaries.

this period, AFDC benefit levels did not keep pace with inflation. This has the effect of making AFDC eligibility more restrictive over time, further limiting the number of poor persons who automatically acquired Medicaid eligibility because of AFDC eligibility.[8] This phenomenon is suggested when comparing the Medicaid beneficiaries with cash assistance payments and the poverty population in figure II-2. The number of Medicaid beneficiaries with cash assistance remained around 16.4 million through 1990, while the poverty population fluctuated, partly as a result of economic downturns and growth. In 1991, the number of beneficiaries also receiving cash assistance payments jumped to 17.2 million reflecting increases in AFDC caseload.

[8]It should be noted that the statistical poverty threshold is adjusted annually to reflect the effect of inflation. A discussion of the relationship between Medicaid eligibility and poverty during this period can be found in: Burwell, Brian O., and Marilyn Rymer. *Trends in Medicaid Eligibility: 1975 to 1985.* Health Affairs, winter 1987. p. 30-45.

FIGURE II-2.
Medicaid Beneficiaries and the Number of Poor
1968-1991

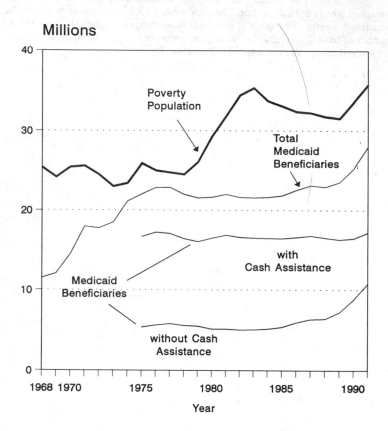

NOTE: Medicaid beneficiary totals include some individuals with incomes in excess of poverty threshold. Medicaid beneficiaries with cash welfare payment totals unavailable before 1975.
Source: Figure prepared by Congressional Research Service based on data from HCFA.

**TABLE II-2. A Comparison of the Size of the Poverty Population
and the Number of Medicaid Beneficiaries, 1975-1991[a]
(poverty and beneficiary estimates are in thousands)**

Year	Medicaid beneficiaries		Total Medicaid beneficiaries[b]	Poverty population
	w/cash asst.	w/o cash asst.		
1975	16,678	5,329	22,007	25,877
1976	17,222	5,593	22,815	24,975
1977	17,067	5,764	22,831	24,720
1978	16,423	5,542	21,965	24,497
1979	16,056	5,464	21,520	26,072
1980	16,497	5,108	21,605	29,272
1981	16,872	5,108	21,980	31,822
1982	16,594	5,009	21,603	34,398
1983	16,519	5,035	21,554	35,303
1984	16,478	5,129	21,607	33,700
1985	16,459	5,355	21,814	33,064
1986	16,596	5,922	22,515	32,370
1987	16,787	6,322	23,109	32,221
1988	16,547	6,360	22,907	31,745
1989	16,321	7,190	23,511	31,528
1990	16,467	8,788	25,253	33,585
1991	17,188	10,779	27,967	35,708

Average annual rate of change:

1975-1980	-0.2%	-0.8%	-0.4%	2.5%
1980-1985	*	0.9	0.2	2.5
1985-1991	0.7	12.4	4.2	1.1
1975-1991	0.2	4.4	1.5	1.9

[a]Medicaid beneficiary estimates represent the number of individuals who had services paid for during the fiscal year. The poverty estimates represent the number of individuals with individual or family annual incomes below the appropriate poverty threshold during the calendar year.

[b]Total number of Medicaid beneficiaries include a number of individuals with cash income in excess of the poverty thresholds.

*Annual rate of change less than .1 percent.

NOTE: Medicaid beneficiary estimates represent the number of Medicaid beneficiaries for 49 States (all States except Arizona), the District of Columbia, Puerto Rico and the Virgin Islands. Poverty population estimates represent individuals in all 50 States and the District of Columbia. Prior to 1982 Arizona did not provide Medicaid services to its residents. Since 1982 Arizona has operated a Medicaid program under a waiver authority. In FY 1991, there were about 313,000 beneficiaries in Arizona. The 5- and 6-year intervals chosen for the average annual rate of change calculations are somewhat arbitrary, and some of the trends shown may be affected by the years picked in computing these averages.

Source: Table prepared by the Congressional Research Service based on data provided by the Bureau of the Census and the Health Care Financing Administration.

Analyses of Medicaid's spending trend in the mid- to late 1970s have pointed to rapid increases in overall medical prices and the rising use of new or previously little-used services as the primary reasons for the program's spending growth. In particular, this period saw an increased use of institutional services. For example, the establishment of Medicaid reimbursement for services in intermediate care facilities for the mentally retarded (ICFs/MR) is directly associated with this rapid increase in vendor payments.[9] Since many beneficiaries require long stays in this type of institutional facility, payments for institutional services are a relatively expensive service category.

3. A Moderate Period of Program Spending Growth, 1982-1988

Growth in program spending moderated between 1982 and 1988. Over this 6-year period the program grew at an annual average of 8.9 percent. Legislative emphasis in the early 1980s tried to limit increases in both Federal and State outlays. For example, the Omnibus Budget Reconciliation Act of 1981 (P.L. 97-35) exempted States from following Medicare's reimbursement rules for hospitals and gave States additional flexibility in designing and administering their programs. Additionally, between FY 1982 and FY 1984, the act reduced Federal payments to States unless certain conditions were met (see *Chapter IX, Recent Legislative History* for a detailed account of these financing changes). The effect of these and other legislative changes on the program's actual spending is difficult to determine. The program's rate of growth in spending was much more moderate over this period. However, it should be noted that: 1) while program spending moderated, a per annum growth rate of 8.9 percent implies the doubling of spending in slightly over 8 years; and 2) over this period there was a parallel moderation in all health spending.

This moderate spending growth coincided with a moderate increase in the number of beneficiaries. The program's total beneficiary count increased from 21.6 million in 1982 to 22.9 million in 1988. This 6 percent increase in beneficiaries represented the largest increase in total beneficiaries since the early to mid-1970s. As can be seen in figure II-2, all of the beneficiary increase in the program is a result of growth in the number of beneficiaries not receiving cash assistance payments. All of this increase in beneficiaries occurred after 1984. Much of this increase in total beneficiaries follows a number of eligibility expansions in the program. Among other changes, these expansions raised maximum allowable income eligibility levels for pregnant women, infants (children under age 1), and young children; and redefined who was categorically eligible for the program (for example, allowing pregnant women to be eligible for the program regardless of family structure).[10]

---

[9]See, Muse, Donald N. *National Annual Medicaid Statistics: Fiscal Years 1973 through 1979.* Health Care Financing Program Statistics. Office of Research and Demonstrations. HCFA Pub. No. 03133, Aug. 1982.

[10]See *Chapter IX, Recent Legislative History*, and *Chapter III, Eligibility* for a detailed description of these changes.

4. Recent Program Spending Growth, 1988-1991

More recently, the rate of change in Medicaid spending has accelerated. Medicaid's 1989 spending total was 13.2 percent larger than in 1988, and its 1990 spending level was more than 18 percent over the 1989 amount. The rate of increase in 1991, 27 percent, is the largest rate of increase in the program in 19 years. Along with this dramatic increase in spending, the number of beneficiaries in the program has also increased. Between 1988 and 1991, the number of Medicaid beneficiaries increased by 5 million. The 1990-1991 increase of 2.7 million beneficiaries is the largest single year increase in the program since the mid-1970s.

5. Projected Program Spending, 1991-1997

The recent increases in the size of program spending and the number of beneficiaries are likely to continue over the next few years. Table II-3 and figure II-3 provide Congressional Budget Office estimates of spending and beneficiaries over the 1991 through 1997 period. These estimates were prepared in August 1992 and will be revised in early 1993.

Between 1991 and 1997, Medicaid spending is projected to increase at a 15.7 percent average annual rate; the number of beneficiaries is projected to increase at a 4.3 percent average annual rate. This steady increase in beneficiaries and spending is largely a result of the program's phased in coverage of poor children between the ages of 6 and 19 contained in the Omnibus Budget Reconciliation Act of 1990 (OBRA 90); the OBRA 90 requirement to mandate Medicare Part B premium payments for the near poor elderly and disabled; continued increases in health care costs; continued reliance of States on provider donations and provider taxes; and increased cash welfare caseloads.[11]

---

[11]Provider donations and provider specific taxes are revenue sources used by States to help finance Medicaid. These controversial revenue plans are described in *Chapter VIII, Financing*. In the fall of 1991 the role of provider donations and taxes in helping to finance the Medicaid program was limited.

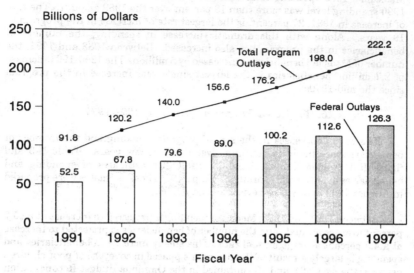

FIGURE II-3.
Projected Trend in Medicaid Spending,
FY 1991 to FY 1997

Billions of Dollars

Total Program Outlays

222.2
198.0
176.2
156.6
140.0
120.2
91.8

Federal Outlays

126.3
112.6
100.2
89.0
79.6
67.8
52.5

| 1991 | 1992 | 1993 | 1994 | 1995 | 1996 | 1997 |

Fiscal Year

NOTE: All figures are projected and subject to the methods and data used in their calculations. CBO projects Federal spending only. Projections were prepared in August 1992. Total outlays assume a 57% Federal matching percent. Limitations on provider donations and taxes and changes in Federal match will affect overall outlay amounts.

Projected Number and Rate of Growth
of Medicaid Beneficiaries,
FY 1991 to FY 1997

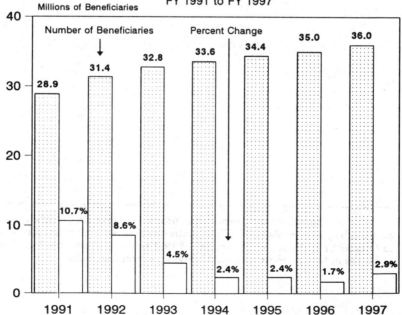

Millions of Beneficiaries

Number of Beneficiaries   Percent Change

36.0
35.0
34.4
33.6
32.8
31.4
28.9

10.7%
8.6%
4.5%
2.4% 2.4% 1.7% 2.9%

| 1991 | 1992 | 1993 | 1994 | 1995 | 1996 | 1997 |

Source: Figure prepared by Congressional Research Service based on CBO estimates as of January and August 1992. Total outlay amounts prepared by CRS. See accompanying text.

TABLE II-3. Projected Medicaid Spending and Beneficiaries, FYs 1991 to 1997

Fiscal year	Federal spending[a] (in billions)	Percent change	Total spending[b] (in billions)	Percent change	Benefi- ciaries[c] (in millions)	Percent change
1991	$ 52.5	27.8	$ 92.4	27.4	28.9	10.7
1992	67.8	29.1	118.8	28.6	31.4	8.6
1993	79.6	17.3	139.4	17.3	32.8	4.5
1994	89.0	11.9	156.0	11.9	33.6	2.4
1995	100.2	12.5	175.5	12.5	34.4	2.4
1996	112.6	12.4	197.2	12.4	35.0	1.8
1997	126.3	12.2	221.3	12.2	36.0	2.7

[a]Federal spending includes spending on benefits and administration and is comparable to the historical outlay spending provided in table II-1.

[b]Total spending is provided to highlight the overall spending trend. The totals provided in this table assume that Federal Medicaid spending will equal approximately 57 percent of total program spending. However, it should be noted that Federal spending has represented a growing share of total program outlays over the last few years.

[c]Beneficiary estimates represent the number of beneficiaries in all 50 States, the District of Columbia, and all outlying territories. As such the estimates are not strictly comparable to the beneficiary totals provided in table II-2. Beneficiary estimates were prepared in Jan. 1992.

NOTE: All figures are estimates and subject to the limitations of the data and methodology employed in their calculations. These spending projections were developed in Aug. 1992 and are likely to change with additional information.

Source: Table prepared by the Congressional Research Service. Federal spending estimates for FY 1992 through 1997 were prepared by the Congressional Budget Office in Aug. 1992, beneficiary estimates were prepared in Jan. 1992. Total spending is estimated by the Congressional Research Service based on a 57 percent overall Federal matching percentage. This matching percentage is likely to change and this,in turn, will affect the total spending estimates.

B. Factors Accounting for Recent Medicaid Spending Growth

The growth in Medicaid spending is affected by a number of complex and interrelated factors. One group of factors is directly related to the scope of Medicaid's services and covered populations. For example, individual State decisions on whether to include optional eligibility categories, optional service categories, and limitations on services all play an important role in the size and rate of the program's spending increases. At the Federal level, legislative changes in the program mandating eligibility expansion play some role. Decisions on the part of the Administration to grant States waivers to provide services in new innovative ways to beneficiaries can also have some effect on spending levels. Additionally, State Medicaid payment rates have been affected by recent court decisions. Medicaid law requires hospitals and nursing home payment rates to be "reasonable and adequate" to meet the costs of "efficiently and economically" operated facilities. In a number of States, providers have sued, claiming that payments failed to meet this test. As a result of these lawsuits, some States have been required to increase payments for inpatient hospital and nursing home services.[12]

Another set of factors are best described as effects of the health sector. The Medicaid program provides services in a sector that has experienced price inflation that is far above general inflation, and that often uses new medical technology to treat patients. These factors may contribute to changes in the amount and intensity of health care services used by Medicaid beneficiaries. Still another set of factors are more demographically or epidemiologically based: the number of single female-headed families is increasing; the overall U.S. population is aging; and the incidence of AIDS has increased. These later factors tend to affect the size of the program's potential eligibility group and/or the intensity and volume of services used.

In the mid-session review of the 1992 Federal budget, the Office of Management and Budget (OMB) reported that:[13]

> most Medicaid spending increases (59 percent) over the 1980-90 time period were due primarily to health care inflation. Federal legislation and waiver programs accounted for 22 percent of the increase; other factors such as intensity of service and State initiatives to increase Federal match, accounted for 15 percent; increased enrollment accounted for only 4 percent of the spending growth.

While the OMB discussion highlights the trend between 1980 and 1990, a number of other factors affect the most recent increases in program spending. These include:

- a significant increase in the size of AFDC caseload. The average monthly number of AFDC recipients has increased from 10.9 million in FY 1988 to over 12 million in the first 9 months of FY 1991;

- mandated and optional expansions determining who is eligible for the program. Financial eligibility requirements for children have become much less restrictive. For example, States can provide coverage to infants and pregnant women up to 185 percent of the Federal poverty level; States must provide coverage to pregnant women and children under age 6 with family incomes below 133 percent of poverty;

- State use of revenue enhancing devices (e.g., provider donations and provider specific taxes) to facilitate increased program spending;[14]

---

[12]See *Chapter V, Reimbursement.*

[13]See U.S. Executive Office of the President. Office of Management and Budget. *Mid-Session Review of the Budget,* July 15, 1991. p. 16.

[14]See *Chapter VIII, Financing* for a description of these devices.

- increases in payments to hospitals and nursing homes; and

- increases in nursing home cost stemming from new quality standards.

C. Overall Medicaid Payments Adjusted for Inflation[15]

The rapid rise in health care prices is well documented. Over the last 25 years medical price inflation, as measured by the Consumer Price Index for Medical Care (CPI-MC), generally has been higher than the overall inflation rate. After adjusting for this rapid rate of medical care inflation, overall Medicaid payments increased from 1966 through 1981 by an average 12.5 percent per annum. However, in 1982 and 1983, overall adjusted Medicaid payments declined. As a result of these declines, the 1983 constant dollar spending amount was about equal to the 1980 total. However, the program's spending pattern in the early 1980s appears to be an aberration. Between 1985 and 1991, adjusted spending increased at an average annual rate of 6.3 percent, the largest average annual rate since the program's early years, 1970 through 1975. Table II-4 and figure II-4 portray the inflation-adjusted spending trend for the program.

As previously noted, the slowing of program spending in the early 1980s may be a reflection of the effects of lowered Federal matching payments and changes in the rules for the State administration of the program.[16] The

---

[15]Adjusting Medicaid spending for price change is difficult. In particular, the adjustment of Medicaid's spending level by the CPI-MC may overstate the impact of price change on program spending. The CPI measure reflects the inflation rate for out of pocket medical payments, not the prices Medicaid programs pay (which may rise more slowly than prices paid by other insurers. (See *Chapter V, Reimbursement*.) Furthermore, it is an aggregate measure that may reflect a mix of health care services and supplies that is different from those provided by the Medicaid program. There are two alternative approaches to this computation. The first approach would be to adjust the spending using a general price measure. This approach adjusts the spending for changes in overall prices. Any sector specific price change is weighted by the change in prices of goods and services outside the health sector. Using this approach would result in a faster rate of growth for constant dollar spending (the average annual rate of increase between 1968 and 1990 using the implicit price deflator for the Gross National Product (GNP) is 5.9 percent as compared to 8.0 percent using the CPI-MC). The second approach would be to construct a price index specifically for the Medicaid program. This program specific index would be a composite index weighted based on the type of Medicaid services used. For an example of this later type of index, see: Chang, Deborah and John Holahan. *Medicaid Spending in the 1980s: The Access-Cost Containment Trade-Off Revisited*. Report No. 90-2. Washington, Urban Institute.

[16]A number of articles exploring Medicaid's spending trends suggest that this is the case. See for instance, Reilly, Thomas W., et al. *Trends in Medicaid Payments and Utilization, 1975-89*. Health Care Financing Review, Supplement 1990.

**TABLE II-4. Medicaid Spending in Constant 1991 Dollars,
Fiscal Years 1966 to 1991
($ in millions)**

Year	Total spending	Percent change	FY 1991 constant dollars	Percent change
1966[a]	$ 1,658	--	$11,250	--
1967[a]	2,368	42.8%	15,067	33.9%
1968[a]	3,686	55.7	22,078	46.5
1969[a]	4,166	13.0	23,419	6.1
1970[a]	4,852	16.5	25,617	9.4
1971	6,176	27.3	30,476	19.0
1972	8,434	36.6	39,809	30.6
1973	9,111	8.0	41,757	4.9
1974	10,229	12.3	44,309	6.1
1975	12,637	23.5	48,671	9.8
1976	14,644	15.9	51,180	5.2
1977	17,103	16.8	53,336	4.2
1978	18,949	10.8	54,404	2.0
1979	21,755	14.8	57,255	5.2
1980	25,781	18.5	61,345	7.1
1981	30,377	17.8	65,465	6.7
1982	32,446	6.8	62,482	-4.6
1983	34,956	7.7	61,332	-1.8
1984	37,569	7.5	61,973	1.0
1985	40,917	8.9	63,628	2.7
1986	44,851	9.6	65,030	2.2
1987	49,344	10.0	66,805	2.7
1988	54,116	9.7	68,915	3.2
1989	61,246	13.2	72,715	5.5
1990	72,492	18.4	79,095	8.8
1991[b]	92,389	27.4	92,389	16.8

Average annual rate of change:

1966-1970		30.8%		22.8%
1970-1975		21.1		13.7
1975-1980		14.5		4.5
1980-1985		9.7		0.7
1985-1991		14.5		6.4

See notes on the following page.

**TABLE II-4. Medicaid Spending in Constant 1991 Dollars,
Fiscal Years 1966 to 1991--Continued**

ᵃSpending amounts for these years represent spending for Medicaid and its predecessor programs, such as Kerr-Mills. Federal matching payments were made for these programs through Dec. 1969.

ᵇ1991 figure is preliminary.

NOTE: Constant dollar spending amounts are based on total program spending and medical care price change as measured using the CPI-MC. The Federal fiscal year began on July 1 until FY 1976 when the beginning of the fiscal year was moved to Oct. 1. Percentage change reported for FY 1976 represents change in spending over 5 quarters. The 5-year intervals chosen for the average annual rate of change calculations are somewhat arbitrary, and some of the trends shown may be affected by the years picked in computing these averages.

Source: Table prepared by the Congressional Research Service based on data obtained from the Health Care Financing Administration and Bureau of Labor Statistics.

FIGURE II-4.
Total Medicaid Spending Adjusted for Inflation, FY 1966-FY 1991

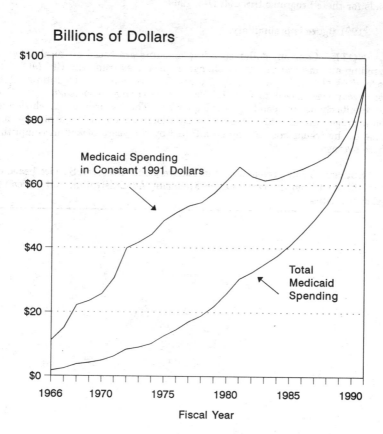

Billions of Dollars

Medicaid Spending in Constant 1991 Dollars

Total Medicaid Spending

Fiscal Year

NOTE: Spending between 1966 and 1972 includes spending on related programs such as the Kerr-Mills and other programs. Spending adjusted using the CPI-medical care.
Source: Figure prepared by Congressional Research Service based on data from HCFA.

Omnibus Budget Reconciliation Act of 1981 lowered Federal matching payments by 3 percent in FY 1982, 4 percent in FY 1983, and 4.5 percent in FY 1984. However, the size of a State's reduction in Federal payments could be modified under certain conditions.[17]

D. Payments Per Beneficiary[18]

Table II-5 and figure II-5 combine the trends in beneficiaries with medical vendor payments. The repercussion of a constant increase in spending combined with a constancy in the number of beneficiaries from the mid-1970s through the early 1980s was a rapid increase in program spending per beneficiary from 1975 through 1981. Between 1975 and 1981, payments per beneficiary increased from $556 to $1,238. The average annual increase for this period equalled 13.7 percent. Between 1981 and 1988, the average increase in payments per beneficiary moderated somewhat, equalling 8.0 percent. While this is a smaller rate of growth it should be noted that an average annual increase of 8.0 percent implies a doubling in payments per beneficiary every 9 years. Furthermore, the 1990 increase in payments per beneficiary once again was in double figures, 10.8 percent, a rate increase that has not been recorded since 1981.

---

[17]See *Chapter IX, Recent Legislative History* for the details on the reduction in State payments.

[18]The analysis in this section of the chapter is based on information contained on the HCFA Form 2082. This statistical data provide information on the size of medical vendor payments. This spending represents all payments to physicians, hospitals, long-term care facilities and other health providers, as well as payments for other covered services and supplies. *Chapter X, Medicaid Payment and Beneficiary Information, Fiscal Year 1991* provides definitions of what is included in this spending data. HCFA Form 2082 data differs from total program spending in that this spending trend excludes administrative spending, any payments provided in capitation plans, and the other adjustments that are a part of total spending. The Medicaid statistical report allows for the analysis of beneficiary and payments relying on a single data source. A detailed discussion of the many issues associated with Medicaid data can be found in: Ku, Leighton, Marilyn Rymer Ellwood, and John Klemm. *Deciphering Medicaid Data: Issues and Needs.* Health Care Financing Review. 1990 Annual Supplement. p. 35-45.

TABLE II-5. Medicaid Payments Per Beneficiary, in Nominal and Constant Dollars, 1968 to 1991

Year[a]	Payments per beneficiary	Percent change	Constant 1991 dollars	
			Payments per beneficiary	Percent change
1968	$ 304	--	$1,766	--
1969	295	-3.0%	1,606	9.0%
1970	297	0.8	1,517	-5.5
1971	307	3.4	1,515	-0.2
1972	358	16.6	1,690	11.5
1973	440	22.9	2,017	19.3
1974	465	5.7	2,014	-0.1
1975	556	19.6	2,141	6.3
1976	618	11.2	2,160	0.9
1977	711	15.0	2,217	2.7
1978	819	15.2	2,351	6.1
1979	951	16.1	2,503	6.4
1980	1,079	13.5	2,567	2.6
1981	1,238	14.7	2,668	3.9
1982	1,361	9.9	2,621	-1.8
1983	1,503	10.4	2,637	0.6
1984	1,569	4.4	2,558	-1.9
1985	1,719	9.6	2,673	3.3
1986	1,821	5.9	2,640	-1.2
1987	1,949	7.0	2,639	-0.1
1988	2,126	9.1	2,707	2.6
1989	2,318	9.0	2,752	1.7
1990	2,568	10.8	2,802	1.8
1991	2,752	7.2	2,752	-1.8
Average annual rate of change:				
1968-1970		8.2%		1.5%
1970-1975		9.6		2.9
1975-1980		13.5		3.5
1980-1985		9.8		0.8
1985-1991		8.2		0.5
1975-1991		10.3		1.6

See notes on the following page.

TABLE II-5. Medicaid Payments Per Beneficiary, in Nominal and
Constant Dollars, 1968 to 1991--Continued

ªFigures represent calendar year spending for years 1968 through 1970. Beginning in 1971 payment amounts represent spending in fiscal years.

NOTE: All figures are estimates. Constant dollar spending is based on fiscal year change in the medical component of the CPI-MC. The use of a different inflation measure will affect the rates of growth depicted in this trend. Spending information represents medical vendor payments for 49 reporting States, the District of Columbia, Puerto Rico and the Virgin Islands. Administrative spending is not included in these estimates. The Federal fiscal year began on July 1 until FY 1976 when the beginning of the fiscal year was moved to Oct. 1. Percentage change reported for FY 1976 represents change in payments over 5 quarters.

Source: Table prepared by the Congressional Research Service for FY 1975 through FY 1990 based on data contained in: Health Care Financing Administration. *Statistical Report on Medical Care Eligibles, Recipients, Payments, and Services, HCFA Form 2082.* For earlier years, estimates are based on data provided by HCFA's Bureau of Data Management Services.

FIGURE II-5.
Medicaid Payments Per Beneficiary, FY 1968-FY 1991

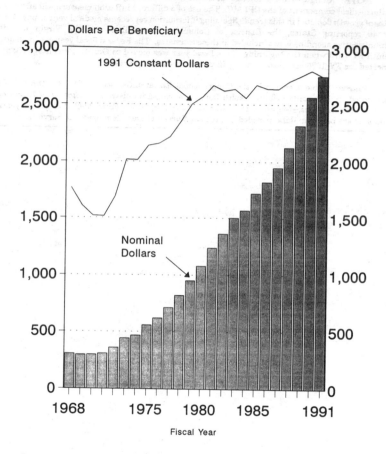

Dollars Per Beneficiary

Fiscal Year

Source: Figure prepared by Congressional Research Service based on data from HCFA.

E. Medicaid Spending in the Context of Overall Health Spending[19]

Another perspective on Medicaid's spending trend can be seen by comparing overall Medicaid spending with the trend in total public and private health care expenditures. Table II-6 and figure II-6 provide this comparison. The table and figure show overall Medicaid spending as a share of total health care expenditures from 1966 to 1990. Over the program's first 8 years, partly as a result of the increase in beneficiaries and program start up, Medicaid grew from 2.9 percent of overall health expenditures to 10 percent. From 1975 through 1989 the program's share of spending fluctuated around the 10 percent level, with spending in the 1970s representing slightly more than 10 percent, and spending in the early 1980s dropping slightly to just under the 10 percent level.

While the previous discussion points out the rapid increase in Medicaid spending, this comparison provides a different perspective. Between 1974 and 1989 Medicaid spending represented roughly 10 percent of all health care expenditures. In other words, while program spending grew rapidly over the 15 years between 1974 and 1989, it did not grow substantially faster than overall health spending. However, in 1990, Medicaid's share of overall health expenditures reached an historical high by jumping to 11.3 percent. A jump in the program's share of health care spending of this magnitude has not taken place since the mid-1970s.

While more than 1 out of every 10 health dollars is spent by Medicaid, the program plays an even more important spending role in some service areas. For instance, in 1990 Medicaid accounted for 45 percent of all nursing home spending, and 31 percent of all home health spending. In other areas, Medicaid's share is closer to the total program's share of overall health spending. In 1990, over 11 percent of all hospital spending (inpatient and outpatient) and over 9 percent of all drug spending were paid for by Medicaid. On the other hand, Medicaid's share of physician spending only equalled about 4 percent. Figure II-7 shows Medicaid's 1990 spending as a share of overall health spending for selected service categories.

---

[19]Trend information in this section relies on data that detail national health expenditures. The data series is prepared by the Health Care Financing Administration, Office of the Actuary. The data are provided on a calendar year basis. In addition, different accounting methods are used than those relied upon for the HCFA Medicaid statistical forms, and the budget data.

TABLE II-6. A Comparison of Medicaid and National Health
Expenditures, Calendar Years 1966 to 1990
($ in millions)

Year	Total Medicaid spending	Annual change	Total health spending	Annual change	Medicaid as % of total spending
1966	$ 1,311	--	$ 45,860	--	2.9%
1967	3,156	140.7%	51,655	12.6%	6.1
1968	3,558	12.7	58,478	13.2	6.1
1969	4,195	17.9	65,739	12.4	6.4
1970	5,315	26.7	74,377	13.1	7.1
1971	6,728	26.6	82,331	10.7	8.2
1972	8,351	24.1	92,307	12.1	9.0
1973	9,463	13.3	102,467	11.0	9.2
1974	11,116	17.5	116,070	13.3	9.6
1975	13,497	21.4	132,944	14.5	10.2
1976	15,258	13.0	152,168	14.5	10.0
1977	17,520	14.8	172,037	13.1	10.2
1978	19,534	11.5	193,654	12.6	10.1
1979	22,404	14.7	217,229	12.2	10.3
1980	26,134	16.6	250,126	15.1	10.4
1981	30,370	16.2	290,219	16.0	10.5
1982	32,131	5.8	326,085	12.4	9.9
1983	35,315	9.9	358,593	10.0	9.8
1984	37,995	7.6	389,637	8.7	9.8
1985	41,750	9.9	422,619	8.5	9.9
1986	45,185	8.2	454,814	7.6	9.9
1987	50,762	12.3	494,098	8.6	10.3
1988	54,873	8.1	546,014	10.5	10.0
1989	62,259	13.5	602,792	10.4	10.3
1990	75,174	20.7	666,187	10.5	11.3

Average annual rate of change:

1966-1970		41.9%		12.8%	
1970-1975		20.5		12.3	
1975-1980		14.1		13.5	
1980-1985		9.8		11.1	
1985-1990		12.5		9.5	

NOTE: All expenditure amounts are in millions. Expenditure information includes program administration costs as well as payments for medical services. Total health spending also includes health related spending on noncommercial research, public health activities and construction. All spending trends are on a calendar year basis rather than a fiscal year basis as in other tables in this chapter. Medicaid spending information from 1966 to 1970 includes spending for Medicaid and its predecessor programs. The 5-year intervals chosen for the average annual rate of change calculations are somewhat arbitrary and some of the trends shown may be affected by the years picked in computing these averages.

Source: Table prepared by the Congressional Research Service based on data obtained from the Health Care Financing Administration, Office of the Actuary, Office of National Health Cost Estimates.

FIGURE II-6.
Medicaid Spending as a Share of Total Health Spending, CY 1966-CY 1990

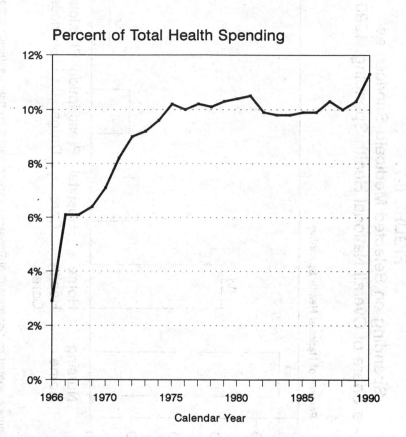

Percent of Total Health Spending

Calendar Year

NOTE: Spending between 1966 and 1970 includes spending on related programs such as the Kerr-Mills and other programs.
Source: Figure prepared by Congressional Research Service based on data from HCFA.

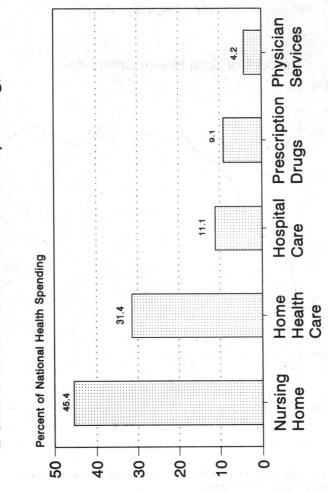

FIGURE II-7.

Spending on Selected Medicaid Services as
a Share of Overall National Health Spending, 1990

Percent of National Health Spending

Nursing Home — 45.4

Home Health Care — 31.4

Hospital Care — 11.1

Prescription Drugs — 9.1

Physician Services — 4.2

Source: Figure prepared by Congressional Research Service based on national health expenditure data obtained from HCFA.

1. *Medicaid vs. Medicare Spending*

The Federal Government plays a pervasive role in health financing. Besides being an important funding source for health services, it also provides funding for health research, the financing of health manpower training, and consumer safety. But this "other" spending is overshadowed by the two major federally supported health programs, Medicaid and Medicare. In CY 1990, Federal health spending totalled $195.4 billion. The largest share of this spending was paid for by Medicare, $111 billion (58.5 percent). Medicaid is the second largest Federal health spending category. The $42.9 billion spent on Medicaid in 1990 represented 21.9 percent of all Federal health spending.[20] Figure II-8 and table II-7 provide information on this spending.

Between 1972 and 1981, Medicaid spending oscillated between 20 and 21 percent of all Federal health spending. The trend in the early 1980s shows a drop in the share of Federal spending (its share ranged between 18 and 19 percent). However, since 1984 Medicaid spending has become a larger share of Federal spending, increasing from 18 percent in 1984 to almost 22 percent in 1990.

In comparison, Medicare has always represented the largest component of Federal health spending. This federally financed and administered program helps pay for health care services of the elderly, disabled, and most persons with end-stage renal disease. The program consists of two parts: hospital insurance (HI) and supplementary medical insurance (SMI). HI helps pay for inpatient hospital care and to a very limited degree nursing home care. SMI helps pay for physician services, hospital outpatient services, and other related health services. As will be described below, this is a different set of covered health services from those covered under the Medicaid program.

Between 1972 and 1988 the growth in Medicare spending outpaced other Federal health spending including Medicaid. As depicted in figure II-8, Medicare's share of Federal health spending increased from 41 percent in 1972 to 59 percent in 1988. However, it should be noted that between 1981 and 1988, Medicare's share of Federal spending essentially remained unchanged. Unlike the Medicaid trend, between 1989 and 1990, Medicare's share of the Federal health total declined to 57 percent. This decline in the share of the health total is primarily a result of the disproportionately large increase in Medicaid spending. All other health spending remained at 21 percent over this 2-year period.

While the 24-year spending trend for both of these programs reflects their dominance in Federal health spending, a number of aspects of the programs are substantially different. The two programs cover different types of beneficiaries, different types of services, and use different payment methods.

In 1990 more than 6 out of every 10 Medicare dollars paid for hospital services. In comparison, Medicaid hospital payments comprised less than 4 of

---

[20]This excludes all State spending in the program.

every 10 Medicaid dollars. Medicare spent about 2 percent of its payments on nursing home services; in contrast, Medicaid dedicated about 32 percent of its spending for these services. While this comparison highlights some of the spending differences between these two programs, it should also be noted that the share of program funds dedicated to a particular service category is affected by the type of beneficiaries who use those services, the intensity of the services used, and the rate of reimbursement for those services.

For example, a large share of Medicaid beneficiaries are children (more than 44 percent in 1990). The health problems of these children are different from the aged and disabled. On average, children are less likely to need expensive institutional care, or be intensive users of inpatient hospital services. In contrast, all of Medicare's beneficiaries are aged and disabled, a subpopulation that has a substantially higher hospital utilization rate.

During the 1980s both Medicare and Medicaid altered their reimbursement methods for hospital services in an attempt to contain costs. Beginning in FY 1984, Medicare changed its hospital reimbursement methods from a retrospective cost based system to a prospective system based on a patient's diagnosis. More recently, Medicare has changed its method of reimbursement for physicians. Likewise, Medicaid's reimbursement mechanisms have also undergone change. For instance, many States have adopted prospective payment systems for hospital reimbursement. However, some studies have shown that Medicaid pays less for hospital and physician services than Medicare.[21]

---

[21]See *Chapter V, Reimbursement.*

TABLE II-7. Medicaid and Medicare as a Share of Federal
and State/Local Health Spending, Calendar Years 1966 to 1990
($ in millions)

Year	Medicaid Federal	Medicaid State/local	Medicaid Total	% of Federal health spending	% of State/local health spending	Medicare	% of Federal health spending
1966	$ 635	$ 676	$ 1,311	8.5%	11.1%	$ 1,728	23.0%
1967	1,532	1,624	3,156	12.5	23.4	5,054	41.3
1968	1,843	1,715	3,558	13.1	22.4	6,164	43.7
1969	2,309	1,886	4,195	14.3	22.1	7,116	44.2
1970	2,856	2,459	5,315	16.1	24.8	7,633	43.0
1971	3,828	2,900	6,728	18.7	26.8	8,495	41.6
1972	4,568	3,783	8,351	19.9	31.0	9,299	40.6
1973	4,954	4,509	9,463	19.7	31.9	10,745	42.7
1974	6,301	4,815	11,116	20.6	29.9	13,458	44.1
1975	7,437	6,060	13,497	20.4	32.4	16,402	45.0
1976	9,165	6,093	15,258	21.3	31.3	19,790	46.1
1977	9,969	7,551	17,520	20.9	33.6	22,832	48.0
1978	10,940	8,594	19,534	20.1	33.8	26,780	49.3
1979	12,755	9,649	22,404	20.8	33.4	31,079	50.6
1980	14,499	11,635	26,134	20.1	35.1	37,533	52.1
1981	17,220	13,150	30,370	20.5	34.8	45,152	53.8
1982	17,487	14,644	32,131	18.7	35.3	52,642	56.4
1983	19,233	16,082	35,315	18.6	36.2	59,906	58.0
1984	20,440	17,555	37,995	18.2	37.4	65,917	58.5
1985	23,149	18,601	41,750	18.7	36.4	72,161	58.4
1986	25,357	19,828	45,185	19.1	34.7	77,383	58.2
1987	27,904	22,858	50,762	19.4	35.5	83,402	57.9
1988	30,982	23,891	54,873	19.8	33.9	90,525	57.8
1989	35,415	26,844	62,259	20.2	34.6	102,590	58.6
1990	42,857	32,317	75,174	21.9	37.0	111,195	56.9

Average annual rate of change:

1966-1970	45.6%	38.1%	41.9%			45.0%	
1970-1975	21.1	19.8	20.5			16.5	
1975-1980	14.3	13.9	14.1			18.0	
1980-1985	9.8	9.8	9.8			14.0	
1985-1990	13.1	11.7	12.5			9.0	

See notes on the following page.

**TABLE II-7. Medicaid and Medicare as a Share of Federal
and State/Local Health Spending, Calendar Years 1966 to 1990--Continued**

NOTE: All spending amounts are in millions. Expenditure information includes program administration costs as well as payments for medical services. Federal and State/local health spending includes health related spending on noncommercial research, public health activities and construction. Medicare spending includes spending for both Part A (hospital insurance) and Part B (supplemental medical insurance). Medicaid spending information from 1966 to 1970 includes spending for Medicaid and its predecessor programs. The 4- and 5-year intervals chosen for the average annual rate of change calculations are somewhat arbitrary and some of the trends shown may be affected by the years picked in computing these averages.

Source: Table prepared by the Congressional Research Service based on data obtained from the Health Care Financing Administration, Office of the Actuary, Office of National Health Cost Estimates.

FIGURE II-8.
Medicaid and Medicare Spending as a Share of Federal and State Spending, 1966-1990

Percent of Spending

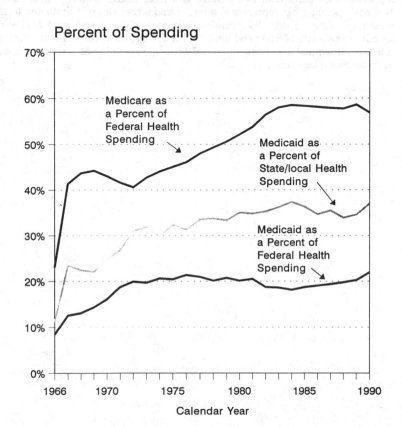

Calendar Year

NOTE: Spending between 1966 and 1970 includes spending on related programs such as the Kerr-Mills and other programs.
Source: Figure prepared by Congressional Research Service based on data from HCFA.

2. *State and Local Medicaid Spending*

State and local expenditures dedicated to Medicaid are a major and growing component of overall State spending.[22] The program represents the single largest category of State and local health spending. In 1990, Medicaid represented 37 percent of every State and local health dollar. Since 1986, Medicaid spending has represented a larger and larger share of State and local health spending. Table II-7 provides estimates of State and local Medicaid spending as a share of State and local health dollars, while table II-8 and figure II-9 provide estimates of State and local Medicaid spending as a share of total State and local expenditures.

---

[22]See *Chapter VIII, Financing* for a State by State description of Medicaid expenditures in State budgets for 1990.

**TABLE II-8. State and Local Medicaid Spending as a Share
of State and Local Expenditures, Calendar Years 1966 to 1990
($ in billions)**

Year	State and local Medicaid spending	State and local expenditures	Medicaid as a percent of expenditures
1966	$ 0.7	$ 66.7	1.0%
1967	1.6	75.0	2.2
1968	1.7	84.0	2.0
1969	1.9	93.0	2.0
1970	2.5	102.8	2.4
1971	2.9	113.8	2.5
1972	3.8	118.8	3.2
1973	4.5	131.3	3.4
1974	4.8	149.6	3.2
1975	6.1	166.4	3.6
1976	6.1	178.2	3.4
1977	7.6	188.8	4.0
1978	8.6	200.9	4.3
1979	9.6	224.9	4.3
1980	11.6	247.9	4.7
1981	13.2	274.4	4.8
1982	14.6	298.2	4.9
1983	16.1	316.2	5.1
1984	17.6	339.7	5.2
1985	18.6	372.3	5.0
1986	19.8	409.4	4.8
1987	22.9	451.4	5.1
1988	23.9	481.7	5.0
1989	26.8	517.7	5.2
1990	32.3	566.6	5.7

Average annual rate of change:

1966-1970	38.1%	11.4%	
1970-1975	19.8	10.1	
1975-1980	13.9	8.3	
1980-1985	9.8	8.5	
1985-1990	11.7	8.8	

ªState and local expenditures net of Federal grants in aid.

NOTE: All figures are estimates. Expenditure information includes program administration costs as well as payments for medical services. Medicaid spending information from 1966 to 1970 includes spending for Medicaid and its predecessor programs. The 4- and 5-year intervals chosen for the average annual rate of change calculations are somewhat arbitrary and some of the trends shown may be affected by the years picked in computing these averages.

Source: Table prepared by the Congressional Research Service based on information obtained from the Health Care Financing Administration, Office of the Actuary, Office of National Health Cost Estimates; and the Bureau of Economic Analysis.

FIGURE II-9.
State and Local Medicaid Spending as a Share of State and Local Expenditures, 1966-1990

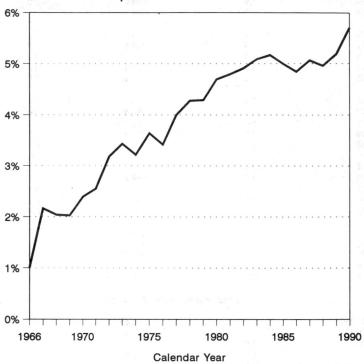

Percent of State
and Local Expenditures

Calendar Year

NOTE: Spending between 1966 and 1970 includes spending on related programs such as the Kerr-Mills
and other programs. State and local expenditures exclude Federal grants in aid.
Source: Figure prepared by Congressional Research Service based on data from HCFA and BEA.

In addition to Medicaid, State and local health spending includes expenditures on items like public health activities, State and local hospitals, vocational rehabilitation, maternal and child health programs, temporary disability medical insurance payments and other items.[23]

Numerous factors affect State Medicaid spending. First, the open-ended nature of Federal matching funds allows States to purchase more health care per State dollar in the Medicaid program than when the State purchases health care services without the Federal matching amount. This may act to stimulate State spending, and can contribute to Medicaid's relatively rapid spending growth. Second, the entitlement nature of Medicaid can make it difficult for States to control expenditures. Since Medicaid is an entitlement, State costs (and Federal matching amounts) are largely determined by the behavior of providers and beneficiaries. States must control program spending by determining and sometimes altering: who is eligible, what medical services are covered, the extent of coverage and payment rates. The optional and mandatory eligibility expansions of the mid- to late 1980s have resulted in States providing Medicaid services to additional people and concomitant increases in State and Federal spending.

Increasing beneficiaries and services are not the sole reason for increased State spending. Many States have begun to seek out new revenue sources to meet Medicaid spending needs, such as provider tax and donation programs. Under these financing mechanisms, providers of Medicaid services (e.g., hospitals and nursing homes) donate funds to the State, or are taxed by the State. These revenues can be used to draw matching funds and thus help to offset program costs. With the additional revenue, State spending has increased. The use of these revenue sources has now been limited by the Medicaid Voluntary Contribution and Provider Specific Tax Amendments of 1991 (P.L. 102-234).[24]

F. State by State Variation in Medicaid Payments and Beneficiaries

Over the entire history of the program, Medicaid spending and beneficiary levels have been dominated by a handful of States. For instance, in FY 1975 Medicaid spending in five States (California, Illinois, Michigan, New York, and Pennsylvania) represented almost 53 percent of the program's vendor payments. Over time other populous States have influenced overall program spending. The Medicaid programs in New Jersey, Ohio and Texas represent a fairly large share of total program spending. More recently these States have been joined by other States including Florida and Massachusetts. In FY 1991, the 10 largest

---

[23]The national health account data series treats as public expenditures any spending that occurs through a program established by public law. This results in spending on workers compensation, although relying on privately collected premiums and providing benefits through private insurers, being counted as public health spending.

[24]See *Chapter VIII, Financing* for a discussion of the controversy surrounding the use of these revenue sources.

Medicaid spending States represented over 59 percent of total program spending.[25] Table II-9 provides FY 1991 total (Federal, State and local) Medicaid vendor payments by State.

Based on this ranking of States, it might appear that State population has an important influence on the size of its spending. However, this is an oversimplification. There is tremendous variability in who is covered by each State's Medicaid program and what services are provided to those who are eligible.

TABLE II-9. State by State Medicaid Payments, Fiscal Year 1991
($ in millions)

State	Total payments	Percent of U.S. total
Alabama	$ 805	1.0
Alaska	160	0.2
Arkansas	688	0.9
California	7,579	9.8
Colorado	673	0.9
Connecticut	1,630	2.1
Delaware	186	0.2
District of Columbia	446	0.6
Florida	2,944	3.8
Georgia	1,799	2.3
Hawaii	238	0.3
Idaho	223	0.3
Illinois	2,731	3.5
Indiana	1,662	2.2
Iowa	766	1.0
Kansas	553	0.7
Kentucky	1,200	1.6
Louisiana	1,723	2.2
Maine	536	0.7
Maryland	1,292	1.7
Massachusetts	2,828	3.7
Michigan	2,540	3.3
Minnesota	1,561	2.0
Mississippi	755	1.0
Missouri	1,118	1.5
Montana	193	0.3
Nebraska	390	0.5
Nevada	178	0.2
New Hampshire	292	0.4
New Jersey	2,725	3.5
New Mexico	342	0.4
New York	13,728	17.8
North Carolina	1,788	2.3
North Dakota	227	0.3
Ohio	3,653	4.7
Oklahoma	814	1.1
Oregon	667	0.9

[25]The 10 largest Medicaid spending States are: New York, California, Ohio, Texas, Pennsylvania, Florida, Massachusetts, Illinois, New Jersey and Michigan.

TABLE II-9. State by State Medicaid Payments, Fiscal Year 1991--Continued
($ in millions)

State	Total payments	Percent of U.S. total
Pennsylvania	$ 3,436	4.5
Rhode Island	657	0.9
South Carolina	910	1.2
South Dakota	196	0.3
Tennessee	1,485	1.9
Texas	3,532	4.6
Utah	311	0.4
Vermont	197	0.3
Virginia	1,218	1.6
Washington	1,131	1.5
West Virginia	542	0.7
Wisconsin	1,471	1.9
Wyoming	90	0.1
Puerto Rico	146	0.2
Virgin Islands	4	0.0
49 reporting States and the District of Columbia	76,814	99.8
U.S. Total	$76,964	100.0

NOTE: Estimates are for State by State spending on medical vendor payments and exclude any administrative payments and capitated payments. Estimates are based on medical vendor payments reported by the States to the Health Care Financing Administration (HCFA), except in the case of Rhode Island, Puerto Rico, and Massachusetts' Blind Agency which were estimated by HCFA.

Source: Table prepared by the Congressional Research Service based on data contained on HCFA Form 2082.

Two of the avenues to Medicaid eligibility (cash welfare criteria and high medical need and costs) lead to an enormous amount of variability in the characteristics of each State's beneficiaries. The program's link to AFDC and SSI means that States with higher than average income eligibility levels are likely to have a larger rate of coverage of low-income children and caretaker adults than in States with below average income eligibility levels.[26] Likewise, whether a State uses the optional medically needy criteria for eligibility will also

---

[26]SSI is a federally administered program and Federal benefit levels are the same in all States. However, State supplementary payments are required by law to maintain the income level of public assistance recipients who were transferred to the SSI program at its inception in the early 1970s. States have the option to provide supplemental payments to other SSI recipients as well. In 1991, all but nine States provided these supplemental payments.

influence what type of individuals are covered by Medicaid in the State.[27] Later this chapter documents the enormous variability in program spending by eligibility type. On a per beneficiary basis, payments for the medically needy (i.e., those individuals who are eligible because they sustain high medical bills) are almost twice that of the categorically needy (chiefly, those who qualify for the program because of their receipt of cash assistance payments). A simple comparison of State Medicaid expenditures is somewhat misleading since some State amounts reflect coverage of the medically needy, individuals who may not be eligible in another State.

Furthermore, as will be described in *Chapter IV, Services*, there are a multitude of optional services that are not covered by all States, including chiropractic services (provided in 27 States in FY 1991), and private duty nursing services (provided in 28 States). The result is that some State spending reflects services that are not even part of another State's program. Additionally, not all services are available to all Medicaid beneficiaries within a State. Again, the decision on what type of services are covered for each eligibility category is determined by each State.

A typical approach to adjust for the number of beneficiaries in a State's program is to present information on Medicaid payments per beneficiary. Table II-10 provides this information for FY 1991. In FY 1991, the five States that spent the most per Medicaid beneficiary included: Connecticut, New York, New Hampshire, the District of Columbia and New Jersey. The five States that spent the least per Medicaid beneficiary were: Mississippi, California, West Virginia, Alabama, and Texas. Overall the program spent $2,752 per beneficiary in 1991. Twenty four States and the District of Columbia spent more per beneficiary, while 25 States spent less.

---

[27]Much of the difference in payments for those eligible for the program because of medical need is a result of the high cost of institutional services. Title XIX allows States to establish a special income level for long-term care eligibility (see *Appendix C, Medicaid, Long-Term Care, and the Elderly*). This special income eligibility level blurs the importance of the medically needy criteria to some extent.

TABLE II-10. Medicaid Payments Per Beneficiary, by State, Fiscal Year 1991

State	Payment per beneficiary
Alabama	$1,997
Alaska	3,123
Arkansas	2,417
California	1,886
Colorado	3,011
Connecticut	5,994
Delaware	3,671
District of Columbia	4,456
Florida	2,358
Georgia	2,411
Hawaii	2,606
Idaho	3,184
Illinois	2,387
Indiana	4,003
Iowa	2,930
Kansas	2,642
Kentucky	2,284
Louisiana	2,690
Maine	3,561
Maryland	3,565
Massachusetts	4,344
Michigan	2,283
Minnesota	3,702
Mississippi	1,607
Missouri	2,221
Montana	3,037
Nebraska	2,915
Nevada	3,005

**TABLE II-10. Medicaid Payments Per Beneficiary,
by State, Fiscal Year 1991--Continued**

State	Payment per beneficiary
New Hampshire	$4,898
New Jersey	4,437
New Mexico	2,113
New York	5,577
North Carolina	2,679
North Dakota	4,319
Ohio	2,812
Oklahoma	2,673
Oregon	2,531
Pennsylvania	2,690
Rhode Island	4,014
South Carolina	2,426
South Dakota	3,435
Tennessee	2,130
Texas	2,043
Utah	2,408
Vermont	2,782
Virginia	2,756
Washington	2,235
West Virginia	1,912
Wisconsin	3,537
Wyoming	2,450
Average for reporting States	2,871
Average for U.S. total	2,752

NOTE: All figures are estimates and subject to the limitations of the data and methods employed in their calculations.

Source: Table prepared by the Congressional Research Service based on data contained on HCFA Form 2082.

While this comparison takes into account the number of Medicaid beneficiaries, it fails to consider the type of beneficiaries in each State. Table II-11 provides another perspective on State spending. In this table, the Medicaid payments per beneficiary are standardized, based on the U.S. average mix of beneficiaries, but allowing State costs per beneficiary to vary between eligibility category.[28] This standardization begins to answer the question: *What would the Medicaid payment per beneficiary be, if each State had the same mix of beneficiaries as the Nation, but provided its own mix of covered services and paid for those services at State reimbursement rates?* The standardization attempts to highlight variation among State payments that can not be attributed to the composition of State Medicaid populations.

This standardization affects the estimated size of payments in many States. After this adjustment, the five states providing the highest payments include: New York, the District of Columbia, Connecticut, New Hampshire, and Minnesota. But a better comparison can be seen in comparing the unadjusted payments per beneficiary with the standardized payments. States like Connecticut, New York, North Dakota, Rhode Island, and Wisconsin experience large declines in their payments per beneficiary after the adjustment when compared to the unadjusted amounts. This suggests that their Medicaid programs have a disproportionately large share of beneficiaries in the more costly eligibility categories.

It is important to note that this standardization only adjusts for patient composition in the State and does not take into account the many other factors that will influence State spending levels. For instance, the price of services will vary from State to State as well as the intensity of use. *Chapter V, Reimbursement* provides State by State tables of reimbursement levels for hospitals, nursing homes, and physician services.

---

[28]This standardization technique attempts to control the mix of beneficiaries within each State by holding the share of recipients in 12 eligibility categories constant across all States. The technique is based on a similar analysis found in: Little, Jane Sneedon. *Medicaid.* New England Economic Review, Jan./Feb. 1991. p. 27-50.

TABLE II-11. Adjusted Medicaid Payments Per Beneficiary, Fiscal Year 1991

State	Categorically needy[a]		Medically needy[b]		Total[c]	
	Adjusted payment per beneficiary	Percent of U.S. average	Adjusted payment per beneficiary	Percent of U.S. average	Adjusted payment per beneficiary	Percent of U.S. average
Alabama	$1,662	0.65			$1,664	0.58
Alaska	4,088	1.61			4,088	1.42
Arkansas	1,953	0.77	$ 805	0.14	1,823	0.63
California	1,633	0.64	3,724	0.67	1,869	0.65
Colorado	3,019	1.19			3,019	1.05
Connecticut	4,128	1.62	5,877	1.05	4,301	1.5
Delaware	3,852	1.51			3,865	1.35
District of Columbia	3,675	1.44	11,826	2.12	4,538	1.58
Florida	2,275	0.89	1,901	0.34	2,226	0.78
Georgia	2,281	0.9	1,499	0.27	2,210	0.77
Hawaii	2,493	0.98	6,118	1.1	2,895	1.01
Idaho	3,252	1.28			3,252	1.13
Illinois	1,906	0.75	4,058	0.73	2,131	0.74

See notes at end of table.

TABLE II-11. Adjusted Medicaid Payments Per Beneficiary, Fiscal Year 1991–Continued

State	Categorically needy[a]		Medically needy[b]		Total[c]	
	Adjusted payment per beneficiary	Percent of U.S. average	Adjusted payment per beneficiary	Percent of U.S. average	Adjusted payment per beneficiary	Percent of U.S. average
Indiana	3,937	1.55			3,951	1.38
Iowa	3,108	1.22	1,388	0.25	2,913	1.01
Kansas	2,784	1.09	3,548	0.64	2,897	1.01
Kentucky	2,106	0.83	3,054	0.55	2,209	0.77
Louisiana	2,580	1.01	2,940	0.53	2,609	0.91
Maine	3,189	1.25	3,556	0.64	3,220	1.12
Maryland	2,583	1.01	6,352	1.14	2,979	1.04
Massachusetts	3,344	1.31	6,608	1.18	3,683	1.28
Michigan	2,046	0.8	4,186	0.75	2,269	0.79
Minnesota	4,080	1.6	5,271	0.94	4,193	1.46
Mississippi	1,494	0.59			1,494	0.52
Missouri	2,127	0.84			2,136	0.74
Montana	2,867	1.13	3,081	0.55	2,949	1.03

See notes at end of table.

TABLE II-11. Adjusted Medicaid Payments Per Beneficiary, Fiscal Year 1991-Continued

State	Categorically needy[a]		Medically needy[b]		Total[c]	
	Adjusted payment per beneficiary	Percent of U.S. average	Adjusted payment per beneficiary	Percent of U.S. average	Adjusted payment per beneficiary	Percent of U.S. average
Nebraska	3,001	1.18	3,074	0.55	2,998	1.04
Nevada	2,910	1.14			2,933	1.02
New Hampshire	4,194	1.65	4,520	0.81	4,223	1.47
New Jersey	4,222	1.66	1,553	0.28	4,007	1.4
New Mexico	2,271	0.89			2,271	0.79
New York	4,058	1.59	9,204	1.65	4,597	1.6
North Carolina	2,334	0.92	4,739	0.85	2,584	0.9
North Dakota	3,100	1.22	6,058	1.09	3,424	1.19
Ohio	3,227	1.27			3,227	1.12
Oklahoma	2,570	1.01	2,470	0.44	2,550	0.89
Oregon	2,808	1.1	1,237	0.22	2,629	0.92
Pennsylvania	2,704	1.06	4,332	0.78	2,869	1.00
Rhode Island	3,208	1.26	3,535	0.63	3,231	1.13

See notes at end of table.

TABLE II-11. Adjusted Medicaid Payments Per Beneficiary, Fiscal Year 1991--Continued

State	Categorically needy[a]		Medically needy[b]		Total[c]	
	Adjusted payment per beneficiary	Percent of U.S. average	Adjusted payment per beneficiary	Percent of U.S. average	Adjusted payment per beneficiary	Percent of U.S. average
South Carolina	2,194	0.86	2,555	0.46	2,225	0.77
South Dakota	3,071	1.21			3,071	1.07
Tennessee	1,972	0.77	1,517	0.27	1,916	0.67
Texas	2,229	0.88	636	0.11	2,050	0.71
Utah	3,213	1.26	2,360	0.42	3,126	1.09
Vermont	2,520	0.99	4,356	0.78	2,713	0.94
Virginia	2,234	0.88	3,713	0.67	2,385	0.83
Washington	2,524	0.99	1,802	0.32	2,439	0.85
West Virginia	1,974	0.78	1,735	0.31	1,941	0.68
Wisconsin	2,898	1.14	2,319	0.42	2,831	0.99
Wyoming	3,062	1.2			3,069	1.07
Average for reporting States	2,546	1.00	5,580	1.00	2,871	1.00

See notes on the following page.

TABLE II-11. Adjusted Medicaid Payments Per Beneficiary, Fiscal Year 1991--Continued

[a]Categorically needy represents spending for those categorically needy for Medicaid, regardless of any receipt of cash assistance payments. Included in this category are individuals who are eligible for Medicaid because of the receipt of AFDC, SSI or other cash assistance payments, individuals who are categorically needy without the receipt of these benefits, individuals who are eligible because their family income is below the income guidelines associated with Federal poverty guidelines.

[b]States with no entry under the *medically needy* column do not use the medically needy option in that State.

[c]Total adjusted payment per beneficiary adjusts a State's payment per beneficiary based on the relative size of the total Medicaid beneficiary population in the categorically needy and medically needy categories and the State payment per beneficiary in each of these categories. Total adjusted payments in States with no medically needy programs have totals lower than in the categorically needy column because these States have no payments for the medically needy (i.e., their medically needy payment is $0). This adjustment takes into account the relative mix of beneficiaries and ignores many additional variables such as differences in utilization and the cost of services.

NOTE: All figures are estimates and subject to the limitations of the data and methods employed in their calculations.

Source: Table prepared by the Congressional Research Service.

G. State Trends, 1975-1991

Table II-12 provides total vendor payment information for FY 1975, FY 1985 and FY 1991, each State's share of total payments, and the average annual growth rate. This table acts as a summary of individual State trends. However, focusing on the beginning and end point of the State spending information hides much of the variation over the 16 years. Figure II-10 is a pictorial representation of State average annual rates of growth over the 16-year period. As noted previously, total Medicaid vendor payments increased at an average annual rate of 12.0 percent over this time period. States with the fastest increase in payments include: Alaska, West Virginia, Florida, Wyoming, and Delaware. States with the slowest average rates of growth include: Illinois, Wisconsin, Michigan, New York, and the District of Columbia. Over the 16-year period, a number of the States with relatively low rates of growth are those States that represent a significant portion of total Medicaid program spending. As a result, the top five States that represented close to 53 percent of FY 1975 spending (California, Illinois, Michigan, New York, and Pennsylvania) represented about 39 percent of the total in FY 1991.

Numerous factors may account for these differences in State growth rates. For instance, the more recent, very rapid growth in program payments has not occurred in all States with equal force. Based on preliminary data from FY 1992 and State projections for FY 1993, the growth rates for a number of Southern States are likely to continue to be relatively high.

TABLE II-12. State by State Medicaid Payments, FY 1975, FY 1985 and FY 1991
($ in millions)

State	FY 1975 payments	Share of total	FY 1985 payments	Share of total	FY 1991 payments	Share of total	Average annual rate of change: FYs 1975-1985	FYs 1985-1991
Alabama	$ 131	1.1%	$ 375	1.0%	$ 805	1.0%	10.8%	13.6%
Alaska	9	0.1	66	0.2	160	0.2	21.5	15.8
Arkansas	93	0.8	358	1.0	688	0.9	14.1	11.5
California	1,491	12.2	4,045	10.8	7,579	9.8	10.2	11.0
Colorado	98	0.8	316	0.8	673	0.9	12.1	13.4
Connecticut	161	1.3	595	1.6	1,630	2.1	13.6	18.3
Delaware	15	0.1	71	0.2	186	0.2	16.4	17.6
District of Columbia	94	0.8	298	0.8	446	0.6	11.9	7.0
Florida	173	1.4	943	2.5	2,944	3.8	18.0	20.9
Georgia	256	2.1	760	2.0	1,799	2.3	11.2	15.5
Hawaii	37	0.3	140	0.4	238	0.3	13.9	9.2
Idaho	24	0.2	76	0.2	223	0.3	11.9	19.6
Illinois	682	5.6	1,653	4.4	2,731	3.5	9.0	8.7
Indiana	172	1.4	747	2.0	1,662	2.2	15.4	14.3
Iowa	82	0.7	360	1.0	766	1.0	15.5	13.4
Kansas	102	0.8	256	0.7	553	0.7	9.4	13.7
Kentucky	100	0.8	540	1.4	1,200	1.6	17.9	14.2
Louisiana	143	1.2	725	1.9	1,723	2.2	17.2	13.5
Maine	60	0.5	232	0.6	536	0.7	14.1	15.0
Maryland	159	1.3	584	1.6	1,292	1.7	13.5	14.2

TABLE II-12. State by State Medicaid Payments, FY 1975, FY 1985 and FY 1991--Continued
($ in millions)

State	FY 1975 payments	Share of total	FY 1985 payments	Share of total	FY 1991 payments	Share of total	Average annual rate of change: FYs 1975-1985	FYs 1985-1991
Massachusetts	$ 494	4.0%	$1,433	3.8%	$ 2,828	3.7%	10.9%	12.0%
Michigan	621	5.1	1,517	4.0	2,540	3.3	9.1	9.0
Minnesota	251	2.1	1,001	2.7	1,561	2.0	14.4	7.7
Mississippi	95	0.8	274	0.7	755	1.0	10.9	18.4
Missouri	99	0.8	525	1.4	1,118	1.5	17.7	13.4
Montana	29	0.2	96	0.3	193	0.3	12.4	12.5
Nebraska	54	0.4	167	0.4	390	0.5	11.6	15.2
Nevada	16	0.1	66	0.2	178	0.2	14.8	18.1
New Hampshire	28	0.2	118	0.3	292	0.4	15.1	16.3
New Jersey	366	3.0	1,145	3.1	2,725	3.5	11.8	15.5
New Mexico	29	0.2	148	0.4	342	0.4	17.2	15.0
New York	2,955	24.1	7,588	20.2	13,728	17.8	9.6	10.4
North Carolina	163	1.3	647	1.7	1,788	2.3	14.4	18.5
North Dakota	23	0.2	117	0.3	227	0.3	17.2	11.7
Ohio	350	2.9	1,767	4.7	3,653	4.7	17.1	12.9
Oklahoma	141	1.2	460	1.2	814	1.1	12.2	10.0
Oregon	74	0.6	239	0.6	667	0.9	12.1	18.7
Pennsylvania	709	5.8	1,797	4.8	3,436	4.5	9.5	11.4
Rhode Island	72	0.6	250	0.7	657	0.9	12.9	17.5
South Carolina	76	0.6	309	0.8	910	1.2	14.7	19.7

TABLE II-12. State by State Medicaid Payments, FY 1975, FY 1985 and FY 1991--Continued
($ in millions)

State	FY 1975 payments	Share of total	FY 1985 payments	Share of total	FY 1991 payments	Share of total	Average annual rate of change: FYs 1975-1985	FYs 1985-1991
South Dakota	$ 22	0.2%	$ 94	0.3%	$ 196	0.3%	15.2%	13.0%
Tennessee	123	1.0	578	1.5	1,485	1.9	16.3	17.0
Texas	461	3.8	1,414	3.8	3,532	4.6	11.6	16.5
Utah	31	0.3	110	0.3	311	0.4	13.2	19.0
Vermont	31	0.3	89	0.2	197	0.3	10.8	14.0
Virginia	160	1.3	547	1.5	1,218	1.6	12.7	14.3
Washington	176	1.4	584	1.6	1,131	1.5	12.4	11.7
West Virginia	29	0.2	173	0.5	542	0.7	19.0	21.0
Wisconsin	361	2.9	942	2.5	1,471	1.9	9.8	7.7
Wyoming	5	0.0	28	0.1	90	0.1	18.3	21.4
Puerto Rico	113	0.9	139	0.4	146	0.2	2.0	0.8
Virgin Islands	2	0.0	4	0.0	4	0.0	7.0	0.3
49 reporting States and District of Col.	$12,127		$37,364		$76,814		11.6%	12.8%
Reporting States and territories	$12,242		$37,508		$76,964		11.5%	12.7%

NOTE: All spending amounts are in millions. Spending represents spending by reporting states for medical vendor payments and excludes any administrative spending. The Federal fiscal year began on July 1 in 1975. Beginning with FY 1976 the fiscal year began on Oct. 1. The 10- and 5-year time intervals chosen for the average annual rate of change calculations are somewhat arbitrary and some of the trends shown may be affected by the years picked in computing these averages.
Source: Table prepared by the Congressional Research Service based on data contained on HCFA Form 2082.

FIGURE II-10. Average Annual Rate of Growth in Total Medicaid Vendor Payments, by State FY 1975-FY 1991

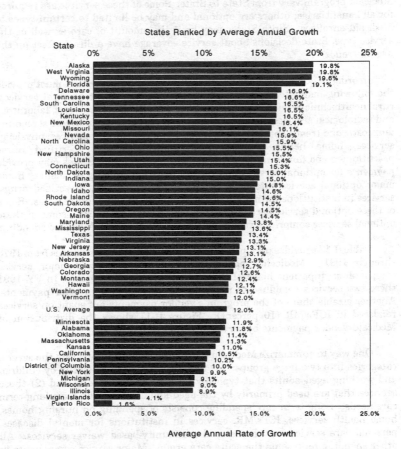

States Ranked by Average Annual Growth

Average Annual Rate of Growth

Source: Figure prepared by Congressional Research Service based on HCFA Form 2082 data.

III. PAYMENTS AND BENEFICIARIES BY SERVICE CATEGORY

A. Payments

As noted in *Chapter IV, Services*, the types of services provided in the Medicaid program vary from State to State. Some of these services are required for all beneficiaries; others are optional and may be limited to certain types of Medicaid enrollees. Since States may limit the amount of care as well as the service type, State decisions about service coverage have a direct effect on the overall trends.

In order to qualify for Federal funds, State Medicaid programs must provide the following mandated services: inpatient and outpatient hospital services, rural health clinic services, federally qualified health center services, laboratory and radiological services, nursing facility services, early and periodic screening, diagnostic and treatment (EPSDT) services, family planning services, physician services, home health services, nurse-midwife services, certified nurse practitioners and family nurse practitioners.[29] In addition, States may provide payments for optional services and receive Federal matching payments. Some major optional service categories include: dental services, prescribed drugs, services in institutions for mental diseases, ICFs/MR, and clinic services. Some of these optional services are offered by every State. As a result, some of these optional services comprise a relatively large share of overall Medicaid spending.

Table II-13 provides total payments for selected service categories from 1975 through 1991. Medicaid's spending is dominated by two major service components: inpatient hospital services and nursing home care. In FY 1991 these two services combined to represent 55 percent of all vendor payments. Another sizable share of the program's vendor payments are spent on services rendered in ICFs/MR (10 percent). Figure II-11 shows the distribution of Medicaid vendor payments by service category in FY 1991.

One way to summarize Medicaid's spending trend is to separate the service categories into two large groups: (1) those services used primarily by children and working aged adults that typically meet acute care needs; and (2) those services that are used primarily by the aged and disabled who have long-term care needs. Long-term care spending consists of spending on nursing homes, home health services, ICFs/MR, services in institutions for mental diseases, personal care services and home- and community-based waiver services. All other spending represents the acute care group. Major service components in this group include: inpatient and outpatient hospital services, physician

---

[29]*Chapter IV, Services* provides definitions for these and the optional services provided by Medicaid.

services, and prescription drugs.[30] Dividing service spending into these two components highlights a number of aspects of service spending.

---

[30]This division of the service categories into two groups does have some limitations. For instance, a large share of prescription drug spending is used by the aged and disabled, groups that account for almost all of long-term care spending.

TABLE II-13. Medicaid Payments by Selected Service Categories, Fiscal Years 1975 to 1991
($ in millions)

Year	Nurs. home care	Inpat. hosp. serv.	Phys. serv.	Prescrib. drugs	Other serv.	ICF/ MR	Outpat. hosp. serv.	Dental serv.	Other practitioner	Lab & x-ray	Home health serv.	Total
1975	$4,319	$3,779	$1,225	$815	$689	$380	$373	$339	$127	$126	$70	$12,24
1976	4,684	4,434	1,369	940	674	634	555	373	147	147	134	14,091
1977	5,328	5,148	1,505	1,018	505	917	877	427	157	177	180	16,239
1978	6,229	5,658	1,554	1,082	516	1,192	835	392	144	180	210	17,992
1979	7,153	6,433	1,635	1,196	678	1,488	847	430	163	186	263	20,472
1980	7,887	7,187	1,875	1,318	841	1,989	1,101	462	198	121	332	23,311
1981	8,542	8,071	2,101	1,535	1,204	2,996	1,409	543	228	147	428	27,204
1982	9,406	8,644	2,086	1,599	1,386	3,467	1,438	492	226	160	496	29,399
1983	10,002	9,746	2,175	1,771	1,571	4,079	1,574	467	226	184	597	32,391
1984	10,633	9,890	2,220	1,968	1,596	4,256	1,646	469	232	207	774	33,891
1985	11,598	10,645	2,346	2,315	1,929	4,719	1,789	458	251	337	1,120	37,508
1986	12,436	11,481	2,548	2,692	2,246	5,081	1,983	532	252	424	1,352	41,027
1987	13,247	12,711	2,776	2,988	2,541	5,591	2,226	541	263	475	1,690	45,050
1988	14,276	13,452	2,953	3,294	2,880	6,022	2,413	577	284	543	2,015	48,710
1989	15,531	14,848	3,408	3,689	3,561	6,649	2,837	498	317	590	2,572	54,500
1990	17,693	18,388	4,018	4,420	4,571	7,354	3,324	593	372	721	3,404	64,859
1991	20,699	21,861	4,946	5,424	5,930	7,680	4,280	709	437	896	4,101	76,964

This division of the service categories into two groups does have some limitations. For instance, a large share of prescription drugs are used by the aged and disabled people that account for almost all of long-term spending.

TABLE II-13. Medicaid Payments by Selected Service Categories, Fiscal Years 1975 to 1991--Continued
($ in millions)

Year	Nurs. home care	Inpat. hosp. serv.	Phys. serv.	Prescrib. drugs	Other serv.	ICF/MR	Outpat. hosp. serv.	Dental serv.	Other practitioner	Lab & x-ray	Home health serv.	Total
					Average annual rates of change (in %):							
1975 to 1980	12.2	13.0	8.4	9.6	3.9	37.1	22.9	6.1	8.8	-0.8	34.5	13.1
1980 to 1985	8.0	8.2	4.6	11.9	18.1	18.9	10.2	-0.2	4.9	22.7	27.5	10.0
1985 to 1991	10.1	12.7	13.2	15.2	20.6	8.5	15.6	7.6	9.7	17.7	24.1	12.7
1975 to 1991	10.1	11.4	9.0	12.4	14.2	20.3	16.2	4.6	7.9	12.8	28.5	12.0

NOTE: All spending amounts are in millions. Spending represents spending by reporting States for medical vendor payments and excludes any administrative spending. Spending information represents medical vendor payments for 49 reporting States, the District of Columbia, Puerto Rico and the Virgin Islands. The Federal fiscal year began on July 1 until FY 1976 when the beginning of the fiscal year was moved to Oct. 1.

Source: Table prepared by the Congressional Research Service based on data contained on HCFA Form 2082.

FIGURE II-11.
Service Payments as a Share of Total Payments, FY 1991

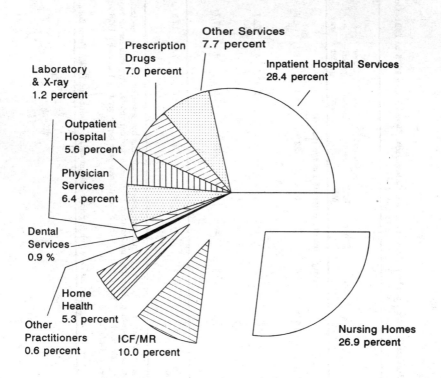

Total Spending = $77.0 Billion

Source: Figure prepared by Congressional Research Service based on HCFA Form 2082 data.

First, over the last 16 years aggregate Medicaid payments for acute care spending have always been larger than spending on long-term care services. However, the rate of growth for long-term care services between 1975 and 1988 was greater than that of acute care services. In 1975 long-term care spending was 73 percent of that for acute care spending. By 1988, long-term care spending had risen to 95 percent of that for acute care. However, since 1988 the rate of growth in acute care service spending has accelerated. By 1991, long-term care spending dropped to 81 percent of the acute care total.

Figure II-12 portrays the pattern in these two spending categories. The top half of the figure highlights the relative size of the two spending categories, while the bottom half of the figure depicts the annual rates of growth. This bottom segment of the figure highlights the changes in the 16-year trend in these two service categories. Generally, between 1976 and 1985, long-term care services experienced annual growth rates that exceeded the annual rate of growth in acute care services. However, since 1985 this trend has been reversed. The rate of growth for acute care services has been greater than that for long-term care. In addition, the bottom figure shows increasing rates of growth in both service areas since 1988.

TABLE II-14. Medicaid Payments for Acute Care and
Long-Term Care Services, Fiscal Years 1975 to 1991
($ in millions)

Year	Acute care spending	Annual change	Long-term care spending	Annual change	Total	Annual change
1975	$ 7,068	--	$ 5,174	--	$12,242	--
1976	8,109	14.7%	5,982	15.6%	14,091	15.1%
1977	9,228	13.8	7,010	17.2	16,239	15.2
1978	9,696	5.1	8,297	18.4	17,992	10.8
1979	10,790	11.3	9,682	16.7	20,472	13.8
1980	12,327	14.2	10,983	13.4	23,311	13.9
1981	14,361	16.5	12,843	16.9	27,204	16.7
1982	15,057	4.8	14,343	11.7	29,399	8.1
1983	16,781	11.4	15,610	8.8	32,391	10.2
1984	17,186	2.4	16,705	7.0	33,891	4.6
1985	18,878	9.8	18,629	11.5	37,508	10.7
1986	21,047	11.5	19,981	7.3	41,027	9.4
1987	23,113	9.8	21,937	9.8	45,050	9.8
1988	25,021	8.3	23,689	8.0	48,710	8.1
1989	28,277	13.0	26,222	10.7	54,500	11.9
1990	34,694	22.7	30,165	15.0	64,859	19.0
1991	42,475	22.4	34,490	14.3	76,964	18.7

Average annual rate of change:

1975-1980		11.2%		15.4%		13.1%
1980-1985		8.9		11.1		10.0
1985-1991		14.5		10.8		12.7
1975-1991		11.7		12.4		12.0

NOTE: Long-term care spending represents spending for all nursing home services, spending in institutions for mental diseases, home health services including personal care services and waiver spending, and payments for ICFs/MR. Acute care spending represents all other payments. Payments represent spending for the 49 reporting States, the District of Columbia, Puerto Rico and the Virgin Islands. The Federal fiscal year began on July 1 until FY 1976 when the beginning of the fiscal year was moved to Oct. 1. The 5-year time intervals chosen for the average annual rate of change calculations are somewhat arbitrary and some of the trends shown may be affected by the years picked in computing these averages.

Source: Table prepared by the Congressional Research Service based on data contained on HCFA Form 2082.

139

FIGURE II-12.
Medicaid Acute Care and Long-Term Care Spending,
FY 1975-FY 1991

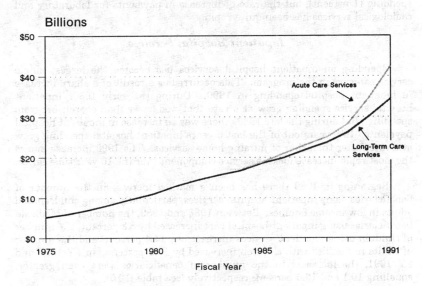

Annual Rate of Change for
Medicaid Acute Care and Long-Term Care Spending,
FY 1975-FY 1991

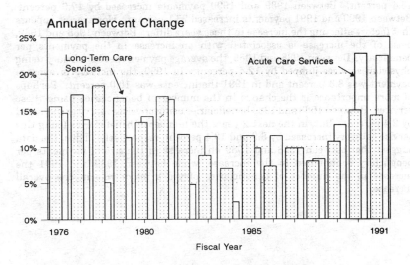

Source: Figure prepared by Congressional Research Service based on data from HCFA.

1. Selected Acute Care Services

Acute care spending is dominated by inpatient hospital spending, physician spending, prescription drug spending, and outpatient hospital services. Laboratory and radiological services represent a small share of program spending (1 percent), but the rate of increase in payments for laboratory and radiological services has been quite rapid.

a. Inpatient Hospital Services

Spending on inpatient hospital services has become the largest single service category in the program. This occurred as a result of a sharp increase in inpatient hospital spending in 1990. During the early 1980s inpatient hospital service spending grew at a rate that was lower than overall program spending. But during the late 1980s there was an increase in inpatient hospital payments. In 5 years out of the last 6 years inpatient hospital spending grew at a rate faster than that of nursing home services. The 1990 increase marks the most rapid increase for this service component over the 16-year time series.

Beginning in 1989 there has been a marked increase in the number of beneficiaries using inpatient hospital services, particularly among children and adults in low-income families. Between 1988 and 1989, the number of Medicaid beneficiaries using inpatient hospital care increased by 8.8 percent; the number of children using inpatient services increased by 14.4 percent; and the number of adults in families with children increased by 13.5 percent. In FY 1990 and FY 1991, the increases in the number of beneficiaries were even greater, equalling 10.1 and 10.6 percent, respectively (see table II-15).

b. Physician Services

Payments for physician services experienced a sharp increase beginning in 1989. Between 1988 and 1989, payments in this service category increased by 15.4 percent. Between 1989 and 1990 payments increased by 17.9 percent. Between 1990 and 1991 payments increased 23.1 percent. However, it appears that factors affecting the increase in these years differ. Between 1988 and 1989, most of the increase is associated with an increase in the payments per beneficiary. Between 1988 and 1989, the average payment per beneficiary using physician services jumped by 12.4 percent. In 1990, the increase in average payment was 8.3 percent and in 1991 the increase was 10.0 percent. Perhaps of more importance is the change in the number of beneficiaries using these services. Between 1988 and 1989 beneficiaries using physician services increased by 2.4 percent. But, in the next 2 years the number of beneficiaries using this service category increased by 8.9 and 13.4 percent, respectively. Thus, the data suggest that between 1988 and 1989 an increase in the size of payments per beneficiary contributed to the increase, while between 1989 and 1991 the increase in the number of beneficiaries played a major role in the overall increase.

c. Outpatient Hospital Services

Over the last 16 years, payments for outpatient hospital services have grown faster than any other acute care service, 16.2 percent. This rapid spending increase is largely a result of very rapid spending increases between 1975 and 1981. Throughout much of the 1980s the rate of growth in outpatient payments moderated. However, as with inpatient services and physician services, 1989 represents the beginning year of a series of marked spending increases. Between 1988 and 1989 outpatient hospital payments increased by 17.6 percent; between 1989 and 1990 payments increased by 17.2 percent; and between 1990 and 1991 payments increased by 28.8 percent. This increase coincides with relatively large increases in the number of beneficiaries using outpatient hospital services. The number of outpatient users increased by 7.7 percent between 1988 and 1989, by 9 percent between 1989 and 1990 and by more than 13 percent between 1990 and 1991.

d. Prescription Drugs

There has been much attention focused on prescription drug payments. OBRA 90 altered the method of reimbursement incorporating a rebate system for State programs.[31] In the fall of 1991 additional changes to Medicaid's prescription drug reimbursements also were made. Between 1975 and 1991, prescription drug spending increased 12.4 percent per annum. Since 1983 this service category has been growing faster than overall Medicaid spending. As with inpatient hospital services and physician services, many more children and adults have prescription drugs paid for by Medicaid than the aged; however, the average Medicaid prescription drug payment per aged and disabled beneficiary is so much greater than for these other groups that aggregate payments for the aged and disabled represent close to three out of every four Medicaid prescription drug dollars.

e. Laboratory and Radiological Services

While prescription drug payments have been the focus of recent reimbursement legislation, laboratory and radiological service payments actually grew at a faster rate in 7 out of the last 8 years. In fact, laboratory and radiological services grew at an average annual rate of 12.8 percent between 1975 and 1991 as compared to a 12.4 percent rate for prescription drugs.

2. Long-Term Care Services

For purposes of this discussion, Medicaid's long-term care services comprise four service categories: nursing home services, institutional services for the mentally retarded (referred to as ICFs/MR), services in institutions for mental diseases and home health care services.[32] The first three categories are

---

[31]See *Chapter V, Reimbursement* for a full description of these provisions.

[32]This last category includes spending on home- and community-based waivers, and personal services.

Medicaid's institutional long-term care spending. The last category represents spending provided by the program for individuals with chronic impairments who remain in the community. Unlike the acute care categories, aged and disabled beneficiaries represent a sizable majority of beneficiaries using these service categories.

a. Nursing Home Services

Until FY 1990 nursing home services represented the largest single service category. While nursing home spending is no longer the largest service category, it still represents more than 27 percent of total service payments. Between 1975 and 1991 nursing home services grew at an average annual rate of 10.1 percent. Between 1990 and 1991 nursing home spending increased by 17.0 percent, an annual rate that is substantially higher than the rates of increase in the mid- to late 1980s. The average annual rate of change between 1985 and 1991 equalled 10.1 percent. This sudden jump in nursing home spending is largely a result of an increase in average payments per beneficiary. The combined number of beneficiaries using skilled nursing services and intermediate care services increased by 38 thousand between 1989 and 1991.[33] OBRA 87 required States to increase Medicaid nursing home rates to reflect costs incurred by nursing facilities in meeting requirements to assure quality nursing home care for Medicaid beneficiaries.[34] These reimbursement requirements are effective beginning in FY 1991 and are likely to affect nursing home payment amounts in the future.

b. Intermediate Care Facilities for the Mentally Retarded

Spending on services in intermediate care facilities for the mentally retarded (ICFs/MR) equalled 10 percent of service payments. This service category is one of the fastest growing categories over the 16-year period. The category grew by 20.3 percent per annum between 1975 and 1991. However, much of this growth occurred in the late 1970s and very early 1980s. Over the last 6 years the ICF/MR rate of growth equalled 8.5 percent, an annual rate that is lower than the overall program's growth rate for this period.

The growth of ICF/MR payments in the early period is the result of an increase in the number of beneficiaries of these services and the average payment per beneficiary. Between 1975 and 1981 increases in ICF/MR beneficiaries were a consequence of the certification of existing State

---

[33]Strictly speaking combining beneficiary counts for the two types of nursing home services, intermediate care facilities and skilled nursing facilities, is inappropriate. This is the case because the same individual may use both services sometime during the year, and therefore be counted more than once. Medicaid law no longer makes a distinction between these two types of nursing facilities. However, in 1990 States still provided HCFA information on the statistical reporting form distinguishing between these two categories.

[34]See *Chapter IX, Recent Legislative History* and *Appendix C, Medicaid, Long-Term Care, and the Elderly* for a full description of these changes.

institutions. Between 1975 and 1981, the number of ICF/MR beneficiaries more than doubled, increasing from about 69,000 to 151,000. Since the early 1980s the number of ICF/MR beneficiaries has hovered between 145 and 150 thousand. However, ICF/MR payments per beneficiary did not level off in the early 1980s. Between 1975 and 1981, the payment per beneficiary increased from 5,538 to 19,312, a 27.5 annual rate of growth. From 1981 to 1991, payments per beneficiary increased from $19,312 to $52,791. Although still high, this 10.6 percent per annum increase is substantially slower than the earlier periods.

c. Home Health Spending

Of all the service categories discussed in this chapter, home health spending grew the most rapidly over the 16-year period. This service category grew at a 28.5 percent annual rate for the 16 years in table II-13. In 1975 this service category represented less than 1 percent of all program service payments; by 1991 it represented more than 5 percent. Furthermore, the growth has been rapid throughout the entire 16 years.

For this discussion, home health spending includes three separate categories of services: 1) home health services; 2) community based waiver services; and 3) personal care services. Over the 16 years, the number of beneficiaries using these services has increased from 343 thousand to 809 thousand. As highlighted in *Chapter VI, Alternate Delivery Options and Waiver Programs*, spending on Medicaid waivers has grown dramatically since the early 1980s. Much of this spending targets the mentally retarded and developmentally disabled (MR/DD). For example, in 1989 more than 63 percent of waiver spending targeted the MR/DD population.

B. Service Category Contributions to Overall Spending Growth

Since individual service categories have grown at substantially different rates, and represent substantially different amounts of program spending, their impact on Medicaid growth in payments will vary. Figure II-13 shows the effect of the growth in each service category on the increase in the program's payments over the 1975-1991 period.

As expected, most of the growth in program spending can be attributed to the current large spending categories: inpatient hospital care, nursing home, and ICF/MR spending. Growth in these three service groups accounts for 65 percent of the payment increase. Since spending on inpatient hospital services and nursing homes has always contributed a large share to program spending, it is not surprising that these service categories played a major role in the program's spending growth. The relatively rapid increase in ICF/MR spending, prescription drug spending, and home health services resulted in these services contributing a disproportionately larger share than expected based on the program's spending pattern in 1975. More than 55 percent of the 16-year spending growth is attributable to the acute care service categories, with the remaining 45 percent a result of long-term care spending increases.

FIGURE II-13.
Contribution of Individual Service Categories to Overall Medicaid Payment Growth, 1975 to 1991

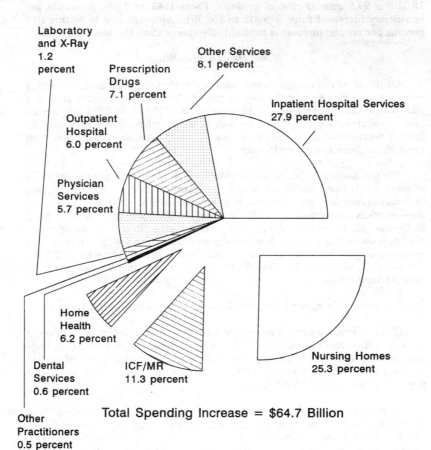

Laboratory and X-Ray 1.2 percent

Prescription Drugs 7.1 percent

Other Services 8.1 percent

Outpatient Hospital 6.0 percent

Inpatient Hospital Services 27.9 percent

Physician Services 5.7 percent

Home Health 6.2 percent

Dental Services 0.6 percent

ICF/MR 11.3 percent

Nursing Homes 25.3 percent

Other Practitioners 0.5 percent

Total Spending Increase = $64.7 Billion

Source: Figure prepared by Congressional Research Service based on HCFA Form 2082 data.

C. Beneficiaries by Service Category

More Medicaid beneficiaries use physician services and prescription drugs than any other service categories (see table II-15). More than 19 million beneficiaries used each of these service categories in 1991. In terms of beneficiary use, the third largest service category was outpatient hospital services. The two largest spending categories, inpatient hospital services and nursing home care, represent a relatively small share of total beneficiaries. About 5.0 million beneficiaries used inpatient hospital care, while 1.5 million beneficiaries used nursing home services.

The rate of increase in beneficiary use for many service categories differs from Medicaid's overall beneficiary trend. The four service categories that have experienced the fastest beneficiary growth rate over the 16-year period are: ICF/MR services; outpatient hospital services; laboratory and radiological services; and home health services. However, the pattern of beneficiary growth for each of these service categories differs. As noted earlier, all of the ICF/MR beneficiary growth occurred between 1975 and 1981. In fact, since 1983 there has been a decline in the number of Medicaid beneficiaries using ICF/MR services. Part of this decline is probably attributable to the "deinstitutionalization" of the developmentally disabled.[35] Home health service beneficiary growth has been relatively rapid over the entire 16-year period, but the number of beneficiaries using these services has increased most rapidly over the last 3 years.

Outpatient hospital services (along with inpatient hospital services and physician service beneficiary trends) experienced modest increases in the mid-1980s, but substantial increases in the number of beneficiaries over the last few years. Since 1988 the number of Medicaid beneficiaries using outpatient services increased by 33 percent.[36] The laboratory and radiological service pattern experienced a dramatic decline in the number of users between 1979 and 1980, followed by a large rate of increase between 1980 and 1985, and a 23 percent increase between 1988 and 1991 coinciding with the recent increases in outpatient hospital services, inpatient hospital services, and physician services.[37]

---

[35]See *Appendix D, Medicaid Services for Persons with Developmental Disabilities* for a complete discussion of this beneficiary trend.

[36] The number of beneficiaries using inpatient hospital services increased by 32 percent, and the number of Medicaid physician service beneficiaries increased by 25 percent over this same time period.

[37]Since this trend data is based on bills paid by Medicaid in any fiscal year, this pattern of large increases in physician services, inpatient and outpatient hospital services, and laboratory and radiological services probably reflects Medicaid's payment of these different services for the same beneficiaries.

TABLE II-15. Medicaid Beneficiaries by Selected Service Categories, Fiscal Years 1975 to 1991
(beneficiaries in thousands)

Year	Nursing home care[a]	Inpatient hospital services	Physician services	Prescribed drugs	ICF/MR	Outpatient hospital services	Dental services	Other practitioner	Lab and x-ray	Home health services	Total
1975	1,312	3,432	15,198	14,155	69	7,437	3,944	2,673	4,738	343	22,007
1976	1,361	3,551	15,624	14,883	89	8,482	4,405	2,848	5,239	319	22,815
1977	1,395	3,768	16,074	15,370	107	8,619	4,656	2,963	5,494	317	22,832
1978	1,379	3,782	15,668	15,188	104	8,628	4,485	3,082	5,684	376	21,965
1979	1,376	3,608	15,168	14,283	114	7,710	4,401	3,011	5,332	359	21,520
1980	1,395	3,680	13,765	13,707	121	9,705	4,652	3,234	3,212	392	21,605
1981	1,372	3,703	14,403	14,256	151	10,018	5,173	3,582	3,822	402	21,980
1982	1,324	3,530	13,894	13,547	149	9,853	4,868	3,223	3,814	377	21,603
1983	1,367	3,696	14,056	13,732	151	10,069	4,940	3,306	4,462	422	21,554
1984	1,355	3,467	14,195	13,935	141	10,035	4,942	3,353	4,822	438	21,607
1985	1,375	3,434	14,387	13,921	147	10,072	4,634	3,357	6,354	535	21,814
1986	1,399	3,544	14,894	14,704	145	10,702	5,162	3,451	7,122	593	22,515
1987	1,421	3,767	15,373	15,083	149	10,979	5,131	3,542	7,596	609	23,109
1988	1,445	3,832	15,265	15,323	145	10,533	5,071	3,480	7,579	569	22,907
1989	1,452	4,170	15,686	15,916	148	11,344	4,214	3,555	7,759	609	23,511
1990	1,461	4,593	17,078	17,294	147	12,370	4,552	3,873	8,959	719	25,255
1991	1,490	5,079	19,119	19,581	145	14,031	5,177	4,271	10,388	809	27,967

See notes at end of table.

TABLE II-15. Medicaid Beneficiaries by Selected Service Categories, Fiscal Years 1975 to 1991–Continued

Year	Nursing home care[a]	Inpatient hospital services	Physician services	Prescribed drugs	ICF/MR	Outpatient hospital services	Dental services	Other practitioner	Lab and x-ray	Home health services	Total
					Average annual rates of change:						
1975 to 1980	1.2%	1.3%	-1.9%	-0.6%	11.3%	5.2%	3.2%	3.7%	-7.1%	2.6%	-0.4%
1980 to 1985	-0.3	-1.4	0.9	0.3	4.0	0.7	-0.1	0.7	14.6	6.4	0.2
1985 to 1991	1.3	6.7	4.9	5.9	-0.2	5.7	1.9	4.1	8.5	7.1	4.2
1975 to 1991	0.8	2.4	1.4	2.0	4.7	4.0	1.7	2.9	4.9	5.4	1.5

[a]Includes all beneficiaries of either intermediate care facility or skilled nursing facility services. Some individuals may transfer from one facility to another. This results in some duplicative counts for this service category. No adjustment has been made.

NOTE: Information represents beneficiaries receiving services in 49 States, the District of Columbia, Puerto Rico and the Virgin Islands. The Federal fiscal year began on July 1 until FY 1976 when the beginning of the fiscal year was moved to Oct. 1. The 5-year time intervals chosen for the average annual rate of change calculations are somewhat arbitrary and some of the trends shown may be affected by the years picked in computing these averages.

Source: Table prepared by the Congressional Research Service based on data contained on HCFA Form 2082.

IV. THE TREND IN PAYMENTS AND BENEFICIARIES BY ELIGIBILITY AND CASH ASSISTANCE STATUS

Eligibility rules and service coverage for Medicaid vary from State to State. Furthermore from State to State, individuals in similar eligibility categories face different income eligibility levels and may use different covered services. While States must cover individuals eligible for AFDC, and most States cover disabled, blind, and aged recipients of SSI, the income eligibility levels for these individuals will vary from State to State (see *Chapter III, Eligibility* and *Appendix A, Medicaid, the Poor, and Health Insurance*). The recent congressionally mandated expansions have uncoupled Medicaid from these cash assistance programs. Low-income children and pregnant women now face mandated eligibility thresholds that are separate than those used for the cash assistance programs. However, States still have options to cover additional categories of persons. These optional categories include the medically needy, and pregnant women and children who have incomes somewhat above mandated eligibility levels.[38]

Trends in Medicaid payments and beneficiaries can be summarized by classifying beneficiaries either by an individual's eligibility status: the aged, the disabled and blind, low-income children, and their caretaker adults; or based on receipt of cash welfare payments: either receiving AFDC or SSI payments, those who qualify for the program because they are medically needy (i.e., they incur substantial out of pocket medical expenses), and those who qualify because they either meet a State's criteria for beneficiaries who do not receive cash assistance or are poor or near-poor pregnant women or young children, aged or disabled. The remaining sections of this chapter look at the spending and beneficiary trends using these two frameworks.[39]

A. Payments and Beneficiaries by Receipt of Cash Assistance

The share of Medicaid payments spent on individuals who are automatically eligible for the program because of receipt of cash assistance has declined since 1975. Table II-16 divides total payments into three categories: (1) payments made on behalf of those who are eligible for Medicaid because of receipt of SSI or AFDC; (2) payments made on behalf of those who are medically needy; and (3) payments made on behalf of those who meet categorical eligibility requirements but do not receive cash assistance payments. Payments for individuals who fall into the optional and mandatory eligibility expansion categories of the late 1980s are found in this last category.

---

[38]States are required to provide coverage to pregnant women and children under age 6 up to 133 percent of poverty. States may opt to cover pregnant women and infants (children under age 1) up to 185 percent of poverty. As detailed in *Chapter III, Eligibility*, there are many additional optional eligibility categories that States may use in determining Medicaid eligibility.

[39]Complete definitions for the type of beneficiaries falling into each of these categories can be found in *Chapter X, Medicaid Payment and Beneficiary Information, Fiscal Year 1991*.

TABLE II-16. Payments by Receipt of Cash Assistance,
Fiscal Years 1975 to 1991
($ in millions)

Year	Beneficiaries receiving cash assistance	Beneficiaries who are medically needy	Beneficiaries not receiving cash assistance	Total
1975	$ 7,188	$ 3,301	$ 1,753	$12,242
1976	8,154	3,848	2,088	14,091
1977	9,577	4,198	2,465	16,239
1978	10,160	4,731	3,101	17,992
1979	11,281	5,334	3,857	20,472
1980	12,344	7,188	3,779	23,311
1981	14,534	7,935	4,736	27,204
1982	15,862	8,127	5,410	29,399
1983	17,112	8,870	6,409	32,391
1984	17,564	9,294	7,033	33,891
1985	19,316	10,359	7,832	37,508
1986	21,039	11,235	8,753	41,027
1987[a]	23,173	12,137	9,723	45,050
1988[a]	24,584	13,068	11,005	48,710
1989[a]	26,927	13,833	13,610	54,500
1990[a]	30,961	14,711	18,981	64,859
1991[a]	35,281	16,141	25,322	76,964

Average annual rate of change:

1975-80	10.8%	16.0%	15.8%	13.1%
1980-85	9.4	7.6	15.7	10.0
1985-91	10.6	7.7	21.6	12.7
1990-91	14.0	9.7	33.4	18.7
1975-91	10.3	10.3	17.9	12.0

[a]Beginning in 1987 total payment estimates include some individuals with unknown cash assistance payment status. In 1987 payments for these beneficiaries equalled $17 million; in 1988 this amount increased to $53 million; in 1989--$130 million; in 1990--$206 million; and in 1991--$220 million.

NOTE: All payment amounts are in millions. Amounts represent spending for 49 reporting States, the District of Columbia, Puerto Rico and the Virgin Islands.

Source: Table prepared by the Congressional Research Service based on data provided by the Health Care Financing Administration.

In 1975, 59 percent of all Medicaid payments were for services rendered to beneficiaries with cash assistance payments. By 1982, this share equalled 54 percent. By 1988, it equalled 50 percent, and in 1991, it equalled 46 percent (see figure II-14). This payment trend is reflective of the trend in beneficiaries. In 1975, almost 76 percent of all Medicaid beneficiaries became eligible for the program as a result of the receipt of SSI or AFDC. In 1981, this group continued to represent about 76 percent of all beneficiaries. But, beginning in 1985, the share of Medicaid beneficiaries who receive cash assistance payments began to decline. The recent eligibility expansions have further reduced this group's share of the total. In 1991, about 61 percent of all Medicaid beneficiaries also received SSI or AFDC. Table II-17 provides trend information for these eligibility groups.

Perhaps the one group of beneficiaries that has had the greatest effect on the cash assistance group's beneficiary and payment trend is the aged. There have been declines in the number of aged cash assistance beneficiaries. Since 1986 the number of aged beneficiaries with cash assistance payments has declined by 11 percent. Declines in the number of aged cash assistance beneficiaries have a large impact on the cash assistance share of overall Medicaid spending because on a per beneficiary basis these individuals are very costly. For instance, in 1991, the payment per aged cash assistance beneficiary ($3,472) was 4.3 times as great as that for children who are in families with cash assistance payments ($814).

The decline in the share of payments for beneficiaries with cash assistance was not offset by increases in the share of payments for the medically needy. The share of Medicaid payments dedicated to individuals who are medically needy peaked in 1980, at 31 percent. By 1982 medically needy payments represented about 27 percent of total payments, and continued at this level until 1988. Between 1988 and 1991 medically needy payments as a share of the total declined, reaching 21 percent in 1991.

The category with a rapidly growing share of Medicaid payments is categorically needy beneficiaries not receiving cash assistance payments. In 1975, payments for these beneficiaries equalled 14 percent of the total increasing to 21 percent by 1984. By 1991, spending on beneficiaries without cash assistance payments increased to 33 percent of the total.

The payment trend for beneficiaries not receiving cash assistance payments occurred across all eligibility categories (i.e., for the aged, disabled and children). The number of disabled persons on the Medicaid rolls who do not also receive cash assistance payments has been increasing. For example, in 1986, 353 thousand people were in this category, and by 1991, 661 thousand were in this category.[40] The number of low-income children who are eligible for Medicaid without the receipt of cash assistance payments has increased consistently over the course of the last 16 years. Between 1975 and 1981, these beneficiaries

---

[40] 1990 figures include those eligible for Medicaid as a result of eligibility expansions in the late 1980s. Almost 31 percent of the 1990 beneficiary count are eligible as a result of these eligibility expansions.

FIGURE II-14.
Medicaid Payments by Receipt of Cash Assistance Payments, FY 1975-FY 1991

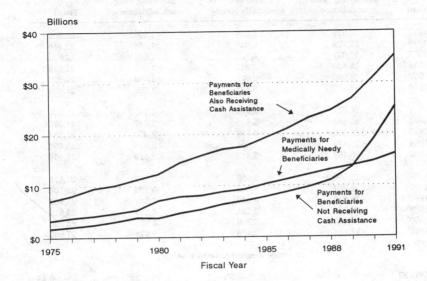

Billions

Payments for Beneficiaries Also Receiving Cash Assistance

Payments for Medically Needy Beneficiaries

Payments for Beneficiaries Not Receiving Cash Assistance

Fiscal Year

Medicaid Payments by Receipt of Cash Assistance Payments as a Share of Total Payments, FY 1975-FY 1991

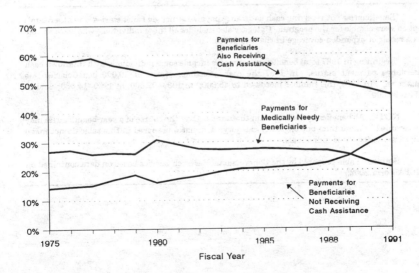

Payments for Beneficiaries Also Receiving Cash Assistance

Payments for Medically Needy Beneficiaries

Payments for Beneficiaries Not Receiving Cash Assistance

Fiscal Year

Source: Figure prepared by Congressional Research Service based on data from HCFA.

TABLE II-17. Beneficiaries by Receipt of Cash Assistance,
Fiscal Years 1975 to 1991
(beneficiaries in thousands)

Year	Beneficiaries receiving cash assistance	Beneficiaries who are medically needy	Beneficiaries not receiving cash assistance[a]	Total
1975	16,678	3,939	1,390	22,007
1976	17,222	4,028	1,564	22,815
1977	17,067	4,124	1,641	22,832
1978	16,423	3,845	1,697	21,965
1979	16,056	3,672	1,793	21,520
1980	16,497	3,832	1,559	21,605
1981	16,872	3,700	1,793	21,980
1982	16,594	3,605	2,037	21,603
1983	16,519	3,582	2,273	21,554
1984	16,478	3,454	2,536	21,607
1985	16,459	3,413	2,610	21,808
1986	16,596	3,656	2,983	22,518
1987[b]	16,787	3,821	3,103	23,109
1988[b]	16,548	3,605	3,305	22,907
1989[b]	16,321	3,431	4,135	23,511
1990[b]	16,468	3,392	5,280	25,255
1991[b]	17,188	3,466	7,217	27,967

Average annual rate of change:

1975-80	-0.2%	-0.5%	2.2%	-0.4%
1980-85	-0.0	-2.3	10.9	0.2
1985-91	0.7	0.3	18.5	4.2
1990-91	4.4	2.2	36.7	10.7
1975-91	0.2	-0.8	10.7	1.5

[a]Beneficiaries not receiving cash assistance payments include beneficiaries who at a State's option were eligible for the program. Category also includes all those individuals who were eligible as a result of expanded coverage in the late 1980s.

[b]Beginning in 1987 total beneficiary estimates include some individuals with unknown cash assistance payment status. In 1987 the cash assistance status of 19,000 beneficiaries was unknown. In 1988, this number increased to 45,000; in 1989--92,000; in 1990--14,000; and in 1991--96,000.

NOTE: All beneficiary counts are in thousands. Over the course of a year beneficiaries may be recorded in more than one eligibility category. Estimates prepared in this table do not make adjustments for these individuals.

Source: Table prepared by the Congressional Research Service based on data contained on HCFA Form 2082.

increased relatively slowly, by about 25 percent. Between 1981 and 1985, the rate of growth began to accelerate, with beneficiaries increasing by 52 percent. However, in the last 6 years, the number increased by 93 percent to 1.4 million beneficiaries in FY 1991. For aged beneficiaries who are eligible for Medicaid without the receipt of cash assistance payments the pattern is somewhat different. Like the other groups, the number of aged beneficiaries not receiving cash assistance payments has shown sudden growth over the last 6 years. Between 1985 and 1991, the number of aged beneficiaries without cash assistance payments increased by 78 percent. But, between 1981 and 1985, the number of beneficiaries in this eligibility category grew by 13 percent.

The shift in who qualifies for the Medicaid program has been recently mollified, somewhat. As noted earlier, AFDC caseloads increased rather rapidly between 1989 and 1991 and this has a direct effect on Medicaid beneficiary estimates. This can be seen in comparing the rate of growth in beneficiaries between 1989 and 1990, and between 1990 and 1991. Between 1989 and 1990, the number of cash assistance beneficiaries increased by less than 1 percent, while the number of beneficiaries without cash assistance payments increased by 27.7 percent. Between 1990 and 1991, the number of beneficiaries with cash assistance increased by 4.4 percent, while the number of beneficiaries without cash assistance increased by 37 percent. The dramatic difference in beneficiary growth between those receiving cash assistance payments and those not receiving cash assistance payments highlights the growing importance of Medicaid beneficiaries who qualify for the program without meeting cash assistance eligibility rules. But the 4.4 percent increase in cash assistance beneficiaries in 1991 marks the largest single year increase in this eligibility group since the early 1970s. The projected beneficiary figures shown earlier include increases in the number of Medicaid beneficiaries receiving cash assistance. However, growth in the number of beneficiaries without cash assistance payments is projected to outpace that of the AFDC and SSI beneficiaries.

B. Payments by Eligibility Status

Payments for the blind and disabled currently account for the largest share of Medicaid payments (37 percent).[41] This eligibility group is closely followed by spending for the aged (33 percent). Much smaller shares of Medicaid payments are dedicated to payments for low-income children and their adult caretakers (15 percent and 14 percent, respectively). Figure II-15 provides information on the share of payments by eligibility status for FY 1991.

Between 1975 and 1988, the growth in total program payments was dominated by rapid increases in spending for the disabled and the aged. Between 1975 and 1988, these eligibility groups accounted for 77 percent of total payment growth. Growth in payments for low-income children and their adult

---

[41]See table II-17.

TABLE II-18. Payments by Beneficiary Eligibility Status, Fiscal Years 1975 to 1991
($ in millions)

Year	Aged	Blind & disabled	Children	Adults	Other	Total
1975	$ 4,358	$ 3,145	$ 2,186	$ 2,062	$ 492	$12,242
1976	4,910	3,920	2,431	2,288	542	14,091
1977	5,499	4,883	2,610	2,606	641	16,239
1978	6,308	5,620	2,748	2,673	643	17,992
1979	7,046	6,882	2,884	3,021	638	20,472
1980	8,739	7,621	3,123	3,231	596	23,311
1981	9,926	9,455	3,508	3,763	552	27,204
1982	10,739	10,405	3,473	4,093	689	29,399
1983	11,954	11,367	3,836	4,487	747	32,391
1984	12,815	11,977	3,979	4,420	700	33,891
1985	14,096	13,452	4,414	4,746	798	37,508
1986	15,100	14,924	5,136	4,877	991	41,027
1987[a]	16,037	16,817	5,508	5,592	1,096	45,050
1988[a]	17,135	18,594	5,848	5,883	1,250	48,710
1989[a]	18,558	20,885	6,892	6,897	1,268	54,500
1990[a]	21,508	24,404	9,100	8,590	1,257	64,859
1991[a]	25,444	28,251	11,600	10,421	1,249	76,964

Average annual rate of change:

1975-80	14.2%	18.4%	7.0%	8.9%	3.7%	13.1%
1980-85	10.0	12.0	7.2	8.0	6.0	10.0
1985-91	10.3	13.2	17.5	14.0	7.8	12.7
1990-91	18.3	15.8	27.5	21.3	-0.6	18.7
1975-91	11.5	14.5	10.8	10.5	5.9	12.0

[a]Beginning in 1987, *other* spending category includes payment amounts for beneficiaries with unknown eligibility status.

NOTE: All payment amounts are in millions. Amounts represent spending for 49 reporting States, the District of Columbia, Puerto Rico and the Virgin Islands. The Federal fiscal year began on July 1 until FY 1976 when the beginning of the fiscal year was moved to Oct. 1. The 5-year time intervals chosen for the average annual rate of change calculations are somewhat arbitrary and some of the trends shown may be affected by the years picked in computing these averages.

Source: Table prepared by the Congressional Research Service based on data contained on HCFA Form 2082.

FIGURE II-15.
Share of Total Medicaid Payments
by Eligibility Status of Beneficiaries, FY 1991

Total Payments = $77.0 Billion

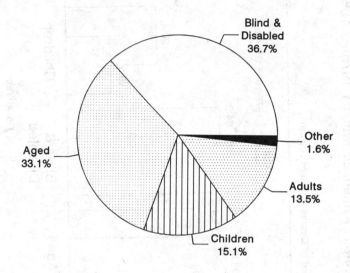

Source: Figure prepared by Congressional Research Service based on data from HCFA.

FIGURE II-16.
Increases in Eligibility Group Payments as a Share of Overall Payment Growth, FY 1975-FY 1988 and FY 1988-FY 1991

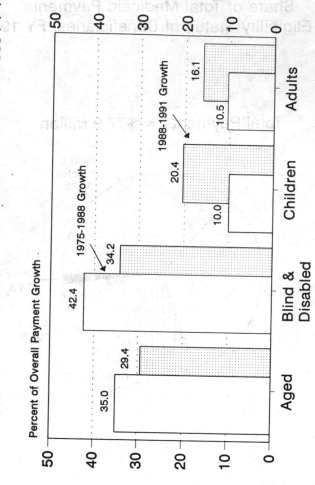

Percent of Overall Payment Growth

1975-1988 Growth

1988-1991 Growth

Aged 35.0 29.4

Blind & Disabled 42.4 34.2

Children 10.0 20.4

Adults 10.5 16.1

Fiscal Year

Source: Figure prepared by Congressional Research Service based on data from HCFA.

caretakers accounted for 20 percent of the growth.[42] However, beginning in 1988 the spending pattern began to change. While growth in payments for the aged and the disabled still dominated payment increases (accounting for 64. percent of the growth between 1988 and 1991), payments for children and adults has rapidly accelerated. Between 1988 and 1991 these two groups contributed 36 percent toward payment growth (see figure II-16).

Historically, ICF/MR payments account for much of the growth in spending on the disabled. Between 1975 and 1984, ICF/MR spending for the disabled accounted for 21 percent of the growth in payments for this eligibility group. Between 1980 and 1985, 48 percent of the growth in payments for the disabled is accounted for by ICF/MR payment growth. However, the importance of ICF/MR payments in explaining payment growth for the disabled has diminished substantially. Between 1985 and 1991, 18 percent of the growth in disabled payments is accounted for by ICF/MR payment growth.

While the rate of increase for ICF/MR spending has slackened, spending on home health services has accelerated. The home health category (which includes spending for personal care services, and home- and community-based waiver) has accounted for 10 percent of the growth in disabled payments between 1985 and 1991. Between 1975 and 1980, this service category accounted for less than 2 percent of the payment growth, and between 1980 and 1985 for less than 6 percent of the growth. This spending trend probably reflects the "deinstitutionalization" of the developmentally disabled from ICF/MR and into community settings.[43]

As will be discussed more thoroughly in *Appendix C, Medicaid, Long-Term Care, and the Elderly*, aged spending is dominated by spending on long-term care services. Historically, payments for nursing facilities have been the major factor behind payment increases in this eligibility category. This trend is consistent throughout the 16-year period. For example, between 1975 and 1980 growth in nursing facility payments for the aged accounted for 68 percent of the total group increase. Between 1989 and 1991 nursing facility payment growth accounted for roughly 67 percent. However, a new development has emerged in this group's spending pattern. As in the case of spending on the disabled, payments for home health services for the aged have grown significantly, and now represent the second largest service spending category for the eligibility group.

Payment for low-income children and adult caretakers is almost exclusively for acute care services. In FY 1991, 46 percent of total payments for children were for inpatient hospital services, outpatient services represented another 11 percent of payments, and physician payments another 13 percent. Payments for caretaker adults present an almost identical distribution, with 47 percent of

---

[42]The remaining 2 percent of growth was made up of spending by all *other* beneficiaries.

[43]See *Appendix D, Medicaid Services for Persons with Developmental Disabilities*.

payments for inpatient hospital services, 12 percent for outpatient hospital services, and 17 percent for physician services. Long-term care payments for low-income children and adult caretakers represent about 1 percent of their respective total payments.[44]

This divergence in the types of services used by each of these categories translates into rather significant differences in payment per beneficiary amounts for each of the eligibility categories. Table II-19 provides payments per beneficiary for 1975 through 1991. As can be seen in the table, on a payment per beneficiary basis, the aged and the disabled received payments that are substantially larger than those for low-income children and adults. In 1975, the payment per aged beneficiary was more than 5 times that of low-income children. By 1989 aged payments were almost 9 times as large. However, in 1990, payments per beneficiary for low-income children and adults increased at a much faster rate than the payments per aged or disabled beneficiary.

C. Beneficiaries by Eligibility Status

Table II-20 provides information on the number of Medicaid beneficiaries by eligibility group. A number of important aspects about the program are highlighted in this table. First, most Medicaid beneficiaries are low-income children and their caretaker adults. Over the last 16 years more than 6 out of 10 beneficiaries have been children or their caretakers. Between 1989 and 1991, the number of beneficiaries in these two categories grew much faster than in any of the others. As has been noted in the previous section, this distribution among beneficiaries is in stark contrast with the distribution of payments. While low-income children represent 46 percent of those receiving Medicaid supported health services, this eligibility group accounted for 15 percent of total payments. Figure II-17 provides the distribution of beneficiaries by eligibility status. This figure can be compared with figure II-15 that provides the distribution of payments for these same eligibility categories.

---

[44]However, it should be noted that this statistic partly stems from the collection of the information on HCFA Form 2082. Children and adults who are eligible for the program because of disability will not be counted in this category. Rather these individuals will be counted in the disabled eligibility group.

TABLE II-19. Payments Per Beneficiary, by Eligibility Group,
Fiscal Years 1975 to 1991
($ in millions)

Year	Aged	Disabled	Children	Adults	Total
1975	$1,205	$1,276	$228	$ 455	$ 556
1976	1,359	1,469	245	479	618
1977	1,512	1,743	270	545	711
1978	1,869	2,068	293	576	819
1979	2,094	2,500	317	661	951
1980	2,540	2,619	335	663	1,079
1981	2,948	3,071	366	725	1,238
1982	3,315	3,600	363	764	1,361
1983	3,545	3,891	402	802	1,503
1984	3,957	4,112	411	789	1,569
1985	4,605	4,459	452	860	1,719
1986	4,808	4,687	512	864	1,821
1987	4,975	4,974	542	999	1,949
1988	5,425	5,332	583	1,069	2,126
1989	5,926	5,817	668	1,206	2,318
1990	6,717	6,564	811	1,429	2,567
1991	7,617	7,005	902	1,555	2,752

Average annual rate of change:

1975-80	15.3%	14.7%	7.6%	7.4%	13.5%
1980-85	12.6	11.2	6.2	5.3	9.8
1985-91	8.7	7.8	12.2	10.4	8.2
1990-91	13.4%	6.7%	11.2%	8.8	7.2
1975-91	12.0	11.0	8.8	7.9	10.3

NOTE: All payment amounts are in millions. Amounts represent spending
for 49 reporting States, the District of Columbia, Puerto Rico, and the Virgin
Islands. The Federal fiscal year began on July 1 until FY 1976 when the
beginning of the fiscal year was moved to Oct. 1. The 5-year time intervals
chosen for the average annual rate of change calculations are somewhat
arbitrary and some of the trends shown may be affected by the years picked in
computing these averages.

Source: Table prepared by the Congressional Research Service based on
data contained on HCFA Form 2082.

TABLE II-20. Medicaid Beneficiaries by Eligibility Status,
Fiscal Years 1975 to 1991
(beneficiaries in thousands)

Year	Aged	Blind & disabled	Children	Adults	Other	Total
1975	3,615	2,464	9,598	4,529	1,800	22,007
1976	3,612	2,669	9,924	4,773	1,836	22,815
1977	3,636	2,802	9,651	4,785	1,959	22,832
1978	3,376	2,718	9,376	4,643	1,852	21,965
1979	3,364	2,753	9,106	4,570	1,727	21,520
1980	3,440	2,911	9,333	4,877	1,500	21,605
1981	3,367	3,079	9,581	5,187	1,364	21,980
1982	3,240	2,891	9,563	5,356	1,434	21,603
1983	3,372	2,921	9,535	5,592	1,129	21,554
1984	3,238	2,913	9,684	5,600	1,187	21,607
1985	3,061	3,017	9,752	5,518	1,214	21,808
1986	3,140	1,382	10,031	5,647	1,366	22,518
1987	3,224	3,381	10,168	5,599	1,418	23,109
1988	3,159	3,487	10,037	5,503	1,388	22,907
1989	3,132	3,590	10,318	5,717	1,175	23,511
1990	3,202	3,718	11,220	6,010	1,105	25,255
1991	3,341	4,033	12,855	6,703	1,035	27,967

Average annual rate of change:

Year	Aged	Blind & disabled	Children	Adults	Other	Total
1975-80	-0.9%	3.2%	-0.5%	1.4%	-3.4%	-0.4%
1980-85	-2.3	0.7	0.9	2.5	-4.1	0.2
1985-91	1.5	5.0	4.7	3.3	-2.6	4.2
1990-91	4.3%	8.5%	14.6%	11.5%	-6.3%	10.7%
1975-91	-0.5	3.1	1.8	2.4	-3.3	1.5

NOTE: Beneficiary counts represent the number of Medicaid beneficiaries for 49 States, the District of Columbia, Puerto Rico, and the Virgin Islands. The Federal fiscal year began on July 1 until FY 1976 when the beginning of the fiscal year was moved to Oct. 1. The 5-year time intervals chosen for the average annul rate of change calculations are somewhat arbitrary and some of the trends shown may be affected by the years picked in computing these averages.

Source: Table prepared by the Congressional Research Service based on data contained on HCFA Form 2082.

FIGURE II-17.
Share of Total Medicaid Beneficiaries
by Eligibility Status of Beneficiaries, FY 1991

Total Beneficiaries = 28.0 Million

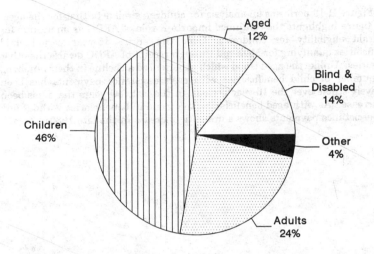

Source: Figure prepared by Congressional Research Service
based on data from HCFA.

A **second** component in the beneficiary trend is that the number of aged beneficiaries has declined from 1975. In 1975, 3.6 million aged beneficiaries received health care services paid for by Medicaid; by 1991 this number had declined to 3.3 million. However, the 1991 aged beneficiary count is the second year with an increase in the aged Medicaid rolls since 1987. It is partly a result of the recent expansion of eligibility to qualified Medicare beneficiaries (QMBs).[45] The long-term trend, however, is influenced by a decline in the number of aged SSI beneficiaries. In 1975 aged beneficiaries who also received SSI payments totalled 2.4 million; in 1984 this number dropped to 1.7 million. However, over the last few years the number of aged Medicaid beneficiaries also receiving SSI has remained around 1.4 million. Figure II-18 portrays the trend in aged beneficiaries.

Figure II-19 performs an analysis for children similar to that for the aged. This figure highlights the continued important role of AFDC as an avenue for Medicaid eligibility for children. Over the entire 16-year period child beneficiaries qualifying for Medicaid through receipt of AFDC dwarfs the other categories. Unlike the aged trend which experienced a decline in their numbers, the number of child beneficiaries with cash assistance payments has been relatively stable over the 16-year period. In the last few years there has been an increase. As with aged beneficiaries, the trend in beneficiaries without any cash assistance payments shows a dramatic increase in the late 1980s.

---

[45]See *Chapter III, Eligibility* for a discussion of QMBs. This discussion is found in the partial coverage section of the chapter. QMBs are poor aged or disabled Medicare beneficiaries on whose behalf Medicaid will pay Medicare's premiums and deductibles.

FIGURE II-18.
Aged Medicaid Beneficiaries by Eligibility Status, FY 1975-FY 1991

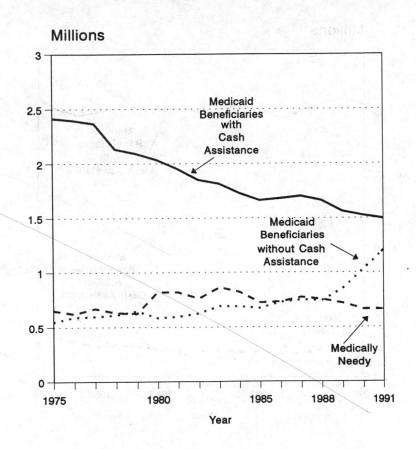

Source: Figure prepared by Congressional Research Service based on data from HCFA.

FIGURE II-19.
Child Beneficiaries by Eligibility Status
FY 1975-FY 1991

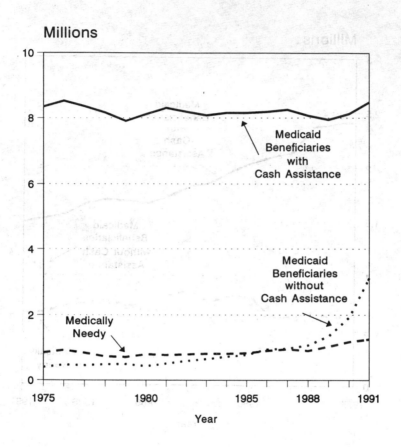

Source: Figure prepared by Congressional Research Service based on data from HCFA.

CHAPTER III. ELIGIBILITY[1]

SUMMARY

The Medicaid program is intended to provide basic medical coverage for certain groups of low-income persons. Traditionally, program eligibility was linked to actual or potential receipt of cash assistance under a welfare program. However, in recent years the program has been expanded to provide protection for low-income pregnant women and children with no ties to the welfare system. It has also been expanded to provide partial coverage for new groups of low-income aged and disabled Medicare beneficiaries. These expansions have increased the population with access to Medicaid coverage. However, the program still offers protection to less than one-half of the noninstitutionalized population with incomes below the Federal poverty line. At the same time, some individuals (primarily nursing home residents) with incomes above this poverty threshold are able to establish eligibility.

The requirements of Federal law, coupled with decisions by individual States in structuring their programs, determine who is actually eligible for Medicaid in a given State. Federal law places limitations on the categories of individuals who can be covered and establishes specific eligibility rules for each category. Within these parameters, States are given certain options. Thus individuals in similar circumstances may be automatically eligible for coverage in one State, be required to assume a certain portion of their expenses before they can gain coverage in a second State and not be eligible at all in a third State.

The Medicaid program can be viewed as offering protection to *three broad population groups of low-income persons*. The *first group includes families, children, and pregnant women*. Recent legislation has extended required coverage to certain pregnant women and children previously not covered, or covered only at State option. The *second population group is the aged*; a significant number of persons in this group do not become eligible until they become institutionalized. The *third population group is the disabled*; this category includes the mentally retarded as well as other citizens with disabling conditions. The program also offers partial protection to certain low-income aged and disabled Medicare beneficiaries who are not otherwise Medicaid eligible. Some poor persons, such as many singles and childless couples, cannot receive Medicaid benefits because they do not fall into one of these coverage categories.

---

[1]This chapter was written by Jennifer O'Sullivan and Richard Price.

Initially coverage of families, children, and pregnant women was linked to the actual or potential receipt by these individuals of cash assistance under the Aid to Families with Dependent Children (AFDC) program. However, in recent years the focus has been on providing increased access to pregnant women and children. Thus, a low-income pregnant woman or child may be covered under Medicaid regardless of the woman's or child's linkage to the welfare system. Specifically, States must cover the following individuals:

- *All pregnant women and children up to age 6 with family incomes below 133 percent of the Federal poverty level* ($1,282 a month ($15,388 a year) for a family of three in 1992). States at their option, may select a maximum income standard up to 185 percent of poverty for pregnant women and infants up to age 1.

- *All children under age 19, born after September 30, 1983, in families with incomes at or below 100 percent of the Federal poverty level* ($964 a month ($11,570 a year) for a family of three in 1992). All poor children under age 19 will be covered by the year 2002.

- *AFDC recipients and AFDC-related individuals.* States set their own income criteria for AFDC coverage; in all cases the maximum benefit is lower than the Federal poverty line. This is the only mandatory coverage category for children older than those included in the poverty-related groups discussed above. Coverage under this category (as distinct from coverage for poverty-related groups) extends to other family members who are considered part of the AFDC assistance unit.

  States may, but are not required to cover so-called *Ribicoff children.* These are children under age 21 (or at State option, under age 20, or under age 19, or under age 18) who would be eligible for AFDC if they met the definition of dependent child.[2] States may limit coverage of Ribicoff children to reasonable subgroups such as those in foster care or those in intermediate care facilities for the mentally retarded.

An infant or child entitled to Medicaid under any of these provisions is entitled to the full range of Medicaid services offered in the State. Pregnant women who are AFDC recipients, who meet the AFDC eligibility criteria, or who would meet such criteria if the child were born are also entitled to the full range of Medicaid services. Coverage for other pregnant women is restricted to services related to pregnancy (including prenatal, delivery, postpartum and family planning services) and other conditions which may complicate the pregnancy.

Medicaid covers additional categories or groups of persons because of its link to another cash welfare program, the Supplemental Security Income (SSI)

---

[2]A *dependent child* is one: (a) who has been deprived of parental support or care because the mother or father is absent from the home continuously, is incapacitated, is deceased, or is unemployed, and (b) who is living with a caretaker relative.

program. SSI provides cash assistance to needy aged, disabled, and blind individuals who have little or no income and resources. Because the elderly, disabled, and blind are groups of persons eligible for SSI, they are also categories of individuals States must cover under their Medicaid programs.

Most States extend Medicaid coverage to all elderly, disabled, and blind persons receiving Federal SSI payments because their income and resources meet the financial standards established for SSI. Medicaid law also gives States the option of using an alternative set of standards that may be more restrictive than SSI policies, but only if those policies were being used for Medicaid eligibility in 1972 when SSI was enacted. Twelve States use alternative standards; these standards may include lower limits on the income or resources a person may have and may include more restrictive definitions of disability.

Under SSI law, States have the option of supplementing the Federal benefit with State supplement payments (SSP) that are made solely with State funds. Many States provide these additional cash assistance payments because they feel the SSI benefit standard to be insufficient to cover a person's living expenses. The SSI benefit for a single individual represents 74 percent of the Federal poverty level. Medicaid allows States to provide automatic coverage to persons receiving SSP on the same basis as persons receiving SSI only, and most States do. When States provide Medicaid coverage to persons receiving SSP, the combined Federal SSI and State benefit payments become the effective eligibility standard.

Medicaid also allows States to extend coverage to another group of elderly, disabled, and blind persons who have too much income to qualify for SSI or SSP and who require care provided by nursing homes or other medical institutions. Income of these persons can not exceed three times the basic SSI payment level ($1,221 per month in 1991 and $1,266 per month in 1992); this rule is sometimes referred to as the *300 percent rule*. States may also apply this financial standard to persons needing long-term care services provided in the community, if these persons would otherwise require institutional care that Medicaid would pay for. Some States use only this rule to cover persons needing long-term care, with the result that if an individual has income in excess of the prescribed standard, they can not receive Medicaid assistance for their care, no matter how insufficient their income may be to cover the costs of their care.

All Medicaid beneficiaries (with the exception of those eligible for only partial coverage) fall into one of two broad coverage categories--the *categorically needy* or the *medically needy*. Initially, the term *categorically needy* referred to actual or potential recipients of cash assistance under the AFDC or SSI programs. More recently, pregnant women and children entitled to poverty-related coverage have been added to this group.

The term *medically needy* refers to persons who, except for income and resources, meet the criteria for categorically needy coverage. These persons become entitled to medically needy protection when their income and resources, after deducting incurred medical expenses, falls below the medically needy standards. States may, but are not required to cover the medically needy.

States having medically needy programs generally use it as a vehicle to cover a significant portion of their institutionalized population.

The distinction between the categorically needy and medically needy is important because the scope of services that States must provide to the categorically needy is much broader than the minimum scope of services that must be offered to the medically needy. In practice, many, but not all, States offer the same service package to both groups.[3]

Medicaid has another set of rules for the treatment of income *after* a person has become eligible for coverage. They apply to eligible beneficiaries who have income in excess of cash assistance programs--those who qualify under a medically needy program or the 300 percent rule--and determine how much of the beneficiary's income must be applied to the cost of care before Medicaid makes its payment. These rules are referred to as the *post-eligibility* rules, or more accurately, the post-eligibility treatment of income rules. Often they apply to persons needing long-term care--both nursing home care and home and community-based care. Special rules exist for the treatment of income and resources of married couples when one of the spouses requires nursing home care and the other remains in the community. These rules are referred to as the "spousal impoverishment" protections of Medicaid law, because they are intended to prevent the impoverishment of the spouse remaining in the community.

The previous discussion has focused on beneficiaries entitled to the full package of Medicaid benefits offered in the State. In recent years, Congress has authorized partial protection for the following defined coverage groups:

- *Qualified Medicare Beneficiaries (QMBs).* QMBs are aged and disabled Medicare beneficiaries with incomes below the Federal poverty line and with resources below 200 percent of the SSI limit. Medicaid is required to pay Medicare premiums and cost-sharing charges for these persons. Medicaid coverage is limited to payment of these charges unless the beneficiary is otherwise eligible for Medicaid.

- *Qualified Disabled and Working Individuals (QDWIs).* Medicare allows certain disabled persons to buy Medicare Part A (Hospital Insurance) protection. These are individuals who were previously entitled to Medicare Part A on the basis of a disability, who lost their entitlement based on earnings from work, but who continue to have the disabling condition. Medicaid is required to pay the Medicare Part A premium for such individuals if their incomes are below 200 percent of the Federal poverty line and their resources are below 200 percent of the SSI limit.

Readers of this chapter should note that the first section discussing Medicaid eligibility for families, children, and pregnant women uses data for 1992. All State-level data presented in this section are routinely updated. The subsequent discussions on Medicaid eligibility for the elderly and the disabled

---

[3]See *Chapter IV, Services* for a discussion of coverage requirements.

and blind, however, use 1991 data. Much of the data presented in these two sections was collected by the National Governors' Association under contract with the Congressional Research Service. These data are not routinely updated, and 1991 is the latest year for which most of this State-level information is available.

I. FAMILIES, CHILDREN AND PREGNANT WOMEN

Medicaid provides coverage for recipients of AFDC. AFDC recipients are low-income dependent children, their caretaker relatives, and certain other individuals residing in the household; they receive a cash welfare payment because they have little or no income. Medicaid is also available for some additional persons meeting or deemed to be meeting AFDC requirements but not actually receiving a cash payment. These persons are designated as categorically needy (that is they fall into one of the categories of persons that Medicaid must cover); they are entitled to the full range of Medicaid services offered in the State.

Medicaid must also be provided to certain low-income pregnant women, infants, and young children who do not otherwise qualify for AFDC, but whose income is nevertheless considered low in relation to Federal poverty guidelines. Coverage under the poverty-related provisions entitles only the individual (and a pregnant woman's newborn child) to benefits. Other members of the household are not covered. The package of services offered to women eligible on the basis of poverty-related coverage is limited to services related to pregnancy and other conditions which may complicate the pregnancy. An infant or child entitled under these provisions is entitled to the full range of services available to the categorically needy.

States may offer protection to some groups of medically needy persons. A medically needy person is one who is in one of the groups covered by Medicaid (i.e., children, pregnant women, or families with dependent children) but who does not meet the income and/or resources requirements for categorically needy eligibility. Individuals are eligible for medically needy coverage if their income and resources, after deduction of incurred medical expenses fall below the State's medically needy standards. A State may offer a more limited package of services for its medically needy population than for its categorically needy population.

A. AFDC-Related Coverage

1. *Mandatory Coverage for AFDC Recipients*

A State is required to cover under Medicaid all persons receiving cash payments under its AFDC program.[4] AFDC payments are made to families with children[5] where one parent is absent from the home continuously, incapacitated, dead, or unemployed and where income is below a specified standard.

Prior to October 1, 1990, States had the option of extending AFDC benefits to two-parent families where the principal breadwinner was unemployed (known as the AFDC-UP program). The Family Support Act of 1988 (FSA, P.L.100-485) made such coverage mandatory as of that date.[6] States that had elected to offer such coverage as of September 26, 1988, are required to continue operating such programs. Other States are permitted to limit cash assistance payments to 6 months in any 13-month period. However, States are required to provide full Medicaid coverage to all members of these families even in months where cash assistance benefits are not paid due to a State-established time limit.[7]

AFDC recipients are required to meet specified income, resources, and other requirements which are outlined below.

a. *AFDC Income Requirements*

State-established income criteria for AFDC (and therefore mandatory Medicaid coverage) differ markedly between the States. The law does, however, specify that the Secretary may not approve any State Medicaid plan if the State AFDC payment levels are less than those in effect on May 1, 1988.[8]

---

[4]For further discussion of the AFDC program see: U.S. Congress. House. Committee on Ways and Means. *1992 Green Book, Background Material and Data on Programs Within the Jurisdiction of the Committee on Ways and Means.* Committee Print, WMCP: 102-44, 102d Cong., 2d Sess. Washington, GPO, May 15, 1992. (Hereafter cited as House Ways and Means, *1992 Green Book*)

[5]The AFDC definition of dependent children generally limits coverage to persons under 18, or in certain instances, under age 19.

[6]The provision is effective Oct. 1, 1992 in the territories.

[7]This AFDC-UP and related Medicaid provision sunset effective Sept. 30, 1998.

[8]The law prohibits States from lowering their AFDC levels. However three States (California, New Jersey, and Wisconsin) have been able to waive this provision in connection with their welfare reform demonstration programs authorized under the general 1115 waiver authority. See *Chapter VI, Alternate Delivery Options and Waiver Programs* for a discussion of section 1115 waivers.

In contrast to the Federal SSI program, AFDC income levels are not automatically increased for inflation each year. Over the 1970-1992 period, benefit levels failed to keep pace with inflation in all but one State. When measured in constant dollars (after adjustment for inflation), the median decline was 43 percent.[9]

Under AFDC, each State establishes a "need standard" and a "payment standard" (which may be equal to or lower than the need standard); these standards are adjusted by family size. To receive AFDC payments, a family must pass two income tests, a gross income test and a countable income test. Families with gross incomes that exceed 185 percent of the State's need standard are ineligible for AFDC. Benefits are generally computed by subtracting countable income (i.e., gross income less certain amounts known as disregards) from the payment standard. The maximum benefit, which is the amount paid to a family with no other income, may be lower than the payment standard; as of January 1, 1992, this was true for 9 States.

Table III-1 shows, by State, the gross income limits (i.e., 185 percent of the need standard), the need standard, the payment standard, and the maximum monthly benefit applicable for 3-person families with no other income, as of January 1, 1992. This table shows that the maximum monthly benefit applicable for 3-person families with no other income ranged from $120 in Mississippi to $924 in Alaska.

[9] *1992 Green Book*, p. 641.

TABLE III-1. Aid to Families With Dependent Children: Gross Income Limit, Need Standard, Payment Standard, and Maximum Benefit by State, January 1992[a][b]

State	185 percent of "need" standard	100 percent of "need" standard	Payment standard	Maximum benefit
Alabama	$1,178	$637	$149	$149
Alaska	1,709	924	924	924
Arizona	1,717	928	334	334
Arkansas	1,304	705	204	204
California	1,284	694	694	663
Colorado	779	421	421	356
Connecticut[c]	1,258	680	680	680
Delaware	625	338	338	338
District of Columbia	1,317	712	409	409
Florida	1,717	928	303	303
Georgia	784	424	424	280
Hawaii	1,974	1,067	666	666
Idaho	1,025	554	315	315
Illinois[c]	1,561	844	367	367
Indiana	592	320	288	288
Iowa	1,571	849	426	426
Kansas	781	422	422	422
Kentucky	973	526	526	228
Louisiana[c]	1,217	658	190	190
Maine	1,060	573	573	453
Maryland	966	522	377	377
Massachusetts	997	539	539	539
Michigan (Wayne Co.)[c]	1,019	551	459	459
Minnesota	984	532	532	532
Mississippi	681	368	368	120
Missouri	577	312	292	292
Montana	884	478	390	390
Nebraska	673	364	364	364
Nevada	1,147	620	372	372
New Hampshire	955	516	516	516
New Jersey	784	424	424	424
New Mexico	599	324	324	324
New York (Suffolk Co.)[c]	1,301	703	703	703
New York (New York City)[c]	1,067	577	577	577
North Carolina	1,006	544	272	272
North Dakota	742	401	401	401
Ohio	1,511	817	334	334
Oklahoma	871	471	341	341
Oregon	851	460	460	460
Pennsylvania[c]	1,136	614	421	421
Rhode Island	1,025	554	554	554
South Carolina	814	440	440	210
South Dakota	747	404	404	404
Tennessee	788	426	426	185
Texas	1,062	574	184	184
Utah	993	537	537	402
Vermont[c]	2,057	1,112	673	673
Virginia[c]	727	393	354	354
Washington	1,876	1,014	531	531
West Virginia	919	497	249	249

See notes at end of table.

TABLE III-1. Aid to Families With Dependent Children: Gross Income Limit, Need, Standard, Payment Standard, and Maximum Benefit by State, January 1992[a][b] --Continued--

State	185 percent of "need" standard	100 percent of "need" standard	Payment standard	Maximum benefit
Wisconsin[c]	$1,197	$647	$517	$517
Wyoming	1,247	674	360	360
Puerto Rico	296	160	180	180
Virgin Islands	555	300	240	240

[a]These calculations assume no child care expenses and work expenses of $90 per month.

[b]Income level at which Medicaid eligibility ends. Because of minimum payment rule, actual AFDC benefits may end at a slightly different income level.

[c]In States with differentials, figure shown is for area with highest benefit.

Source: Table prepared by the Congressional Research Service on the basis of a telephone survey of the States.

Specified amounts of both unearned and earned income are disregarded in calculating AFDC benefits. Unearned income not counted includes the first $50 in child support payments. Earned income not counted is reduced over time, thereby lessening the immediate impact of the transition to work. Earned income disregards during the first 4 months of employment equal $120 plus one-third of remaining earnings. After 4 months, the total disregard is $120. After 12 months the total disregard is $90. The maximum child care allowance is $175 per child per month ($200 for a child under age 2).

Because specified amounts of personal income are disregarded in determining eligibility for AFDC, a person or family with income which exceeds the maximum benefit may still be eligible for cash assistance and therefore automatic Medicaid coverage. Table III-2 shows the income levels at which AFDC eligibility ends for a family of three; the income cutoff levels decline after 4 months and after 12 months due to the lower income disregards. Again, this table demonstrates the wide variations between States. After 12 months, the effective cutoff level for a family of three ranges from $239 in Alabama to $1,014 in Alaska.

**TABLE III-2. Aid to Families With Dependent Children: Income Levels
at Which AFDC Eligibility Ends for a Family of Three,
by State and Period of Receipt, January 1992[a] [b]**

State	First 4 months	Months 8-12	After 12 months
Alabama	$ 344	$ 269	$ 239
Alaska	1,506	1,044	1,014
Arizona	621	454	424
Arkansas	426	324	294
California	1,161	814	784
Colorado	752	541	511
Connecticut[c]	1,140	800	770
Delaware	627	458	428
District of Columbia	734	529	499
Florida	575	423	393
Georgia	756	544	514
Hawaii	1,119	786	756
Idaho	593	435	405
Illinois[c]	671	487	457
Indiana	552	408	378
Iowa	759	546	516
Kansas[c]	753	542	512
Kentucky	909	646	616
Louisiana[c]	405	310	280
Maine	980	693	663
Maryland	686	497	467
Massachusetts	929	659	629
Michigan (Wayne Co.)	809	579	549
Minnesota	918	652	622
Mississippi	672	488	458
Missouri	558	412	382
Montana	705	510	480
Nebraska	666	484	454
Nevada	615	450	420
New Hampshire	894	636	606
New Jersey	756	544	514
New Mexico	606	444	414
New York (New York City)[c]	986	697	667
North Carolina	528	392	362
North Dakota	722	521	491
Ohio	621	454	424
Oklahoma	632	461	431
Oregon	810	580	550
Pennsylvania[c]	752	541	511
Rhode Island	951	674	644
South Carolina	780	560	530
South Dakota	726	524	494
Tennessee	759	546	516
Texas	396	304	274
Utah	926	657	627
Vermont[c]	1,130	793	763
Virginia[c]	651	474	444
Washington	917	651	621
West Virginia	494	369	339
Wisconsin[c]	896	637	607

See notes at end of table.

TABLE III-2. Aid to Families With Dependent Children: Income Levels
at Which AFDC Eligibility Ends for a Family of Three, by
State and Period of Receipt, January 1992[a] [b]--Continued

State	First 4 months	Months 8-12	After 12 months
Wyoming	$660	$480	$450
Guam	615	450	420
Puerto Rico	390	300	270
Virgin Islands	480	360	330

[a]These calculations assume no child care expenses and work expenses of $90 per month.

[b]Income level at which Medicaid eligibility ends. Because of minimum payment rule, actual AFDC benefits may end at a slightly different income level.

[c]In States with differentials, figure shown is for area with highest benefit.

Source: Table prepared by the Congressional Research Service on the basis of a telephone survey of the States.

It should be noted that while AFDC does not make a cash payment where the payment amount would be less than $10, Medicaid must be provided in such cases.

b. AFDC Resource Requirements

AFDC applicants meeting the income criteria are also required to meet resource criteria. By Federal law and regulation, the resource limit for real and personal property cannot exceed $1,000 per family unit. The State must exclude from this calculation the family's home (of any value), up to $1,500 equity value in an automobile, and burial plots and funeral agreements for members of the AFDC assistance unit. In addition, States are permitted, but not required, to exclude basic maintenance items essential to day to day living, such as clothing and furniture.

c. Other AFDC Requirements[10]

FSA requires States, effective October 1, 1990, to have a job opportunities and basic skills (JOBS) program. The purpose of this program is to ensure that needy families with children obtain the education, training, and employment that will help them avoid long-term welfare dependence. States are required to enroll virtually all able-bodied persons whose youngest child is at least age three, provided State resources are available.

Federal law also requires AFDC mothers to assign their child support rights to the State and to cooperate with welfare officials in establishing the paternity of a child and in obtaining support payments from the father.

2. Transitional Coverage for Working Poor Families

An individual who increases his (or her) income from employment faces not only the loss of AFDC but also the potential loss of Medicaid coverage. For individuals and their families who find work that does not include health insurance benefits, the loss of Medicaid coverage could serve as a greater work disincentive than the loss of cash payments. To address this concern, FSA expanded Medicaid protection previously available to families who leave AFDC due to earnings.[11]

States are required to provide 6 months of extended Medicaid coverage to each family that received AFDC in at least 3 of the 6 months preceding the month the family lost such assistance due to either increased hours of employment, increased income of the caretaker relative, or the family member's loss of one of the time limited earned income disregards (as described above). States are required to provide full Medicaid coverage or alternatively provide "wrap around" coverage." Under the "wrap around" option, States could pay the family's expenses for premiums, deductibles, and coinsurance for any health care coverage offered by the employer of the caretaker relative.

FSA further provides that families covered during the entire 6-month period, and earning below 185 percent of the poverty line, qualify for a second 6-month extension period. States have a number of coverage options during this coverage period. They may offer regular Medicaid benefits or limit coverage to acute care services. They may also offer "wrap around" coverage. Additionally,

---

[10]A State's AFDC plan may require a minor pregnant woman or a minor with a dependent child to reside in a place of residence maintained by an adult relative or guardian. The fact that an individual may be denied AFDC on this basis may not be construed as permitting a State to deny Medicaid to the individual if such individual is eligible for Medicaid on another basis. Further, if a State terminates an individual's AFDC coverage on the basis of this AFDC provision, Medicaid coverage may not be discontinued until it is determined that the individual is not otherwise eligible.

[11]This expanded protection will sunset, effective Sept. 30, 1998.

they may offer to enroll families in alternative coverage such as an employer or State employee plan, a State uninsured plan, or a health maintenance organization (HMO). If a State offers alternative coverage, it must assure that maternity care and ambulatory preventive pediatric care is available without charge to the families.

States are permitted to impose premiums for the second 6-month extension period if the family's income (excluding average necessary child care expenses) exceeds the poverty line. Premiums may not exceed three percent of the family's average gross monthly earnings (less average necessary child care expenses). Premiums are to be calculated based on quarterly reports from families on earnings and child care expenses.

The General Accounting Office reports that 11 States selected one or more of the available coverage options in the April 1990-June 1991 period.[12] Three States (Colorado, Minnesota, and Oregon) provided wrap around coverage with States supplementing employer coverage if the employer package provided fewer benefits than the State Medicaid plan. The six States that used the HMO option (D.C., Massachusetts, Minnesota, New York, Washington, and Wisconsin) were using an extension of what was already offered to Medicaid recipients in the State. Two States imposed a premium. Maine required a payment equal to three percent of the family's income, while South Dakota imposed a premium of approximately $6-$20 a week.

3. Mandatory Coverage of Other AFDC-Related Persons

States are also *required* to extend categorically needy protection to additional AFDC-related groups of persons, though the individuals in such groups are not actually receiving a cash payment. States must provide coverage to the following population groups. (For a discussion of the required coverage of pregnant women and children, see subsection B below.)

States are required to extend Medicaid for 4 months to a family losing AFDC coverage because of increased child or spousal support. Families eligible for this extension must have been receiving AFDC in at least 3 of the preceding 6 months.

States must extend coverage to the following groups for an unlimited period, provided the individuals in the group continue to meet the requisite criteria.

- *Persons whose cash payment would be less than $10.* Persons denied an AFDC cash payment solely because the payment amount would be less than $10 must be covered under Medicaid.

---

[12]U.S. General Accounting Office. *Welfare to Work: Implementation and Evaluation of Traditional Benefits Need HHS Action.* GAO/HRD 92-118, Sept. 29, 1992. p. 37.

- *Persons whose AFDC payments are reduced to zero because of recovery of overpayments of AFDC funds.*

- *Work supplementation participants.* States may establish a work supplementation program (WSP) under the JOBS program. Under WSP, the State reserves the amount that would otherwise be payable to an AFDC family and uses it instead to provide and subsidize a job for the program participant. States may make work supplementation either mandatory or optional. States are required to provide Medicaid to program participants (and other family members) if such persons would be eligible for AFDC in absence of the supplementation program.

- *Adoption assistance.* Title IV-E of the Social Security Act authorizes Federal matching for State adoption assistance programs intended to lessen the barriers to adoption of children with special needs. Medicaid coverage is required if at the time the adoption assistance proceedings were initiated, the child was: eligible for AFDC (or would have met the requirements except for removal from the home because of voluntary placement or court order), eligible for SSI, in foster care, or receiving AFDC (or would have been receiving assistance if the child had been living with a relative). A child for whom an adoption agreement is in effect is eligible for assistance in the State where he or she resides.

- *Foster care.* Title IV-E of the Social Security Act authorizes Federal matching funds for State expenditures for foster care maintenance payments for certain children. Medicaid coverage is mandatory for such children and must be provided by the State in which the child resides. Further, when an individual in foster care is a minor parent of a child in the same home or institution, the individual's child is considered to be a foster care child for purposes of Medicaid eligibility.

- *Individuals ineligible for AFDC because of a requirement prohibited under Medicaid.*[13]

- *Individuals eligible for Medicaid except for the 1972 Social Security increase.* This applies to persons who were receiving both Social Security and cash assistance in August 1972.

4. Optional Coverage of Additional Persons

States are *permitted*, but not required, to provide Medicaid protection to certain additional groups of AFDC-related persons though these persons are not actually receiving a cash payment. These persons are sometimes referred to as the "optional categorically needy." The benefit package available to the optional categorically needy is the same as that made available to the mandatory categorically needy.

a. Ribicoff Children

An important optional category for older children is known as "Ribicoff children".[14] This coverage category originally included all children under age 21 who would be eligible for AFDC if they met the definition of dependent child. However, recent legislation has provided other paths to eligibility for younger children. As discussed in subsection B below, States are required to provide Medicaid coverage to children under age 6 with family incomes below 133 percent of poverty. They are also required to cover children under age 19, born after September 30, 1983, with family incomes at or below 100 percent of poverty.

The category known as Ribicoff children has been superseded as a coverage path for children born after September 30, 1983 but remains a coverage path for children born prior to that date. The Ribicoff coverage category will gradually diminish in importance as more children are included under the poverty related coverage categories.

Ribicoff children are children under age 21 (or at State option, under age 20, or under age 19, or under age 18) who would be eligible for AFDC if they met the definition of dependent child. States may limit coverage of Ribicoff children to reasonable subgroups such as those in foster care, in intermediate care facilities for the mentally retarded, or receiving active treatment as inpatients in psychiatric facilities. All States cover some Ribicoff children. Table III-3 shows (based on information available March 1992) that 29 States cover all Ribicoff children below a State selected age (i.e., 18, 19, or 21), while the remaining States limit coverage to specified categories of children.

---

[13]A number of State courts have found that the AFDC rules for deeming the availability of income of an applicant's siblings and/or nonparental caretakers cannot be used for Medicaid purposes.

[14]This group is named after former Senator Ribicoff, sponsor of legislation authorizing coverage for this group.

TABLE III-3. Coverage of *Ribicoff Children*, March 1992

State	All under age	Limited to specified reasonable categories under age
Alabama	--	21
Alaska	21	--
Arizona	18	--
Arkansas[a]	18	21
California	21	--
Colorado	--	21
Connecticut	21	--
Delaware	--	21
District of Columbia	21	--
Florida	--	18/21[b]
Georgia	--	18
Hawaii	--	19/21[c]
Idaho	--	18/21[b]
Illinois[a]	18	21
Indiana	--	21
Iowa	21	--
Kansas	--	18/21[b]
Kentucky	18/19[d]	--
Louisiana	--	18/21[b]
Maine	21	--
Maryland	21	--
Massachusetts	21	--
Michigan	21	--
Minnesota	21	--
Mississippi[a]	18	21
Missouri	--	18/21[b]
Montana	21	--

See notes at end of table.

TABLE III-3. Coverage of *Ribicoff Children*, March 1992--Continued

State	All under age	Limited to specified reasonable categories under age
Nebraska	20	--
Nevada	--	19
New Hampshire	--	19
New Jersey	21	--
New Mexico	--	18
New York	21	--
North Carolina	21	--
North Dakota	21	--
Ohio	21	--
Oklahoma	21	--
Oregon	--	21
Pennsylvania	21	--
Rhode Island	--	19
South Carolina	18/19[d]	21
South Dakota	--	21
Tennessee	--	21
Texas	--	18/19[d]
Utah	18	--
Vermont	21	--
Virginia	--	21
Washington[c]	18	21
West Virginia	--	18/21[a]
Wisconsin[c]	18	21
Wyoming	--	19/21[b]

[a]State covers all children under age 18 and some reasonable categories under age 21.

[b]State covers one or more reasonable categories of children under age 18 and one or more reasonable categories of children under age 21.

[c]State covers one or more reasonable categories of children under age 19 and one or more reasonable categories of children under age 21.

[d]State covers children under age 18, except that children under 19 may be covered if in secondary school.

Source: Table prepared by the Congressional Research Service based on information reported by: U.S. Dept. of Health and Human Services. Health Care Financing Administration. *Medicaid State Profile Data (spDATA) System: Characteristics of Medicaid State Programs,* May 1992; and the *Medicare and Medicaid Guide* (published by the Commerce Clearing House), as updated through Sept. 1992.

b. Other Persons

Other optional category needy groups are:

- *Individuals eligible for AFDC but not receiving it.*

- *Individuals who would be eligible for AFDC if child care costs were paid from earnings.* This group includes persons for whom work-related child care expenditures are paid by a State agency as a service expenditure.

- *Individuals who would be eligible if the State's AFDC plan were as broad as allowed under the law.*

- *Institutionalized individuals who would be eligible for cash assistance if they left the institution.*

- *Children under certain adoption assistance agreements.* As noted above, States are required to provide Medicaid coverage to certain children covered under Title IV-E adoption assistance agreements. In addition, a State may provide Medicaid coverage for children for whom State adoption assistance agreements (other than under Title IV-E) are in effect.

  To be covered under this provision, certain conditions must be met. The State must determine that the child has special needs. Before the adoption agreement went into effect, the child must have been covered under Medicaid, or would have been eligible for Medicaid if the standards and methodologies of the Title IV-E program were applied rather than the AFDC standards and methodologies. Children covered under this option may be under age 21, 20, 19, or 18, as selected by the State.

- *Disabled children age 18 or younger who would be eligible if they were in a medical institution.* This group, sometimes referred to as the Katie Beckett group is discussed in subsection III-A below.

- *Health maintenance organization enrollees.* States may provide for an extension period for beneficiaries enrolled in HMOs who lose their Medicaid eligibility. The extension period may not exceed 6 months from the date of initial enrollment.

B. Special Provisions Applicable for Pregnant Women and Young Children[15]

The program offers several ways for both pregnant women (including those without other children in the home) and young children not receiving AFDC to attain Medicaid eligibility.

A pregnant women may qualify on the basis that if her unborn child were born and living with her, she would be eligible for AFDC. This woman is a "qualified pregnant woman" and entitled to the full range of Medicaid services offered in the State. A pregnant woman not otherwise eligible for Medicaid (either because of income or family structure) may qualify for poverty-related coverage. States are required to offer poverty-related coverage to pregnant women with incomes below 133 percent of poverty ($15,388--$1,282 a month--for a family of three in 1992). States may extend this poverty-related coverage up to 185 percent of the poverty line ($21,404--$1,784 a month--for a family of three in 1992). The package of services offered to women eligible on the basis of poverty-related coverage is limited to services related to pregnancy and other conditions which may complicate the pregnancy.

The program also offers several ways to cover children not receiving (or deemed to be receiving) cash assistance. An infant under age one may be covered under the poverty-related provisions. States must cover infants and children under age 6 with incomes under 133 percent of poverty; a State may extend this coverage for an infant under age 1 up to 185 percent of poverty. States must also cover all children under age 19, born after September 30, 1983, in families with incomes below 100 percent of poverty ($11,570--$964 a month--for a family of three in 1992). An infant or child entitled to Medicaid under any of these provisions is entitled to the full range of Medicaid services offered in the State.

Unlike AFDC benefit levels (and the accompanying automatic Medicaid eligibility), poverty-related coverage levels are increased for inflation each year.

These coverage provisions are discussed in more detail below.

1. Qualified Pregnant Women

A State may provide cash assistance under AFDC to pregnant women (without other children in the home) meeting AFDC income and resources requirements. AFDC benefits may begin with the sixth month of pregnancy. Regardless of the State's decision under its AFDC program, Medicaid coverage must begin for all pregnant women meeting AFDC income and resources requirements from the medical verification of pregnancy. A women entitled to

---

[15]States may take a number of actions to streamline the eligibility determination process. These include establishing presumptive eligibility for pregnant women and shortening Medicaid application forms. These strategies are discussed in *Chapter VII, Administration.*

Medicaid as a qualified pregnant woman is entitled to the full range of Medicaid benefits.

2. Poverty-Related Coverage

A pregnant woman or child whose income and resources are in excess of the AFDC standards in the State may qualify under one of two "poverty-related" coverage categories.

The first coverage category is *pregnant women, infants, and children up to age 6 with family incomes below 133 percent of the Federal poverty level* ($15,388 for a family of three in 1992). A State may select an income standard up to 185 percent of poverty for pregnant women and infants *up to* age 1; the law specifies that a State may not elect this option if its AFDC payment levels are lower than those in effect on July 1, 1987. However, the 133 percent level is applicable for all children age under age 6.

The 133 percent level is the minimum level applicable for pregnant women and infants under age 1. Some States are required to use an income level higher than 133 percent of poverty for these groups. These are States who, under the optional coverage provisions of prior law, used an income level between 133 and 185 percent of poverty. Specifically, any State which, as of December 19, 1989, had implemented or approved a higher level must continue to use that higher standard for pregnant women and infants.[16]

Table III-4 shows the poverty level used by each State for coverage of pregnant women and infants, effective January 1, 1992.

TABLE III-4. Poverty Level Coverage for Pregnant Women
and Infants, January 1992

State	Percentage of poverty
Alabama	133%
Alaska	133
Arizona	140
Arkansas	185
California	185
Colorado	133
Connecticut	185
Delaware	160
District of Columbia	185
Florida	150
Georgia	133
Hawaii	185
Idaho	133
Illinois	133

See notes at end of table.

---

[16]The National Governors' Association reports that as of Sept. 1989, 17 States used a level higher than 133 percent of poverty.

TABLE III-4. Poverty Level Coverage for Pregnant Women
and Infants, January 1992--Continued

State	Percentage of poverty
Indiana	150
Iowa	185
Kansas	150
Kentucky	185
Louisiana	133
Maine	185
Maryland	185
Massachusetts	185
Michigan	185
Minnesota	185
Mississippi	185
Missouri	133
Montana	133
Nebraska	133
Nevada	133
New Hampshire	133
New Jersey	185
New Mexico	185
New York	185
North Carolina	185
North Dakota	133
Ohio	133
Oklahoma	133
Oregon	133
Pennsylvania	133
Rhode Island	185
South Carolina	185
South Dakota	133
Tennessee	185
Texas	185
Utah	133
Vermont	185
Virginia	133
Washington	185
West Virginia	150
Wisconsin	155
Wyoming	133

Source: National Governors' Association, Jan. 1992.

A State using a standard above 150 percent of poverty may impose a premium; however, in no case can the premium exceed 10 percent of the amount by which family income (after deducting child care expenses) exceeds 150 percent of the Federal poverty line. There is no indication that any State has actually imposed such a premium.

A second broad poverty-related coverage category is that of *older children who do not otherwise qualify for Medicaid*. These are children who are at least 6 years old, under age 19, born after September 30, 1983, and with incomes at or below the poverty level. This coverage group continuously expands over time so that after the year 2002 all poor children under age 19 will be covered.[17]

Methodologies used for assessing income for AFDC purposes (including deductions for child care and work expenses) are generally used for both poverty-related coverage categories. There is no "spenddown" for poverty-related coverage; thus costs that are incurred for medical care cannot be deducted from income in determining eligibility.

States are permitted, but are not required, to apply a resource test for poverty-related coverage. For pregnant women, the resource standard and the method of valuing resources may be no more restrictive than that used for SSI; for infants and children, the standard and the method of valuation may be no more restrictive than that applied under AFDC. The NGA reports that as of January 1, 1992 48 States, including the District of Columbia, had dropped assets tests for pregnant women and children; only California, Iowa, and North Dakota still had the tests.[18]

States can not require pregnant women to apply for AFDC benefits in order to be able to apply for and receive Medicaid.

Pregnant women whose eligibility is based on poverty-related coverage are not entitled to the full Medicaid benefit package. Their coverage is restricted to services related to pregnancy (including prenatal, delivery, postpartum and family planning services) and other conditions which may complicate pregnancy. Specific services meeting this requirement are not identified. However, the DHHS Medicaid Manual notes that "reasonable interpretation related to a successful pregnancy outcome is expected."

The benefits available for poverty-related infants and children include all services covered under the individual State's Medicaid program. A special continuation provision applies to an infant or child receiving inpatient services on the day that he or she would lose eligibility due to reaching the maximum age limit (i.e., age 1, 6, or 19). In this case, benefits must be continued through the end of the inpatient stay.

---

[17]The law also includes a coverage category known as "qualified children." These are children under age 19, born after Sept. 30, 1983 (or such earlier date as the State may select), who meet the income and resources criteria of the State's AFDC plan. As of July 1, 1991, this group was effectively subsumed under the new category requiring coverage of all children under age 19, born after Sept. 30, 1983, with incomes below poverty. However, if a State elects to cover a child born before this date, this child would be a "qualified child."

[18]See *Chapter VII, Administration* for additional discussion of additional actions to streamline eligibility determinations for this population group.

3. Eligibility Extensions

The law includes certain requirements that ensure a minimum period of Medicaid coverage for pregnant women and newborns. These requirements are applicable regardless of what eligibility group the pregnant woman or infant is classified under.

An eligible pregnant woman who would lose eligibility because of a change in family income is deemed to continue to be eligible as a poverty related individual throughout the pregnancy and postpartum period. This provision applies only after actual eligibility has been established; it does not apply to women who have only been determined presumptively eligible for the program.

Services for pregnant women must be provided for 60 days postpartum, and the remaining days of the month in which the 60th day falls. This requirement is applicable only if during the pregnancy the woman applied for and received Medicaid services.

Medicaid establishes deemed eligibility for certain newborns. A child born to a woman eligible for and receiving Medicaid on the date of the child's birth is deemed eligible for Medicaid for 1 year provided that the child resides continuously in the mother's household and the mother remains eligible for Medicaid or (for a child born on or after January 1, 1991) would have remained eligible if she were still pregnant. Since a pregnant woman cannot lose Medicaid eligibility based on a change in income, neither can the newborn. An infant is deemed eligible only in the State where the mother was eligible on the date of the birth.

4. Possible Expansions

As noted above, the methodology used in evaluating income and resources for determining eligibility for pregnant women and children not receiving cash assistance can be no more restrictive but may be more liberal than that which would be applied under the most closely related cash assistance program. This is known as the Section 1902(r)(2) provision.[19] Recent analyses have suggested that States may use this section to allow for more types and greater amounts of income and resource disregards. Under this approach, States could structure their eligibility policies so that more children and pregnant women could qualify for Medicaid coverage (and accompanying Federal matching). A July 1992 analysis by the Maternal and Child Health Policy Research Center showed that 47 States were aware of the 1902(r)(2) option. Fifteen States had made changes in their methodologies; but only two of these could be considered significant. The majority of States using the option revised their methodologies to disregard parental income of pregnant women living in their parents' home. Washington effectively expanded coverage to all children under 19 with incomes below poverty. Effective July 1, 1993, Minnesota is slated to increase its coverage to

---

[19]See also the discussion of income and resources standards for the medically needy, below.

all pregnant women and children under 19 with incomes below 275 percent of poverty.

C. Medically Needy Coverage

Families with children, and low-income pregnant women and children may potentially be included under a States's medically needy plan if a State elects to offer such coverage. However, this eligibility path will become less significant for these persons, due to the significant expansions in required poverty-related coverage for pregnant women and children. Some families with older children or with very large medical expenses, who are otherwise ineligible for Medicaid, may still qualify for medically needy coverage. The medically needy program remains a very significant coverage category for the aged and disabled, particularly for the institutionalized population. (See discussion in subsection III-B below.)

1. Coverage Groups

States are permitted, but not required, to cover the medically needy. These are persons: (1) who, except for income and resources, fall into one of the categories covered by the State (i.e., families with dependent children, pregnant woman, certain children, the aged, the blind, and the disabled); and (2) whose income and/or resources are in excess of the standards for categorically needy coverage, but below medically needy standards established by the State.

A State having a medically needy program must, as a minimum provide coverage to the following:

- Pregnant women who, except for income and resources, would be eligible as categorically needy; and

- Individuals under age 18 who, but for income and resources, would be covered as mandatory categorically needy.

As a minimum, a State is required to offer ambulatory services (i.e., noninstitutional services) to these children and to any other medically needy persons entitled to institutional services in the State. It is also required to provide prenatal and delivery services for pregnant women. Further, it is required to offer home health services to any individual entitled to nursing facility care. A special minimum requirement applies if a State provides coverage for medically needy persons under age 21 or over 65 in institutions for mental diseases or coverage for medically needy persons in intermediate care facilities for the mentally retarded. In this case, the State is required to cover either the same services as those which are mandatory for the categorically needy or alternatively the care and services listed in at least 7 of the first 21 paragraphs in the law defining covered mandatory and optional services.[20]

---

[20]See *Chapter IV, Services* for a discussion of mandatory and optional services.

The mandatory eligibility extensions described above, for categorically needy pregnant women and certain newborns who would otherwise lose coverage, are also applicable for medically needy pregnant women and newborns of medically needy pregnant women who are in the same circumstances. The services available to these pregnant women are restricted to pregnancy-related and postpartum services; the package available to newborns is the same as that available to other medically needy infants.

As of March 1992, 37 States (including the District of Columbia) had medically needy programs in place; however, Florida dropped its program in April 1992. Most of these programs offered broader coverage than the minimum mandated by law. Many States included children over 18; 7 States used age 19 as the age limit while 23 States used the maximum age limit of 21. Thirty States covered the caretaker relatives of these children. All but one State (Texas) covered the aged, blind, and disabled. (See table III-5.)

TABLE III-5. Characteristics of State Medically Needy Programs, March 1992

State	Presence of medically needy program	Age limit for medically needy children	Care-taker relative	Optional coverage groups		
				Aged	Blind	Disabled
Alabama	No	--	--	--	--	--
Alaska	No	--	--	--	--	--
Arizona[a]	NA	--	--	--	--	--
Arkansas	Yes	18[b]	Yes	Yes	Yes	Yes
California	Yes	21	Yes	Yes	Yes	Yes
Colorado	No	--	--	--	--	--
Connecticut	Yes	21	Yes	Yes	Yes	Yes
Delaware	No	--	--	--	--	--
District of Columbia	Yes	21	Yes	Yes	Yes	Yes
Florida	Yes[c]	21	Yes	Yes	Yes	Yes
Georgia	Yes	18	No	Yes	Yes	Yes
Hawaii	Yes	19	No	Yes	Yes	Yes
Kansas	Yes	21	Yes	Yes	Yes	Yes
Kentucky	Yes	19	Yes	Yes	Yes	Yes
Louisiana	Yes	18[b]	Yes	Yes	Yes	Yes
Maine	Yes	21	Yes	Yes	Yes	Yes
Maryland	Yes	21	Yes	Yes	Yes	Yes
Massachusetts	Yes	21	Yes	Yes	Yes	Yes
Michigan	Yes	21	Yes	Yes	Yes	Yes
Minnesota	Yes	21	Yes	Yes	Yes	Yes
Mississippi	No	--	--	--	--	--
Missouri	No	--	--	--	--	--
Montana	Yes	21	No	Yes	Yes	Yes

See notes at end of table.

TABLE III-5. Characteristics of State Medically Needy Programs, March 1992--Continued

State	Presence of medically needy program	Age limit for medically needy children	Optional coverage groups			
			Care-taker relative	Aged	Blind	Disabled
Nebraska	Yes	21	Yes	Yes	Yes	Yes
Nevada	No	--	--	--	--	--
New Hampshire	Yes	19	Yes	Yes	Yes	Yes
New Jersey	Yes	21	No	Yes	Yes	Yes
New Mexico	No	--	--	--	--	--
New York	Yes	21	Yes	Yes	Yes	Yes
North Carolina	Yes	21	Yes	Yes	Yes	Yes
North Dakota	Yes	21	Yes	Yes	Yes	Yes
Ohio	No	--	--	--	--	--
Oklahoma	Yes	21	Yes	Yes	Yes	Yes
Oregon	Yes	21	No	Yes	Yes	Yes
Pennsylvania	Yes	21	Yes	Yes	Yes	Yes
Rhode Island	Yes	19	Yes	Yes	Yes	Yes
South Carolina	Yes	19[b]	Yes	Yes	Yes	Yes
South Dakota	No	--	--	--	--	--
Tennessee	Yes	21	Yes	Yes	Yes	Yes
Texas	Yes	18	Yes	No	No	No
Utah	Yes	18	Yes	Yes	Yes	Yes
Vermont	Yes	21	Yes	Yes	Yes	Yes
Virginia	Yes	21	No	Yes	Yes	Yes
Washington	Yes	18[b]	Yes	Yes	Yes	Yes
West Virginia	Yes	19	Yes	Yes	Yes	Yes

See notes at end of table.

TABLE III-5. Characteristics of State Medically Needy Programs, March 1992—Continued

State	Presence of medically needy program	Age limit for medically needy children	Optional coverage groups			
			Care-taker relative	Aged	Blind	Disabled
Wisconsin	Yes	19	No	Yes	Yes	Yes
Wyoming	No	–	–	–	–	–
Totals	37	–	30	36	36	36

[a]Arizona's Medicaid program is authorized under section 1115 waiver authority and is not comparable to other States.

[b]States also include coverage for some categories of children under age 21.

[c]Medically needy program eliminated Apr. 1992.

Source: HCFA, *Medicaid State Profile Data (spDATA) System: Characteristics of Medicaid State Programs,* May 1992.

2. Income and Resource Standards

States having medically needy programs establish a single income and resource standard for all covered population groups. The methodology used in evaluating income and resources for the medically needy can be no more restrictive, but may be more liberal, than that which would be applied under the most closely related cash assistance program. The use of such methodology may not bar otherwise eligible persons from coverage.[21][22]

a. Income Standards

States establish medically needy income standards based on family size. For purposes of Federal matching payments, the income standard cannot exceed 133-1/3 percent of the maximum payment for a similarly sized family, with no income or resources, under the State's AFDC plan.[23] Table III-6 shows, effective January 1, 1992, the medically needy income levels by State, by family size. (This table does not reflect any income disregards that may be applicable.) As would be expected, given its link to the AFDC program, the levels vary considerably by State.[24] For a family of three, the level ranged from $250 per month in Tennessee to $934 per month in California.

---

[21]As noted earlier, these rules also apply to methodologies used for determining categorically needy eligibility for pregnant women and children not receiving cash assistance and for optional categorically needy coverage groups.

[22]This requirement, included in the Medicare Catastrophic Coverage Act of 1988 (MCCA, P.L.100-260), represents the culmination of several years of legislative activity. This began with the enactment of a provision in DEFRA which prohibited HCFA from imposing penalties based on a State using more liberal standards than those used under the most closely related cash assistance program. (This was known as the "DEFRA moratorium.")

[23]OBRA 90 permits certain States to continue to base their medically needy income limit for a family of one on the maximum limit for an AFDC family of two. This provision applies in States which provided for such a policy as of June 1, 1989.

[24]The maximum medically needy income level is the same for all medically needy groups. See subsection II-B below for a discussion of the implications of this requirement on the aged and disabled populations.

TABLE III-6. Medically Needy Monthly Protected Income Levels,
Family Size One Through Four, January 1992

	Family of one	Family of two	Family of three	Family of four
Alabama	NA	--	--	--
Alaska	NA	--	--	--
Arizona	NA	--	--	--
Arkansas	$108	$217	$275	$ 333
California	600	750	934	1,100
Colorado	NA	--	--	--
Connecticut	473	629	773	908
Delaware	NA	--	--	--
District of Columbia	407	428	545	665
Florida[a]	180	241	303	364
Georgia	208	317	375	442
Hawaii	396	531	666	802
Idaho	NA	--	--	--
Illinois	283	358	492	558
Indiana	NA	--	--	--
Iowa	483	483	566	666
Kansas	422	466	470	488
Kentucky	217	267	308	383
Louisiana	100	192	258	317
Maine	315	341	458	575
Maryland	359	400	442	484
Massachusetts	522	650	775	891
Michigan	408	541	567	593
Minnesota	467	583	709	828
Mississippi	NA	--	--	--
Missouri	NA	--	--	--
Montana	407	417	443	469
Nebraska	392	392	492	584
Nevada	NA	--	--	--
New Hampshire	436	608	616	623
New Jersey	350	433	566	658
New Mexico	NA	--	--	--
New York	509	742	750	850
North Carolina	242	317	367	400
North Dakota	345	400	435	530
Ohio	NA	--	--	--
Oklahoma	284	359	459	567
Oregon	413	526	613	753
Pennsylvania	425	442	467	567
Rhode Island	558	600	741	850
South Carolina	225	225	283	341
South Dakota	NA	--	--	--

See notes at end of table.

TABLE III-6. Medically Needy Monthly Protected Income Levels,
Family Size One Through Four, January 1992--Continued

	Family of one	Family of two	Family of three	Family of four
Tennessee	$175	$192	$250	$ 308
Texas	100	211	267	301
Utah	350	430	536	626
Vermont	758	758	900	1,008
Virginia	250	308	358	400
Washington	458	575	650	725
West Virginia	200	275	290	312
Wisconsin	510	592	689	823
Wyoming	NA	--	--	--

[a]Medically needy program eliminated Apr. 1992.

NOTE: NA = not applicable; no medically needy program.

Source: National Governors' Association, 1992.

An individual with income above the applicable medically needy income level may reduce his or her income to the requisite level by spending on medical care. The process by which an individual reduces his or her income to the medically needy income standard is known as the "spenddown." For example, if an individual has monthly income of $550 and the State's income standard is $450, the applicant would be required to incur $100 in medical expenses (i.e., spend-down) before he or she would be eligible for Medicaid. When Medicaid eligibility is triggered, the program will not pay for any of these spenddown expenses.[25]

Medical expenses which are considered spenddown expenses include Medicare premiums and cost sharing charges (for persons eligible for both programs), and expenses for necessary medical and remedial services which are either included under the State's Medicaid program or recognized under State law but not included in the program. The State Medicaid agency may set reasonable limits on the amounts deducted. Excluded from the amounts deducted are expenses subject to payment by a third party, unless the third party is a public program of a State or political subdivision of a State.

States use a time period from 1 month to 6 months in calculating the spenddown. Generally a shorter time period is more beneficial to the applicant. Using the above example, if the State has a 1 month spenddown calculation period, the individual would be required to incur $100 in medical expenses in a month, after which covered services would be paid for by Medicaid. The same calculation and spenddown requirements would apply in the following month. On the other hand, if the State had a 6 month calculation period, the individual would have to incur $600 ($100 x 6) in medical expenses before Medicaid would begin coverage; coverage would continue for the remainder of the 6-month

[25]See also the discussion of the *209(b)* spenddown, subsection II-A-2 below.

period. The length of the calculation period does not significantly affect total out-of-pocket expenditures for persons with predictable and recurring medical expenses. However, individuals faced with acute nonrecurring problems generally benefit more from a shorter calculation period.

OBRA 90 established a "pay-in" option. States may allow applicants, at their option, to establish medically needy eligibility by making payments equal to the difference between their income and the medically needy standard. As of November 1991, DHHS had not issued policy guidelines for this option; one State, Utah, was using this approach to establish eligibility.

b. Resource Standards

States also establish resource standards based on family size. The methodology used in evaluating resources can be no more restrictive than that used for the most closely related cash assistance program (i.e., AFDC or SSI). In March 1992, the resources standard for a family of three ranged from $1,000 in Texas to $10,000 in Iowa. (See table III-7.) Persons with resources in excess of these levels may become eligible if they reduce their resources to these levels. Many persons reduce their resources to these levels by spending the excess amount on medical care.

TABLE III-7. **Medically Needy Resource Standard Levels, Family Size One Through Four, March 1992**

	Family of one	Family of two	Family of three	Family of four
Alabama	NA	--	--	--
Alaska	NA	--	--	--
Arizona	NA	--	--	--
Arkansas	$ 2,000	$ 3,000	$ 3,100	$ 3,200
California	2,000	3,000	3,150	3,300
Colorado	NA	--	--	--
Connecticut	2,000	3,000	3,100	3,200
Delaware	NA	--	--	--
District of Columbia	2,600	3,000	3,100	3,200
Florida[a]	5,000	6,000	6,000	6,500
Georgia	2,000	4,000	4,100	4,200
Hawaii	2,000	3,000	3,250	3,500
Idaho	NA	--	--	--
Illinois	2,000	3,000	3,050	3,100
Indiana	NA	--	--	--
Iowa	10,000	10,000	10,000	10,000
Kansas	2,000	3,000	3,000	3,000
Kentucky	2,000	4,000	4,050	4,100
Louisiana	2,000	3,000	3,025	3,050
Maine	2,000	3,000	3,100	3,200
Maryland	2,500	3,000	3,100	3,200
Massachusetts	2,000	3,000	3,100	3,200
Michigan	2,000	3,000	3,200	3,400
Minnesota	3,750	6,450	6,650	6,850
Mississippi	NA	--	--	--

TABLE III-7. Medically Needy Resource Standard Levels,
Family Size One Through Four, March 1992--Continued

	Family of one	Family of two	Family of three	Family of four
Missouri	NA	--	--	--
Montana	$2,000	$3,000	$3,100	$3,200
Nebraska	4,000	6,000	6,025	6,050
Nevada	NA	--	--	--
New Hampshire	2,500	4,000	4,000	4,000
New Jersey	4,000	6,000	6,100	6,200
New Mexico	NA	--	--	--
New York	3,000	4,300	4,350	5,100
North Carolina	1,500	2,250	2,350	2,450
North Dakota	3,000	6,000	6,025	6,050
Ohio	NA	--	--	--
Oklahoma	2,000	3,000	3,100	3,200
Oregon	2,000	3,000	3,050	3,100
Pennsylvania	2,400	3,200	3,500	3,800
Rhode Island	4,000	6,000	6,100	6,200
South Carolina	4,000	6,000	6,000	6,000
South Dakota	NA	--	--	--
Tennessee	2,000	3,000	3,100	$3,200
Texas	1,000	1,000	1,000	1,000
Utah	2,000	3,000	3,025	3,050
Vermont	2,000	3,000	3,150	3,300
Virginia	2,000	3,000	3,100	3,200
Washington	2,000	3,000	3,050	3,100
West Virginia	2,000	3,000	3,050	3,100
Wisconsin	2,000	3,000	3,300	3,600
Wyoming	NA	--	--	--

ªMedically needy program eliminated Apr. 1992.

NOTE: NA = not applicable; no medically needy program.

Source: HCFA, *Medicaid State Profile Data (spDATA) System: Characteristics of Medicaid State Programs,* May 1992.

D. Capsule Summary

As can be seen from the preceding discussion, there are a variety of ways that pregnant women and children may become eligible for Medicaid protection. Table III-8 presents in capsule form the income levels applicable for key coverage groups by State, as of January 1, 1992. As can be seen from these tables, the mandated coverage of the poverty-related population is a significant factor in expanding program access to pregnant women and young children. Coverage of older children is also improving with the required coverage of all children under age 19, born after September 30, 1983, in families with incomes at or below poverty.

TABLE III-8. Capsule Summary: Monthly Income Eligibility Levels (for a Family of Three) for Pregnant Women and Children, by State, January 1992

State	Payment standard[a]	AFDC levels — Effective eligibility levels for persons with income[b]			Medically needy levels	Poverty level coverage[c]		
		First 4 months	Months 8-12	After 12 months		Pregnant women and infants	Children under age 6	Children born after 9/30/83
Alabama	$149	$ 344	$ 269	$ 239	NA	$1,282	$1,282	$ 964
Alaska	924	1,506	1,044	1,014	NA	1,603[d]	1,603[d]	1,205[d]
Arizona	334	621	454	424	NA	1,350	1,282	964
Arkansas	204	426	324	294	275	1,784	1,282	964
California	694	1,161	814	784	934	1,784	1,282	964
Colorado	421	752	541	511	NA	1,282	1,235	964
Connecticut[e]	680	1,140	800	770	773	1,784	1,282	964
Delaware	338	627	458	428	NA	1,543	1,283	964
District of Columbia	409	734	529	499	545	1,784	1,282	964
Florida	303	575	423	393	303	1,446	1,282	964
Georgia	424	756	544	514	375	1,282	1,282	964
Hawaii	666	1,119	786	756	666	2,052[d]	1,475[d]	1,109[d]
Idaho	315	593	435	405	NA	1,282	1,282	$964
Illinois[e]	367	671	487	457	492	1,282	1,282	964
Indiana	288	552	408	378	NA	1,446	1,282	964
Iowa	426	759	546	516	566	1,784	1,282	964
Kansas[e]	422	753	542	512	470	1,446	1,282	964
Kentucky	526	909	646	616	308	1,784	1,282	964
Louisiana[e]	190	405	310	280	258	1,282	1,282	964
Maine	573	980	693	663	458	1,784	1,282	964
Maryland	377	686	497	467	442	1,784	1,282	964

See notes at end of table.

TABLE III-8. Capsule Summary: Monthly Income Eligibility Levels (for a Family of Three) for Pregnant Women and Children, by State, January 1992—Continued

State	AFDC levels Payment standard[a]	Effective eligibility levels for persons with income[b]			Medically needy levels	Poverty level coverage[c]		
		First 4 months	Months 8-12	After 12 months		Pregnant women and infants	Children under age 6	Children born after 9/30/83
Massachusetts	$539	$929	$659	$629	$775	$1,784	$1,282	$964
Missouri	292	558	412	382	NA	1,282	1,282	964
Montana	390	705	510	480	443	1,282	1,282	964
Nebraska	364	666	484	454	492	1,282	1,282	964
Nevada	372	678	492	462	NA	1,282	1,282	964
New Hampshire	516	894	636	606	616	1,282	1,282	964
New Jersey	424	756	544	514	566	1,784	1,282	964
New Mexico	324	606	444	414	NA	1,784	1,282	964
New York[e]	577	986	697	667	750	1,784	1,282	964
North Carolina	272	528	392	362	367	1,784	1,282	964
North Dakota	401	722	521	491	435	1,282	1,282	964
Ohio	334	621	454	424	NA	1,282	1,282	964
Oklahoma	341	632	461	431	459	1,282	1,282	964
Oregon	460	810	580	550	613	1,282	1,282	964
Pennsylvania[e]	421	752	541	511	467	1,282	1,282	964
Rhode Island	554	951	674	644	741	1,784	1,282	964
South Carolina	440	780	560	530	263	1,784	1,282	964
South Dakota	404	726	524	494	NA	1,282	1,282	964
Tennessee	426	759	546	516	250	1,784	1,282	964
Texas	184	396	304	274	267	1,784	1,282	964

See notes at end of table.

TABLE III-8. Capsule Summary: Monthly Income Eligibility Levels (for a Family of Three) for Pregnant Women and Children, by State, January 1992--Continued

State	AFDC levels					Poverty level coverage[c]		
	Payment standard[a]	Effective eligibility levels for persons with income[b]			Medically needy levels	Pregnant women and infants	Children under age 6	Children born after 9/30/83
		First 4 months	Months 8-12	After 12 months				
Utah	$537	$ 926	$657	$627	$536	$1,282	$1,282	$964
Vermont[e]	673	1,130	793	763	900	1,784	1,282	964
Virginia[e]	354	651	474	444	358	1,282	1,282	964
Washington	531	917	651	621	650	1,784	1,282	964
West Virginia	249	494	369	339	290	1,446	1,282	964
Wisconsin[e]	517	896	637	607	689	1,494	1,282	964
Wyoming	360	660	480	450	NA	1,282	1,282	964

[a]The maximum benefit for persons with no other income is lower than the payment standard in nine States. (See table III-1.)

[b]Assumes no child care expenses and work expenses of $90 per month.

[c]Figures based on annual poverty guidelines published in the *Federal Register*, v. 56, no. 34, Feb. 20, 1991.

[d]Alaska and Hawaii have higher poverty levels than the other States.

[e]In States with different payment levels, the figure shown is for the area with the highest benefit.

NOTE: NA = not applicable; no medically needy program in the State.

Source: Congressional Research Service and the National Governors' Association.

II. AGED[26]

Eligibility for Medicaid is linked to another cash welfare program, the Supplemental Security Income (SSI) program, that defines additional "categories" or groups of persons for whom States must provide health care coverage. One such group is the elderly. Medicaid law generally requires that States cover persons receiving SSI. SSI provides cash assistance to needy aged, blind, and disabled individuals who have little or no income and resources.[27] Since the elderly (defined as persons 65 years of age and older) are one of the groups eligible for SSI, they are also one of the groups States must cover under their Medicaid programs.

This seemingly straightforward "categorical" requirement for eligibility, however, becomes complicated by a variety of different financial standards that States may use in determining whom among their elderly population they actually cover. Medicaid is above all a program of exception and variation, with the result that generalization about eligibility as it applies to a particular individual or the Nation as a whole is difficult.

For example, as already noted, States must *generally* provide coverage to persons receiving SSI; that is, they must cover persons who receive cash assistance because their income and resources meet the nationwide eligibility standards established for SSI. However, Medicaid law gives States the option of using an alternative set of eligibility standards that may be more restrictive than SSI policies, but only if those policies were being used for Medicaid eligibility in 1972 when SSI was enacted. Currently 12 States use these alternative eligibility standards.

Under SSI law, States have the option of supplementing the Federal benefit standard with *State supplement payments* (SSP) that are made solely with State funds. Many States provide these additional cash assistance payments because they feel the SSI benefit standard to be insufficient to cover a person's living expenses; in 1991, the SSI benefit for a single individual represented 74 percent of the Federal poverty level. Medicaid allows States to provide automatic coverage to persons receiving SSP on the same basis as they do for persons receiving SSI only.

The preceding groups might be considered welfare-related paths to eligibility. Medicaid also allows States to cover persons who are not poor by SSI standards, but who need assistance with medical expenses.

---

[26]Tables in the previous section of this chapter were based on 1992 data. This section's tables use 1991 data. Much of the data presented in this section was collected by the National Governors' Association under contract with the Congressional Research Service. These data are not routinely updated, and 1991 is the latest year for which most of this State-level information is available.

[27]For further discussion of the SSI program see: House Ways and Means, *1992 Green Book.*

One of these groups is known as the medically needy. These are persons who have incomes too high to qualify for SSI, but who have incurred medical expenses that deplete their income and resources to levels that make them needy. States are permitted, but not required, to cover the medically needy under their plans. If they decide to cover the medically needy, they must also decide whether they will include the elderly under their programs. In 1991, 37 States had medically needy programs and 35 elected to provide Medicaid coverage to elderly medically needy persons. Many elderly persons meet the financial standards for medically needy coverage as the result of needing nursing home care; not all States, however, cover nursing home care under their medically needy programs. Twenty-nine States with medically needy programs for the elderly included nursing home care as a covered service in 1991. Other States may have decided not to include nursing home care as part of their medically needy programs because to do so would mean an expanded pool of persons eligible for coverage and also because of the cost of this care.

Medicaid also allows States to extend coverage to another group who are not poor by SSI standards, but only if their income does not exceed a certain level *and* they reside in nursing homes or other medical care institutions. The provision in Medicaid law that allows States to cover these persons is often referred to as the "300 percent rule" because the income level used for coverage cannot exceed three times the basic SSI payment level (in 1991, $1,221 per month, and in 1992, $1,266). Some States use only this rule to cover persons needing nursing home care, with the result that if an individual has income in excess of the prescribed standard, they can not receive Medicaid assistance for their care, no matter how insufficient their income may be to cover the costs of their care. This means that a person with monthly income of $1,222 in 1991 and living in a State using only the 300 percent rule would not be able to qualify for Medicaid coverage of their care, even though the cost of their nursing home care was $3,000 a month. The consequences of the 300 percent rule for this person are discussed later in this section.

These varying financial standards for eligibility mean that Medicaid serves a more diverse elderly population than may appear at first to be the case. In addition, because States may elect certain options and not others, the mix of elderly persons actually covered can vary from State to State.

A. Welfare-Related Coverage

1. *Coverage of Persons Receiving SSI*

Most States have decided to provide Medicaid coverage to all elderly persons receiving Federal SSI payments, and in so doing, they use SSI rules as the basis for Medicaid eligibility. In order to qualify for SSI, persons must meet two tests. They must have income, as well as resources, below standards that apply uniformly throughout the Nation.

For 1991, individuals were considered eligible for SSI if their countable income (which includes certain disregards or deductions from gross income, such as the first $20 of monthly Social Security benefits) did not exceed the Federal

SSI benefit of $407 a month, or 74 percent of the Federal poverty level. For couples, income could not exceed $610 a month, or 82 percent of the Federal poverty level. In 1992, these amounts increased to $422 and $633 for individuals and couples, respectively.[28]

In addition, SSI limits the countable resources persons may have in order to qualify for benefits. Countable resources generally refer to liquid assets such as money in bank accounts, stocks and bonds, mutual fund investments, and certificates of deposit. Currently the limit for these resources is $2,000 for an individual and $3,000 for a couple.

Countable resources do not, however, include all resources that an individual or couple may own. They exclude the following:

- a home of any value, as long as it is used as the applicant's principal place of residence;

- up to $2,000 of household goods and personal effects (a wedding ring and an engagement ring are excluded from this limit);

- an automobile with a market value of $4,500 or less;

- the cash surrender value of life insurance to the extent that the total face value of all life insurance policies does not exceed $1,500;

- burial spaces and up to $1,500 per person for burial expenses (reduced by the face value of any excluded life insurance policies);

- certain amounts of property that are essential to self-support; and

- housing assistance provided under certain programs.[29]

Thirty-nine States and the District of Columbia provide Medicaid coverage to persons eligible for SSI. In 32 States, application for SSI also represents an application for Medicaid; if an individual is found eligible for SSI, then that person becomes entitled to Medicaid benefits without any additional action required on the applicant's part. Seven States use SSI rules in determining

---

[28]As is discussed below, many States supplement the basic Federal SSI benefit with a State-funded State supplement payment (SSP). The combined Federal SSI/SSP is the amount that is used for determining eligibility.

[29]Countable resources also exclude: resources of a blind or disabled individual which are necessary to fulfill an approved plan for achieving self-support; certain stock in regional or village corporations held by natives of Alaska; restricted allotted land owned by an enrolled member of an Indian tribe; payments or benefits provided under a Federal statute, other than SSI, where exclusion is required by statute; disaster relief assistance; and SSI and Social Security retroactive payments.

eligibility for Medicaid but require persons to file a separate application for Medicaid.

2. Coverage in 209(b) States

States have an alternative to extending Medicaid coverage to persons receiving SSI. They may use instead the standards they had in place for Medicaid eligibility in 1972 prior to the enactment and implementation of SSI. When SSI was enacted in 1972, certain States expected that the number of elderly and disabled cash assistance recipients would grow significantly. To protect States from potentially large increases in their Medicaid expenditures for the aged and disabled population, section 209(b) of the Social Security Amendments of 1972 (P.L. 92-603) permitted States, at their option, to continue using the financial standards and definitions for disability they had in effect in January 1972 to determine Medicaid eligibility for their aged, blind, and disabled residents, rather than making all SSI recipients automatically eligible for Medicaid.[30]

Currently 12 States use the 209(b) option. Table III-9 shows these "209(b)" States.

TABLE III-9. States Using the 209(b) Option for Medicaid Eligibility, December 1, 1991

Connecticut	Minnesota	North Dakota
Hawaii	Missouri	Ohio
Illinois	New Hampshire	Oklahoma
Indiana	North Carolina	Virginia

Often the financial standards used by 209(b) States are more restrictive than SSI's. For example, 209(b) States may require persons to meet a lower income standard than SSI's or may use more restrictive policies for defining countable income. They may also have lower limits for the amounts of resources a person may have. In certain other cases, a State's standards may be the same as SSI's or even more liberal. When a State's criteria are not particularly more restrictive than SSI's, electing the "more restrictive" 209(b) option allows a State to determine eligibility in a way that corresponds more closely to other State

---

[30]U.S. Library of Congress. Congressional Research Service. *Medicaid Eligibility for the Elderly in Need of Long Term Care.* CRS Report for Congress No. 87-986 EPW, by Edward Neuschler with the assistance of Claire Gill. 152 p. Prepared under Contract No. 86-26 with the National Governors' Association. Center for Policy Research. Health Policy Studies. Washington, Sept. 1987. p. 6. (Hereafter cited as *Medicaid Eligibility for the Elderly in Need of Long Term Care*)

programs and policies, and also does not require the State to adopt all SSI program rules for Medicaid eligibility.[31]

States electing the 209(b) option must allow applicants to deduct medical expenses from income in determining eligibility. This is sometimes referred to as the "209(b) spend-down." For example, if an applicant has a monthly income of $400 (not including any SSI or SSP payments) and the State's income standard is $350, the applicant would become eligible for Medicaid after incurring $50 in medical expenses that month. As will be discussed later, the spend-down process is also used in establishing medically needy eligibility.

3. Coverage of Persons Receiving State Supplement Payments

Many States, recognizing that the SSI benefit standard may provide too little income to meet an individual's living expenses, supplement SSI with additional cash assistance payments. States use a variety of different policies for providing these State supplement payments (SSP).

Some States provide supplemental payments to all persons who receive SSI.[32] States may also make payments to elderly persons living independently in the community without special needs, while others may require that the elderly have special needs, such as requiring in-home personal care assistance or home-delivered meals as the result of impairment or frailty. Many States provide SSP to elderly persons residing in some kind of protected living arrangement, which can range from adult foster care to domiciliary care in a large congregate care facility. Many persons eligible for SSP receive that payment only and do not receive SSI because their other income is too high. In all these cases, States may extend Medicaid coverage to persons receiving SSP on the same basis as they do persons receiving SSI only.

When States provide Medicaid coverage to persons receiving SSP, the combined Federal SSI and State SSP benefit payments can become the effective income eligibility standard. Table III-10 provides an example of what this benefit standard was in 1991 for certain persons receiving SSI/SSP; in this case, elderly persons who had no other income and who lived independently in the community without special needs. Because specified amounts of income are disregarded in determining eligibility for SSI and most State SSP programs, a person with income which exceeds the maximum benefit may still be eligible for cash assistance and Medicaid. For 209(b) States, however, the effective Medicaid income eligibility standards may be below the SSI/SSP standard, because the State uses a more restrictive policy. Note that amounts in table III-10 will be different for persons receiving SSP because they are living in a protected living arrangement, since States generally provide higher supplemental payments to these persons than they do to persons living at home.

---

[31]Ibid., p. 92.

[32]Ibid., p. 80.

TABLE III-10. Maximum Potential SSI and SSP Benefits for Elderly Individuals and Couples Living Independently, January 1991[a]

State	Maximum SSI benefit	
	Individuals	Couples
Alabama	$407	$610
Alaska	756	1,120
Arizona	407	610
Arkansas	407	610
California	630	1,167
Colorado	465	919
Connecticut	766[b]	1,132[b]
Delaware	407	610
District of Columbia	422	640
Florida	407	610
Georgia	407	610
Hawaii	412	619
Idaho	477[c]	654[c]
Illinois	NA[d]	NA[d]
Indiana	407	610
Iowa	407	610
Kansas	407	610
Kentucky	407	610
Louisiana	407	610
Maine	417[e]	625[e]
Maryland	407	610
Massachusetts	536	802
Michigan	438	656
Minnesota	488[f]	742[f]
Mississippi	407	610
Missouri	407	610
Montana	407	610
Nebraska	431	644
Nevada	443	684
New Hampshire	434[g]	631[g]
New Jersey	438	635
New Mexico	407	610
New York	493	713
North Carolina	407	610
North Dakota	407	610
Ohio	407	610
Oklahoma	471	738
Oregon	409	610
Pennsylvania	439	659
Rhode Island	471	731
South Carolina	407	610
South Dakota	422	625
Tennessee	407	610
Texas	407	610
Utah	413	622
Vermont	472[h]	728[h]
Virginia	407	610
Washington	435[i]	632[i]
West Virginia	407	610
Wisconsin	510	776
Wyoming	427	650

TABLE III-10. **Maximum Potential SSI and SSP Benefits for Elderly Individuals and Couples Living Independently, January 1991[a]--Continued**

[a]In most States these maximums apply also to blind or disabled SSI recipients who are living in their own households; but some States provide different benefit schedules for each category.

[b]Individual budget process.

[c]State disregards $20 of SSI payment in determining the State supplementary payment.

[d]State decides benefits on case-by-case basis.

[e]State disregards $55 monthly of SSI payment in determining the State supplementary payment.

[f]Payment level for Hennepin County. State has two geographic payment levels--one for Hennepin County and the other for the remainder of the State.

[g]State disregards $13 of an individual's income in determining the supplementary payment.

[h]State has two geographic payment levels--highest are shown in table.

[i]Sum paid in King, Pierce, Kitsap, Snohomish, and Thurston Counties.

Source: Table prepared by the Congressional Research Service based on data from the Social Security Administration.

States may extend Medicaid coverage to persons who receive SSP only. These persons must meet all SSI eligibility criteria, other than income, and SSP must be available statewide. Table III-11 shows that 34 States, as of January 1, 1991, provided automatic Medicaid coverage to persons receiving only SSP. For those States providing coverage to persons living independently, all but two covered the elderly. All States providing Medicaid to persons living in a group arrangement cover the elderly. Note that States may also cover other population groups eligible for SSI and SSP, namely the blind and disabled, and these groups will be discussed below.

TABLE III-11. States Choosing Medicaid Coverage of State Supplementary
Payments (SSP-Only) Recipients, Covered Populations,
and Living Arrangement Options, January 1991[a]

		Population Covered		
	States choosing optional Medicaid coverage for SSP-only recipients	Living independently	Living in a group arrangement	Individuals receiving federally-administered optional State supplement[b]
Alabama	No			
Alaska[c]	Yes	A,B,D	A,B,D	
Arizona	No			
Arkansas	No			
California	Yes	A,B,D		
Colorado	Yes	A,B,D		
Connecticut	Yes	A,B,D		
Delaware	Yes		A,B,D	
District of Columbia	Yes			X[d]
Florida	No			
Georgia	No			
Hawaii	Yes	A,B,D	A,B,D	
Idaho	Yes	A,B,D		
Illinois	Yes	A,B,D		
Indiana	Yes		A,B,D	
Iowa	Yes	B	A,B,D	
Kansas	No			
Kentucky	Yes	A,B,D	A,B,D	
Louisiana	No			
Maine	Yes	A,B,D	A,B,D	
Maryland	Yes		A,B,D	
Massachusetts	Yes	A,B,D	A,B,D	
Michigan	Yes	A,B,D	A,B,D	
Minnesota	Yes	A,B,D	A,B,D	
Mississippi	No			
Missouri	No	B	A,B,D	
Montana[e]	Yes	A,B,D	A,D	
Nebraska	Yes	A,B,D		
Nevada	Yes	A,B	A,B	

See notes at end of table.

TABLE III-11. States Choosing Medicaid Coverage of State Supplementary Payments (SSP-Only) Recipients, Covered Populations, and Living Arrangement Options, January 1991[a]--Continued

	Population Covered			
	States choosing optional Medicaid coverage for SSP-only recipients	Living independently	Living in a group arrangement	Individuals receiving federally-administered optional State supplement[b]
New Hampshire	Yes	A,B,D		
New Jersey	Yes	A,B,D	A,B,D	
New Mexico	No			
New York	Yes	A,B,D	A,B,D	
North Carolina	Yes		A,B,D	
Texas	No			
Utah	Yes			X[g]
Vermont	Yes	A,B,D	A,B,D	
Virginia	Yes	A,B,D	A,B,D	
Washington	Yes	A,B,D	A,B,D	
West Virginia	No			
Wisconsin	Yes	A,B,D	A,B,D	
Wyoming	No			

[a]States may define specific living arrangements within these broad categories.

[b]All descriptions of federally administered optional State supplement were taken from: Social Security Administration. *State Assistance Programs for SSI Recipients.* Baltimore, Maryland, Jan. 1990.

[c]Alaska does not cover blind and disabled under 18.

[d]Optional supplement provided to all aged, blind and disabled persons who are eligible for SSI payments or would be eligible except for income. No statutory minimum age requirement for receiving adult foster care supplementation, but children receive Medicaid through child welfare services provisions. Recipients in medical facilities who are eligible for Federal payments under section 1611 (e)(1)(E) receive State optional supplementation for up to 2 months.

[e]Montana covers individuals living independently only if they meet the Federal definition for developmental disability.

[f]Optional State supplement provided to SSI recipients living alone or living in household of another. Blind and disabled children are eligible for State supplementation. Recipients in medical facilities who are eligible for Federal payments under section 1611(e)(1)(E) receive State optional supplementation for up to 2 months.

ᵍOptional State supplement provided to SSI recipients who are living alone or with others. Persons living in the household of another receive the same State optional supplement as those living alone. Blind and disabled children are eligible for optional supplementation.

NOTE: A = aged; B = blind; and D = disabled.

Source: National Governors' Association, Jan. 1991.

B. Medically Needy Coverage

The preceding groups might be considered welfare-related paths to eligibility. Medicaid provides States an option for covering elderly persons who are not poor by SSI or SSP standards, but who need assistance with medical care expenses. These persons are referred to as medically needy. They become medically needy by "spending down" or depleting their income and resources on the cost of needed care.

In order to qualify for medically needy coverage, a person must first live in a State that exercises the medically needy option. Thirty-seven States had medically needy programs in January 1991.[33] States are not required to cover the elderly under their medically needy programs, and, in 1991, two States, Arkansas and Texas, did not.[34] In addition to the 35 States covering the elderly under medically needy option, three 209(b) States, which did not have general medically needy programs (Indiana, Missouri, and Ohio), were required as a condition of their electing the more restrictive 209(b) option to have very similar spend-down programs for the elderly. Thus, in 1991, a total of 38 States provided Medicaid coverage to elderly persons who had too much income to qualify for cash assistance but whose income was insufficient to cover their medical expenses.

Persons seeking medically needy coverage for their medical expenses must also deplete their income and resources to specified levels before they can qualify. In practice, persons qualifying for medically needy coverage generally first deplete their resources to the State's eligibility standard, and then continue to incur medical expenses that reduce their income to the level required by the State.[35]

---

[33]Table III-5 in the first section of this report provides information on States' medically needy programs as of Mar. 1992.

[34]Table III-5 indicates that Arkansas began covering the elderly under its medically needy program in 1992.

[35]Tables III-6 and III-7 indicate what these levels were in States with medically needy programs in 1992.

In 1991, the countable resource level for medically needy coverage was often the same as SSI's--$2,000 for an individual and $3,000 for a couple. This means that a person can not have, for example, more than $2,000 in a bank account before qualifying for medically needy coverage.

Income standards for medically needy coverage, however, were often different from SSI's 1991 benefit standard of $407 for a single individual and $610 for a couple. In fact, very often they were lower than SSI's benefit standard. Because States must use a single eligibility standard for all medically needy applicants--families and children as well as the elderly--and because the medically needy income standard by Federal law may be no more than one-third higher than the AFDC payment, the medically needy standard is often lower than the SSI benefit standard for the elderly, and especially for couples. The gap between medically needy income standards and SSI's benefit standard can be expected to grow over time, since the Federal SSI benefit is updated annually for inflation and States are not required, and generally do not, adjust their AFDC payments for inflation.

Many elderly persons qualify for medically needy coverage because they need nursing home care (Medicaid's term for this care is nursing facility care). At an average cost of $30,000 a year, nursing home costs can quickly deplete the resources of an elderly individual, especially after prolonged stays, and they also exceed the monthly income of most persons. States, however, are not required to include nursing facility care among the services covered under their medically needy programs. As a result not all States with medically needy programs covering the elderly provide coverage to persons in nursing homes. Table III-12 indicates that 29 States with medically needy programs for the elderly included nursing home care as a covered service in January 1991. Five other 209(b) States allowed a similar spend-down process for elderly persons in nursing homes.

TABLE III-12. Determining Medicaid Eligbility for Institutionalized Individuals Whose Income Exceeds Cash Assistance Levels, January 1991

State	Qualifies for institutional care through the medically needy program	Income standard used for determining institutional eligibility	States determine eligibility using:		
			Special income eligibility threshold (gross income)	Income eligibility threshold for medically needy (net income)	Income eligibility threshold for 209 (b) States
Alabama	NA	300% SSI	$1,221.00		
Alaska	NA	300% SSI	1,221.00		
Arizona	NA	300% SSI	1,221.00		
Arkansas	NA	300% SSI	1,221.00		
California	Yes	MNIL		$600	
Colorado	NA	300% SSI	1,221.00		
Connecticut	Yes	300% SSI or MNIL	1,221.00	473	
Delaware	NA	210% SSI	854.70		
District of Columbia	Yes	MNIL		407	
Florida	No	300% SSI	1,221.00		

See notes at end of table.

TABLE III-12. Determining Medicaid Eligibility for Institutionalized Individuals Whose Income Exceeds Cash Assistance Levels, January 1991.-Continued

State	Qualifies for institutional care through the medically needy program	States determine eligibility using:		
		Income standard used for determining institutional eligibility	Special income eligibility threshold (gross income)	Income eligibility threshold for medically needy (net income)	Income eligibility threshold for 209 (b) States
Georgia	Yes	300% SSI or MNIL	$1,221.00	$317[a]	
Hawaii	Yes	MNIL		376	
Idaho	NA	300% SSI	1,221.00		
Illinois	No	NMN-SD			NH Rate
Indiana	NA	NMN-SD			NH Rate
Iowa	No	300% SSI	1,221.00		
Kansas	Yes	MNIL		407	
Kentucky	Yes	300% SSI or MNIL	1,221.00	217	
Louisiana	No	300% SSI	1,221.00		

See notes at end of table.

TABLE III-12. Determining Medicaid Eligibility for Institutionalized Individuals Whose Income Exceeds Cash Assistance Levels, January 1991—Continued

State	Qualifies for institutional care through the medically needy program	Income standard used for determining institutional eligibility	States determine eligibility using:		
			Special income eligibility threshold (gross income)	Income eligibility threshold for medically needy (net income)	Income eligibility threshold for 209 (b) States
Maine	Yes	300% SSI or MNIL	1,221.00	416	
Maryland	Yes	MNIL		384	
Massachusetts	Yes	MNIL		522	
Michigan	Yes	MNIL		400	
Minnesota	Yes	MNIL		420[b]	
Mississippi	NA	300% SSI	1,221.00		
Missouri	NA	NMN-SD			NH Rate
Montana	Yes	MNIL		386	
Nebraska	Yes	MNIL or NMN-SD		392	NH Rate
North Dakota	Yes	MNIL		345	

See notes at end of table.

TABLE III-12. Determining Medicaid Eligibility for Institutionalized Individuals Whose Income Exceeds Cash Assistance Levels, January 1991–Continued

State	Qualifies for institutional care through the medically needy program	Income standard used for determining institutional eligibility	States determine eligibility using:		
			Special income eligibility threshold (gross income)	Income eligibility threshold for medically needy (net income)	Income eligibility threshold for 209 (b) States
Ohio	NA	300% SSI or NMN-SD	1,221.00		$350
Oklahoma	No	300% SSI or NMN-SD	1,221.00	275	
Oregon	Yes	300% SSI or MNIL	1,221.00	395	
Pennsylvania	Yes	300% SSI or MNIL	1,221.00	425	
Utah	Yes	300% SSI or MNIL	1,221.00	350	

See notes at end of table.

TABLE III-12. Determining Medicaid Eligibility for Institutionalized Individuals Whose Income Exceeds Cash Assistance Levels, January 1991--Continued

State	Qualifies for institutional care through the medically needy program	Income standard used for determining institutional eligibility	States determine eligibility using:		
			Special income eligibility threshold (gross income)	Income eligibility threshold for medically needy (net income)	Income eligibility threshold for 209 (b) States
West Virginia	Yes	300% SSI or MNIL	1,221.00	200	
Wisconsin	Yes	300% SSI or MNIL	1,221.00	510	
Wyoming	NA	300% SSI	1,221.00		

[a]Georgia uses the medically needy income threshold for a family size of two.

[b]Medically needy income threshold for aged, blind, and disabled individuals.

[c]Tennessee's medically needy program for the aged does not use a single income threshold. Instead the State uses different thresholds for different facilities.

TABLE III-12. Determining Medicaid Eligibility for Institutionalized Individuals Whose Income Exceeds Cash Assistance Levels, January 1991 –Continued

Key

Medically Needy Coverage:

YES   Institutional care is available through the medically needy program.

NO   The State has a medically needy program for aged individuals but does not cover institutional care.

NA   The State does not have a medically needy program for aged individuals.

Income Standard:

MNIL   Medically Needy Income Level.–The institutionalized individual's income is reduced by the cost of institutional care and other allowable medical expenses (i.e., spend-down). If the net income is less than the medically needy income threshold, the individual is Medicaid eligible.

% SSI   A special income standard has been established to determine Medicaid eligibility for institutionalized individuals with income in excess of cash assistance program standards. Under Federal law the special income standard can be no more than 300 percent of the basic SSI payment level.

NMN-SD   Non-Medically Needy Spend-Down.–Nursing home residents who do not qualify for a cash payment may be covered under the "spend-down" process the State is required to implement because it uses Medicaid eligibility rules more restrictive than those used by SSI.

NH Rate   Nursing Home Rate.–The State uses the Medicaid nursing home rate to determine Medicaid eligibility and the individual's contribution to the cost of care in the institution.

% SSI   In some States, an individual may qualify through the medically needy or 209(b) spend-down processes or through a special MNIL or income standard. This enables States to avoid the complex spend-down computation and makes automatically eligible those NMN-SD persons with incomes below the special income standard.

Source: National Governors' Association, 1991.

C. Optional Coverage of Institutionalized Persons Under a Special Income Level--the 300 Percent Rule

States have another option for covering certain individuals with incomes too high to qualify for SSI or SSP. These persons must (1) require care provided by a nursing home or other medical institution, (2) meet the State's resource standard, and (3) have income that does not exceed a specified level. Medicaid law requires that income for these persons be no more than three times the basic SSI payment level. This provision in Medicaid law is often referred to as the *300 percent rule*. For 1991, the limit was $1,221 (3 times $407) and for 1992, it was $1,266. States may use a level that is lower than the maximum of 300 percent of SSI, if they wish.

In order to qualify for coverage under this rule, the applicant's gross income, with no disregards or deductions permitted, must be below the prescribed level. Table III-12 shows States providing coverage for institutional care under the special income rule. In 1991, 35 States used the 300 percent rule or some lower special income level for making persons eligible for institutional care.

Table III-12 indicates that a number of States using the special income rule also had medically needy programs for making persons eligible for institutional care. This enables States to make those persons with incomes below the specified level automatically eligible for coverage, so as to avoid the spend-down computation necessary under medically needy programs when medical expenses and income must be estimated for a 1 to 6 month time period.[36]

Seventeen States used only the 300 percent rule for making persons eligible for institutional care.[37] In these States, without either medically needy programs or medically needy programs covering nursing home care, persons with incomes above the State specified level cannot qualify for Medicaid assistance for the cost of their care, no matter how insufficient their income may be to cover the costs. Depending on the particular State and circumstances of the individual, these persons might end up being discharged from the nursing home or relying on family members to pay the balance of the cost of their care. Alternatively, they might find a nursing home willing to accept available income as payment in full, or be referred to other State or local assistance programs or State-owned nursing homes. In other cases, persons may remain in the community, with or without receiving the care they need.[38]

---

[36]Persons with incomes above the special income level may qualify as medically needy after meeting the spend-down requirements.

[37]These States were: Alabamá, Alaska, Arizona, Arkansas, Colorado, Delaware, Florida, Idaho, Iowa, Louisiana, Mississippi, Nevada, New Jersey, New Mexico, South Dakota, Texas, and Wyoming.

[38]For information about the impact of the 300 percent rule on Florida residents, see: Quadagno, Jill, et al. *Falling into the Medicaid Gap: The Hidden Long-Term Care Dilemma*. Gerontologist, v. 31, no. 4, 1991.

All States, therefore, provide coverage of institutional care for persons with incomes higher than the SSI/SSP levels generally required for coverage of services provided in the community. They do so either through medically needy programs or the 300 percent rule.

D. Optional Coverage for Persons Needing Home and Community-Based Care

States have an option of covering persons needing home and community-based care services, if these persons would otherwise require institutional care that would be paid for by Medicaid. These services are provided under waiver programs authorized in section 1915(c) of Medicaid law.[39] The programs, often referred to as home and community-based care waiver programs, require States to make special application to HCFA for the programs they wish to operate. With approval, they may provide a wide variety of nonmedical, social, and supportive services that have been shown to be critical in allowing chronically ill and disabled persons to remain in their homes. States are using waiver programs to provide services to a diverse long-term care population, including the elderly, and others who are disabled or who have chronic mental illness, mental retardation and developmental disabilities, and AIDS. Waiver programs serving the elderly generally also cover the disabled. As of December 1991, 40 States had waiver programs serving aged/disabled persons. These and other waiver programs covering home and community-based care are discussed in greater detail in *Chapter VI, Alternate Delivery Options and Waiver Programs*.

Under their waiver programs, States may use any or all of the major paths to eligibility that have just been discussed. They may limit coverage to those persons receiving SSI and/or SSP. Alternatively, they may cover persons as medically needy because they incur expenses for home and community-based care services that deplete their financial resources. In addition, they may use the 300 percent rule for persons needing waiver services just as they do for persons requiring institutional care. States may also apply to waiver beneficiaries the spousal impoverishment protections that are discussed below for couples when one of the spouses requires Medicaid coverage of long-term care expenses.

E. Mandatory and Optional Coverage for Additional Elderly Persons

1. Mandatory Coverage for Additional Elderly Persons

States are required to extend Medicaid eligibility to additional groups of elderly persons who may not actually receive SSI, but who are deemed to meet SSI standards. These include:

- *Recipients of Social Security increases after April 1977.* A State must cover former SSI recipients who receive Social Security benefits, butlose their SSI or SSP payments following a Social Security cost-of-

---

[39]Section 1915(d) of Medicaid law also allows States to provide home and community-based care to elderly persons at risk of needing nursing home care.

living increase (COLA), if they would still be eligible for SSI or SSP but for the COLA increase. In a 209(b) State, Medicaid must be provided to these persons when their income (after disregard of the COLA and deduction of incurred medical expenses) falls below the State standard. This provision is sometimes referred to as the Pickle Amendment (P.L. 94-566, section 503).

- *Individuals receiving mandatory State supplements.* States are required to make mandatory State supplementary payments to any individual who would otherwise receive less under SSI than he or she received under the old Federal/State cash assistance programs.

- *Grandfathered 1973 recipients.* Persons eligible in December 1973 (according to rules in effect in that month) as essential spouse, or institutionalized must continue to be covered under Medicaid provided they have continued to meet the December 1973 criteria.

- *Individuals eligible for Medicaid except for the 1972 Social Security increase.* Medicaid must cover individuals who would be eligible for SSI except for the 20 percent increase in Social Security benefits occurring in August 1972. Persons covered under this provision must have been entitled to Social Security and receiving cash assistance on that date.

2. Optional Coverage of Additional Groups

States have the option of extending coverage to certain additional elderly persons. These include:

- *Individuals eligible for SSI but not receiving it.*

- *Institutionalized individuals who would be eligible for cash assistance if they left the institution.*

- *HMO enrollees.* Individual who lose their eligibility while enrolled in certain HMOs or other prepaid plans may be covered for an additional period specified by the State not exceeding 6 months from the date of initial enrollment.

- *Hospice beneficiaries.* States may cover hospice services under their Medicaid programs. In States covering this service, terminally ill individuals who have voluntarily elected to receive hospice care must be covered if they would be eligible for Medicaid if they were in a medical institution.

- *Elderly poor individuals.* States may provide Medicaid coverage to elderly and disabled persons whose incomes do not exceed 100 percent of the Federal poverty level and whose resources do not exceed SSI's standard.[40]

F. Other Eligibility Considerations for the Elderly

1. Personal Needs Allowance

Medicaid has another set of rules for the treatment of income *after* a person has become eligible for coverage. They apply to eligible beneficiaries who have income in excess of cash assistance programs--those who qualify under a medically needy program or the 300 percent rule--and determine how much of the beneficiary's income must be applied to the cost of care before Medicaid makes its payment. These rules are commonly referred to as the *post-eligibility* rules, or more accurately, the post-eligibility treatment of income rules. Often they apply to persons needing long-term care--both nursing home care and home and community-based care.

Post-eligibility rules require that an individual's payment for care equal total income from all sources in a month, minus certain amounts that are set-aside for the personal needs of the beneficiary, the living expenses of a spouse and minor children if those family members have little or no income of their own, and medical care and medical insurance expenses.

For persons in nursing homes and other institutions, Medicaid requires that States reserve from a beneficiary's income a personal needs allowance. This is an amount that is considered reasonable to cover incidental expenses for items not included in the institution's basic charge, e.g., clothing and other personal needs items. Medicaid law requires that States set aside a minimum of $30 per month for individuals and $60 per month for couples.[41] States may set aside

---

[40]According to the *Medicare and Medicaid Guide* published by the Commerce Clearing House and updated through Jan. 1992, the following States were exercising this option for elderly *or* disabled persons: District of Columbia, Florida, Hawaii, Maine, Massachusetts, Nebraska, New Jersey, Pennsylvania, South Carolina. It should be noted that certain States providing Medicaid coverage to persons receiving SSP may end up covering persons with incomes at 100 percent of the Federal poverty level or higher, to the extent that SSP payments provide income at those levels.

[41]Under the Department of Veterans Affairs income-based pension program, the maximum amount of pension payable to Medicaid-eligible veterans who are in nursing homes that participate in Medicaid and who have no dependents was limited to $90. In addition, this $90 monthly pension payment was exempt from State Medicaid rules for personal needs allowances; the full amount of the pension payment was protected for personal needs. These provisions expired Sept. 30, 1992. P.L. 102-568, the Veterans Dependency and Indemnity Compensation Reform Act of 1992, extends these provisions through Sept. 30, 1997, and expands their scope to include Medicaid-eligible surviving spouses with no children.

**TABLE III-13. Amounts Protected for Personal Needs of a
Nursing Home Resident on Medicaid, January 1991**

State	Protected out of resident's income
Alabama	$30.00
Alaska	75.00
Arizona	61.05
Arkansas	30.00
California	35.00
Colorado	34.00
Connecticut	42.00
Delaware	36.00
District of Columbia	60.00
Florida	35.00
Georgia	30.00
Hawaii	30.00
Idaho	30.00
Illinois	30.00
Indiana	30.00
Iowa	30.00
Kansas	30.00
Kentucky	40.00
Louisiana	38.00
Maine	40.00
Maryland	40.00
Massachusetts	45.00
Michigan	32.00
Minnesota	52.00
Mississippi	40.00
Missouri	30.00
Montana	40.00
Nebraska	30.00
Nevada	35.00
New Hampshire	40.00
New Jersey	35.00
New Mexico	30.00
New York	50.00
North Carolina	30.00
North Dakota	45.00
Ohio	30.00
Oklahoma	30.00
Oregon	30.00
Pennsylvania	30.00
Rhode Island	40.00
South Carolina	30.00
South Dakota	30.00
Tennessee	30.00
Texas	30.00
Utah	30.00
Vermont	40.00
Virginia	30.00
Washington	41.62
West Virginia	30.00
Wisconsin	40.00
Wyoming	30.00

Source: National Governors' Association, 1991.

higher amounts if they choose.[42] Table III-13 shows the amount each State protects for an institutionalized resident's personal needs, as of January 1, 1991.

2. Medicaid's Treatment of Income and Resources of Institutionalized Persons with Spouses Still Living at Home

The Medicare Catastrophic Coverage Act of 1988 established new rules for the treatment of income and resources of married couples when one of the spouses requires nursing home care and the other remains in the community. These rules are referred to as the *spousal impoverishment* protections of Medicaid law, because they are intended to prevent the impoverishment of the spouse remaining in the community. Under prior Medicaid law, the spouse remaining at home could actually be impoverished by the institutionalization of the other spouse because the income and resources that belonged to the nursing home spouse were considered available for the cost of care. In addition, amounts that could be set aside for the community spouse often were inadequate to cover basic living expenses and personal needs.[43]

For example, today the income of many elderly couples comes largely from the Social Security and pension benefits that the husband receives because of his work history in the labor force. The wife, who may have had limited or no attachment to the work force, may receive only a small Social Security benefit in her own name. If the husband requires nursing home care and seeks Medicaid coverage for his care under a State's medically needy program, for instance, most States, prior to spousal impoverishment protections, considered the husband's income his for purposes of determining eligibility. They also considered resources held in the husband's name, as well as jointly held resources, to be fully available to him and would require that these resources be spent down to the State's resource standard before considering him Medicaid eligible. In most States, this could mean that the community spouse would have been left only $2,000.

Following eligibility, post-eligibility rules considered the husband's income to be available for the cost of his care, and allowed a deduction to be made for his wife's living expenses only to the extent that her own income did not exceed the standard specified by the State. In most States, this standard was the basic SSI benefit level, or less. This meant that a wife with little or no income of her

---

[42]Institutionalized Medicaid beneficiaries who have no income automatically receive a $30 monthly allowance from SSI, which States may supplement.

[43]In determining how much income and resources belonged to each spouse, Medicaid used SSI's "name on the instrument" rule. Income belonged to the person whose name was on the check and resources to the person whose name was on the account or deed, unless there was evidence to the contrary. Burwell, Brian. *Middle-Class Welfare: Medicaid Estate Planning for Long-Term Care Coverage.* Lexington, Massachusetts, SysteMetrics/McGraw-Hill, Sept. 1991. p. 11.

own would have available for her living expenses an amount less than the Federal poverty level.

Spousal impoverishment law established new income and resource *eligibility* rules as well as *post-eligibility* treatment of income rules for couples when one spouse requires nursing home care and the other remains in the community.

Spousal impoverishment eligibility rules. The new income eligibility rules do not permit income of community spouses to be used in determining the nursing home spouse's eligibility unless the income is actually made available to the institutionalized spouse. Under prior law, income of the community spouse could be counted for up to one month, or indefinitely in a few States.

Spousal impoverishment resource eligibility rules provide for a new method of counting a couple's resources in initial eligibility determinations. They apply to persons entering nursing homes on or after September 30, 1989. Under the new rules, States must assess a couple's combined countable resources, when requested by either spouse, at the beginning of a continuous period of institutionalization, defined as at least 30 consecutive days of care.[44] The Health Care Financing Administration's (HCFA) guidance on implementing spousal impoverishment law requires that nursing homes advise people entering nursing homes and their families that resource assessments are available upon request. The couple's home, household goods, and personal effects are excluded from countable resources. In addition, 209(b) States may not use more restrictive policies for defining these resources under spousal impoverishment law.

From the combined resources, an amount is protected for the spouse remaining in the community. This amount is the greater of an amount equal to *one-half* of the couple's resources *at the time the institutionalized spouse entered the nursing home,* up to a maximum of $66,480 in 1991, or the State standard. As of January 1, 1991, Medicaid law required the State resource standard to be no lower than $13,296 and no greater than $66,480. These amounts are adjusted to reflect increases in the Consumer Price Index (CPI).[45] On January 1, 1992, the minimum became $13,740 and the maximum $68,700. Table III-14 shows State spousal resource standards for 1991. When the community spouse's half of the couple's combined resources is less than the State standard, the institutionalized spouse may transfer resources to the community spouse to bring that spouse up to the State standard. In other cases,

---

[44]States may charge a reasonable fee for making assessments of a couple's resources when assessments are not made in conjunction with an application for Medicaid eligibility.

[45]These minimum and maximum amounts are increased for each calendar year after 1989 by the percentage increase in the CPI for all urban consumers between September 1988 and the September before the calendar year involved. Higher amounts than the maximum can be protected if required under a court order.

the community spouse may be required to apply resources to the nursing home spouse's cost of care.

TABLE III-14. Spousal Impoverishment: State Protected Income and Resource Amounts, January 1, 1991

State	Community spouse's monthly protected income allowance minimum[a]		Community spouse's protected resource minimum
	Income	Percent of poverty	
Alabama	$ 856	122	$25,000
Alaska	1,662	237	66,480
Arizona	856	122	13,296
Arkansas	856	122	13,296
California	1,662	237	66,480
Colorado	856	122	13,296
Connecticut	856	122	13,296
Delaware	1,662	237	13,296
District of Columbia	856	122	13,296
Florida	985	141	66,480
Georgia	1,662	237	66,480
Hawaii	1,662	237	66,480
Idaho	856	122	13,296
Illinois	1,662	237	66,480
Indiana	856	122	13,296
Iowa	1,662	237	24,000
Kansas	856	122	13,296
Kentucky	1,662	237	66,480
Louisiana	1,662	237	66,480
Maine	856	122	13,296
Maryland	856	122	13,296
Massachusetts	856	122	13,296
Michigan	856	122	13,296
Minnesota	857	122	13,296
Mississippi	1,662	237	66,480
Missouri	856	122	13,296
Montana	856	122	13,296
Nebraska	856	122	13,296
Nevada	856	122	13,296
New Hampshire	856	122	13,296
New Jersey	856	122	13,296
New Mexico	856	122	31,290
New York	1,662	237	66,480
North Carolina	856	122	13,296
North Dakota	1,662	237	66,480
Ohio	856	122	13,296
Oklahoma	1,662	237	25,000
Oregon	856	122	13,296
Pennsylvania	856	122	13,296
Rhode Island	856	122	13,296
South Carolina	1,662	237	66,480
South Dakota	1,662	237	20,000
Tennessee	856	122	13,296
Texas	1,662	237	13,296

See notes at end of table.

TABLE III-14. Spousal Impoverishment: State Protected Income
and Resource Amounts, January 1, 1991--Continued

State	Community spouse's monthly protected income allowance minimum[a]		Community spouse's protected resource minimum
	Income	Percent of poverty	
Utah	$ 856	122	$13,296
Vermont	1,200	171	66,480
Virginia	856	122	13,296
Washington	1,258	179	66,480
West Virginia	856	122	13,296
Wisconsin	1,662	237	66,480
Wyoming	1,662	237	66,480

[a]The minimum income amount a State protects for the community spouse when determining the institutionalized individual's contribution to institutional care. The minimum required by Federal law is 122 percent of the Federal poverty level for a couple, or $856. However, in all States the minimum may be set as high as $1,662. On July 1, 1991, the minimum protected income allowance increased to 133 percent, and on July 1, 1992, it increased to 150 percent of the Federal poverty level for a couple.

[b]The minimum resource amount protected for the community spouse when determining the couple's contribution to institutional care. The minimum allowed by Federal law is the greater of $13,296 or one-half the couples assets, up to $66,480. However, a State may set a minimum as high as $66,480. These amounts are adjusted for increases in the Consumer Price Index.

Source: National Governors' Association, 1991.

Three examples will help illustrate how resources are protected for the spouse in the community. One couple, living in a State that protected $13,296 for the community spouse in 1991, had total countable resources of $20,000. One-half of the couple's total resources is attributed to each spouse, and in this case, the community spouse's share equals $10,000. This amount is less than the State's standard of $13,296, and is also less than the maximum of $66,480. In this example, the nursing home spouse may transfer to the community spouse $3,296 to bring that spouse up to the State's standard. The nursing home spouse must spend down his (or her) remaining share of $6,704 ($10,000 minus $3,296) to the State's resource standard for a single individual, generally $2,000, before he (or she) may become resource eligible.[46]

---

[46]In this example, spousal impoverishment law could be more restrictive than previous policy. If the couple's $20,000 of resources were jointly owned, as a bank account, for instance, either party could withdraw any amount on his or her own signature without the other party's consent. When ownership was in this form, Medicaid (through SSI rules) considered the account to be fully available to the applicant, because the applicant had access to the entire amount in the account. However, the nonapplicant co-owner also had full access to the
(continued...)

The protected amount for the community spouse would be different for a couple having $20,000 of combined resources and living in a State that had established its standard at $20,000, as opposed to $13,296. The community spouse's share of $10,000 is less than the State's standard of $20,000. In this case, all of the nursing home spouse's share of resources could be transferred to the community spouse, because the State had decided to protect $20,000 for the community spouse. The nursing home spouse would become resource eligible for Medicaid coverage with the transfer.

Another couple had total resources of $150,000 in 1991 and lived in a State that protected $66,480. One-half of their combined resources equals $75,000. However, the State's standard protected only $66,480 for the community spouse, the maximum that may be protected under Medicaid law. In this case, the community spouse would be required to transfer to the nursing home spouse $8,520 ($75,000 minus $66,480), to be applied to the cost of nursing home care. The nursing home spouse would have to spend down this amount and most of the other half of their combined resources before becoming eligible for Medicaid.

Spousal impoverishment post-eligibility rules. Spousal impoverishment law also established new post-eligibility rules for determining how much of the nursing home spouse's income must be applied to the cost of care. The new rules require that States recognize a minimum maintenance needs allowance for the living expenses of the community spouse. As of January 1, 1991, this minimum was set at 122 percent of the Federal poverty level for a couple, or $856 per month. On July 1, 1991, the minimum protected income allowance increased to 133 percent of the Federal poverty level ($984 per month at that time and $1,019 per month beginning January 1, 1992), and on July 1, 1992, it increased again to 150 percent of the Federal poverty level for a couple ($1,149 per month). These amounts may be increased, depending on the amount of the community spouse's actual shelter costs and whether minor or dependent adult children or certain other persons are living with the community spouse.[47]

---

[46](...continued)
account. If the nonapplicant co-owner withdrew any or all of the $20,000 of funds from the account, SSI would not consider the withdrawal to be a potentially disqualifying transfer (discussed below) unless the applicant took part in or consented to the transfer. Thus the community spouse could retain the full $20,000, rather than the $13,296 of this example.

[47]The minimum monthly maintenance needs allowance for the community spouse equals or exceeds the sum of (1) effective Sept. 30, 1989, 122 percent of the Federal poverty level for a family of two; effective, July 1, 1991, 133 percent of the Federal poverty level for a family of two; and effective July 1, 1992, 150 percent of the Federal poverty level for a family of two; and (2) an excess shelter allowance, defined as the amount by which rent or mortgage expenses, taxes and insurance, and in the case of a condominium or cooperative, required maintenance charge, plus utility costs, exceed 30 percent of the preceding amount. Additional amounts may be protected for family members (a minor or dependent child, dependent parent or dependent sibling residing with the community spouse). Higher amounts may be protected when ordered by a court.

However, the total amount that may be recognized for the maintenance needs allowance could not exceed $1,662 as of January 1, 1991.[48] Table III-14 indicates amounts States recognized for the monthly maintenance needs of the community spouse in January 1991.

To the extent that income of the community spouse does not meet the State's maintenance need standard and the institutionalized spouse wishes to make part of his or her own income available to the community spouse, the nursing home spouse may supplement the income of the community spouse to bring that spouse up to the State standard. For example, the husband of a couple was institutionalized in 1991 and received Social Security and pension income amounting to $900 a month. His wife received a Social Security check of $350 a month. They resided in a State with a maintenance needs standard of $856 a month. Under spousal impoverishment rules, income paid solely to one spouse or the other is considered as belonging to that respective spouse.[49] Because the community spouse's income was less than the State's income standard, the nursing home spouse may have deducted from his income $506 ($856 minus $350) to bring the community spouse up to the State's maintenance need standard.[50]

3. Maintenance Needs Standards for Persons Receiving Home and Community-Based Care Services

As noted above, States may apply more liberal income eligibility standards, e.g., the 300 percent rule, to persons qualifying for home and community-based waiver services. When that is the case, beneficiaries may become responsible for paying some portion of the costs of their care, after deductions are made for living expenses in the community. Table III-15 shows amounts of income and resources that States protected, as of January 1, 1991, for persons receiving waiver services.

For individuals, five States protected less income than the 1991 SSI benefit standard of $407, eight States protected the SSI benefit level, and 27 States protected amounts greater than SSI's standard. For resources, States generally protected SSI levels.

Note that in a number of States, the beneficiary and ineligible spouse are not treated as a couple, and the spouse's income is treated separately from the applicant's income. In this case, the ineligible spouse's income is not "deemed" to the other spouse requiring home and community-based care services. Under

---

[48]This amount increases for each calendar year after 1989 by the percentage increase in the CPI for all urban consumers between September 1988 and the September before the calendar year involved. As of Jan. 1, 1992, this maximum became $1,718.

[49]If income is paid in both names, half is considered available to each spouse.

[50]This deduction would be made after a deduction had been made for the nursing home spouse's personal needs allowance.

SSI and Medicaid eligibility rules, income and resources of the applicant's spouse are automatically considered available, or deemed, to the individual requiring care when that person is living in the same household as the ineligible spouse. If the spouse requiring care were institutionalized, on the other hand, only the applicant's own financial resources would be considered available for care after the first month in the institution. These deeming rules have presented eligibility barriers for persons who need long-term care and who can be served in the community. Under waiver programs, States may waive the deeming requirements that would otherwise apply to couples.

States also have the option of applying spousal impoverishment protections to the ineligible spouse of a beneficiary receiving waiver services. As of January 1, 1991, five States--Iowa, Kentucky, New York, Ohio, and Rhode Island--used spousal impoverishment rules for couples when one spouse receives waiver services. More States may choose to do so as they seek renewals for their waiver programs.[51]

TABLE III-15. Amount of Income and Resources Individuals Receiving
Home and Community-Based Services Are Permitted To Retain
for Maintenance Needs, January 1991

| State | Program standard | Maintenance needs | | | |
| | | Income family size | | Resources family size | |
		One	Two	One	Two
Alabama	SSI	$ 407.00	$814.00	$2,000.00	$4,000.00
Alaska	NA				
Arizona[a]	300% SSI	1,221.00		2,000.00	
Arkansas	NA				
California	MNIL	600.00	750.00	2,000.00	3,000.00
Colorado	SSI + St. supp.	452.00	681.00	2,000.00	3,000.00
Connecticut[a]	State est. rate	1,662.00		1,600.00	
Delaware[a]	SSI + St. Supp.	547.00		2,000.00	3,000.00
District of Columbia	NA				

See notes at end of table.

___

[51]Conversation with HCFA officials in Oct. 1991.

TABLE III-15. Amount of Income and Resources Individuals Receiving
Home and Community-Based Services Are Permitted To Retain
for Maintenance Needs, January 1991--Continued

State	Program standard	Maintenance needs			
		Income family size		Resources family size	
		One	Two	One	Two
Florida[a]	100% FPIL	523.33		2,000.00	3,000.00
Georgia	SSI	407.00	610.00	2,000.00	3,000.00
Hawaii	100% FPIL	603.00	850.00	2,000.00	3,000.00
Idaho[a]	NH rate	819.00		2,000.00	
Illinois	MNIL + $25	308.00	383.00	2,000.00	3,000.00
Indiana	SSI[b]	387.00	579.00	1,500.00	2,250.00
Iowa[a]	300% SSI	1,221.00	c	2,000.00	3,000.00[c]
Kansas	SSI	407.00	460.00	2,000.00	3,000.00
Kentucky	SSI + St. supp.	427.00	610.00[c]	2,000.00	4,000.00[c]
Louisiana	SSI	407.00	610.00	2,000.00	3,000.00
Maine	SSI + St. supp.	417.00	834.00	2,000.00	3,000.00
Maryland	NA				
Massachusetts	NR				
Michigan	NA				
Minnesota	MNIL	466.00	582.00	3,000.00	6,000.00
Mississippi	SSI	407.00	610.00	2,000.00	3,000.00
Missouri	SSI	407.00	610.00	999.99	2,600.00
Montana[a]	MNIL	400.00		2,000.00	
Nebraska[a]	MNIL	433.00		2,000.00	3,000.00
Nevada[a]	200% SSI	814.00		2,000.00	
New Hampshire[a]	300% SSI[b]	1,028.00		1,500.00	
New Jersey[a]	300% SSI	1,221.00		2,000.00	
New Mexico[a]	State est. rate	1,043.00		2,000.00	
New York[a]	State est. rate	500.00	c	3,000.00	c

See notes at end of table.

TABLE III-15. Amount of Income and Resources Individuals Receiving Home and Community-Based Services Are Permitted To Retain for Maintenance Needs, January 1991--Continued

State	Program standard	Income family size One	Income family size Two	Resources family size One	Resources family size Two
North Carolina	MNIL	242.00	317.00	1,500.00	2,250.00
Rhode Island	MNIL	558.33	600.00[c]	2,000.00	4,000.00[c]
South Carolina[a]	300% SSI	1,221.00		2,000.00	
South Dakota[a]	SSI + St. supp.	422.00	829.00	2,000.00	3,000.00
Tennessee[a]	SSI	407.00		2,000.00	
Texas	NA				
Utah	NA				
Vermont[a]	MNIL	766.00		2,000.00	3,000.00
Virginia[a]	SSI	407.00		2,000.00	3,000.00
Washington[a]	MNIL	458.00		2,000.00	
West Virginia[a]	300% SSI	1,221.00		2,000.00	
Wisconsin[a]	SSI + St. supp.	611.00		2,000.00	
Wyoming	NA				

[a]For the purpose of determining eligibility for home and community-based waiver recipients, these States treat the waiver recipient as an individual, regardless of family size.

[b]1990 SSI standard.

[c]Spousal impoverishment rules apply for waiver recipients living with a noneligible spouse. Income and resource amounts, if shown, apply only to a family of two consisting of a recipient and dependent.

NA = No waiver for the aged.
NR = No response.
SSI = 1991 SSI income level.
MNIL = The State's threshold for their medically needy program.
FPIL = Federal poverty income level.
St. Supp. = State supplement to SSI.
NH Rate = The State's nursing home rate calculated monthly.

Source: National Governors' Association, 1991.

4. Transfer of Assets

Medicaid requires States to prohibit persons seeking Medicaid coverage of their institutional or home and community-based care costs from transferring resources for less than fair market value during the 30-month period prior to their application for coverage. Spouses of such persons are also prohibited from transferring resources for less than fair market period during this same period. If a transfer has occurred, States must establish a period of ineligibility beginning with the month the resources were transferred. The actual length of the period of ineligibility is determined by comparing the cost of care and the value of the assets transferred. The number of months in the period equals 30 months, or a shorter period if fewer months result when the total uncompensated value of the transferred resource is divided by the average monthly cost to a private patient of nursing facility services in the State, or in the community in which the person is institutionalized. For purposes of the prohibition on transfer of assets, resources mean cash or other liquid assets or any real or personal property that an individual (or spouse, if any) owns and could convert to cash to be used for support and maintenance.

The transfer prohibition does not apply if:

- The transfer was that of the applicant's home to: his or her spouse; child under 21; blind or disabled adult child; or sibling who has an equity interest in the home and who was residing in the home for at least a year prior to the individual's admission to the institution; or a son or daughter who was residing in the home for at least 2 years prior to the beneficiary's admission to the nursing home and was providing care that delayed institutionalization of the beneficiary.

- Resources were transferred to the community spouse or to the individual's child who is blind or permanently and totally disabled.

- A satisfactory showing is made either that the individual intended to dispose of resources at fair market value or for other valuable consideration or that resources were transferred for a purpose other than to qualify for Medicaid.

- The State determines that the denial of eligibility would work an undue hardship.

States are not permitted to have a more restrictive or less restrictive policy on transfer of assets than that just described.

5. Liens

A lien is a legal right to hold property or have it sold or applied for payment of a claim. States are barred, except under certain circumstances, from placing a lien on the property of a Medicaid beneficiary prior to his death because of Medicaid claims correctly paid on his behalf. However, States may place a lien at any time on both real and personal property following a court judgment that claims were incorrectly paid (e.g., for a person who should not have been eligible for Medicaid).

A State may place a lien on real property of institutionalized Medicaid beneficiaries who, when the State determines after notice and opportunity for hearing, are reasonably likely to remain in a nursing home for the remainder of their lives. States may not place a lien on the home of a beneficiary if the spouse or child under 21 or blind or disabled child is residing in the home. Further, the State may not place a lien if the beneficiary has a sibling in the home who has an equity interest in the home and was residing there continuously for at least 1 year prior to the beneficiary's admission to the facility. Any lien dissolves if the individual is discharged from the medical institution and returns home.

A State may not make an adjustment or recover funds in satisfaction of a claim against a recipient's property except: (a) from the estate of a beneficiary who was 65 or older at the time the service was rendered; or (b) from the estate or upon the sale of the property subject to a lien when the individual is institutionalized. A foreclosure action may not be taken until after the death of the surviving spouse and/or any children who are under 21 or are blind or disabled. Further, when a lien has been imposed on an individual's home, the State may not foreclose on the property if: (a) a sibling residing in the home has lived there for at least 1 year prior to the beneficiary's institutionalization; or (b) a beneficiary's adult child residing in the home has lived there for at least 2 years prior to the beneficiary's admission to the nursing home and was providing care that delayed institutionalization of the beneficiary. The lien provisions allow States to recoup certain expenses only when the beneficiary no longer needs the resources.

III. THE DISABLED AND BLIND[52]

In addition to the elderly, Medicaid covers two other groups of persons because of their link to the SSI program. SSI provides cash assistance to needy disabled and blind individuals who have little or no income and resources. Because the disabled and blind are groups of persons eligible for SSI, they are also categories of individuals States must cover under their Medicaid programs.

SSI law defines disabled individuals as those who are unable to engage in any substantial gainful activity by reason of a medically determined physical or mental impairment expected to result in death, or that has lasted or can be expected to last for a continuous period of at least 12 months. The blind are persons with 20/200 vision or less with the use of a correcting lens in the person's better eye, or those with tunnel vision of 20 degrees or less.

---

[52]This section makes reference to tables based on 1991 data. Much of the data in these tables was collected by the National Governors' Association under contract with the Congressional Research Service. These data are not routinely updated, and 1991 is the latest year for which most of this State-level information is available.

In addition, SSI law provides that certain persons may be considered presumptively disabled or blind and authorizes SSI benefits for a period of 3 months before a final judgement on disability or blindness has been made. Examples of impairments which may warrant a finding of presumptive disability or presumptive blindness include amputation of two limbs, allegations of total deafness, blindness, bed confinement, stroke, Down's syndrome, and certain manifestations of HIV infection (but not asymptomatic infection).

The general rules for coverage of the disabled and blind under Medicaid are exactly the same as those described above for the elderly. If persons meet SSI's definitions for disability or blindness and have income that does not exceed the Federal SSI benefit standard and countable resources that do not exceed $2,000 for an individual and $3,000 for a couple, then they are eligible for SSI cash payments. States may provide Medicaid coverage to all disabled and blind individuals receiving SSI. States may also exercise the 209(b) option of using more restrictive eligibility standards for the disabled and blind, if these standards were in place for Medicaid eligibility in 1972 prior to the enactment of SSI. These standards may include more restrictive definitions of disability or blindness, as well as lower thresholds or more restrictive definitions of income and resources.

States may also extend Medicaid coverage to disabled and blind persons qualifying for SSP. Table III-11 above shows that, among those States providing Medicaid coverage to persons receiving SSP only and living independently, most cover all aged, blind, and disabled persons. Two States (Iowa and Missouri) however, provide coverage only for blind persons and one State (Nevada) covers only the blind and elderly. For persons in a group living arrangement and receiving SSP only, one State (Montana) covers only the disabled and elderly, and another State (Nevada) covers only the blind and elderly.

States may also provide Medicaid coverage to medically needy disabled and blind persons, that is, persons who have income in excess of SSI/SSP standards, but who need assistance with medical care expenses. In 1991, 35 States covered the disabled and blind under their medically needy programs, and three 209(b) States, which did not have general medically needy programs, were required to allow the disabled and blind to spend down for coverage. (See table III-5 above.)

Finally States may use the 300 percent rule for extending Medicaid coverage to disabled and blind persons. Persons qualifying under this rule must require care provided by a nursing home or other medical institution and can not have income that exceeds three times the SSI benefit standard. They may also qualify for coverage because they can be served with home and community-based care under a waiver program.

A. Special Eligibility Rules for the Disabled and Blind

1. Mandatory Continuation Coverage of Working Blind and Disabled Persons

SSI and Medicaid law contain provisions that are intended to remove work disincentives for the disabled and blind receiving SSI.

Under SSI, the Secretary of DHHS is required to prescribe criteria for determining when employment or earnings from employment demonstrate an individual's ability to engage in substantial gainful activity (SGA). Current regulations provide that average countable earnings of over $500 a month over an extended period, generally not less than 6 months, indicate that an individual is able to engage in SGA. If persons *applying* for SSI have demonstrated the ability to engage in SGA, they will not be able to establish SSI disability status.[53]

SSI, however, applies special rules to disabled and blind persons who are already *receiving SSI and who are also working*. These provisions are contained in section 1619 of SSI law. Section 1619(a) provides for the continuation of special SSI cash benefits for those persons receiving SSI on the basis of *disability* even if they are working at the SGA level, as long as there is not a medical improvement in the disabling condition. The amount of their special cash benefits is gradually reduced as their earnings increase under an income disregard formula until their countable earnings reach the SSI benefit standard or what is known as the *break even point*. For these persons, the earned income eligibility limit was $899 per month in 1991.[54] People who receive special SSI benefits under this provision continue to be eligible for Medicaid on the same basis as regular SSI recipients.

Under section 1905(q) of Medicaid law, States must also continue Medicaid coverage for "qualified severely impaired individuals under the age of 65." These are *disabled and blind* individuals whose earnings would take them past the SSI income disregard breakeven point.[55] This special eligibility status applies as long as the individual: (1) continues to be blind or have a disabling impairment; (2) except for earnings, continues to meet all the other requirements for SSI eligibility; (3) would be seriously inhibited from continuing or obtaining employment if Medicaid eligibility were to end; and (4) has earnings that are not sufficient to provide a reasonable equivalent of benefits from SSI, SSP (if

---

[53]Current law, however, provides for a deduction from earnings of extraordinary impairment-related work expenses, for purposes of determining whether an individual is able to engage in SGA.

[54]In addition to the earned income disregards, impairment-related work expenses of disabled persons are not counted in determining regular SSI or special SSI benefits.

[55]A virtually identical provision is contained in section 1619(b) of SSI law.

provided), Medicaid, and publicly funded attendant care that would have been available in the absence of those earnings.

In implementing the fourth criterion, the Social Security Administration decided to compare the individual's gross earnings to a "threshold" amount that represents average expenditures for Medicaid benefits for disabled SSI cash recipients in the individual's State of residence. The impact of this provision is to establish a higher income standard for continued Medicaid eligibility.

2. *Optional Coverage of Noninstitutionalized Disabled Children*

Medicaid's deeming rules have presented eligibility barriers for disabled children who could be provided needed care in their homes. For a child under the age of 21 and living at home, the income and resources of the child's parents are automatically considered available for medical care expenses; they are "deemed" to the child. If the same child is institutionalized, however, after the first month away from home, the child no longer is considered to be a member of the parents' household and only the child's own financial resources are considered available for care. The child then is able to qualify for Medicaid.

To obtain Medicaid coverage, some individuals remained in institutions, even though their medical needs could be met in the home. This situation was dramatized in 1982 by the case of Katie Beckett. Katie Beckett was a ventilator-dependent institutionalized child who was unable to go home, not because of medical reasons but because she would no longer have been eligible for Medicaid.

Medicaid law contains a provision, sometimes referred to as the *Katie Beckett provision*, that allows States to extend Medicaid coverage to certain disabled children under 18 who are living at home and who would be eligible for Medicaid if in a hospital, nursing facility, or intermediate care facility for the mentally retarded. The State must determine that: (1) the child requires the level of care provided in an institution; (2) it is appropriate to provide care outside the facility; and (3) the cost of care at home is no more than institutional care.

States electing this option are required to cover on a statewide basis all disabled children who meet these criteria. As of January 1992, the following States offered this coverage: Arkansas, Delaware, Georgia, Idaho, Maine, Massachusetts, Michigan, Minnesota, Nebraska, Nevada, Pennsylvania, Rhode Island, South Dakota, Vermont, West Virginia, and Wisconsin.[56]

States may also cover disabled and blind children and adults under home and community-based care waivers, as discussed above and in *Chapter VI, Alternate Delivery Options and Waiver Programs*.

---

[56]Data compiled from the *Medicare and Medicaid Guide*, Commerce Clearing House, Medicaid State charts updated through Jan. 1992.

B. Mandatory Coverage for Additional
Disabled and Blind Persons

States are required to extend Medicaid eligibility to additional groups of disabled and blind persons who may not actually receive SSI, but who are deemed to meet SSI standards. These include:

- *Recipients of Social Security increases after April 1977.* A State must cover former SSI recipients who receive Social Security benefits, but lose their SSI or SSP payments following a Social Security cost-of-living increase (COLA), if they would still be eligible for SSI or SSP but for the COLA increase. In a 209(b) State, Medicaid must be provided to these persons when their income (after disregard of the COLA and deduction of incurred medical expenses) falls below the State standard. This provision is sometimes referred to as the Pickle Amendment.

- *Disabled widows and widowers receiving increases under 1983 amendments.* The Social Security Amendments of 1983 made certain changes with respect to calculation of benefits for certain disabled widows and widowers; as a result, payments were increased for some persons. A State must cover under Medicaid disabled widows and widowers whose benefits were increased and who would be eligible for SSI and/or optional SSP payments except for the revised calculation and subsequent COLA adjustments. Persons affected by this provision were required to file a Medicaid application prior to July 1, 1988.

- *Retention of Medicaid for certain widows and widowers.* An individual who would otherwise qualify for SSI on the basis of disability or blindness, but beginning at age 60 qualifies for Social Security early widow's or widower's benefits may lose SSI. Effective July 1, 1988, these persons are deemed eligible for Medicaid until they qualify for Medicare.

- *Disabled adult children.* Effective July 1, 1987, States are required to cover persons who: (a) are at least 18 years old and received SSI benefits on the basis of blindness or disability that began before age 22; (b) become entitled to Social Security child's benefits or an increase in such benefits on the basis of disability; and (c) cease to be eligible for their SSI benefits (and related Medicaid eligibility) because of insurance benefits or increase in benefits.

- *Individuals receiving mandatory State supplements.* States are required to make mandatory State supplementary payments to any individual who would otherwise receive less under SSI than he or she received under the old Federal/State cash assistance programs.

- *Grandfathered 1973 recipients.* Persons eligible in December 1973 (according to rules in effect in that month) as disabled, blind, essential spouse, or institutionalized must continue to be covered under

Medicaid provided they have continued to meet the December 1973 criteria.

- *Individuals eligible for Medicaid except for the 1972 Social Security increase.* Medicaid must cover individuals who would be eligible for SSI except for the 20 percent increase in Social Security benefits occurring in August 1972. Persons covered under this provision must have been entitled to Social Security and receiving cash assistance on that date.

C. Optional Coverage of Additional Groups

States have the option of extending coverage to certain additional disabled and blind persons. These include:

- *Individuals eligible for SSI but not receiving it.*

- *Institutionalized individuals who would be eligible for cash assistance if they left the institution.*

- *HMO enrollees.* Individual who lose their eligibility while enrolled in certain HMOs or other prepaid plans may be covered for an additional period specified by the State not exceeding 6 months from the date of initial enrollment.

- *Hospice beneficiaries.* States may cover hospice services under their Medicaid programs. In States covering this service, terminally ill individuals who have voluntarily elected to receive hospice care must be covered if they would be eligible for Medicaid if they were in a medical institution.

- *Disabled poor individuals.* States may provide Medicaid coverage to elderly or disabled persons whose incomes do not exceed 100 percent of the Federal poverty level and whose resources do not exceed SSI's standard.[57]

---

[57]According to the *Medicare and Medicaid Guide* published by the Commerce Clearing House and updated through Jan. 1992, the following States were exercising this option for elderly *or* disabled persons: District of Columbia, Florida, Hawaii, Maine, Massachusetts, Nebraska, New Jersey, Pennsylvania, South Carolina. It should be noted that certain States providing Medicaid coverage to persons receiving SSP may end up covering persons with incomes at 100 percent of the Federal poverty level or higher, to the extent that SSP payments provide income at those levels.

IV. PARTIAL COVERAGE

Medicaid provides partial coverage for three defined population groups: qualified Medicare beneficiaries (QMBs), qualified disabled and working individuals (QDWIs), and COBRA continuation beneficiaries. An additional population group--specified low-income Medicare beneficiaries--will be added in 1993. Persons meeting the qualifications for coverage under one of these categories, but not otherwise eligible for Medicaid, are not entitled to the regular Medicaid benefit package. Instead, they are entitled to have Medicaid make specified payments in their behalf.

A. Qualified Medicare Beneficiaries (QMBs)

A qualified Medicare beneficiary (QMB) is an aged or disabled Medicare beneficiary whose income is at or below 100 percent of poverty, and whose resources are at or below 200 percent of the SSI limit. Medicaid is required to pay Medicare premiums and cost sharing charges for these persons. Medicaid protection is limited to payment of these charges, unless the beneficiary is otherwise eligible for benefits under the program.

Persons meeting the QMB definition must be entitled to Medicare Part A (hospital insurance) coverage. Included is the relatively small group of aged persons who are not automatically entitled to Part A coverage, but who have bought Part A protection by paying a monthly premium. Not included are working disabled persons who have exhausted Medicare Part A entitlement but who have extended their coverage by payment of a monthly premium.

To be eligible as a QMB, an individual must have income at or below 100 percent of the Federal poverty line for a family of the same size.[58] The determination of income is made in the same manner as is made for SSI. Individuals with income above the threshold are not permitted to spenddown to meet the eligibility criteria.

In 1992, the Federal poverty level is $6,810 for a single and $9,190 for a couple. The Federal poverty level is published annually (usually in mid-February) in the *Federal Register*. Cost-of-living increases (COLAs) in Social Security benefits are disregarded in determining QMB eligibility through the month following the month in which the annual update is published. Thus, in most years COLAs are disregarded through March. For QMBs without Social Security income, the poverty levels are effective as of the date of publication.

A QMB must also meet specified resources standards, namely resources cannot exceed 200 percent of that allowed under SSI. For the QMB program, the limits are $4,000 for an individual and $6,000 for a couple. SSI rules govern

---

[58] A 209(b) State which as of Jan. 1, 1987 used an income level lower than the SSI level was allowed an extra year to phase-in coverage of persons up to 100 percent of poverty. These States were required to cover persons at or below 95 percent of poverty in 1991 and at or below 100 percent of poverty beginning in 1992.

the determination of countable resources; thus certain items such as an individual's home and household goods are always excluded from the calculation.

Medicaid pays Medicare premiums and cost-sharing charges for QMBs, as follows:

- Medicare Part B monthly premiums ($31.80 in 1992). Medicare Part B pays for physicians' services and other medical services. Almost all persons entitled to Medicare Part A are also enrolled in Medicare Part B.[59]

- Medicare Part A monthly premium paid by the limited number of aged not automatically entitled to Part A protection. The premium is $192 in 1992.

- Coinsurance and deductibles under Medicare Part A and Part B. This includes the Medicare hospital deductible ($652 in 1992), the Part B deductible ($100) and the Part B coinsurance (20 percent of Medicare's approved payment amount). The State sets the actual amount of Medicaid payment. (See discussion of payment rules in *Chapter V, Reimbursement*.) A State may require QMBs to pay nominal cost-sharing charges, subject to the same restrictions as are applicable to cost-sharing charges imposed on the categorically needy. (See *Chapter IV, Services*.) Medicaid's actual payment plus any Medicaid copayment paid by the QMB is considered payment in full for Medicare coinsurance and deductibles.

  A QMB may not be billed for any physicians' charges which exceed Medicare's recognized payment amount (so-called *balance billing*).

- Coinsurance and deductibles that HMOs and competitive medical plans (CMPs) charge their enrollees. These are in lieu of the Medicare coinsurance and deductibles which would be paid if the individuals were not enrollees of these plans. States, at their option may also pay the HMO and CMP enrollment premiums.

Many persons meeting QMB criteria are also eligible for regular Medicaid coverage. These persons are entitled both to Medicaid payment for Medicare premiums and cost-sharing charges and to the full range of Medicaid services otherwise available to them (as either categorically needy or medically needy).

---

[59]States may enroll QMBs and pay Medicare Part B premiums under the State buy-in process. (See *Chapter V, Reimbursement* for a discussion of the buy-in.) They may also pay any applicable Part A premiums for QMBs in this manner. Payment of premiums through the buy-in process is advantageous to the State because premiums paid in this manner are not subject to any penalties for late enrollment or reenrollment which might otherwise apply.

A May 1991 survey of the implementation of the QMB program by Families USA indicated that many potentially eligible seniors were not receiving program benefits because they were not aware of its existence. The organization stated that QMB benefits were reaching less than half of the four million seniors with incomes below poverty. At the time, DHHS indicated that it was attempting to expand QMB public awareness activities.[60]

As of October 1992, Medicare reported that there were 189,914 Medicare Part A beneficiaries for whom QMB payments were being made. As of the same date, States reported a total of 3,962,175 Part B buy-ins[61] of which 1,329,998 were separately identified as QMBs; however this later number is low due to reporting problems. (See table III-16.) The QMB numbers include many persons who were eligible for the full Medicaid benefit package.

TABLE III.16. Qualified Medicare Beneficiaries by State, October 1992

State	Part A QMBs	Part B buy-ins	Part B QMBs only
Alabama	1,606	106,259	19,096
Alaska	324	5,028	2
Arizona	174	33,832	23,609
Arkansas	4,751	71,324	9,155
California	20,753	674,710	38,513
Colorado	192	39,710	15,034
Connecticut	520	28,431	17,690
Delaware	441	4,970	881
District of Columbia	495	12,937	51
Florida	39,734	216,417	24
Georgia	10,971	140,895	34,259
Hawaii	1,403	12,403	1,305

[60]Application for QMB benefits must be made at the State office that determines Medicaid eligibility. Some observers have suggested that if Social Security offices performed this function, more potential eligibles would enroll in the QMB program. However, DHHS has noted that while the Social Security Administration can assist in public awareness activities, it does not have the capability of making complete income eligibility determinations.

[61]This number includes *all* Part B buy-ins. Some Part B buy-ins are not QMBs. For a discussion of the dual eligible population, see *Chapter V, Reimbursement*.

TABLE III.16. Qualified Medicare Beneficiaries by State, October 1992
--Continued--

State	Part A QMBs	Part B buy-ins	Part B QMBs only
Idaho	320	10,506	6,210
Illinois	2,385	109,601	87,315
Indiana	2,548	67,784	40,765
Iowa	1,676	43,999	21,031
Kansas	57	29,804	8,617
Kentucky	991	82,791	21,463
Louisiana	4,305	96,730	20,775
Maine	2	24,252	8,008
Maryland	5,510	52,100	46,939
Massachusetts	8,513	91,111	77,827
Massachusetts Bl.	18	2,048	14
Michigan	1,424	102,190	2
Minnesota	1,997	43,844	29,469
Mississippi	6,912	95,859	78,029
Missouri	336	61,221	47,042
Montana	397	9,002	3,955
Nebraska	1	13,313	0
New Hampshire	4	4,326	1,154
New Jersey	616	101,972	70,427
New Mexico	30	25,513	4,016
New York	56	268,306	24,016
North Carolina	6,813	133,032	50,403
North Dakota	3	4,997	1,001
Ohio	4,436	13,654	84,651
Oklahoma	5,527	54,700	53,857
Oregon	14	33,200	20,115
Pennsylvania	14,301	137,002	114,502
Rhode Island	1,205	12,282	1,638
South Carolina	110	86,261	26,931

TABLE III.16. Qualified Medicare Beneficiaries by State, October 1992
--Continued--

State	Part A QMBs	Part B buy-ins	Part B QMBs only
South Dakota	725	10,446	4,339
Tennessee	9,189	124,155	44,290
Texas	15,514	259,664	65,839
Utah	25	11,646	5,172
Vermont	356	9,360	2,896
Virgin Islands	0	836	3
Virginia	525	88,249	21,973
Washington	3,783	60,450	34,739
West Virginia	4,004	32,282	12,669
Wisconsin	3,107	68,778	19,098
Wyoming	213	4,101	1,308
Northern Marianas	0	318	0
Guam	0	552	0
Total	189,914	3,962,175	1,329,998

Source: Based on State level data contained in: Health Care Financing Administration. *Medicare Premium Billing File.* Billing Cycle, Oct. 1992.

B. Specified Low-Income Medicare Beneficiaries

Beginning in 1993, States will be required to pay Medicare Part B premiums for persons meeting the QMB criteria except for income. The income limit for these specified low-income beneficiaries is 110 percent of the Federal poverty line in 1993, rising to 120 percent of the Federal poverty line beginning in 1995. Medicaid protection is limited to payment of monthly Part B premiums unless the beneficiary is otherwise eligible for benefits under the program. Medicare Part B premiums are set at $36.60 in 1993, $41.10 in 1994, and $46.10 in 1995.

C. Qualified Disabled and Working Individuals (QDWIs)

Medicare allows certain disabled persons to buy Medicare Part A (Hospital Insurance) protection. These are individuals who were previously entitled to Medicare Part A on the basis of a disability, who lost their entitlement based on earnings from work, but who continue to have the disabling condition. Medicaid is required to pay the Medicare Part A premium for such individuals if their incomes are below 200 percent of the Federal poverty line, their resources are below 200 percent of the SSI limit, and they are not otherwise eligible for

Medicaid. These persons are known as qualified disabled and working individuals (QDWIs).

Income and resources eligibility is determined using the methodologies of the SSI program. States are permitted to impose a premium for individuals with incomes between 150 percent and 200 percent of the poverty level. The premium is to be based on a percentage of the Medicare Part A premium according to a sliding scale increasing in reasonable increments as an individual's income increases.

Medicaid benefits for QWDIs are limited to payment of Medicare Part A premiums.

D. Qualified COBRA Continuation Beneficiaries

Federal law requires employers (with 75 or more employees) that offer a group health plan to offer employees the option to elect continuation coverage under certain conditions, such as termination of employment. The premium for such coverage may generally not exceed 102 percent of the amount otherwise applicable. This option was originally established under the Consolidated Omnibus Budget Reconciliation Act of 1985, and is therefore known as the COBRA continuation provision.

State Medicaid programs have the option of paying COBRA continuation premiums in the case of individuals with incomes below poverty and with resources below 200 percent of the SSI limit.[62] Medicaid payment may only be made if the State determines that the cost of COBRA premiums is likely to be less than the Medicaid expenditures for an equivalent set of services. The methodology for making this cost effectiveness determination must be approved by DHHS.

Medicaid benefits for this population group are limited to payment of COBRA premiums, unless the individual is otherwise eligible for Medicaid.

V. OTHER CONDITIONS AND CRITERIA

A. Citizenship

1. *General Requirements*

A State's Medicaid program must cover otherwise eligible residents if they are either citizens or aliens lawfully admitted for permanent residence or permanently residing in the United States under color of law (e.g., certain aliens admitted pursuant to the discretionary authority of the Attorney General).

A State's Medicaid plan is also required to cover treatment for emergency medical conditions for illegal aliens and for persons in lawful temporary resident

---

[62]Unlike the case for QMBs and QWDIs, 209(b) States are permitted to use their more restrictive eligibility methodologies for this population.

status who otherwise meet the program's eligibility criteria. An emergency medical condition is defined as a medical condition (including emergency labor and delivery) manifesting itself by acute symptoms of sufficient severity (including severe pain) such that the absence of immediate medical attention could reasonably be expected to result in placing the patient's health in serious jeopardy, serious impairment to bodily functions, or serious dysfunction of any bodily organ or part.

Effective October 1, 1988, all Medicaid applicants must declare in writing, under penalty of perjury, that they are a citizen or national of the U.S., or an alien in a satisfactory immigration status. In addition, States are required to verify with the Immigration and Naturalization Service (INS), the immigration status of all aliens applying for Medicaid through the INS's designated system, Systematic Alien Verification for Eligibility (SAVE). This requirement does not apply to aliens seeking treatment for emergency medical conditions.

2. Lawful Temporary Resident Aliens

The Immigration Reform and Control Act of 1986 (IRCA, Public Law 99-603) provides that aliens who have lived continuously in the U.S. since January 1, 1982 may apply for legalization. If their status is adjusted to lawful temporary resident status (LTR), they are not immediately eligible for Medicaid unless the following conditions are met. They must meet all the financial and categorical criteria for Medicaid coverage. Further, they must be under 18, or a Cuban-Haitian entrant, or aged, or blind, or disabled as defined under the SSI program.

An LTR alien who meets the financial and categorical criteria, but does not fall into one of these specified groups, is only eligible for emergency services or services for pregnant women. These persons may be eligible for the full range of benefits beginning 5 years after the date they are granted LTR status.

B. Residence

A State's Medicaid program must cover otherwise eligible residents of the State. An individual is generally considered a resident of a State if he or she is living in it with the intention of remaining there permanently or indefinitely. Eligibility may not be denied because an individual has not resided in the State for a specified period or because the individual is temporarily absent from the State. A State is also prohibited from denying coverage to an individual who satisfies the residency rules but who did not establish residence in the State before entering an institution.

A State is required to reimburse for services provided to its residents in another State in the following circumstances:

• Medical services are needed because of a medical emergency;

• Medical services are needed and the beneficiary's health would be endangered if he were required to travel to his State of residence;

- The State determines, on the basis of medical advice, that the needed medical services or necessary supplementary resources are more readily available in another State; or

- It is general practice for beneficiaries in a particular locality to use medical resources in another State.

C. Homeless

Homelessness does not automatically qualify an individual for Medicaid. A homeless person must still meet the program's eligibility criteria. However, a State may not exclude from coverage any otherwise eligible individual who resides in the State, regardless of whether or not the residence is maintained permanently or at a fixed address. States are required to provide a method of making eligibility cards available to eligible individuals who do not reside in a permanent dwelling or do not have a permanent home or mailing address.

CHAPTER IV. SERVICES[1][2]

SUMMARY

State Medicaid programs provide payments for a specified group of medical services when these are provided to program beneficiaries. As noted in the previous chapter, within Federal guidelines, each State defines the eligible population. Similarly, within Federal guidelines, each State defines its own benefit package. Thus, there is considerable variation among the States in types of services covered and the amount of care provided under specific service categories.

Medicaid law draws a distinction between services States are required to cover and those they may elect to cover. In order to receive any Federal matching payments for any Medicaid services, States are required to offer coverage for a core group of services (including hospital and physicians' services) provided to the categorically needy. These services are referred to as "mandatory services." In addition, States may receive Federal matching funds for additional services offered to the categorically needy; these services are referred to as "optional services."[3] Federal law also places certain requirements on the types of services States are required to cover if they have elected to have a medically needy program. These requirements are different from those applicable for the categorically needy. The services States cover under their Medicaid plans are generally medical in nature. Personal care or supportive services are generally not included unless they are provided under a waiver.

States may place certain limits on the coverage of all services. For example, they may place limits on the number of covered hospital days[4] or the number of covered physician visits.

---

[1]This chapter was written by Jennifer O'Sullivan.

[2]The discussion in this chapter is based on the requirements contained in Federal law (section 1905 of the Social Security Act) and regulations (42 C.F.R. Part 440).

[3]The distinction between mandatory and optional services may not necessarily reflect the relative importance of a particular service for a particular beneficiary.

[4]Public Law 100-360 prohibits States (effective July 1, 1989) from imposing limits on the number of covered hospital days with respect to infants receiving services in hospitals serving a disproportionate number of low-income patients.

Despite this flexibility, States do have to meet the following four additional requirements in designing their benefit packages:

Amount, duration, and scope. Each covered service must be sufficient in amount, duration, and scope to reasonably achieve its purpose. The State may not arbitrarily deny or reduce the amount, duration, or scope of services solely because of the type of illness or condition. The State may place appropriate limits on a service based on such criteria as medical necessity.[5]

Comparability. The services available to any categorically needy beneficiary in a State must generally be equal in amount, duration, and scope to those available to any other categorically needy beneficiary in the State. Similarly, services available to an individual in a covered medically needy group must be equal in amount, duration, and scope to those available to all persons in the covered medically needy group.

Statewideness. Generally, a State plan must be in effect throughout an entire State, that is the amount, duration, and scope of coverage must be the same statewide.

Freedom-of-Choice. Beneficiaries may obtain services from any institution, agency, pharmacy, person, or organization that undertakes to provide the services and is qualified to perform the services.

The Secretary may waive applicability of these requirements under certain circumstances.[6]

States are permitted to impose nominal cost-sharing charges, with certain major exceptions, in connection with the use of covered services.

I. REQUIRED COVERAGE

A. General Requirements

All States are required to offer coverage to the categorically needy for a specified group of services which are referred to as "mandatory services." The following are mandatory services:

---

[5]The Medicaid law authorizes Federal matching for "necessary medical services." It also requires States to provide methods and procedures to safeguard against unnecessary utilization of care and services. (See *Chapter VII, Administration*). Unlike Medicare, the Medicaid statute does not contain a specific exclusion of services not "medically necessary" for diagnosis and treatment.

[6]See discussion of waivers in *Chapter VI, Alternate Delivery Options and Waiver Programs*.

- inpatient hospital services,
- outpatient hospital services,
- rural health clinic services,
- federally qualified health center services,
- other laboratory and x-ray services,
- nursing facility (NF) services for individuals 21 or older,
- early and periodic screening, diagnostic and treatment (EPSDT) services for individuals under age 21,
- family planning services,
- physicians' services,
- home health services for any individual entitled to NF care,
- nurse-midwife services (to the extent nurse midwives are authorized to practice under State law or regulation), and
- services of certified nurse practitioners and certified family nurse practitioners (to the extent these individuals are authorized to practice under State law or regulation).

States may also offer coverage to the categorically needy for any of a broad range of additional services which are referred to as "optional services." Optional services include such items as prescribed drugs, dental services, clinic services, eyeglasses, and physical therapy. (See section II in this chapter for a description of both mandatory and optional services.)

Federal law also places certain requirements on the types of services States are required to cover if they have elected to have a medically needy program. These requirements are different from those applicable to the categorically needy.[7] States having medically needy programs are required, at a minimum, to offer the following:

- Prenatal and delivery services for pregnant women;
- Ambulatory services for individuals under 18 and individuals entitled to institutional services;
- Home health services for individuals entitled to NF services; and
- If the State provides coverage for medically needy persons over age 65 or under 21 in institutions for mental diseases or coverage for the medically needy in intermediate care facilities (ICFs) for the mentally retarded, it is required to cover either the same services as those which are mandatory for the categorically needy (except certified nurse practitioners' services) or alternatively the care and services listed in 7 of the 21 paragraphs in the law defining covered mandatory and optional services.

The coverage available to the categorically needy may not be less than that offered to the medically needy. States do, however, have the option of offering a more restrictive package for this latter group.

---

[7]A service which is mandatory for the categorically needy population is almost always labelled "mandatory," even if it is not mandatory for the medically needy population in the State.

Federal matching is not available for services provided to inmates of public institutions (except for medical institutions). Further, Federal matching is not available for services provided in a mental hospital to individuals aged 22-64.

B. Special Provisions

Special requirements are applicable for the scope of services which must be offered to certain population groups.[8]

"Qualified Medicare beneficiaries" (QMBs) are aged and disabled Medicare beneficiaries with incomes below the Federal poverty line and countable resources below $4000 for an individual. State Medicaid programs are required to pay Medicare's cost-sharing charges for this population group. States are not required to provide additional services to a QMB unless the individual is otherwise eligible for Medicaid in the State.

"Qualified disabled and working individuals" (QDWIs) are disabled, but employed individuals, who are entitled to enroll in the Medicare part A hospital insurance program. Medicaid coverage of these persons is limited to payment of Medicare's part A premium charge for QDWIs with incomes below 200 percent of the Federal poverty line and countable resources below $4,000 for an individual.

State Medicaid programs have the option of paying Consolidated Omnibus Budget Reconciliation Act (COBRA) continuation premiums in the case of individuals with incomes below poverty and with resources below 200 percent of the supplemental security income (SSI) limit. Medicaid payments may only be made if the State determines that the cost of COBRA premiums is likely to be less than the Medicaid expenditures for an equivalent set of services.

II. COVERED SERVICES

This section includes a brief description of the types of services covered under State Medicaid programs. The first subsection describes the mandatory services, while the second section describes the optional services.

A. Mandatory Services

The following services are "mandatory services" and are defined in law and regulations as follows:[9]

- *Inpatient hospital services* (other than services in an institution for mental diseases). Federal regulations specify that: (1) the services must be of the type ordinarily furnished in a hospital to inpatients; (2) the facility must be licensed or formally approved as a hospital by an

---

[8]See *Chapter III, Eligibility* for a description of these population groups.

[9]The services in this section are generally listed in the order they appear in the law.

officially designated authority for State standard-setting; (3) the facility must meet the requirements for participation in Medicare (except in the case of medical supervision of nurse mid-wife services); (4) the care and treatment of inpatients must be under the direction of a physician or dentist (except in the case of nurse mid-wife services); and (5) the facility must have in effect an approved utilization review plan, applicable to all Medicaid patients (unless a waiver has been granted by the Secretary).

- *Outpatient hospital services.* Federal regulations specify that: (1) the services are preventive, diagnostic, therapeutic, rehabilitative, or palliative services that are furnished to outpatients; (2) the services must be provided under the direction of a physician or dentist (except in the case of nurse mid-wife services; (3) the facility must be licensed or formally approved as a hospital by an officially designated authority for State-standard setting; and (4) the facility must meet the requirements for participation in Medicare (except in the case of medical supervision of nurse mid-wife services).

- *Rural Health Clinic (RHC) services.* A RHC is a facility providing health services in a rural area with a shortage of personal health services or a shortage of primary medical care manpower. RHC services are mandatory consistent with State law permitting such services. Each RHC must be under the medical direction of a physician and must have a nurse practitioner or physician assistant on its staff. Services may be furnished by a physician, physician assistant, nurse practitioner, nurse midwife, or other specialized nurse practitioner. Part-time or intermittent visiting nurse care and related medical supplies are included if the Secretary determines there is a shortage of home health agencies in the area, the services are furnished by nurses employed by the clinic, and the services are furnished under a written plan of treatment to a homebound recipient. Also covered are other ambulatory services furnished by a rural health clinic.

- *Federally Qualified Health Center (FQHC) services.* A FQHC is a center receiving a grant under Section 329, 330 or 340 of the Public Health Service Act (migrant and community health centers and health centers for the homeless) or an entity receiving funds through a contract with a grantee. The term also includes an entity determined by the Secretary to meet the requirements for receipt of Federal funds with respect to need and community impact, the health services provided, governance, and management and finance. The term FQHC includes an outpatient health program or facility operated by a tribe or tribal organization under the Indian Self-Determination Act.

The FQHCs provide comprehensive primary and preventive health services to medically underserved populations. They may also provide supplemental services such as health education or mental health services appropriate to the needs of the population served.

The FQHCs are required to serve Medicaid beneficiaries. State Medicaid programs are required to cover ambulatory services that are offered by a FQHC and included in a State's plan. As of January 1992, 73 nonfederally funded health centers had been designated FQHCs.

- *Other laboratory and x-ray services.* These are professional and technical laboratory and radiologic services which are: (1) ordered and provided by or under the direction of a physician or other licensed practitioner of the healing arts within the scope of his practice as defined by State law or ordered and billed by a physician but provided by an independent laboratory; (2) provided in an office or similar facility other than a hospital outpatient department or clinic; and (3) provided by a laboratory that meets Medicare conditions for coverage.

- *Nursing Facility (NF) services.*[10] The NFs are institutions which provide (1) skilled nursing care and related services for residents who require medical or nursing care; (2) rehabilitation services for the rehabilitation of injured, disabled or sick persons; or (3) on a regular basis, health-related care and services to individuals who because of their mental or physical condition require care and services (above the level of room and board) which can be made available to them only through institutional facilities. Nfs are required to meet a number of requirements relating to provision of services, residents' rights, and administration. (See *Chapter VII, Administration* for a discussion of these requirements.)

  The NF services, other than services in an institution for mental disease, are mandated for individuals age 21 or older.

- *Early and Periodic Screening, Diagnostic, and Treatment (EPSDT) services.* States must offer EPSDT services to persons under age 21. Under the EPSDT benefit, a State must provide screening, vision, hearing and dental services at intervals which meet recognized standards of medical and dental practice established after consultation with recognized medical and dental organizations involved in child health care. The State must also provide for medically necessary screening, vision, hearing and dental services at such other intervals indicated as medically necessary to determine the existence of certain physical or mental illnesses or conditions.

---

[10]Prior to October 1, 1990, Medicaid covered services in skilled nursing facilities (SNFs) and ICFs. The Omnibus Budget Reconciliation Act of 1987 (OBRA 87) eliminated, effective October 1, 1990, the distinction between SNFs and ICFs and established a new NF benefit. Nursing services, including what were previously optional ICF services, are mandatory. All nursing facilities participating in Medicaid must meet a single set of requirements relating to the provision of services, resident's rights, administration, and other matters. OBRA 87 made no changes in Medicaid law requirements for ICFs for the mentally retarded (ICFs/MR) or institutions for mental disease.

Minimum screening services include a comprehensive health and developmental history (including assessment of both physical or mental illnesses or conditions), comprehensive unclothed physical exam, appropriate immunizations according to age and health history, and laboratory tests (including lead blood level assessment appropriate for age and risk factors), and health education. Minimum vision services and hearing services include diagnosis and treatment for defects including eyeglasses or hearing aids. Minimum dental services include relief of pain and infection, restoration of teeth and maintenance of dental health.

Any service which a state may cover under Medicaid that is necessary to treat or ameliorate a defect, physical or mental illness, or a condition identified by a screen must be provided to EPSDT participants regardless of whether the service is otherwise included under the State's Medicaid plan.

- *Family planning services.* This category includes services and supplies for women of child bearing age, including minors who can be considered to be sexually active, who desire such services and supplies.[11] (Abortions are excluded from family planning services.)[12]

- *Physicians' services.* Physicians' services must be furnished by or under the personal supervision of a licensed doctor of medicine or osteopathy, and must be within the scope of practice of medicine or osteopathy as defined under State law. The services are covered whether provided in the office, patient's home, a hospital, NF, or elsewhere. Also included are medical and surgical services furnished by a dentist: (1) to the extent such services may be performed under State law either by a physician or by a doctor of dental surgery or dental medicine; and (2) if they would be covered as a physician's service if furnished by a physician.

- *Home health services.* These services must be provided to any individual entitled to NF care. They are defined as services provided at an individual's place of residence (not including a hospital or NF). Services must be provided on a physician's orders as part of a written plan of care that is reviewed by a physician every 60 days. Home health services include three mandatory services (part-time nursing, home health aide, and medical supplies and equipment) and one

---

[11]Medicaid coverage for sterilizations is only available if: the individual is 21, is not mentally incompetent, and has voluntarily given informed consent for the procedure. Hysterectomies are not covered if the purpose of the procedure is to render the woman permanently incapable of reproducing.

[12]As noted, abortions are not covered as family planning services. Federal matching payments for abortions have been limited, by language in the Department's appropriations bills, to cases where the life of the mother is in danger.

optional service (physical therapy, occupational therapy, and speech pathology and audiology services) as follows:

- *Part-time nursing.* These are nursing services provided on a part-time or intermittent basis by a home health agency. If there is no agency in the area, the services may be provided by a registered nurse who is currently licensed to practice in the State, receives written orders from the patient's physician, documents the care and services provided, and has had orientation to acceptable clinical and administrative record keeping from a health department nurse.

- *Home-health aide.* These services are provided by a home health agency.

- *Medical supplies and equipment.* These are items suitable for use in the home. Medical supplies include catheters, syringes, and surgical dressings. Equipment includes oxygen equipment.

- *Physical therapy, occupational therapy, and speech pathology and audiology services.* These services may be provided by a home health agency or by a facility licensed by the State to provide medical rehabilitation services.

A home health agency is defined as an agency or organization that meets the requirements for participation in Medicare.

Effective October 1, 1994, the term home health services will include personal care services which are: (1) prescribed by a physician to an individual in accordance with a written plan of care; (2) provided by a person qualified to provide the service who is not a member of the individual's family; (3) supervised by a registered nurse; and (4) furnished in a home or other location, excluding services provided to an inpatient or a NF resident.

- *Nurse-midwife services.* States are required to provide coverage for these services to the extent the nurse-midwife is authorized to practice under State law or regulation. The services are covered whether or not the nurse-midwife is under the supervision of or associated with a physician or other health care provider.

- *Certified pediatric nurse practitioner or certified family nurse practitioner.* States are required to provide coverage for these services to the extent the practitioner is authorized to practice under State law or regulation. The services are covered whether or not the certified pediatric nurse practitioner or certified family nurse practitioner is under the supervision of or associated with a physician or other health care provider.

B. Optional Services

In addition to those services which have been labelled mandatory, States may offer coverage for a broad range of other medical services. The Health Care Financing Administration (HCFA) has identified a total of 31 optional service categories. Table IV-1 shows, effective October 1991, the number of States electing to provide each service for their categorically needy population, and, if applicable, for both their categorically needy and medically needy populations. As can be seen from the table, virtually all States cover certain service categories such as prescription drugs, clinic services, ICF services for the mentally retarded, and optometrists' services. A more limited number of States have elected to provide coverage under some other service categories, for example, respiratory care services. Table IV-2 shows, as of October 1991, the optional services covered by each State both for their categorically needy and, if applicable, their medically needy populations.

TABLE IV-1. Optional Medicaid Services and Number of
States[a] Offering Each Service as of October 1, 1991

Service	States offering service to categorically needy only	States offering service to both categorically and medically needy	Total
Podiatrists' services	12	33	45
Optometrists' services	14	36	50
Chiropractors' services	8	19	27
Other practitioners' services	13	32	45
Private duty nursing	8	20	28
Clinic services	15	40	55
Dental services	12	36	48
Physical therapy	11	31	42
Occupational therapy	8	26	34
Speech, hearing and language disorder	11	29	40
Prescribed drugs	16	38	54
Dentures	8	31	39
Prosthetic devices	14	38	52
Eyeglasses	16	33	49
Diagnostic services	5	21	26
Screening services	4	19	23
Preventive services	3	20	23
Rehabilitative services	12	33	45
Services for age 65 or older in mental institution:			
A. Inpatient hospital services	14	26	40
B. NF services	11	22	33
ICF services for mentally retarded	21	28	49
Inpatient psychiatric services for under age 21	10	29	39
Christian Science nurses	1	2	3
Christian Science sanitoria	4	11	15
NF for under age 21	20	30	50
Emergency hospital services	14	28	42
Personal care services	9	19	28
Transportation services	14	37	51
Case management services	10	33	43
Hospice services	9	24	33
Respiratory care services	3	11	14

[a]Includes the territories. Thus, maximum number is 56.

Source: U.S. Dept. of Health and Human Services, 1991.

MEDICAID SERVICES STATE BY STATE

October 1, 1991

Basic Required Medicaid Services

Medicaid recipients receiving federally-supported financial assistance must receive at least these services:
- Inpatient hospital services
- Outpatient hospital services
- Rural health clinic (including federally-

qualified health center) services
- Other laboratory and x-ray services
- Nurse Practitioners' services
- Nursing facility (NF) services and home health services for individuals age 21 and older

- Early and periodic screening, diagnosis, and treatment (EPSDT) for individuals under age 21
- Family planning services and supplies
- Physicians' services
- Nurse-Midwife services

Federal financial participation (FFP) is also available to States electing to expand the Medicaid programs to cover additional services, and individuals eligible for medical but not for financial assistance.

Although States must assure the availability of necessary transportation, they may seek FFP as an optional service and/or administrative cost. Definitions and limitations on eligibility and services vary from State to State.

Details are available from local welfare offices and State Medicaid agencies. Services provided only under the Medicare buy-in agreement or the EPSDT program are not shown on this chart.

Optional Services in State Medicaid Programs*

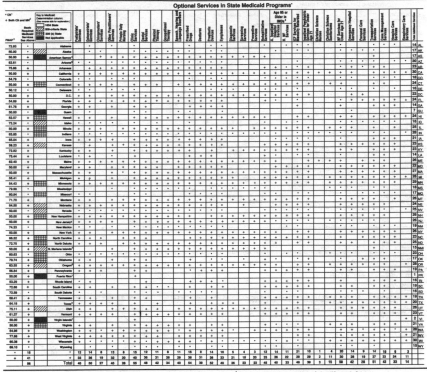

[1] Categorically Needy (CN): Individuals receiving federally-supported financial assistance.
   Medically Needy (MN): Individuals who are eligible for medical but not for financial assistance.
[2] Federal Medical Assistance Percentage (FMAP): Rate of Federal Participation in a State's Medical Assistance Program under Title XIX of the Social Security Act. Effective October 1, 1991 through September 30, 1992 (Fiscal Year 1992).
[3] American Samoa and the Northern Mariana Islands operate special Medicaid waivered programs.
[4] Arizona operates a federal assistance program under a Section 1115 Demonstration Project.
[5] Services indicated as available to the Medically Needy are not available to all Medically Needy groups.
[6] All services are provided through public health facilities.
[7] IMDs – Institutions for Mental Diseases

The data shown were supplied by individual Regional Offices and compiled by the Intergovernmental Affairs Office, Medicaid Bureau
HCFA Pub. No. 02155-92

U.S. Department of Health and Human Services
Health Care Financing Administration
Intergovernmental Affairs Office, Medicaid Bureau

STATE MEDICAID PROGRAM CHANGES

ALABAMA
Added: Rehabilitative Services for CN

CALIFORNIA
Added: Private Duty Nursing for CN and MN
Respiratory Care Services for CN and MN

COLORADO
Added: Hospice Care Services for CN

DISTRICT OF COLUMBIA
Added: NF Services for Under Age 21 for MN

FLORIDA
Added: NF Services for Under Age 21 for CN
Personal Care Services for CN and MN
Respiratory Care Services for CN and MN

HAWAII
Added: Case Management Services for CN and MN

IDAHO
Added: Personal Care Services for CN

INDIANA
Added: Case Management Services for CN

IOWA
Deleted: Rehabilitative Services for CN and MN

KANSAS
Deleted: Podiatrists' Services for CN and MN
Chiropractors' Services for CN and MN

MAINE
Deleted: ICF Services for Mentally Retarded for CN and MN

MARYLAND
Added: NF Services for Age 65 or Older in IMDs for MN

MASSACHUSETTS
Deleted: Chiropractors' Services for CN and MN
Private Duty Nursing Services for MN

MICHIGAN
Deleted: Chiropractors' Services for CN and MN

MISSISSIPPI
Deleted: ICF Services for Mentally Retarded for CN

NEBRASKA
Added: Screening Services for CN and MN

NEVADA
Added: Inpatient Psychiatric Services for Under Age 21 for CN

NEW MEXICO
Added: Occupational Therapy for CN
Speech, Hearing and Language Disorders for CN
Deleted: Rehabilitative Services for CN

NORTH CAROLINA
Added: Prosthetic Devices for CN and MN

OHIO
Added: Case Management Services for CN
Deleted: Inpatient Hospital Services for Age 65 or Older in IMDs for CN
Personal Care Services for CN

OREGON
Added: Screening Services for CN and MN
Inpatient Hospital Services for Age 65 or Older in IMDs for MN
ICF Services for Mentally Retarded for MN
Inpatient Psychiatric Services for Under Age 21 for MN
Christian Science Sanitorium Services for MN
NF Services for Under Age 21 for MN

PENNSYLVANIA
Added: Dentures for MN
Rehabilitative Services for CN and MN
Emergency Hospital Services for CN and MN
Deleted: Respiratory Care Services for CN and MN

SOUTH CAROLINA
Expanded Medicaid to include Medically Needy individuals. Except for Physical and Occupational Therapy, all services currently covered are provided for both CN and MN.

SOUTH DAKOTA
Added: Rehabilitative Services for CN

TENNESSEE
Added: Hospice Care Services for CN and MN
Deleted: Physical Therapy for CN and MN
Dentures for CN and MN
Eyeglasses for CN and MN
Diagnostic Services for CN and MN
Screening Services for CN and MN
Preventive Services for CN and MN
Christian Science Nurses for CN and MN

UTAH
Added: Screening Services for CN and MN
Preventive Services for CN and MN

VERMONT
Deleted: Private Duty Nursing for CN and MN

VIRGINIA
Deleted: Private Duty Nursing for CN and MN
Inpatient Hospital Services for Age 65 or Older in IMDs for MN
NF Services for Age 65 or Older in IMDs for MN
ICF Services for Mentally Retarded for Under Age 21 for MN

WASHINGTON
Added: Chiropractors' Services for CN

WISCONSIN
Added: Emergency Hospital Services for MN

WYOMING
Added: Other Practitioners' Services for CN
Speech, Hearing and Language Disorders for CN

---

* NOTES

1. States may choose either to determine the categorical Medicaid eligibility of their aged, blind, and disabled residents, or have the Social Security Administration (SSA) make these determinations for them. The "Medicaid Determination" column reflects the selected option.

☐ The State has an agreement with SSA under section 1634 of the Social Security Act. SSA makes Medicaid eligibility determination for supplemental security income (SSI) recipients. (31 States and the District of Columbia)

▨ The State makes its own Medicaid eligibility determination for SSI recipients using the SSI eligibility criteria. (7 States and the Northern Mariana Islands)

▦ The State uses more restrictive criteria than those of the SSI program to determine Medicaid eligibility for SSI recipients. A State that selects this option is commonly referred to as a "209 (b) State". Section 209 (b) of Public Law 92–603 later became Section 1902 (f) of the Social Security Act. (12 States)

■ The Medicaid determination option is not applicable.

2. The Omnibus Budget Reconciliation Act of 1990 (OBRA '90) authorized the selection of up to eight States to provide community-supported living arrangements (CSLA) services as an optional State plan service. The States selected to provide CSLA services are: California, Colorado, Florida, Illinois, Maryland, Michigan, Rhode Island, and Wisconsin.

3. Also as a Medicaid option, OBRA '90 allows for the provision of home and community care to functionally disabled, elderly individuals who are either medically needy or eligible for Medicaid due to receipt of SSI benefits. To date, no State has received approval to operationalize this service.

Optional services are defined in law and regulations as follows:[13]

- *Medical care or any other type of remedial care recognized under State law, furnished by licensed practitioners within the scope of their practice as defined by State law.* Included within this definition are services provided by chiropractors, podiatrists, and optometrists. Coverage for care provided by chiropractors is limited, by regulation, to treatment by means of manual manipulation of the spine that the chiropractor is legally licensed by the State to perform.

- *Private duty nursing services.* These are nursing services for persons who require more individual and continuous care than is available from a visiting nurse or routinely provided by the nursing staff of a hospital or NF. The services must be provided by a registered nurse or licensed practical nurse, be under the direction of a physician, and be provided to an individual in his home, hospital or NF.

- *Clinic services.* Clinic services are preventive, diagnostic, therapeutic, rehabilitative, or palliative items or services that are provided to outpatients under the direction of a physician or dentist without regard to whether the clinic itself is administered by a physician. The services are provided by a facility that is not part of a hospital but is organized and operated to provide medical care to outpatients. Clinic services for the homeless may be provided outside the clinic by clinic personnel.

- *Dental services.* Dental services are defined as diagnostic, preventive or corrective procedures provided by or under the supervision of a dentist in the practice of his profession including treatment of the teeth and associated structures of the oral cavity and treatment of disease, injury, or impairment that may affect the oral or general health of the recipient.

- *Physical therapy and related services.* This category includes the following services (including necessary equipment and supplies):

    - *Physical therapy.* Physical therapists plan and administer treatment to relieve pain, improve functioning mobility, maintain cardiopulmonary functioning, and limit the disability of people suffering from a disabling injury or disease.

      Covered physical therapy services are those which are prescribed by a physician and provided by or under the direction of a qualified physical therapist. A qualified therapist is one who is licensed by the State, where

---

[13]The services listed in this section are generally listed in the order they appear in the law and on HCFA's chart of optional Medicaid services (table IV-2).

applicable, and a graduate of a physical therapy program approved by both the Council on Medical Education of the American Medical Association and the American Physical Therapy Association, or its equivalent.

- *Occupational therapy.* Occupational therapists direct their patients in activities designed to help them learn the skills necessary to perform daily tasks, diminish or correct pathology, and promote and maintain health.

  Covered services are those prescribed by a physician and provided by or under the direction of a qualified occupational therapist. A qualified therapist is one who is registered by the American Occupational Therapy Association or who is a graduate of an occupational therapy program approved by the Council on Medical Education of the American Medical Association and engaged in supplemental clinical experience required by the American Occupational Therapy Association.

- *Services for persons with speech, hearing and language disorders.* These are diagnostic, screening, preventive or corrective services, provided by or under the direction of a speech pathologist or audiologist, for which a patient is referred by a physician. A speech pathologist or audiologist is one who has a certificate of clinical competence from the American Speech and Hearing Association, has completed the equivalent educational requirements and work experience, or has completed the academic program and is acquiring supervised work experience to qualify for the certificate.

- *Prescribed drugs.* Prescribed drugs are simple or compound substances or mixtures of substances prescribed for the cure, mitigation, or prevention of disease or health maintenance. They must be: (1) prescribed by a physician or other licensed practitioner of the healing arts within the scope of his practice as defined and limited by Federal and State law; (2) dispensed by a licensed pharmacist or a licensed authorized practitioner in accordance with the State Medical Practice Act; and (3) dispensed on a written prescription that is recorded and maintained in the pharmacist's or practitioner's records.

  Federal matching funds are not available for drugs determined by the Food and Drug Administration to be less than effective, or for drugs that are identical, similar, or related to drugs for which such a determination has been made.

  Generally, the Omnibus Budget Reconciliation Act of 1990 (OBRA 90) requires States to cover the drugs of a manufacturer who complies with a rebate agreement.[14] The statute includes exceptions for some

---

[14]See *Chapter V, Reimbursement* for a discussion of rebates.

classes of products and permissive limitations for others. States may exclude from coverage or otherwise restrict the following classes of drugs:

- anorexia or weight gain drugs;
- fertility drugs;
- drugs used for cosmetic purposes or hair growth;
- drugs used for the symptomatic relief of cough and colds;
- smoking cessation drugs;
- prescription vitamin and mineral products, except prenatal vitamins and fluoride preparations;
- nonprescription drugs;
- covered outpatient drugs for which the manufacturer seeks to require, as a condition of sale, that associated tests or monitoring services be purchased exclusively from the manufacturer or its designee; and
- barbiturates; and
- benzodiazepines.

The law authorizes HCFA to update the list by regulation on the basis of whether a drug is subject to clinical abuse or inappropriate use.

- *Dentures.* These must be made by or under the direction of a dentist to replace a full or partial set of teeth.

- *Prosthetic devices.* These are replacement, corrective, or supportive devices prescribed by a physician or other licensed practitioner of the healing arts within the scope of his practice as defined by State law to: (1) artificially replace a missing portion of the body; (2) prevent or correct a physical deformity or malfunction; or (3) support a weak or deformed portion of the body. Within this category, States may include hearing aids, orthopedic shoes, and durable medical equipment.

- *Eyeglasses.* These are lenses, including frames, and other aids to vision prescribed by a physician skilled in diseases of the eye or by an optometrist.

- *Diagnostic, screening, preventive, and rehabilitative services.* Diagnostic services are medical procedures or supplies recommended by a physician or other licensed practitioner of the healing arts, within the scope of practice under State law, to enable him to identify the existence, nature, or extent of illness, injury or other health deviation.

Screening services means the use of standardized tests given under medical direction in the mass examination of a designated population to detect the existence of one or more particular diseases or health deviations or to identify for more definitive studies those suspected of having certain diseases.

Preventive services are those provided by a physician or other licensed practitioner of the healing arts within the scope of his practice under State law to: (1) prevent disease, disability, and other health conditions or their progression; (2) prolong life; and (3) promote physical and mental health and efficiency.

Rehabilitation services means (except as otherwise included under another service definition) medical or remedial services recommended by a physician or other licensed practitioner of the healing arts (within the scope of his or her practice under State law) for maximum reduction of physical or mental disability and restoration of a beneficiary to the best possible functional level.

- *Inpatient hospital services and NF services for individuals age 65 or older in Institutions for Mental Diseases (IMDs).* A State may choose to provide services at either of these levels of care to persons 65 or over in a mental institution. An institution for mental disease is defined as one that meets Medicare requirements except that the requirement for utilization review may be waived.[15] Covered services include diagnosis, treatment and care of individuals with mental diseases including medical care, nursing care and related services.

- *Services in an Intermediate Care Facility for the Mentally Retarded (ICF/MR).* Services in an institution for the mentally retarded or persons with related conditions may be covered if: (1) the primary purpose of the institution is to provide health or rehabilitative services for such persons; (2) the institution meets requisite certification requirements; and (3) the individual is receiving active treatment. The institution must provide in a protected residential setting ongoing evaluation, planning, 24-hour supervision, coordination, and integration of health or rehabilitative services to help each individual function at his greatest ability.

  Each client must receive a continuous active treatment program which includes aggressive, consistent implementation of a program of specialized and generic training, treatment, health services and related services that is directed toward: (1) the acquisition of the behaviors necessary for the client to function with as much self determination and independence as possible; and (2) the prevention or deceleration of regression or loss of current optimal functional status. Active treatment does not include services to maintain generally independent clients who are able to function with little supervision or in the absence of a continuous active treatment program.

- *Inpatient psychiatric hospital services for individuals under age 21.* These are inpatient services provided in a psychiatric hospital or distinct part thereof or in another inpatient setting designated by the

---

[15]See *Appendix E, Medicaid Services for the Mentally Ill* for a discussion of IMDs.

Secretary. The services must be provided under the direction of a physician by an accredited facility or accredited program in the facility. A team, consisting of physicians and other personnel qualified to make determinations with respect to mental health conditions and treatment, must certify that services are necessary on an inpatient basis and can reasonably be expected to improve the patient's condition to the extent that eventually such services will no longer be necessary. Active treatment requirements specify that services must be provided pursuant to a professionally developed and supervised individual plan of care which is designed to achieve the beneficiary's discharge from the facility at the earliest practical time.

If the individual is receiving services on the date he or she turns 21, coverage may be extended until the individual no longer needs such care, or turns 22, whichever is earlier.

- *Hospice care.* States may offer coverage for hospice care provided to a terminally ill individual who has voluntarily elected to have payment made for such care in lieu of having payment made for certain other services. The definitions for covered services and the definition of a hospice program are the same as those under Medicare. Covered services include nursing care, physical or occupational therapy or speech language pathology, medical social services under the direction of a physician, home health aide and homemaker services, medical supplies and the use of medical appliances, physicians' services, short-term inpatient care and counseling. The services must be provided under a written plan of care. A hospice program is a public agency or private organization which is primarily engaged in providing such services directly or under arrangement, makes services available as needed on a 24 hour basis, and meets applicable licensing requirements. Beneficiaries' elections of hospice care may be for a period or periods established by the State and may be revoked by them.

- *Case management services.* Case management services are defined as services which will assist eligible individuals in gaining access to needed medical, social, educational and other services. States may provide these services without regard to the statewideness requirement or the requirement that Medicaid services be equal in amount, duration, and scope for all categorically needy beneficiaries. The provision of case management services may not restrict the beneficiaries' freedom-of-choice to select a provider of services.

A State may limit the provision of case management services to individuals with acquired immune deficiency syndrome (AIDS), or with AIDS-related conditions, or with either. A State may also limit the provision of case management services to individuals with chronic mental illness.

- *Respiratory care services.* Respiratory therapists are employed under medical supervision in a wide range of services from providing emergency care to relief for patients with emphysema or asthma.

  Covered respiratory care services are defined as those which are provided on a part-time basis in the home of an individual by a respiratory therapist or other health care professional trained in respiratory therapy, as determined by the State. Respiratory care payments are those that are not otherwise included within other items and services for such persons under the State's program. Covered individuals must: (1) be medically-dependent on a respirator for life support at least 6 hours a day; (2) have been so dependent as inpatients for at least 30 consecutive days, or the maximum number of days authorized under the State plan, whichever is less; (3) require respiratory care on an inpatient basis and be eligible for Medicaid for the inpatient care; and (4) have adequate social support services to be cared for at home and (5) wish to be cared for at home. States are permitted to limit coverage of respiratory services to ventilator-dependent individuals.

- *Any other medical care or remedial care recognized under State law, specified by the Secretary.* The following items have been specified by the Secretary:

  - *Services of Christian Science sanitoria nurses.* These are services provided by nurses who are listed and certified by the First Church of Christ, Scientist, Boston, Massachusetts.

  - *Services in Christian Science sanitoriums.* These are services provided in sanitoriums operated by or listed and certified by the First Church of Christ, Scientist, Boston, Massachusetts.

  - *Nursing facility (NF) services for individuals under age 21.*

  - *Emergency hospital services.* These are services that are necessary to prevent the death or serious impairment to the health of a beneficiary and because of the threat to life or health, necessitates the use of the most accessible hospital available that is equipped to furnish the services. The services are covered even if the hospital does not meet Medicare conditions of participation or the definition of inpatient or outpatient hospital services.

  - *Personal care services in a beneficiary's home.* These are services which are prescribed by a physician in accordance with the beneficiary's plan of care and provided by an individual who is qualified to provide the services, supervised by a registered nurse, and not a member of the beneficiary's family. A State which has been granted a home and community based services waiver may define personal care services differently for purposes of that waiver.

As noted earlier, effective October 1, 1994, the term home health services will include personal care services, provided certain requirements are met.

- *Transportation.* Transportation services may be covered as an optional service or as a mandated administrative expense.[16] The optional service category includes expenses for transportation and other related travel expenses determined to be necessary to secure medical examinations and treatment. Covered services include only those furnished by a provider to whom a direct vendor payment can be made, for example, an ambulance company. (Other services may be covered as administrative expenses.) Travel expenses include the costs of transportation, the cost of meals and lodging enroute and while receiving medical care, and the cost of an attendant, if necessary, to accompany the beneficiary including his or her meals, lodging, and transportation.

The OBRA 90 established two capped entitlement programs which permits states to offer the following services:

- *Home and community care for functionally disabled elderly individuals.* Home and community care services may be provided to functionally disabled individuals age 65 or over. These are persons who are unable to perform two out of three specified activities of daily living (toiletting, transferring, and eating) or who have Alzheimer's disease and meet specified tests of functional disability. States are permitted to limit eligibility based on reasonable classifications such as age, functional disability and need for services.

Services which may be furnished in accordance with an individual community care plan developed by a case manager are: homemaker/home health aide services, chore services, personal care services, nursing care services, respite care, training for family members, adult day care, and, under certain circumstances, other services. The Secretary is to establish minimum quality standards for providers.

---

[16]Federal regulations include an administrative requirement that States must specify that its Medicaid agency will assure necessary transportation for beneficiaries to and from providers. If covered as an administrative expense, Federal matching is at the appropriate administrative rate--generally 50 percent. If covered as an optional service, Federal matching is at the Federal Medical Assistance Percentage rate (see *Chapter VIII, Financing*).

Federal matching payments are capped at $40 million in FY 92, $70 million in FY 93, $130 million for FY 94, $160 million for FY 95, and $180 for FY 96; funds are to be allocated to the States that choose to provide these optional services. During each State's election period for providing this service (which is four calendar quarters, at a minimum), the State is required to provide services, regardless of the availability of Federal matching.

- *Community-supported living arrangement services.* Community-supported living arrangement services may be provided to persons with mental retardation or related conditions. Individuals eligible for services are those who live in their own or their family's home, apartment, or other rental unit in which no more than three individuals receiving these services reside. Covered services are personal assistance, training and rehabilitation, emergency assistance, assistive technology, adaptive equipment, support services, and other services.

Federal expenditures are capped at $100 million over 5 years. Between two and eight States will be permitted to elect the option. States electing the option are required to develop a state plan, including quality assurance standards, which must be subject to public hearing and approved by the Secretary.

III. REQUIREMENTS APPLICABLE FOR ALL SERVICES

States have to meet four additional requirements in designing their benefit packages. These relate to: amount, duration, and scope of services; comparability; statewideness; and freedom-of-choice. The Secretary may waive applicability of these requirements under certain circumstances.[17]

A. Amount, Duration, and Scope

A State is required to specify the amount, duration, and scope of each service that it provides for the categorically needy and for each covered medically needy group. Each service must be sufficient in amount, duration, and scope to reasonably achieve its purpose. The Medicaid agency may place limits on services. Program regulations provide that the agency may not arbitrarily deny or reduce coverage of a required service solely because of the diagnosis, type of illness, or condition.

B. Comparability

The services available to any categorically needy beneficiary under a State program must generally be equal in amount, duration, and scope to those available to any other categorically needy beneficiary in the State. For example, if a State provides unlimited physician visits for the aged, it may not restrict the

---

[17]See discussion of waivers in *Chapter VI, Alternate Delivery Options and Waiver Programs.*

allowed number of physician visits to six per year for the Aid to Families With Dependent Children (AFDC) population. Similarly, services available to an individual in a covered medically needy group must be equal in amount, duration and scope to those available to all persons in the covered medically needy group.

The coverage available to the categorically needy may not be less than that offered to the medically needy. States do however, have the option of offering a more restrictive package for this latter group.[18]

There are a number of exceptions to the comparability requirements, primarily tied to a beneficiary's age or coverage category. For example, NF services may be limited to persons over 21. EPSDT services are limited to persons under 21. Further, States may limit additional benefits available under Medicare to dual Medicare/Medicaid beneficiaries. In addition, States covering case management services as an optional benefit are exempted from the comparability requirement for such services.

C. Statewideness

Generally, a State plan must be in effect throughout an entire State, that is the amount, duration, and scope of coverage must be the same statewide. However, certain limited exceptions are authorized. For example, a State does not have to offer any additional services which are offered by a prepaid health plan to its enrollees, to other beneficiaries in the State. Also, a State operating a home and community-based services waiver does not have to offer all services covered under the waiver to other beneficiaries. Further, a State covering case management services as an optional benefit is not subject to the statewideness requirement for such services.

D. Freedom-of-Choice

Beneficiaries may obtain services from any institution, agency, pharmacy, person, or organization that undertakes to provide the services and is qualified to perform the services, (including an organization that provides these services or arranges for the provision of these services on a prepaid basis). This is known as the "freedom-of-choice" requirement. The freedom-of-choice requirement is not applicable in Puerto Rico, the Virgin Islands, and Guam. Further this requirement may be waived under certain circumstances.[19]

---

[18]Information reported by the Commerce Clearing House Guide as of August 1991, shows that 24 of the 36 States (including D.C., but excluding the territories) which had medically needy programs offered the same package of services to both their categorically needy and medically needy populations.

[19]See discussion of waivers in *Chapter VI, Alternate Delivery Options and Waiver Programs.*

IV. UTILIZATION CONTROLS AND SERVICE LIMITATIONS

States may adopt various methods to attempt to control the costs of Medicaid services. One approach involves setting limits on payments; these reimbursement controls are discussed in detail in *Chapter V, Reimbursement*. Another approach attempts to curtail payments for inappropriate services or services which are not medically necessary. Using this approach, States may place limits on the amount, duration, and scope of covered services, such as inpatient hospital services and physician services. In certain cases, extensions are granted based on documentation of medical necessity.

A. Hospital Services[20]

In general, States may place limits on the number of covered days of inpatient care. However, they are prohibited from imposing such limits on the number of covered days of hospital care for infants under age one and for children under age six receiving services in hospitals serving a disproportionate number of low-income patients.

Durational limits may be calculated on a per year, per admission, or per spell of illness basis. States may also limit coverage based on a percentile of the length-of-stay data from the Professional Activity Study (PAS) or another average length of stay measure. The PAS, which presents the average length of stay calculated by diagnosis and region, is collected by the Commission on Professional Hospital Activities.

The National Governors' Association reports that as of January 1, 1991, 22 States had imposed length of stay limits on inpatient hospital services; five used PAS limits for some portion of their inpatient population. A number of States had policies under which an extension from the specified limit could be granted based on documentation of medical necessity. (See table IV-3.)

The Federal Government may not require States to establish preadmission screening programs. However, States may choose to establish such programs on their own.

---

[20]See also discussion of certification requirements in *Chapter VII, Administration*.

TABLE IV-3. Inpatient Hospital Length of Stay Restrictions, in Effect as of January 1, 1991

| State | Limits on covered days: | | Extensions of stay |
	Number of days	Percentile of PAS* or other related length of stay measure	
Alabama	14/CY; for dual eligible, non-QMB recipients, the Medicare and Medicaid days run concurrently.		
Alaska		75	If 75th percentile is surpassed, prior authorization must be obtained for a stay up to 90th percentile. Beyond 90th percentile, prior authorization is again required. Additional days may be authorized for deliveries.
Arizona [a]			
Arkansas	25/FY	50	Exceptions to the 25-day limit will be considered for medically necessary days for EPSDT beneficiaries. PAS does not apply to beneficiaries under 21.
California [b]			
Colorado			
Connecticut			
Delaware			
District of Columbia			
Florida	45/FY for beneficiaries 21 years and older		

See notes at end of table.

TABLE IV-3. Inpatient Hospital Length of Stay Restrictions, in Effect as of January 1, 1991--Continued

| State | Limits on covered days: | | Extensions of stay |
	Number of days	Percentile of PAS* or other related length of stay measure	
Georgia	30/admission, psychiatric only		Based on medical necessity, prior approval is required to extend psychiatric stay beyond 30 days.
Hawaii			
Idaho	40		
Illinois[c]			
Indiana	day limit is based on diagnosis		
Iowa			
Kansas			
Kentucky	14/admission		
Louisiana	15/CY		Medical necessity documentation is required.
Maine			
Maryland			
Massachusetts	Maximum length of stay is determined during the preadmission screening		

See notes at end of table.

TABLE IV-3. Inpatient Hospital Length of Stay Restrictions, in Effect as of January 1, 1991--Continued

State	Limits on covered days: Number of days	Percentile of PAS* or other related length of stay measure	Extensions of stay
Michigan			
Minnesota			
Mississippi	30/FY; beneficiaries under age 21 in a disproportionate share hospital for a special diagnosis are exempt from limits		Children under 21 can be approved for additional medically necessary days under an expanded EPSDT program.
Missouri		75	Disproportionate share hospitals and EPSDT cases with prior authorization
Montana			
Nebraska		75	
Nevada	4 day limit for detoxification for alcohol and drug abuse		
New Hampshire			
New Jersey			
New Mexico			
New York			
North Carolina			

See notes at end of table.

TABLE IV-3. Inpatient Hospital Length of Stay Restrictions, in Effect as of January 1, 1991.--Continued

State	Limits on covered days:		Extensions of stay
	Number of days	Percentile of PAS* or other related length of stay measure	
North Dakota			
Ohio	30/spell of illness		Exceptions when certified medically necessary; the beneficiary is jointly eligible under Medicaid and Crippled Children's Program; or the hospital is paid on a prospective basis.
Oklahoma	20/FY for individuals 21+; 60/FY for individuals under 21		Extensions may be granted for catastrophic illness.
Oregon	18/FY for individuals over age 21.		Extensions are available when the patient enters the hospital with at least 1 day remaining in the 18 day limit. If the stay exceeds 18 day limit, the patient is allowed to complete the stay. Extensions for adults are also given for rehabilitative treatment in a Certified Acute Rehabilitative Facility (CARF)--hospital based spinal cord injury center.
Pennsylvania			
Rhode Island			
South Carolina			

See notes at end of table.

TABLE IV-3. Inpatient Hospital Length of Stay Restrictions, in Effect as of January 1, 1991–Continued

State	Limits on covered days:		Extensions of stay
	Number of days	Percentile of PAS[*] or other related length of stay measure	
South Dakota			
Tennessee	Limits apply to following transplants: Heart 43/FY; Liver 67/FY; Bone marrow 40/FY.		
Texas	30/spell of illness[d]		
Utah			
Vermont			
Virginia	21/admission for coverage within a 60-day period for the same diagnosis beginning with the date of the first admission. Children under age 21 are exempt.		
Washington		75[e]	
West Virginia	25/FY		Extensions are available for medically necessary services for beneficiaries under age 21.
Wisconsin			
Wyoming		X[f]	

See notes at end of table.

TABLE IV-3. Inpatient Hospital Length of Stay Restrictions, in Effect as of January 1, 1991.-Continued

Footnotes

ᵃPAS=Professional Activity Study, which is the average length of stay, calculated by diagnosis and region, as collected and prepared by the Commission on Professional Hospital Activities.

ᵃArizona operates a demonstration program under which contractors are at risk for cost of unnecessary patient stay; thus, there is no need for the State to require covered day limits.

ᵇCalifornia operates a selective contracting program for inpatient hospital services. There are no specific length of stay limits. However, there is a preadmission screening of all elective admissions, and concurrent review of all emergency admissions and extensions of hospital stays based on medical necessity.

ᶜIllinois established a selective contracting program, whereby a statewide limit of covered hospital days is set and allocated among the hospitals. An individual hospital can exceed its day limit, but once the statewide limit is reached, all hospitals receive 65 percent reimbursement for excess days.

ᵈTexas requires an individual to be out of the hospital 60 consecutive days between stays.

ᵉWashington adopted a diagnosis related group (DRG) reimbursement system. Only non-DRG inpatient services are subject to a 75th percentile of PAS length of stay limit.

ᶠWyoming requires all hospital admissions (including emergency care) and length of stay, except routine maternity and newborn care, to be approved by PRO.

Source: National Governors' Association, 1991.

B. Physicians' Services

Many States have elected to place specific limits on the number of physician visits covered by the program during a specified time period. These limits are frequently linked to the visit site, for example limits on inpatient hospital visits, long term care facility visits, or office visits. Some States apply limits based on broader categories. Table IV-4 shows, effective January 1, 1991 which States imposed numerical limits on covered physician visits. As of that date, 22 States had limits on inpatient visits, 25 States had limits on visits to long-term care facilities, 16 States had limits on office visits, and 12 States imposed combined limits on two or more categories of visits.

TABLE IV-4. Limits on Physician Service Coverage by State, in Effect as of January 1, 1991

State	Inpatient hospital visits	Location of physician visit:		
		Long-term care facility visits	Office visits	Combination of visits
Alabama	1 day; 14/CY/per physician			12/CY in any combination of office, nursing home, or hospital outpatient visits.
Alaska		1/month		
Arizona				
Arkansas	1/day;25/FY/per physician			12/CY noninpatient visits in any combination of office, home, long-term care facilities, and outpatient hospital visits. Also, physician consultations are limited to 2/CY if provided in a physician's office, patient's home or hospital.[a]
California				
Colorado				
Connecticut	42/year for psychiatrists visits	12 routine visits/year		
Delaware				
District of Columbia				
Florida	1/day, with the exception of emergencies	1/month	1/provider/day is allowed for supervision of chronic illness.	

See notes at end of table.

TABLE IV-4. Limits on Physician Service Coverage by State, in Effect as of January 1, 1991--Continued

State	Inpatient hospital visits	Long-term care facility visits	Office visits	Combination of visits
		Location of physician visit:		
Georgia	1/day; critical visits are unlimited if medically necessary.	12/FY[b]	12/FY[b]	
Hawaii		2/month, with the exception of acute episodes with prior authorization		
Idaho				
Illinois				
Indiana	1/day	1/27 days	4/mo; 20/yr/provider[b]	
Iowa				
Kansas	1/month for confirmatory consultation limits; 1/10 days/provider[a]	1 routine visit/month	12 or 24/year. Absolute limit of 12 office visits/yr. for adults; for EPSDT beneficiary, 24/yr. with prior authorization for additional visits.[c]	

See notes at end of table.

TABLE IV-4. Limits on Physician Service Coverage by State, in Effect as of January 1, 1991–Continued

State	Inpatient hospital visits	Location of physician visit:			
		Long-term care facility visits	Office visits	Combination of visits
Kentucky			1 comprehensive visit/12-month period/physician.	
Louisiana	15/yr; 1/day for each day of admission without surgery			12/yr. for physician's office, beneficiary's home, nursing facilities or hospital outpatient.
Maine				
Maryland				
Massachusetts	1/day	1/day	1/day	
Michigan		1/30 days		
Minnesota		1/30 days[b]	1/day/physician[b]	7/7 day period
Mississippi	1/day;30/FY. An exception to the limit is made for intensive or coronary care units, for which 2/day are allowed.	36/year		12/FY in any combination of physician office visits and rural health clinic visits.
Missouri		1/month		
Montana				
Nebraska				

See notes at end of table.

TABLE IV-4. Limits on Physician Service Coverage by State, in Effect as of January 1, 1991--Continued

| State | Location of physician visit: | | | |
	Inpatient hospital visits	Long-term care facility visits	Office visits	Combination of visits
Nevada			5/month; maximum of 3 visits per provider	5/month in any combination of office or nursing home visits.
New Hampshire		18/year	18/year with exceptions for children under 19.	18/FY in any setting other than inpatient hospital. Children under 19 are exempt from this limit.
New Jersey				
New Mexico	2/day/provider or provider group	2/day	1/day^d	
New York				
North Carolina				24/year in any combination of physician's office, hospital outpatient (emergency rooms excluded), freestanding clinics,podiatric, optometric, and chiropractic visits. Exempt are EPSDT, pregnancy-related services, life threatening conditions (hemophilia, unstable diabetes, and cancer therapy). State also covers 1 adult health screening (preventive) exam/year for beneficiaries 21 year and older.

See notes at end of table.

TABLE IV-4. Limits on Physician Service Coverage by State, in Effect as of January 1, 1991.--Continued

| State | Location of physician visit: | | | |
	Inpatient hospital visits	Long-term care facility visits	Office visits	Combination of visits
North Dakota	1/day	1/month; more are allowed if medically necessary.		
Ohio	10/month; 1 critical care visit/day.	24/CY		24/CY for all providers of physician services including outpatient hospital visits.[a]
Oklahoma	1/day; additional visits are allowed for individuals under 21.	2/month	4/month; additional visits may be allowed in connection with an acute physical injury, family planning and EPSDT.	4/month in any combination of physician office, home, organized outpatient hospital clinic, and any other physician visits except nursing homes, inpatient hospital, and inpatient psychiatric. Exceptions are treatment for acute physical injury, family planning, or EPSDT.
Oregon	2/day, 8/day for critical care	2/day	2/day	
Pennsylvania	$1,000/stay/hospitalization/ physician service; also 2 consultations/specialty/ hospitalization.			Outpatient: $500/day on all physician services. 1/provider/day for hospital, home, office, emergency room, clinic, inpatient care, nursing home, or screening visits.
Rhode Island	37/stay			

See notes at end of table.

TABLE IV-4. Limits on Physician Service Coverage by State, in Effect as of January 1, 1991--Continued

State	Inpatient hospital visits	Location of physician visit:		
		Long-term care facility visits	Office visits	Combination of visits
South Carolina		5/month		18/year for beneficiaries age 21+ in any combination of physician office, podiatric, dental, chiropractic, opthomology, and psychiatric evaluation. Exceptions are patients with cancer, allergies, AIDS, on dialysis or insulin, or using psychiatric services.
South Dakota				
Tennessee	1/day	1/month for level I care[e]; 4/month for level II care[e]	24/FY	
Texas				
Utah				
Vermont	1/day for acute hospital care	1/week for NFs; additional visits must be adequately substantiated.	5/month	
Virginia	1/day; for adults 21+, 21 visits/60 day period for the same diagnosis			
Washington	1/day; exceptions: surgery reimbursed with global fee that includes follow up visits.	2/month; exception: additional visits justified by diagnosis.	1/day	

See notes at end of table.

TABLE IV-4. Limits on Physician Service Coverage by State, in Effect as of January 1, 1991--Continued

State	Inpatient hospital visits	Long-term care facility visits	Office visits	Combination of visits
		Location of physician visit:		
West Virginia		1/30 days; exception: documented acute condition.		
Wisconsin	1/day	1/month for routine visit	1/year only applies to the procedure code for annual checkup.	
Wyoming		1/month for routine visit		

ªAdditional visits are available if medically necessary.

ᵇMore visits are available with prior authorization.

ᶜNonemergency visit to the hospital now counts as an office visit.

ᵈNew Mexico limits office visits to one per day unless referred to another physician or if the claim documents a change in the client's condition.

ᵉTennessee has two levels of NF care and distinguishes between them for service limits.

Source: National Governors' Association, 1991.

As of 1989, 13 States also had implemented mandatory second surgical opinion programs. (See table IV-5.) Under these programs, the need for certain specified procedures or groups of procedures must be confirmed in advance by another physician before payment will be made.

TABLE IV-5. States Having Mandatory Second Surgical Opinion Programs, 1989

State	Number of procedures
Colorado	19
Indiana	18
Massachusetts	7
Michigan	17
Minnesota	NA
Missouri	13
New Jersey	7
Oregon	NA
South Carolina	3
Tennessee	4
Virginia	10
Washington	4
Wisconsin	9

NOTE: NA = Not available.

Source: U.S. Dept. of Health and Human Services. Health Care Financing Administration. *High Volume and High Payment Procedures in the Medicaid Population.* Report to Congress. HCFA Pub. No. 03289, Sept. 1989. Washington, 1989.

In response to a congressional directive contained in OBRA 86, HCFA reviewed various aspects of these second surgical opinion programs. It found that for 11 reporting States, a total of 43 procedures had been targeted for second opinion review. (Information was not obtained for Minnesota or Oregon.) One procedure was covered by all 11 States--hysterectomies. Procedures covered by at least five States included cholecystectomy, tonsillectomy/adenoidectomy, hernia repair, hemorrhoidectomy, cataract extraction, and laminectomy/laminotomy. Twenty-one procedures were covered by only one State.[21]

The HCFA analysis also compared the list of procedures subject to second opinion review against certain yardsticks. It noted that the procedures were those the States believed could be postponed without undue risk. Many of the procedures, particularly those identified by three or more States, also appeared on the lists of high volume or high payment procedures which had been developed by HCFA based on analysis of 1984 claims data. Data on the rates of nonconfirmation upon examination by a second physician were limited; 6 of the 13 procedures for which such information was available showed nonconfirmation rates of 10 percent or more.

The OBRA 86 had directed the Department of Health and Human Services (DHHS) to examine State programs with a view toward identifying procedures appropriate for a mandatory second opinion program. The HCFA analysis concluded that the procedures selected by the States represented a reasonable pool of potential procedures that might be appropriate for a mandatory second surgical opinion program. However, OBRA 86 (as modified by OBRA 90) prohibits the Secretary from issuing final regulations requiring States to implement mandatory second surgical opinion programs.

C. Nursing Facility (NF) Services

Federal Medicaid rules require that a physician must personally approve a recommendation that an individual be admitted to a NF. In addition, the NF must make a comprehensive evaluation, shortly after admission, of the resident's functional capacity.

A number of States have also instituted formal preadmission screening programs. These programs apply to persons already eligible for Medicaid. In some States they also are applied to private patients expected to become eligible for Medicaid in the near future. Thirty States had instituted such programs as of Fall 1985 (the latest period for which such information is available).

In addition, OBRA 87 required that States establish preadmission screening and annual resident review (PASARR) programs to determine for all persons with mental illness and mental retardation whether they require the level of services provided by nursing homes. PASARR requirements are intended to prevent the inappropriate placement of people with mental illness or mental retardation in nursing facilities where they do not receive the care and specialized services they need for their conditions.

The PASARR has two components. First, it requires States to screen persons with mental illness and mental retardation **prior** to their admission to

---

[21]U.S. Dept. of Health and Human Services. Health Care Financing Administration. *High Volume and High Payment Procedures in the Medicaid Population.* Report to Congress. HCFA Pub. No. 03289, Sept. 1989. Washington, 1989.

a nursing home. Since January 1, 1989, nursing homes participating in Medicaid have been prohibited from admitting any individual with mental illness or mental retardation unless the person is determined by the State to require the level of services provided by the NF.

The PASARR also requires that States review, on an annual basis, all nursing home residents with mental illness and mental retardation to determine whether NF placement continues to be appropriate. The first round of these annual reviews was to be completed April 1, 1990. The law requires that certain residents be discharged if their placement in a NF is found to be inappropriate. OBRA 87 allowed States to submit to the Secretary of DHHS alternative disposition plans (ADPs) for persons needing to be discharged. At least 46 States submitted ADPs which were approved by the Secretary.

D. Prescription Drugs

Many States place limitations on prescription drug coverage. They may limit the quantity of drugs dispensed by limiting the number of prescriptions that can be filled or refilled in a certain time period. They may also place limits on the quantity per prescription (for example, a 30 day supply or 100 unit limit). These quantity limits are generally maximums, though minimums are also applied in certain cases, such as for maintenance drugs. States may also restrict (or not cover at all) over-the-counter drugs. Table IV-6 shows limits placed by States on prescription drug coverage.

TABLE IV-6. Limits on Prescription Drugs, by State, in Effect as of July 1, 1991

State	Prescription limit per month	Type of limit: Refill limit	Type of limit: Quantity limit	Type of limit: Limit on over-the-counter (OTC) drugs
Alabama	None	5 refill limit	4 Rx's/month	Few OTC drugs reimbursed
Alaska	None	None	30-34 day supply or 100 units	Few OTC drugs reimbursed
Arizona[a]				
Arkansas	6 per month	5 refill limit	30-34 day supply or 100 units	Few OTC drugs reimbursed
California	Maintenance drugs: maximum of 3 claims in 75 days, coupled with minimum dispensing quantity of 100.	Yes	100 day supply	Most OTC drugs reimbursed
Colorado	None	None	None	Few OTC drugs reimbursed
Connecticut	None	6 drugs/ month	None	Few OTC drugs reimbursed
Delaware	None	None	30-34 day supply or 100 units	Few OTC drugs reimbursed
District of Columbia	None	3 drugs/month	30-34 day supply or 100 units	Few OTC drugs reimbursed
Florida	6 drugs/month	None	None	Few OTC drugs reimbursed
Georgia	6 drugs/month	None	30-34 day supply or 100 units	Few OTC drugs reimbursed
Hawaii	None	None	Yes	Most OTC drugs reimbursed
Idaho	None	None	30-34 day supply or 100 units	Few OTC drugs reimbursed

See notes at end of table.

TABLE IV-6. Limits on Prescription Drugs, by State, in Effect as of July 1, 1991—Continued

State	Prescription limit per month	Type of limit: Refill limit	Type of limit: Quantity limit	Limit on over-the-counter (OTC) drugs
Illinois	None	2 refill limit	30-34 day supply or 100 units	Few OTC drugs reimbursed
Indiana	In long-term care facilities only: 2 dispensing fees/ drug/beneficiary/month	None	None	Most OTC drugs reimbursed
Iowa	None	None	None	Few OTC drugs reimbursed
Kansas	None	None	30-34 day supply or 100 units	Few OTC drugs reimbursed
Kentucky	None	After initial filling, one dispensing fee per 30 day period for designated maintenance drugs.	30-34 day supply or 100 units	Few OTC drugs reimbursed
Louisiana	None	5 refill limit	30-34 day supply or 100 units	Few OTC drugs reimbursed
Maine	None	5 refill limit	30-34 day supply or 100 units	Few OTC drugs reimbursed
Maryland	None	2 refill limit	30-34 day supply or 100 units	Few OTC drugs reimbursed
Massachusetts	None	5 refill limit	30-34 day supply or 100 units	Few OTC drugs reimbursed
Michigan	None	5 refill limit	None	Few OTC drugs reimbursed
Minnesota	None	None	30-34 day supply or 100 units	Most OTC drugs reimbursed
Mississippi	5 drugs/month	5 refill limit	30-34 day supply or 100 units	Few OTC drugs reimbursed

See notes at end of table.

TABLE IV-6. Limits on Prescription Drugs, by State, in Effect as of July 1, 1991–Continued

State	Prescription limit per month	Type of limit: Refill limit	Type of limit: Quantity limit	Limit on over-the-counter (OTC) drugs
Missouri	None	None	None	Most OTC drugs reimbursed
Montana	None	None	30-34 day supply or 100 units	Few OTC drugs reimbursed
Nebraska	None	None	100 day supply	Most OTC drugs reimbursed
Nevada	5 drugs/month	None	30-34 day supply or 100 units	Few OTC drugs reimbursed
New Hampshire	None	5 refill limit	30-34 day supply or 100 units	Most OTC drugs reimbursed
New Jersey	None	None	30-34 day supply or 100 units	Few OTC drugs reimbursed
New Mexico	None	None	180 day supply	Few OTC drugs reimbursed
New York	Some, but not all drugs	5 refill limit	Benzodiazepines: Triplicate drug 30 day supply	Few OTC drugs reimbursed
North Carolina	6 drugs/month	None	None	Few OTC drugs reimbursed
North Dakota	None	5 refill limit	None	Few OTC drugs reimbursed
Ohio	None	None	Yes	Few OTC drugs reimbursed
Oklahoma	3 drugs/month	None	30-34 day supply or 100 units	Few OTC drugs reimbursed
Oregon	None	None	100 day supply	Few OTC drugs reimbursed
Pennsylvania	None	5 refill limit	30-34 day supply or 100 units	Most OTC drugs reimbursed

See notes at end of table.

TABLE IV-6. Limits on Prescription Drugs, by State, in Effect as of July 1, 1991–Continued

| State | Prescription limit per month | Type of limit: | | Limit on over-the-counter (OTC) drugs |
		Refill limit	Quantity limit	
Rhode Island	None	5 refill limit	30-34 day supply or 100 units	Few OTC drugs reimbursed
South Carolina	3 drugs/month	None	100 day supply	Few OTC drugs reimbursed
South Dakota	None	None	30-34 day supply or 100 units	Few OTC drugs reimbursed
Tennessee	7 drugs/month	5 refill limit	30-34 day supply or 100 units	Few OTC drugs reimbursed
Texas	3 drugs/month	5 refill limit	None	Most OTC drugs reimbursed
Utah	None	None	30-34 day supply or 100 units	Few OTC drugs reimbursed
Vermont	None	5 refill limit	60 day or 100 units	Few OTC drugs reimbursed
Virginia	None	None	None	For nursing home patient only-- most drugs reimbursed
Washington	None	2 refill limit	30-34 day supply or 100 units	Most OTC drugs reimbursed
West Virginia	None	5 refill limit	30-34 day supply or 100 units	Few OTC drugs reimbursed
Wisconsin	None	Yes	30-34 day supply or 100 units	Few OTC drugs reimbursed
Wyoming	None	5 refill limit	30-34 day supply or 100 units	Few OTC drugs reimbursed

aArizona's operates under a demonstration program.

Source: National Pharmaceutical Council. *Pharmaceutical Benefits under State Medical Assistance Programs,* Sept. 1991. p. 96-97.

Prior authorization involves obtaining State approval of a drug before it is dispensed. States are permitted to impose prior authorization requirements on any drug except in the first 6 months following approval of the drug by the Food and Drug Administration. OBRA 90 specified that effective July 1, 1991, States that use prior authorization for prescription drugs must provide for telephone response within 24 hours of an inquiry and permit dispensing a 72-hour supply of the drug in an emergency.

Table IV-7 shows that as of May 1991, 36 States and the District of Columbia had prior authorization programs in effect. This information was collected prior to the effective date of the OBRA 90 requirements.

TABLE IV-7. States With Medicaid Prior Authorization Prescription Drug Procedures, May 1991

State	Procedure in place
Alabama	Yes
Alaska	Yes
Arizona	AHCCCS[a]
Arkansas	Yes
California	Yes
Colorado	Yes
Connecticut	Yes
Delaware	No
District of Columbia	Yes
Florida	Yes
Georgia	Yes
Hawaii	Yes
Idaho	Yes
Illinois	Yes
Indiana	No
Iowa	Yes
Kansas	Yes
Kentucky	Yes
Louisiana	No
Maine	Yes
Maryland	Yes
Massachusetts	Yes
Michigan	Yes
Minnesota	Yes
Mississippi	Yes
Missouri	Yes

TABLE IV-7. States With Medicaid Prior Authorization Prescription Drug Procedures, May 1991--Continued

State	Procedure in place
Montana	No
Nebraska	Yes
Nevada	Yes
New Hampshire	No
New Jersey	Yes
New Mexico	Yes
New York	No
North Carolina	No
North Dakota	No
Ohio	Yes
Oklahoma	No
Oregon	Yes
Pennsylvania	No
Rhode Island	No
South Carolina	Yes
South Dakota	No
Tennessee	Yes
Texas	Yes
Utah	Yes
Vermont	Yes
Virginia	Yes
Washington	Yes
West Virginia	Yes
Wisconsin	Yes
Wyoming	No

*Arizona operates a demonstration program known as the Arizona Health Care Cost Containment System (AHCCCS). Under AHCCCS, the State contracts with prepaid health plans. These plans are paid on a capitation basis and are responsible for providing all of the services covered by the program, including prescription drugs. An individual prepaid plan may impose its own prior authorization requirements.

Source: National Pharmaceutical Council. *Pharmaceutical Benefits Under State Medical Assistance Programs*, Sept. 1991. p. 102.

V. EXPERIMENTAL ITEMS/TRANSPLANTS

Public health programs and private health insurance plans generally decide whether or not to reimburse for a particular medical procedure based on whether it is safe and effective. Generally, they will pay for items that are classified as accepted medical practice, but not for those classified as "experimental" or "investigational." The Federal Medicare program, whose reimbursement decisions often guide other insurance or medical program payers, precludes payment for experimental items.

Individual States can make their own decisions with respect to coverage of transplants under Medicaid, provided certain requirements are met. Federal law prohibits Federal matching for organ transplant procedures unless: (1) the State plan provides written standards for coverage; and (2) the standards provide that similarly situated individuals are treated alike and any restrictions placed on providers who could provide the care are consistent with access to high quality care. If a State covers organ transplants, such services must be sufficient in amount, duration, and scope to achieve their purpose.[22]

A recent analysis by the Intergovernmental Health Policy Project (IHPP)[23] showed that all States, except for Wyoming, offered coverage for some solid organ transplants in 1990. Virtually all States covered kidney and liver transplants. Heart transplants were available in the majority of States while combined heart/lung transplants were only covered in about one-half of the States. Coverage for lung transplants and pancreas transplants was limited. (See table IV-8.) Only three States (Nevada, New Mexico and Tennessee) failed to cover organ procurement costs associated with Medicaid transplants, while every State paid for immunosuppressive drugs.

The IHPP analysis suggested that most States did not impose significant restrictions on the availability of covered organ transplant services. With the exception of liver transplants, age was rarely used as a criteria; ten States limited coverage of liver transplants to children. States covering their medically needy populations generally allowed this group the same coverage for organ transplants as was available for the categorically needy. Several States imposed special payment restrictions or caps.

---

[22]Despite these requirements, courts may require States to fund transplants in individual cases. For example, in *Velia Montoya vs. Marlin W. Johnston* (DC WD Tex 1987) 654 F.Supp.511, the district court enjoined the State from enforcing a payment limit which had the effect of excluding medically necessary liver transplants for two children.

[23]U.S. Dept. of Health and Human Services. Health Resources and Services Administration. *A Guide to State Organ Transplant Activities in the United States*. Report prepared by Susan Laudicina, Contract No. HRSA 90-747, Intergovernmental Health Policy Project, George Washington University, Dec. 1990. Washington, 1990.

The IHPP review found that most State Medicaid programs used specific medical criteria to select patients for transplant surgery and frequently used independent medical advisory committees to make the determinations. Approximately half of the States had developed their own standards that medical transplant centers were required to meet while others adopted Medicare standards.

TABLE IV-8. Medicaid Coverage of Solid Organ Transplants, by Procedure, by State, 1990

	Heart	Heart/ Lung	Kidney	Liver	Lung	Pancreas
Alabama			X	X		
Alaska			X	X		
Arizona	X		X	X		
Arkansas	X		X	X		
California	X		X	X		
Colorado	X	X	X	X		
Connecticut	X	X	X	X		
Delaware	X	X	X	X		X
District of Columbia	X		X	X		
Florida	X		X	X		
Georgia			X	X		
Hawaii			X	X		
Idaho			X			
Illinois	X		X	X		
Indiana	X	X	X	X		X
Iowa	X		X	X		
Kansas	X		X	X		
Kentucky	X	X	X	X	X	X
Louisiana	X	X	X	X	X	X
Maine	X	X	X	X	X	
Maryland	X	X	X	X	X	
Massachusetts	X	X	X	X	X	X
Michigan	X	X	X	X	X	X
Minnesota	X		X	X		
Mississippi	X	X	X	X	X	X
Missouri	X		X	X		
Montana	X		X	X		
Nebraska	X		X	X		
Nevada			X	X		
New Hampshire			X	X		
New Jersey	X	X	X	X		
New Mexico	X	X	X	X	X	
New York	X	X	X	X		
North Carolina	X	X	X	X	X	
North Dakota	X	X	X	X	X	X

TABLE IV-8. Medicaid Coverage of Solid Organ Transplants,
by Procedure, by State, 1990--Continued

	Heart	Heart/ Lung	Kidney	Liver	Lung	Pancreas
Ohio	X	X	X	X	X	X
Oklahoma			X	X		
Oregon[a]	X	X	X	X		
Pennsylvania	X	X	X	X	X	X
Rhode Island	X	X	X	X		
South Carolina	X		X	X		
South Dakota	X		X	X		
Tennessee	X		X	X		
Texas	X		X	X		
Utah			X	X		
Vermont	X	X	X	X	X	X
Virginia			X			
Washington[a]	X	X	X	X	X	
West Virginia	X		X	X		
Wisconsin	X	X	X	X	X	X
Wyoming						
TOTALS	40	23	50	48	15	12

[a]Oregon and Washington cover pancreas/kidney transplants but not pancreas transplant procedures.

Source: IHPP, 1990.

VI. COST SHARING

States are permitted to impose cost-sharing charges with certain major exceptions. These cost-sharing charges may serve as a means of utilization control.

States may not impose deductible or coinsurance charges on either the categorically needy or the medically needy under the following circumstances:

- No such charges may be imposed on services provided to children under age 18; States may provide that no cost-sharing charges will be imposed for children aged 18 to 21;

- States are barred from imposing cost-sharing charges on services related to pregnancy (including prenatal, delivery, and post-partum services) or to any other medical condition which may complicate the pregnancy. States may provide that no cost-sharing charges will be imposed for any services provided to pregnant women;

- States may not impose cost-sharing charges on services provided to inpatients in hospitals, nursing facilities, ICFs/MR, or other medical institution if such individuals are required to spend all their income for medical expenses except for the amount exempted for personal needs;

- States may not impose cost-sharing charges on emergency, family planning, or hospice services; and

- States are precluded from imposing cost-sharing charges on categorically needy enrollees in health maintenance organizations (HMOs). They may also exempt the medically needy from such charges.

States may impose charges on restricted groups under a waiver, but only if the waiver is for a demonstration project that the Secretary finds meets certain conditions (including testing a unique and previously untested use of copayments).

Cost sharing charges must be "nominal" in amount as defined under regulations. In the case of noninstitutional services, the maximum deductible cannot exceed $2.00 per month; coinsurance charges may range from $0.50 to $3.00 (depending on the amount Medicaid pays for the service). In the case of institutional services, the maximum charge per admission cannot exceed 50 percent of the payment the program makes for the first day of care.

The Secretary may waive the nominality requirement in the case of nonemergency services in emergency rooms where the State has established, to the satisfaction of the Secretary, that alternative sources of nonemergency services are actually available and accessible. When the Secretary is satisfied that such conditions have been met and a waiver has been granted, the State may impose a charge up to twice the amount defined as nominal.[24]

States may also impose an enrollment fee, premium, or similar charge on the medically needy though States generally have not availed themselves of this option.

States may impose a monthly premium charge on pregnant women and infants whose income exceeds 150 percent of the Federal poverty line. The amount of the premium may not exceed 10 percent of the amount by which the

---

[24]In March 1992, the Inspector General of DHHS issued two reports on Medicaid emergency room use. The report examined a variety of approaches that nine States had tried to curtail the use of emergency rooms by Medicaid patients in nonemergency situations. The report noted that the most successful approaches focused on providing Medicaid recipients with alternative more appropriate access to care. A few States had developed copayment (including nominal) copayment approaches. The report noted that:

Copayment programs were generally not successful due to opposition. Two of the four copayment procedures were either never implemented or terminated and one of the two remaining copayment programs has been judged to be unsuccessful.

family's income, less childcare expenses, exceeds 150 percent of the poverty line for a comparable sized family.

States are required to pay Medicare Part A premiums for certain working disabled persons not otherwise eligible for Medicaid whose income is below 200 percent of the Federal poverty line. States may impose a monthly premium for persons with incomes above 150 percent of the poverty level. The premium is to be set based on a sliding scale from 0 percent (at 150 percent of poverty) to 100 percent (at 200 percent of poverty).

No provider participating under Medicaid may deny services to an individual because of his inability to pay cost-sharing charges; however, this does not exclude the beneficiary from liability for paying such charges. As a practical matter, many cost-sharing obligations are uncollectible; in effect the cost-sharing requirement represents a reduction in provider payments in such cases.

The National Governors' Association reports that as of January 1, 1991, 25 States imposed cost-sharing charges on one or more Medicaid services. (See table IV-9.) Many of these States imposed such charges on a broad range of services. The service category for which cost sharing charges were imposed most frequently was drugs.

TABLE IV-9. State Co-payment Policies, in Effect as of January 1, 1991

State	Service category	Co-pay amount[a]
Alabama	Ambulatory surgical center services	$3.00
	Durable medical equipment	3.00
	Federally qualified health centers	1.00
	Inpatient hospital	$50/admission
	Outpatient hospital[b]	3.00
	Supplies/appliances	1.00
	Physician office visits (including optometric)	1.00
	Prescription drugs	varies[c d]
	Rural health clinics[b]	1.00
Alaska	None	
Arizona	Office visits	$1.00
	Elective surgery	$5.00
	Nonemergency use of emergency room	$5.00
Arkansas	None	
California	Prescription drugs	$1.00[c]
	Emergency room (inappropriate use)	$5.00
	Outpatient hospital	$1.00
Colorado[e]	Physician services	$2.00

See notes at end of table.

TABLE IV-9. State Co-payment Policies, in Effect as of
January 1, 1991--Continued

State	Service category	Co-pay amount[a]
Colorado[e]--continued	Community mental health centers	$2.00
	Inpatient hospitals	$15/stay
	Outpatient hospital	3.00
	Prescription drugs	1.00
	Physician visit	2.00
	Rural health clinics	2.00
Connecticut	None	
Delaware	None	
District of Columbia	Prescription drugs	$ .50[d] [f]
	Eyeglasses	2.00
Florida	Dentures	Varies[f] [g]
	Prosthetic devices--hearing aids	Varies[f] [g]
Georgia	None	
Hawaii	None	
Idaho	None	
Illinois	Inpatient hospital	Varies[h]
Indiana	None	
Iowa	Chiropracty	$1.00
	Dental	3.00[f]
	Prescription drugs	1.00
	Eyeglasses--optician services	2.00
	Medical equipment and supplies	2.00
	Optometry	2.00
	Podiatry	1.00
	Prosthetic devices	
	• hearing aids	3.00
	• orthopedic shoes	2.00
	Psychologist	2.00
	Psychotherapy (CMHC only)	2.00
	Rehabilitation agency	2.00
	Transportation--ambulance	2.00
Kansas	Ambulatory surgery center services	$3.00
	Audiology	3.00
	Chiropracty	.50
	Dental	2.00
	Prescription drugs	1.00
	Freestanding psychiatric hospital (private)	$25/stay
	Home health agency (skilled nursing)	2.00

See notes at end of table.

TABLE IV-9. State Co-payment Policies, in Effect as of
January 1, 1991--Continued

State	Service category	Co-pay amount[a]
Kansas--continued	Hospital:	
	• inpatient	25/admission
	• nonemergency outpatient	1.00
	• outpatient surgery	3.00
	Medical equipment	3.00
	Mental health center	2.00
	Optometrist	2.00
	Physician office visit	1.00
	Podiatry	1.00
	Psychology	2.00
	Transportation--nonemergency ambulance	1.00
Kentucky	None	
Louisiana	None	
Maine	Prescription drugs	$0.75[i]
Maryland	Prescription drugs	$0.50
Massachusetts	None	
Michigan[j]	Chiropracty	$1.00
	Dental	3.00[f]
	Prescription drugs	0.50
	Optometry	2.00
	Podiatry	2.00
	Prosthetic devices--hearing aids	3.00
Minnesota	None	
Mississippi	Dental	$2.00
	Prescription drugs	1.00[d k]
	Home health visit	2.00
	Hospital:	
	• emergency room	2.00
	• inpatient	5.00
	Optometry	2.00
	Rural health clinic--office visit	1.00
	Transportation--ambulance	2.00
Missouri	Audiology	Varies[l]
	Dental	Varies[l]
	Dentures	Varies[g]
	Prescription drugs	Varies[l]
	Hospital	
	• inpatient	$10/admission
	• outpatient	3.00
	Optometry	Varies[l]
	Podiatry	Varies[l]

See notes at end of table.

TABLE IV-9. State Co-payment Policies, in Effect as of
January 1, 1991--Continued

State	Service category	Co-pay amount[a]
Montana	Audiology	$0.50[f]
	Clinic services	1.00
	Clinical social worker	0.50
	Dental	1.00
	Prescription drugs	1.00
	Eyeglasses	1.00
	Home dialysis for ESRD	0.50
	Home health	
	(not including durable medical equipment)	1.00
	Hospital:	
	• inpatient	$3/day[m]
	• outpatient	1.00
	Nurse specialist service	1.00
	Occupational therapy	0.50
	Optometry	1.00
	Physical therapy (outpatient)	0.50
	Physician	1.00
	Podiatry	1.00
	Private duty nursing	0.50
	Prosthetic devices:	
	• hearing aids	0.50
	• medical equipment and supplies	0.50
	Psychological	0.50
	Speech pathology	0.50
Nebraska	None	
Nevada	None	
New Hampshire	Prescription drugs:	
	• generic	$0.50
	• brand names	1.00
New Jersey	None	
New Mexico	None	
New York	None	
North Carolina	Chiropracty	$0.50
	Clinic	0.50
	Dental	2.00[k]
	Eyeglasses (each pair and repair of $4+)	2.00
	Hospital--outpatient	1.00
	Optometry	1.00
	Physician	0.50
	Podiatry	1.00
	Prescription drugs	0.50
North Dakota	Eyeglasses--replacement lenses & frames within 1 year of original prescription	$3.00

See notes at end of table.

TABLE IV-9. State Co-payment Policies, in Effect as of
January 1, 1991--Continued

State	Service category	Co-pay amount[a]
Ohio	None	
Oklahoma	None	
Oregon	None	
Pennsylvania	Prescription drugs	$0.50
	Hospital:	
	• inpatient	$3/day[n]
	• nonemergency service in a hospital	Varies[o]
	• emergency room	Varies[o]
	All other allowable services	Varies[p]
Rhode Island	None	
South Carolina	Prescription drugs	$1.00[d] [f]
South Dakota	Ambulatory surgical center	Varies[g]
	Chemical dependency treatment	Varies[g]
	Chiropracty	$0.50
	Dental	1.00
	Dentures	3.00
	Durable medical equipment	Varies[g]
	EPSDT screening	1.00
	Hospital--outpatient (except lab)	Varies[g]
	Mental health centers	Varies[g]
	Optometry	0.50
	Physician	3.00
	Podiatry	2.00
	Prescription drugs	1.00[d]
	Psychotherapy	2.00
	Rehabilitation hospital outpatient (except lab)	Varies[g]
Tennessee	None	
Texas	None	
Utah	None	
Vermont	Prescription drugs	$1.00
Virginia	Clinic	$1.00[d] [f]
	Hospital:	
	• inpatient	$30/admission[d] [f]
	• outpatient, nonemergency	2.00[d] [f]
	Optometry--eye exams	1.00[d] [f]
	Physician	1.00[d] [f]
	Prescription drugs	1.00[d] [f]
Washington	None	
West Virginia	Prescription drugs	Varies[q]

See notes at end of table.

TABLE IV-9. State Co-payment Policies, in Effect as of
January 1, 1991--Continued

State	Service category	Co-pay amount[a]
Wisconsin	Audiological testing	$1.00
	Chiropracty	1.00
	Day treatment service	0.50
	Dental	Varies[r]
	Prescription drugs	0.50[s]
	Durable medical equipment	1.00
	Eyeglasses	Varies[t]
	Hospital:	
	• inpatient, general	$3/day[u]
	• inpatient, mental disease	$3/day[u]
	• outpatient	3.00
	• surgery	3.00
	Optometry	Varies[l]
	Oral surgery	1.00
	Orthodonty	Varies[v]
	Physician visits:[w]	
	• consultation	3.00
	• diagnostic procedure in office	1.00
	• eye exams	2.00
	• home	1.00
	• lab procedure in office	1.00
	• radiology procedure in office	2.00
	• office	1.00
	• outpatient hospital	1.00
	Prosthetic devices--hearing aids	Varies[l]
	Prosthodonic appliance	3.00
	Psychotherapy	Varies[t x]
	Rural health clinics	2.00
	Speech/hearing/language	Varies[y]
	Physical and occupational therapy	$.50/15 min.[z]
	Transportation-ambulance/nonemergency	$2/trip
Wyoming	Prescription drug	$1.00

Key: CMHC--Community Mental Health Center
DME--Durable Medical Equipment
ESRD--End Stage Renal Disease

[a]Unless otherwise specified, co-pay amounts are paid per service visit. They apply to all population groups allowed under the law except where otherwise noted.

[b]For these services the State requires the co-payment be paid per claim for all Medicaid beneficiaries who are also Medicare eligible. All other Medicaid beneficiaries--the co-payment is per visit.

[c]Applies to persons age 19 and over.

[d]Applies to pregnant women for nonpregnancy related services.

[e]Medicaid beneficiaries are subject to a maximum of $120 in co-payments per year.

[f]Applies to persons age 21 and over.

[g]Co-pay is 5 percent of reimbursement for these services.

[h]$2 for per diem of $275 to $325; $3 for per diem over $325.

[i]$4.50 per month limit on prescriptions.

[j]These co-pay policies are not applicable to individuals who enroll in physician-sponsored plans.

TABLE IV-9. State Co-payment Policies, in Effect as of
January 1, 1991--Continued

[k]Applies to persons age 18 and over.
[l]$.50 to $3.00.
[m]Maximum co-pay charge of $66 per stay.
[n]Maximum co-pay charge of $21 per stay.
[o]In Pennsylvania the co-payments for services range from $1 to $6 based on the Medicaid fee for the services provided. If the Medicaid fee is:
$ 1.00--10.00 the co-pay is $1;
$10.01--25.00 the co-pay is $2;
$25.01--50.00 the co-pay is $4;
$50.01 or more the co-pay is $6.
[p]For all other services Pennsylvania has established a co-payment based on the Medicaid fee for the service provided. If the Medicaid fee is:
$ 1.00--10.00 the co-pay is $0.50;
$10.01--25.00 the co-pay is $1.00;
$25.01--50.00 the co-pay is $2.00;
$50.01 or more the co-pay is $3.00.
[q]$0.50 on $10.00 or less; $1.00 on 10.01 or more.
[r]$0.50 to $1.00.
[s]Co-payment limited to $5 per month per pharmacy.
[t]$0.50 to $2.00.
[u]Maximum co-payment of $75 per stay.
[v]$2.00 to $3.00.
[w]A cap of $30 cumulative limit per calendar year per physician for all physician services (physician visits surgery, lab and x-ray services, and diagnostic tests) applies.
[x]Co-payment may be charged only on the first 15 visits or $500 per year.
[y]$0.50 per 15 minutes for some services; $1.00 per procedure for others.
[z]Co-payment is limited to the first 30 hours or $1,500 of accumulated services per beneficiary, per calendar year.

Source: National Governors' Association, 1991.

CHAPTER V. REIMBURSEMENT[1]

SUMMARY

Under Medicaid law, States now have considerable freedom to develop their own methods and standards for reimbursement of Medicaid services. This chapter reviews States' methods for determining provider payment and for collecting amounts due from other potential sources of payment for Medicaid beneficiaries.

Before 1980, Medicaid programs were required to use the same methods as Medicare in paying for hospital and nursing facility services. Facilities were paid on the basis of the actual costs they incurred in providing care. Legislative changes in 1980 and 1981 permitted States to develop their own reimbursement methodologies for these services. Most States have now moved to "prospective" payment systems, under which the amount of payment for a defined unit of service (such as a day of care in a nursing facility or full treatment of an inpatient hospital case) is established in advance. Some of these systems are comparable to Medicare's prospective payment system (PPS), under which reimbursement varies according to the classification of each case into a diagnosis related group, or DRG. In other States, hospitals are paid a flat rate, for each day of care or for total care for each patient, without regard to diagnosis. Finally, States may develop rates through negotiation with hospitals. In a number of States, the Medicaid program participates in an "all-payer" system, under which most insurers in the State agree to a single method for paying hospitals.

States are required to make additional payments to "disproportionate share" hospitals (DSHs), those that serve a higher than average number of Medicaid and other low-income patients. State DSH payments have grown dramatically in recent years, from an estimated $831 million in FY 1990 to a projected $16.5 billion in FY 1992, over 12 percent of total Medicaid spending. The Medicaid Voluntary Contribution and Provider-Specific Tax Amendments of 1991 (P.L. 102-234) limits national aggregate spending for DSH payment adjustments to 12 percent of total Medicaid program spending, roughly the level projected for FY 1992. States with DSH payments already exceeding 12 percent may not increase those payments faster than the rate of growth in their overall Medicaid spending. Other States may raise their DSH payments, subject to an allocation system that will keep aggregate national payments within the cap.

Data collected by the American Hospital Association (AHA) indicate that most States are paying less than the full cost incurred by hospitals in serving

---

[1]This chapter was written by Mark Merlis.

Medicaid beneficiaries. In the median State in 1990, Medicaid covered 84.5 percent of estimated costs; in the aggregate, AHA estimates that Medicaid nationally covered 80.3 percent of hospital costs. Courts have found Medicaid reimbursement inadequate in several States, and litigation is pending in several more. As a result, many States increased their Medicaid payments in 1991 (whether for DSHs or for all hospitals). More recent data might therefore show smaller shortfalls in Medicaid payments.

For nursing facility services, Medicaid law formerly distinguished between two types of facilities: skilled nursing facilities (SNFs) and intermediate care facilities (ICFs). The distinction between the two types of care was eliminated effective October 1, 1990. Nearly all States have adopted PPSs for nursing facility services, although they may pay on a retrospective basis for certain cost components. Rates may be set for individual facilities or for peer groups (based on such factors as size and location). As of 1989, 12 States have adopted "case mix" reimbursement systems, under which higher payments are made to facilities that accept more severely ill patients.

For services of physicians or other individual practitioners, payment amounts are usually the lesser of the provider's actual charge for the service or a maximum allowable charge established by the State. Payments may be determined through "prevailing charge" screens, under which the maximum is set at a fixed percentile of the customary charges of area providers for comparable services. Or the State may use a fee schedule, specifying a flat maximum payment amount for each service. In 1989, 41 States and the District of Columbia used fixed fee schedules. The Physician Payment Review Commission (PPRC) has estimated that State payment rates for physician services in that year averaged 73.7 percent of what would have been allowed under Medicare for the same services.

States use a wide variety of methods for reimbursing hospital outpatient services. Hospitals may be paid their actual costs for providing outpatient care, or the State may pay fixed rates. These may be based on a hospital's historic costs or may involve a fee schedule comparable to those used for physician services. As of 1989, only 10 States were still paying on the basis of actual costs; the rest had adopted some form of prospective rates or a fee schedule.

For prescription drugs, States are required to establish a system that pays a pharmacy's cost for acquiring a drug plus a fixed dispensing fee. Payment for drugs that exist in both brand-name and generic versions is generally limited to the price of the least expensive readily available generic equivalent. The pharmacy thus has an incentive to substitute the generic drug unless the physician specifically requests that the brand-name version be furnished. The Omnibus Budget Reconciliation Act of 1990 (OBRA 90) requires pharmaceutical manufacturers to grant rebates to Medicaid programs for the drugs they purchase, thus giving Medicaid discounts comparable to those offered to other high-volume purchasers.

Although Medicaid programs cover numerous other kinds of services, the law establishes specific payment rules for only a few of them. Payment to rural health clinics, hospices, and clinical laboratories must generally follow Medicare rules.   For some services, including laboratory services, durable medical equipment, and eyeglasses, States are permitted to establish "volume purchasing" programs, selecting a sole source for the service through competitive bidding or other means.

Medicaid payments to health maintenance organizations (HMOs) and similar entities are generally in the form of a fixed monthly per capita amount for each beneficiary enrolled. Regulations limit this amount to 100 percent of the amount that the State would have spent to provide the services covered by the contract to an equivalent group of non-enrolled beneficiaries. With a single exception, payments to federally qualified health centers (FQHCs), the amounts paid by HMOs to their subcontractors for services to Medicaid beneficiaries are not subject to Medicaid rules.

With minor exceptions, Medicaid is the payer of last resort, secondary to any other insurance coverage a beneficiary may have or to any other third party who may be liable for medical payments or medical support on the beneficiary's behalf.

Most aged Medicaid beneficiaries and many of the disabled are also eligible for Medicare benefits.   States enter into "buy-in" agreements with the Department of Health and Human Services (DHHS) for these dual eligibles. The State pays Medicare premiums on the beneficiaries' behalf. Medicare pays for the services it covers, with Medicaid paying beneficiary cost-sharing, the deductibles and coinsurance required under Medicare. States are now required to buy in for most aged and disabled Medicare beneficiaries with incomes below 100 percent of the poverty line, and will have to pay premiums for those below 120 percent of the poverty line by 1995. For many dual eligibles, Medicaid also pays for services that Medicare does not cover but that are included in the State's Medicaid plan, such as prescription drugs and most nursing facility care. Provisions of the Medicare Catastrophic Coverage Act of 1988 will require all States to buy in for most aged and disabled Medicare beneficiaries with incomes below 100 percent of the poverty line.

OBRA 90 requires States, effective January 1, 1991, to pay premiums and cost-sharing on behalf of beneficiaries eligible for enrollment in a group health plan when it is cost-effective to do so. For example, a beneficiary who is employed might be eligible for coverage under an employer health plan, but might be required to pay a monthly premium to join. Medicaid will pay that premium, as well as deductibles and coinsurance required under the plan, if the cost is less than the cost of the services that the employer plan will cover and that would otherwise have been paid directly by Medicaid.   Some Medicaid beneficiaries may also have private health insurance for other reasons, or may be eligible for payments through automobile or liability insurance or workers' compensation. Finally, an absent parent may be responsible for medical support payments.   Applicants for Medicaid benefits are required to disclose any potential payment sources, and Medicaid programs must have a system for pursuing third party claims. For most services, States have adopted a "cost avoidance" system, denying payment of claims for which third party liability is

known to exist. For a few types of services, Medicaid programs pay the claims
and then seek to collect from the responsible party.

I. INTRODUCTION

Under Medicaid law, States have considerable freedom to develop their own
methods and standards for reimbursement of Medicaid services. In recent years,
partly in response to concerns about maintaining access to care, Congress has
begun to impose more specific requirements relating to adequacy of payment
levels for certain services. Actual payment methodologies, however, are still left
largely to the discretion of the States.

Four basic statutory requirements apply to all types of services.

- Providers must accept Medicaid reimbursement as payment
  in full, except for any beneficiary cost-sharing amounts
  provided for by the State plan or any amount due from a
  medically needy beneficiary with a spend-down liability (see
  Chapter III, Eligibility and *Chapter IV, Services* for a
  discussion of these provisions).

- Medicaid is secondary to any other health coverage or third
  party payment source available to beneficiaries, including
  Medicare.

- "Methods and procedures" for making payments must be such
  as to assure that payments will be "consistent with efficiency,
  economy, and quality of care." (The Health Care Financing
  Administration (HCFA) relies on this provision as a general
  authority to regulate State reimbursement methodologies
  and to establish upper limits for State payments.)

- The State's payment rates must be sufficient to attract
  enough providers so that covered services will be as available
  to Medicaid beneficiaries as they are to the general
  population. This rule was codified by the Omnibus Budget
  Reconciliation Act of 1989 (OBRA 89) but had previously
  been established by regulation.

The law imposes more specific tests on the adequacy of payment rates for
certain services, including hospital and nursing facility care and obstetrical and
pediatric physician services. Actual payment rules or methodologies are
prescribed by law for only a few types of providers: federally qualified health
centers (FQHCs, which are Public Health Service grantees and similar entities),
rural health clinics, independent laboratories, and hospices. The Omnibus
Budget Reconciliation Act of 1990 (OBRA 90) has added requirements relating
to payment for prescription drugs. However, Federal Medicaid regulations go
beyond the statute in establishing payment ceilings or other tests of the
reasonableness of State reimbursement methodologies for services not
specifically covered by the statute.

Part II of this chapter describes the legal requirements governing Medicaid reimbursement for specific types of providers or services, including the new requirements for prescription drug reimbursement. It also provides an overview of the variety of payment methodologies adopted by States for four major service types: physician services, hospital inpatient and outpatient care, and nursing facility care.[2] To the extent possible, Medicaid payments for these major services are compared to providers' costs or to payments made by other patients or insurers. The greatest attention is devoted to hospital payments, partly because these are currently the subject of numerous court challenges and partly because more comprehensive payment data are available for hospitals than for physicians or nursing facilities.

Part III discusses the coordination of Medicaid payments with other payments that may be available for services furnished to Medicaid beneficiaries, including Medicare and other insurance plans. The discussion concludes with an explanation of the relationship between Medicaid and the Indian Health Service.

II. MEDICAID REIMBURSEMENT RULES AND METHODOLOGIES

A. Inpatient Services

For services to inpatients, including those of hospitals, nursing facilities, and intermediate care facilities for the mentally retarded (ICFs/MR), two basic payment methodologies are in use: retrospective and prospective.

In a *retrospective system*, payment amounts are determined after services are rendered and are based on the actual costs incurred by the provider in furnishing those services. Commonly, the State will make periodic interim payments, with final reimbursement amounts determined after an annual audit.[3] The costs ultimately reimbursed may be limited to "reasonable" costs, as defined by the State. States may establish ceilings, above which a provider's costs will not be considered reasonable. In a fully *prospective system*, payment amounts are determined in advance. The provider receives a specified rate for each service rendered, regardless of whether the provider's actual costs are more or less than that rate.

Until 1980, State Medicaid programs were required to follow Medicare reimbursement principles in paying for inpatient services. Under the Medicare

---

[2]Information on Arizona's payment methodologies has been omitted from these discussions, because services under Arizona's demonstration medical assistance program are furnished almost entirely through capitated, HMO-like arrangements. See *Appendix G, Managed Care* for a discussion of the Arizona program.

[3]The Omnibus Budget Reconciliation Act of 1987 (OBRA 87, P.L. 100-203) repealed a requirement that State audits be coordinated with audits of the same providers conducted by Medicare.

rules in effect at that time, this meant that nearly every State used a retrospective reasonable cost system (a few States had waivers to operate "all-payer" hospital systems; see section *b* below). In what is known as the "Boren amendment," the Omnibus Reconciliation Act of 1980 (OBRA 80 P.L. 96-499) repealed this requirement for nursing facility services, freeing States to establish new methodologies of their own. The Omnibus Budget Reconciliation Act of 1981 (OBRA 81, P.L. 97-35) applied the amendment to inpatient hospital services.

The law now provides simply that payment rates for hospitals and nursing facilities must be "reasonable and adequate" to meet the costs of "efficiently and economically operated" facilities in providing care that meets Federal and State quality and safety standards. For hospital inpatient care the rates must also be sufficient to assure reasonable access to services and must include adjustments for DSHs, those serving a high proportion of low-income patients. Payments may not exceed the hospital's customary charges to the public.[4] For nursing facilities, rates must take into account the costs of compliance with the nursing home reform provisions of the Omnibus Budget Reconciliation Act of 1987 (OBRA 87). For both hospitals and nursing facilities there are also limits on Medicaid reimbursement for costs relating to transfer of the facility to new ownership.

Nearly all States have responded to the new flexibility by shifting from retrospective to prospective payment systems (PPSs) for both hospital and nursing facility services. States' interest in prospective payment has stemmed from concerns that providers paid on a full cost basis have no incentive to perform efficiently and may furnish unnecessary services. Critics of PPSs contend that quality may be compromised if providers are forced to provide care within a fixed budget, and that providers may refuse care to patients whose costs are likely to exceed the predetermined payment. (The possible impact of Medicaid reimbursement levels on access to care is discussed further in *Appendix H, Medicaid as Health Insurance: Measures of Performance.*)

While the Boren amendment gave States the flexibility to develop new payment systems, it also established a benchmark against which those systems were to be measured: the State must find, and must provide assurances satisfactory to the Secretary, that its Medicaid rates are reasonable and adequate.[5] In 1990, the Supreme Court affirmed that facilities had a right to

---

[4]In the case of a public hospital that provides free care or imposes only nominal charges, Medicaid reimbursement is not limited by this "customary charge" rule. The State may provide reasonable compensation for services to Medicaid beneficiaries.

[5]Conference report language accompanying the 1981 extension of the Boren language to hospitals restated this benchmark but also suggested that States might "limit increases to the increases that result from price increases for goods and services purchased by hospitals." U.S. Congress. House. Conference Report on the Omnibus Budget Reconciliation Act of 1981. House Report. No. 97-208,
(continued...)

seek judicial review of the reasonableness and adequacy of Medicaid rates (*Wilder* v. *Virginia Hospital Association*. 110 S.Ct. 2510, 1990). The *Wilder* decision merely settled the question of whether the Boren amendment conferred rights on providers that could be enforced in court. Even before this decision, hospitals in some States had obtained court judgments that Medicaid payments were inadequate.

Earlier in 1990, for example, Temple University won an injunction compelling Pennsylvania to comply with requirements for extra payments to DSHs (*Temple University* v. *White*. 729 F.Supp. 1093, 1990, affirmed CA-3, 90-1112, 1991). In Michigan, a Federal court ruled the State's hospital rates inadequate simply because the State had never made the required internal finding that its rates were reasonable; because the State had failed to follow the proper procedures, the court did not need to examine whether the rates were actually reasonable (*Michigan Hospital Association* v. *Babcock*. 736 F.Supp. 759, 1990). Other rulings have focused more directly on the rates themselves. In 1989, the U.S. Court of Appeals for the Tenth Circuit ruled that, while Colorado made the required findings about the adequacy of rates, its process for doing so was a mere formality and the rates themselves were inadequate (*Amisub (PSL), Inc.* v. *Colorado*, 879 F.2d 789 (10th Cir., 1989), cert denied, 110 S.Ct. 3212 (1990)). Colorado had imposed a 46 percent across-the-board cut in hospital rates and was not meeting the full costs of any facility. Similarly, in 1991, a Federal court in the State of Washington enjoined the use of the State's DRG payment system, under which the average hospital received only 80 percent of its costs (*Multicare Medical Center* v. *State of Washington*, W.D.Wa. C88-421Z, 1991). There have also been cases applying the Boren amendment to nursing facility reimbursement.[6]

A July 1991 review of Boren amendment cases found that litigation was pending in 12 States, while hospitals in another 10 States were considering filing suit.[7] There are also likely to be further suits by nursing facilities, based not only on the Boren amendment but also on an OBRA 87 requirement that

---

[5](...continued)
97th Cong., 1st Sess. Washington, GPO, July 29, 1981. p. 962. Hospital costs per admission have grown about 50 percent faster than input prices since 1981, as measured by HCFA's market basket index. A State that paid full costs in 1981 and adopted the conferees' suggestion beginning in that year would have been paying about 66 percent of cost by 1990. At least one Federal court has held, however, that States may not limit rate increases to increases in input prices. *Multicare Medical Center* v. *State of Washington*, W.D.Wa. C88-421Z (1991).

[6]For example, *Pinnacle Nursing Home* v. *Axelrod*, 719 F.Supp. 1173 (1990); *Health Care Association of Michigan* v. *Babcock*, W.D.Mi, K89-50063 CA (1990).

[7]U.S. Library of Congress. Congressional Research Service. *Medicaid: Recent Trends in Beneficiaries and Spending*. CRS Report for Congress No. 92-365 EPW, by Kathleen King, Richard Rimkunas, and Dawn Nuschler. Washington, 1992.

rates be revised to reflect the costs of complying with new and more stringent quality requirements.

1. Inpatient Hospital Services

Although the Boren amendment eliminated the statutory limit on Medicaid hospital payments, Medicaid regulations provide that the aggregate amount spent by a State for inpatient services during a year may not exceed the aggregate amount which would have been spent if the State had used the current Medicare system.[8] (The Secretary is prohibited from using this requirement to limit a State's payments to DSHs. Newly enacted limits on these payments are discussed below.) Beginning in 1983, Medicare shifted to a prospective payment system (PPS) for inpatient services. This has altered the benchmark against which a State's Medicaid reimbursement system is measured, but has not changed the basic rule.

a. Basic Systems

As of July 1, 1991, all but four States had adopted some form of prospective system for inpatient hospital reimbursement. Table V-1 shows the basic system in use in each State, as reported in a 1991 survey conducted for the Prospective Payment Assessment Commission (ProPAC).[9] It should be noted that the systems described in the table and in the following discussion are those used for most acute general hospitals in the State. States may use different modes of payment for particular classes of facilities. For example, States may follow Medicare in using a PPS for acute general hospitals and a reasonable cost system for psychiatric and other specialized hospitals. In addition, States that negotiate rates with preferred providers under a selective contracting system may have a separate payment methodology for emergency or other services obtained outside that system.

---

[8]Note that this requirement applies only in the aggregate. Reimbursement for specific facilities or patients may exceed Medicare levels, so long as overall average reimbursement for the State does not. The Secretary is prohibited from using this requirement to limit a State's payments to disproportionate share hospitals.

[9]Much of the information in this section is from: Prospective Payment Assessment Commission. *Medicaid Hospital Payment*. Congressional Report C-91-02, Oct. 1, 1991. Washington, 1991.

TABLE V-1. Medicaid Inpatient Hospital Payment Systems, by State, 1991

State	Retrospective/ reconciled — Cost	Prospective limit on costs — Cost to trend limit	Prospective limit on costs — Cost to peer and trend limit	Prospective rates — Hospital level	Prospective rates — Hospital level with peer groups	Prospective rates — Diagnosis specific	Prospective rates — Negotiated
Alabama					Yes		
Alaska				Yes			
Arizona[a]	Yes						
Arkansas	Yes						
California[b]			Yes				Yes
Colorado						Yes	
Connecticut	Yes	Yes					
Delaware		Yes					
District of Columbia				Yes			
Florida				Yes			
Georgia				Yes			
Hawaii				Yes			

See notes at end of table.

TABLE V-1. Medicaid Inpatient Hospital Payment Systems, by State, 1991--Continued

State	Retrospective/ reconciled	Prospective limit on costs		Prospective rates			
	Cost	Cost to trend limit	Cost to peer and trend limit	Hospital level	Hospital level with peer groups	Diagnosis specific	Negotiated
Idaho		Yes					
Illinois[b]					Yes	Yes	
Indiana		Yes					
Iowa						Yes	
Kansas						Yes	
Kentucky					Yes		
Louisiana		Yes					
Maine				Yes			
Maryland				Yes			
Massachusetts				Yes			
Michigan						Yes	
Minnesota						Yes	

See notes at end of table.

TABLE V-1. Medicaid Inpatient Hospital Payment Systems, by State, 1991--Continued

State	Retrospective/ reconciled	Prospective limit on costs		Prospective rates			
	Cost	Cost to trend limit	Cost to peer and trend limit	Hospital level	Hospital level with peer groups	Diagnosis specific	Negotiated
Mississippi					Yes		
Missouri		Yes					
Montana						Yes	
Nebraska				Yes			
Nevada						Yes	
New Hampshire						Yes	
New Jersey						Yes	
New Mexico						Yes	
New York						Yes	
North Carolina				Yes			
North Dakota						Yes	
Ohio						Yes	

See notes at end of table.

TABLE V-1. Medicaid Inpatient Hospital Payment Systems, by State, 1991--Continued

State	Retrospective/ reconciled Cost	Prospective limit on costs		Prospective rates			
		Cost to trend limit	Cost to peer and trend limit	Hospital level	Hospital level with peer groups	Diagnosis specific	Negotiated
Oklahoma					Yes		
Oregon						Yes	
Pennsylvania						Yes	
Rhode Island							Yes
South Carolina						Yes	
South Dakota						Yes	
Tennessee				Yes			
Texas						Yes	
Utah						Yes	
Vermont							Yes
Virginia					Yes		
Washington[b]						Yes	Yes

See notes at end of table.

TABLE V-1. Medicaid Inpatient Hospital Payment Systems, by State, 1991--Continued

State	Retrospective/ reconciled		Prospective limit on costs		Prospective rates			
	Cost		Cost to trend limit	Cost to peer and trend limit	Hospital level	Hospital level with peer groups	Diagnosis specific	Negotiated
West Virginia	Yes							
Wisconsin							Yes	
Wyoming	Yes							
Total number of States using payment system[d]	4		6	1	10	6	22	4

[a]Arizona operates the Arizona Health Care Cost Containment System (AHCCCS) as an alternative to Medicaid.

[b]Two systems are in effect.

[c]Illinois shifted from a negotiated to a DRG system after the survey on which this table is based.

[d]Sum of total is greater than the number of States because some States employ more than one payment system.

Source: Table prepared by the Congressional Research Service based on information from Abt Associates Incorporated, under contract to ProPAC.

Of the 45 States and the District of Columbia using prospective payment for inpatient hospital services in 1991, 40 based reimbursement solely on prospective rates. These States pay a fixed amount for each case. Others pay actual costs, subject to prospective limits. That is, payment to a hospital is limited to the lesser of a prospectively determined cap and the hospital's actual costs or charges for treating each patient. Limits are based on each hospital's historic costs, updated for inflation. Three States have never shifted to prospective payment (Delaware, West Virginia, and Wyoming), while one other (Arkansas) has recently returned to a retrospective system. In these States, payment is based entirely on a percentage of costs or charges.

Of the States using fully prospective rates, 20 have adopted a system comparable to Medicare's prospective payment system (PPS), under which reimbursement varies according to the classification of each case into a diagnosis related group, or DRG (Washington also uses DRGs for some hospitals). One State, Nevada, groups cases into five classes, each with its own prospective rate.

Fourteen other States pay a flat rate per day or per case, regardless of diagnosis. Maryland has established a rate for each individual service furnished by the hospital (one rate for each day of routine care, one rate for each x-ray and lab test, and so on). The flat rates are established for each individual facility but may be subject to overall limits for classes or "peer groups" of facilities, established through such factors as bed size, presence of teaching programs, or location. Of the States using flat-rate prospective systems, 10 established rates on a hospital specific basis; the other 5 States used peer group rating systems.

Finally, four States negotiate rates with hospitals. As will be discussed below, two of these States (California and Washington, for part of the State) generally restrict beneficiaries to facilities with negotiated rates. Rhode Island and Vermont also negotiate rates, but do not impose such restrictions.

Diagnosis Related Group (DRG) Systems. Under a DRG system, the reimbursement rate for services to a particular patient is based on the patient's diagnosis and/or the nature of the services furnished. Each case is classified into one of a set of diagnosis related groups (the Medicare system uses 487 DRGs, but some States use fewer in their Medicaid systems). Each DRG is assigned a weighting factor, which measures the relative resources required by a typical patient with a particular problem or complaint, as compared to all other patients. Under Medicare, the factors range from a low of 0.1 for false labor to a high of 15.3 for a liver transplant; an average case would have a DRG weight of 1.0.[10] A single all-inclusive payment is made for each case in a particular DRG, by multiplying a fixed predetermined rate by the weighting factor for the applicable DRG. (Medicare's system makes a number of additional adjustments in the payment for certain hospitals.)

---

[10]Because of changes over time in the mix of cases treated by hospitals, the average weight for a Medicare case is now closer to 1.3.

In Medicaid DRG systems, the rates paid for each DRG may vary by hospital, or there may be different rates for specified classes of facilities, defined by size, geographic area, or other factors. The State's system may allow additional reimbursement for "outliers," patients whose costs or length of inpatient stay are significantly higher than the average for other patients in the same DRG. (Medicaid law requires States with prospective systems to make outlier adjustments for certain services to infants and young children; see below.)

Because Medicaid patients may tend to enter the hospital for different reasons than Medicare patients, the weighting factors established for DRGs under Medicare may not be appropriate for Medicaid reimbursement. (Medicare weights may be especially inappropriate for pediatric cases, because of the very small number of children receiving Medicare benefits.) Most States using DRGs have developed their own weights on the basis of Medicaid-specific data; some have used Medicare weights temporarily while collecting their own data.

Flat Rate Systems. In a typical flat rate system, the payment rate for each hospital is equal to that hospital's average costs, per day or per case, in a base year, plus some allowance for inflation. Many States using this approach have imposed "ceilings," under which the costs used for developing an individual hospital's rate may not exceed a fixed percentile of the costs for other comparable hospitals. Some States, instead of applying ceilings to base year costs, use class ceilings in computing their inflation adjustments. The hospital's annual increase in costs may not exceed that of typical hospitals in its peer group.

If the State sets flat rates per case, rather than per day, the hospital may be overpaid or underpaid if the average length of the hospital stay for each case is significantly different from that in the base year. A number of States have provided for some form of adjustment in these situations. In Nevada, for example, the basic per-case rate for each patient is expected to cover the first 15 days of care. The hospital may receive additional daily payment for days beyond that limit.

Some States, instead of establishing rates on the basis of historic cost, use a budgetary method: rates are based on projections of probable utilization and hospital revenue requirements in the current year. States using this approach in 1989 included Alaska, Maryland, Massachusetts, and Rhode Island. While rates in a budgeted system are developed individually for each hospital, they may be subject to overall ceilings. Rhode Island, for example, has used a Statewide "maxi-cap" to limit the annual percentage increase in any hospital's rates. A budgeted system may provide for rate adjustments if a hospital's cost or revenue experience differs significantly from the estimates used in budgeting.

b. Special Payment Issues

Selective Contracting Systems. OBRA 81 gave States the option of developing selective contracting systems for Medicaid services. Section 2175 of the Act allowed States to apply for waivers of Medicaid requirements, including the requirement that beneficiaries be allowed a free choice of medical providers, in order to allow the development of innovative delivery or reimbursement systems (the waiver rules are discussed more fully in *Chapter VI, Alternate Delivery Options and Waiver Programs*). One of the available options for States is to limit program participation (except for emergency services) to providers who meet reimbursement, quality, and utilization standards approved by the State. Certain payment rules cannot be waived under this option, including requirements for additional payment to disproportionate share hospitals (see below) and requirements for prompt payment to providers.

California and Washington have used this authority to restrict the inpatient hospitals from which beneficiaries may obtain services (Washington's waiver applies only in certain counties). Illinois operated a similar system until 1991, when it shifted to a DRG system.[11] Except in emergencies or other exceptional cases, beneficiaries may use only those hospitals selected for participation through a system of competitive negotiation. Reimbursement rates for the participating hospitals are established in the course of the negotiation.[12] In Illinois' system, the State and the hospital also projected the total number of days of care to be used by Medicaid patients. Reimbursement rates were reduced for days in excess of the projected limits.

All-Payer Systems. Beginning in the 1970s, several States established "all-payer" hospital rate-setting systems. In these systems, all insurers or other payers in the State, including Medicare and Medicaid, agreed to pay uniform rates or use a standard reimbursement methodology for inpatient services. Medicare and Medicaid involvement in an all-payer system was permitted only on a demonstration basis, through waivers approved by the Secretary under a general authority to conduct tests of program improvements. The original all-payer States thus served as proving grounds for alternatives to the traditional Medicare/Medicaid reasonable cost system.

Two of these original systems, Maryland's and Massachusetts', were budget based. New Jersey's was the first to experiment with DRGs and served as a forerunner for the current Medicare prospective payment system (PPS) for inpatient hospital services. New York set all-inclusive rates for each hospital on a per day basis, using historic cost and a variety of ceilings based on peer group comparisons.

Since the enactment of Medicare's PPS in 1983, continued participation of Medicare in an all-payer system has depended on a showing by the State that costs under its system were rising no faster than they would if the State had conformed to the Medicare PPS rules. As of 1991, only Maryland continues to operate a full all-payer system on a statewide basis; one part of New York, the Finger Lakes area, also maintains an all-payer system. Several other States

---

[11]Kentucky also received a waiver for this purpose in 1984, but terminated its project shortly thereafter.

[12]Other States may set hospital rates through a process of negotiation, but do not restrict the providers from which beneficiaries may obtain services.

maintain partial all-payer systems, including Medicaid and private insurers but excluding Medicare. States with such systems in 1990 included the former Medicare waiver States (Massachusetts, New Jersey, and New York) along with Alaska, Connecticut, and Maine.[13] In Rhode Island, Medicaid and Blue Cross jointly negotiate rates with hospitals; other payers are not affected.

A Medicaid program may continue to participate in a partial all-payer system so long as it complies with the general rules governing Medicaid reimbursement, including the Secretary's regulatory requirement that aggregate Medicaid reimbursement not exceed Medicare levels. Federal waivers are required only if the State wants Medicare to participate in the system as well.[14]

Administrative Days/Swing Beds. Under Medicare, small rural hospitals may enter into "swing bed" agreements with HCFA, under which beds may be used either for inpatient hospital care or for care equivalent in intensity to that furnished by a nursing facility. Costs are allocated and reimbursement adjusted to reflect the level of care furnished to each patient. A Medicaid program may also allow for swing beds, but only in hospitals that have entered into a Medicare swing bed arrangement. The State may develop a specific payment methodology for swing bed days of care at the nursing facility level or may pay at a rate based on average payments for comparable services in freestanding nursing facilities. The swing bed program assists hospitals that are underused and also helps to meet local shortages of nursing facility beds.

Sometimes a hospital which is not a swing bed facility will provide care to a patient at the nursing facility level of intensity because a place cannot be found for the patient in an appropriate facility and the patient cannot be discharged. (See *Appendix H, Medicaid as Health Insurance: Measures of Performance* for a discussion of nursing facility placement problems.) The days of inpatient care received by patients in this situation are known as "administrative days." Medicaid payment for an administrative day is limited by statute to the statewide average Medicaid payment rate for a day of care in a skilled nursing facility.[15]

c. Disproportionate Share Hospitals (DSHs)

Basic Requirements. OBRA 81 required that States' Medicaid reimbursement systems "take into account the situation of hospitals which serve a disproportionate number of low-income patients with special needs." Plans in some States to meet this requirement by making additional payments to DSHs potentially conflicted with the Secretary's regulation capping aggregate Medicaid

---

[13]American Hospital Association. Postcard survey of States, Nov. 5, 1990.

[14]Maine developed a system that took hospitals' Medicare revenues into account when determining what hospitals could charge other payers, thus achieving overall budgetary control without direct Medicare participation.

[15]This provision has not been amended to reflect the elimination of the distinction between skilled nursing facilities and intermediate care facilities.

reimbursement at Medicare levels. The Consolidated Omnibus Budget Reconciliation Act of 1985 (COBRA 85, P.L. 99-272) prohibited the Secretary from limiting States' payment adjustments to disproportionate share hospitals.

Prior to 1987, States were free to establish their own criteria for classifying facilities as DSHs and to develop their own reimbursement methods for these hospitals. OBRA 87 (P.L. 100-203) established minimum criteria which all States' systems had to meet beginning in July 1, 1988; these requirements have been amended several times since their enactment.

A hospital is eligible for additional payment if (a) its Medicaid utilization rate is more than one standard deviation above the average Medicaid utilization rate for all Medicaid-participating hospitals in the State, or (b) its low-income utilization rate is at least 25 percent.[16] In addition to meeting one of these two tests, the hospital must have on staff at least two obstetricians who are prepared to accept Medicaid patients. This requirement does not apply to children's hospitals or to those that do not furnish non-emergency obstetrical care; rural hospitals may use other attending physicians for obstetrical care.

In computing the amount of the supplementary payment, the State must use one of three methods. It may (a) use the formula for comparable payment adjustments under Medicare, with special adjustments for children's hospitals; (b) provide for a fixed payment increase or percentage increase for DSHs plus an additional increase for hospitals whose Medicaid utilization is more than one standard deviation above the statewide mean; or (c) develop its own methodology which may vary payments to different types of hospitals, so long as all hospitals of each type are treated equally and adjustments are reasonably related to hospitals' Medicaid or low-income volume. The payment adjustments are required even if they result in Medicaid payments to a hospital in excess of the hospital's usual charges to the public for similar services.

The new requirements were phased in over a 3 year period and were fully effective for inpatient services furnished on or after July 1, 1990. Certain alternative State systems for compensating DSHs are temporarily or permanently exempt from the requirements, provided that the aggregate increased payments under those systems are equal to the aggregate amounts that would be paid if the States complied with the requirements. However, no State may be exempted under a section 2175 waiver for selective contracting.

---

[16]The Medicaid utilization rate is defined as the number of days of care furnished to Medicaid beneficiaries during a given period divided by the total number of days of care provided during the period. The low-income utilization rate is the sum of two fractions: Medicaid payments plus State and local subsidies divided by total patient care revenues, and inpatient charges attributable to charity care (other than charity care subsidized by State or local government) divided by total inpatient charges. (The "standard deviation" used in the first criterion is a statistical measure of the dispersion of hospitals' utilization rates around the average; the use of this measure identifies hospitals whose Medicaid utilization is unusually high.)

Public Laws 100-360 and 101-508 (OBRA 90) require States to modify certain reimbursement practices for inpatient services provided by designated disproportionate share hospitals to children under 6 and by any hospital to infants under 1 year old. Reimbursement for such services must be made without regard to any durational limits in the State Medicaid plan (such as a provision that the State covers only a certain number of days of care per admission or per year). In States that pay hospitals on a prospective basis, the payment systems must provide for "outlier" adjustments, to compensate disproportionate share hospitals for infants whose hospital stays are unusually long or costly. For services to infants, no dollar limits may be imposed, other than under a prospective payment system (such a system remains subject to the requirement for outlier adjustments).

Limits on DSH Payments. Beginning in 1990, State payment adjustments for DSHs rose sharply. In 1989, 41 States surveyed by the National Association of Public Hospitals (NAPH) reported total adjustments of $569 million, or an average of $327,893 for each of the 1,547 facilities receiving the additional payments. Projected payments were $831 million for 1990 and $1.1 billion for 1991.[17] By late 1991, however, States projected that FY 1992 DSH payments would reach $8 billion, or 12 percent of total Medicaid spending. (Later estimates are much higher; see below.)

The Administration viewed this development as tied to the increasing State reliance on provider donations and provider-specific taxes as sources of Medicaid financing (see *Chapter VIII, Financing* for a discussion of this issue).[18] A State could increase DSH payments by any amount it chose, tax away the increase, and thus draw unlimited Federal funds. In addition, HCFA contended that States were designating hospitals as DSHs inappropriately, with some States designating nearly every facility in the State as a DSH. In conjunction with the issuance of final rules restricting the use of donations and taxes, HCFA also issued a proposed rule on October 31, 1991, that would have forbidden a State from designating a hospital as a DSH unless the hospital's Medicaid utilization rate or low-income utilization rate was at least equal to the statewide average.

The Medicaid Voluntary Contribution and Provider-Specific Tax Amendments of 1991 (P.L. 102-234) prohibited the Secretary from restricting State designations of DSHs and instead set limits on DSH payments. Effective January 1, 1992, national aggregate DSH payment adjustments during each fiscal year are limited to 12 percent of total Medicaid spending for that year.

---

[17]National Association of Public Hospitals. *Revised State Medicaid Policies for Disproportionate Share Hospitals: An Updated Status Report.* Washington, 1991.

[18]Some of the States relying most heavily on donation or tax programs also had very high DSH payments. Overall, however, the connection is not a strong one. In FY 1992, DSH payments in States with donation or tax programs were projected to equal 13.2 percent of total Medicaid spending, only slightly more than the projected 12.6 percent for all States.

Individual States' payments in January through September 1992 are generally limited to those made under methodologies in effect by the end of FY 1991. For FY 1993 and subsequent fiscal years, each State will have its own DSH limit. "High DSH" States, those whose payments are already above the 12 percent limit, will be allowed to increase their payments by no more than the projected growth in their overall Medicaid spending. Other "non-high DSH" States will be allowed larger increases, so long as aggregate national payments do not exceed the national cap. If projected DSH payments for a year under States' current rules are less than 12 percent of total projected Medicaid spending, the difference will constitute a pool of funds that may be divided among the non-high DSH States. Each State will receive the lesser of: (a) a share of the pool proportionate to the State's share of all Medicaid spending by non-high DSH States, or (b) the amount that would raise the State's allowable payment adjustments to 12 percent of its Medicaid spending.

The Act allows an exception to the DSH limits beginning January 1, 1996, but only if Congress has taken certain action by that date. States would not be subject to the limits if they designate as DSHs only hospitals that have above-average Medicaid or low-income utilization rates, account for at least 1 percent of all Medicaid days in the State, or meet other criteria established by the Secretary. However, this alternative will become available only after Congress enacts legislation limiting DSH payments in the States that elect the option.

The 12 percent national limit was based on the amount States projected they would spend for DSH payments in FY 1992 at the time the legislation was enacted. More recent State reports indicate that States have actually spent considerably more. Unaudited submissions by States in August 1992 showed DSH FY 1992 payments of $19.7 billion, 16.1 percent of total estimated Medicaid payments. The final FY 1992 base DSH amounts computed by HCFA (after disallowances and other adjustments) total $16.5 billion. HCFA projects that the same amount would equal slightly more than 12 percent of projected spending for FY 1993. Accordingly, FY 1993 DSH spending for all States will be limited to the FY 1992 base amounts. No increases are allowed for low-DSH States. Table V-2 shows the preliminary FY 1993 DSH allocations by State.

TABLE V-2. Preliminary Medicaid Disproportionate Share
Allocations, Fiscal Year 1993

| State | Disproportionate share allocations FY 1993 | |
	Allotment (in thousands)	State designation as a high or low DSH State
Alabama	$412,952	high
Alaska	15,611	low
Arizona[a]		
Arkansas	3,600	low
California	1,600,000	high
Colorado	332,764	high
Connecticut	393,969	high
Delaware	4,800	low
District of Columbia	32,902	low
Florida	191,400	low
Georgia	296,703	low
Hawaii	38,052	low
Idaho	1,141	low
Illinois	298,933	low
Indiana	140,708	low
Iowa	4,633	low
Kansas	182,896	high
Kentucky	265,433	high
Louisiana	1,021,390	high
Maine	274,301	high
Maryland	117,481	low
Massachusetts	478,632	low
Michigan	543,423	high
Minnesota	17,240	low
Mississippi	154,964	low
Missouri	699,112	high
Montana	1,000	low
Nebraska	2,500	low

See notes at end of table.

TABLE V-2. Medicaid Disproportionate Share Allocations,
Fiscal Year 1993--Continued

| State | Disproportionate share allocations FY 1993 | |
	Allotment (in thousands)	State designation as a high or low DSH State
Nevada	$ 73,560	high
New Hampshire	391,113	high
New Jersey	1,092,356	high
New Mexico	8,484	low
New York	2,784,477	high
North Carolina	332,661	low
North Dakota	1,000	low
Ohio	451,834	low
Oklahoma	25,867	low
Oregon	17,312	low
Pennsylvania	967,407	high
Rhode Island	40,336	low
South Carolina	422,651	high
South Dakota	1,000	low
Tennessee	440,944	high
Texas	1,513,029	high
Utah	7,453	low
Vermont	22,693	low
Virginia	104,555	low
Washington	230,929	low
West Virginia	66,355	low
Wisconsin	8,020	low
Wyoming	1,000	low
U.S. Total	**$16,531,576**	

[a]Arizona's medical assistance demonstration project is exempt from DSH payment limits.

NOTE: Allocations are preliminary and will likely change with additional information. All allocation amounts are reported in thousands. High or low disproportionate share designation is based on HCFA's estimate that a State's DSH base allotment for FY 1993 is above 12 percent (high) or below 12 percent (low) of medical assistance payments (excluding administrative costs).

Source: Table prepared by the Congressional Research Service based on data supplied by HCFA. Estimates are based on data supplied by the States in June 1992.

d. Hospital Reimbursement Levels

Medicaid hospital reimbursement in most States appears to be less than the cost hospitals incur in treating Medicaid beneficiaries. The only comprehensive source of data on Medicaid costs and payments is an annual survey of community hospitals conducted by the American Hospital Association (AHA).[19] The survey includes questions about gross Medicaid charges and actual Medicaid payments received by each hospital. Hospitals' charges are generally in excess of their actual costs. AHA estimates actual costs for Medicaid patients at each hospital by using that hospital's overall cost-to-charge ratio; the estimate may be inaccurate if the ratio is actually different for Medicaid and non-Medicaid patients.

[19]"Community hospitals" are nonfederal, short-term general hospitals and "other special" hospitals (short-term special hospitals that are not psychiatric or tuberculosis facilities) that are not units of institutions (such as prison or college infirmaries) and that are open to the public.

**TABLE V-3. American Hospital Association Estimates
of Medicaid Hospital Payments as a Percent
of Medicaid Hospital Expenses, 1989 and 1990**

	Medicaid payment as a percent of Medicaid cost		Percent change
	1989	1990	1989-90
Alabama	81.6	73.1	-10.4
Alaska	89.5	87.8	-1.9
Arizona	104.4	98.8	-5.4
Arkansas	70.8	72.0	1.7
California	63.4	66.7	5.2
Colorado	60.8	56.4	-7.2
Connecticut	71.3	71.1	-0.3
Delaware	101.4	80.8	-20.3
District of Columbia	81.5	69.5	-14.7
Florida	85.8	82.6	-3.7
Georgia	74.0	86.1	16.4
Hawaii	65.0	73.6	13.2
Idaho	78.6	82.1	4.5
Illinois	53.0	56.8	7.2
Indiana	94.4	95.1	0.7
Iowa	93.6	88.1	-5.9
Kansas	77.7	87.0	12.0
Kentucky	87.8	93.7	6.7
Louisiana	82.4	88.4	7.3
Maine	92.4	85.0	-8.0
Maryland	105.1	106.3	1.1
Massachusetts	78.8	87.1	10.5
Michigan	82.0	86.2	5.1
Minnesota	85.7	88.0	2.7
Mississippi	105.0	104.1	-0.9
Missouri	69.7	68.3	-2.0
Montana	92.4	90.6	-1.9
Nebraska	72.3	73.4	1.5
Nevada	68.2	46.8	-31.4

**TABLE V-3. American Hospital Association Estimates
of Medicaid Hospital Payments as a Percent
of Medicaid Hospital Expenses, 1989 and 1990--Continued**

	Medicaid payment as a percent of Medicaid cost		Percent change
	1989	1990	1989-90
New Hampshire	95.5	84.5	-11.5
New Jersey	106.2	104.8	-1.3
New Mexico	79.4	96.2	21.2
New York	85.1	88.9	4.5
North Carolina	69.7	61.7	-11.5
North Dakota	97.3	95.9	-1.4
Ohio	89.9	94.4	5.0
Oklahoma	85.0	83.3	-2.0
Oregon	56.0	62.5	11.6
Pennsylvania	68.2	65.6	-3.8
Rhode Island	91.5	94.6	3.4
South Carolina	67.0	83.5	24.6
South Dakota	91.3	91.1	-0.2
Tennessee	94.6	93.5	-1.2
Texas	75.9	82.1	8.2
Utah	68.1	78.7	15.6
Vermont	73.2	75.5	3.1
Virginia	77.2	79.5	3.0
Washington	76.3	81.6	6.9
West Virginia	86.7	84.8	-2.2
Wisconsin	74.5	77.6	4.2
Wyoming	91.1	92.8	1.9
Total U.S.	78.3	80.3	2.6

NOTE: Arizona has been included, despite the fact that the State does not pay hospitals directly for most services, because AHA included figures reported by Arizona hospitals in computing the U.S. total estimates shown.

Source: American Hospital Association. *Unsponsored Hospital Care and Medicaid Shortfalls, 1980-1990: A Fact Sheet Update.* Washington, 1992.

Table V-3 shows Medicaid payments as a percent of estimated Medicaid costs by State in 1989 and 1990.[20] Note that the figures represent costs and payments for both inpatient and outpatient care; costs for the two types of care are not reported separately in the AHA survey. Nationally, aggregate Medicaid payments were 80.3 percent of estimated costs for Medicaid beneficiaries in 1990. The percentage in the median State was 84.5 percent.[21] The aggregate national figure represents a slight improvement over the same figure for 1989. However, the ratio of payment to expenses dropped in 23 States while rising in the other 28.

Hospitals in three States are shown as receiving payments in excess of their Medicaid costs; this may be the result of AHA's method for converting charges into costs or other survey problems, rather than any actual overpayment. In seven other States (California, Colorado, Illinois, Nevada, North Carolina, Oregon, and Pennsylvania) payments were equal to two thirds or less of estimated Medicaid costs. California and Illinois are the States that had selective contracting systems in 1990, under which the State chose hospitals to furnish most Medicaid services, with the selection based in part on the hospitals' willingness to grant discounts. Colorado, as noted earlier, imposed a 46 percent across-the-board payment cut in mid-1988 and was successfully sued under the Boren amendment; suits are also pending or have been resolved in most of the other States.

While comparable data for 1991 are not yet available, it is probable that the ratio of Medicaid payments to costs rose significantly. Total Medicaid payments for inpatient and outpatient hospital services grew 42 percent from FY 1990 to FY 1991. Some of this growth may have been related to increases in the number of beneficiaries receiving hospital services, rather than to improved payment levels. Still, the dramatic increases in DSH payments and reimbursement changes resulting from Boren amendment litigation are likely to have reduced Medicaid shortfalls in many States, although these effects may have been partially offset by revenue reductions resulting from provider donation and tax programs.

---

[20]The figures are sorted by the State where each hospital is located, not by the State whose Medicaid program paid the bills. While these are generally the same, States do pay for services obtained by Medicaid beneficiaries in out-of-State hospitals. In some areas (such as multi-State metropolitan area), it may be common for beneficiaries to cross State lines for care. Thus the AHA State data do not exactly reflect relative State Medicaid reimbursement levels.

[21]This is slightly higher than the national total, because some of the States covering the most hospital care (e.g., California and Illinois) had among the lowest payment/cost ratios.

**TABLE V-4. American Hospital Association Estimates
of Medicaid Hospital Expenses and Medicaid
Payment Shortfalls as a Percent of
Total Hospital Expenses, 1990**

State	Medicaid expenses	Medicaid shortfall/ (surplus)
Alabama	7.5%	2.0%
Alaska	15.0	1.8
Arizona	10.2	0.1
Arkansas	9.6	2.7
California	16.2	5.4
Colorado	7.8	3.4
Connecticut	9.2	2.7
Delaware	9.0	1.7
District of Columbia	11.9	3.6
Florida	8.6	1.5
Georgia	11.0	1.5
Hawaii	14.1	3.7
Idaho	6.3	1.1
Illinois	13.3	5.7
Indiana	7.6	0.4
Iowa	8.2	1.0
Kansas	7.5	1.0
Kentucky	11.6	0.7
Louisiana	11.1	1.3
Maine	11.4	1.7
Maryland	11.7	(0.7)
Massachusetts	8.2	1.1
Michigan	12.3	1.7
Minnesota	10.5	1.3
Mississippi	11.7	(0.5)
Missouri	8.5	2.7
Montana	10.2	1.0
Nebraska	7.1	1.9
Nevada	6.8	3.6
New Hampshire	4.6	0.7
New Jersey	8.4	(0.4)
New Mexico	9.5	0.4
New York	19.3	2.1
North Carolina	9.3	3.6
North Dakota	9.2	0.4
Ohio	11.3	0.6
Oklahoma	10.6	1.8
Oregon	8.4	3.2
Pennsylvania	9.4	3.2

TABLE V-4. American Hospital Association Estimates
of Medicaid Hospital Expenses and Medicaid
Payment Shortfalls as a Percent of
Total Hospital Expenses, 1990--Continued

	Medicaid expenses	Medicaid shortfall/ (surplus)
Rhode Island	9.8	0.5
South Carolina	10.3	1.7
South Dakota	7.7	0.7
Tennessee	11.8	0.8
Texas	9.5	1.7
Utah	10.2	2.2
Vermont	8.2	2.0
Virginia	7.8	1.6
Washington	14.0	2.6
West Virginia	10.7	1.6
Wisconsin	5.6	1.3
Wyoming	9.0	0.6
Total U.S.	11.2	2.3

NOTE: Arizona has been included, despite the fact that the State does not pay hospitals directly for most services, because AHA included figures reported by Arizona hospitals in computing the U.S. total estimates shown.

Source: American Hospital Association. *Unsponsored Hospital Care and Medicaid Shortfalls, 1980-1990: A Fact Sheet Update.* Washington, 1992.

Table V-4 shows estimated Medicaid costs and what AHA terms "Medicaid payment shortfalls" (the difference between Medicaid payments and costs) as a percent of total hospital costs in each State in 1990. Medicaid accounted for 19.3 percent of total costs in New York and just 4.6 percent in New Hampshire. Nationally, 11.2 percent of hospital expenses were for Medicaid beneficiaries, compared to 10.6 percent in 1989. A number of factors may account for the wide variation in Medicaid share, including differences in State's eligibility policies, in the characteristics of beneficiaries and the services they use, and in hospitals' admission policies. (This issue will be discussed further in *Appendix H, Medicaid as Health Insurance: Measures of Performance*.) The last column of the table shows the Medicaid shortfall in each State, again expressed as a percent of total costs in the State.[22] In AHA's view, this is the share of total hospital costs that should have been paid by Medicaid but was not. The national total of 2.3 percent of costs is unchanged from 1989; while Medicaid payments relative to costs improved slightly, Medicaid's share of total costs also grew. The estimated Medicaid losses totalled $4.6 billion.

Hospitals and private insurers contend that Medicaid losses must be made up through higher charges to other payers, a phenomenon known as cost-shifting. Private insurers pay more than the costs of treatment for their enrollees, while both Medicaid and Medicare pay less than cost. Figure V-1 shows the Prospective Payment Assessment Commission's estimates of the ratio of payments to costs for Medicaid, Medicare, and private payers at the average hospital in 1989. Medicare's payments covered 90.5 percent of cost, and Medicaid covered 74.1 percent of cost. (This figure is for an average hospital and is thus different from the national aggregate of 78.3 percent reported by AHA for 1989.) Private payers paid 28.1 percent more than the costs of treating their enrollees.

---

[22]In Alabama, for example, Medicaid payments equalled 73.1 percent of Medicaid costs; these in turn represented 7.5 percent of total hospital expenses. The Medicaid shortfall was 26.9 percent (100 percent minus 73.1 percent) of Medicaid costs, or 2.0 percent of total costs (26.9 percent times 7.5 percent).

FIGURE V-1. Average Inpatient Hospital Payments as a Share of Costs by Payer, 1989

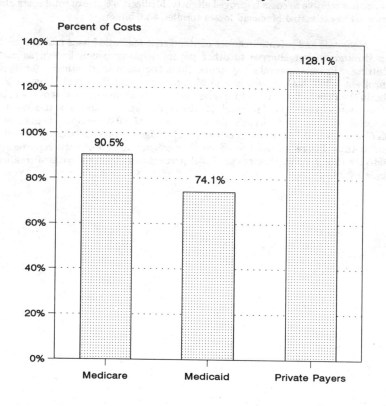

Source: Figure prepared by Congressional Research Service based on ProPAC analysis of American Hospital Association 1989 Annual Survey.

Table V-5, based on 1990 AHA data, places unreimbursed Medicaid costs in the context of overall community hospital financial performance in 1990. Expenses are divided among Medicaid, uncompensated care (total bad debt and charity care), and all other (including expenses for privately insured and Medicare patients). Patient-related revenues may be defined as consisting of net patient revenue (Medicaid and other patient and insurer payments) and State and local subsidies. The latter are not usually considered patient revenues, but are included here because they are generally intended to help cover the cost of uncompensated care.[23]   After the patient-related revenues are applied to expenses, hospitals are left with a 1990 deficit of $4.6 billion for Medicaid and $9.5 billion for bad debt and charity care. In the aggregate, hospitals had a surplus of $9.0 billion for all other patient care. (This surplus reflects an even larger surplus for private patients and a deficit under Medicare.)

TABLE V-5. Community Hospital Revenues and Expenses, 1990
(in billions of dollars)

	Medicaid	Uncompensated	All other	Total
Expenses	23.0	12.1	168.1	203.2
Net patient revenue	18.4	0.0	177.1	195.5
State/local subsidy	0.0	2.6	0.0	2.6
Sum, patient-related revenue --	18.4	2.6	177.1	198.1
Patient-related surplus (deficit)	(4.6)	(9.5)	9.0	(5.1)
Net other revenue--				13.7
Final surplus--				8.6

Source: Table prepared by the Congressional Research Service based on analysis of data from the American Hospital Association 1990 survey of community hospitals.

Hospitals also have revenues in addition to patient and insurer payments and government subsidies. These include interest on endowments or other funds, private contributions, and income from activities other than patient care (such as parking garages). These "non-patient revenues" totalled $13.7 billion

---

[23]AHA uses the term "unsponsored care" to describe the amount of uncompensated care remaining after these State and local government subsidies have been applied.

in 1990 and turned an aggregate deficit into an aggregate surplus for community hospitals in that year. Hospitals could cover all but $400 million of their costs for uncompensated care and Medicaid shortfalls through this additional resource before drawing on the surplus generated by other patients. However, the remaining deficit would still have had to be made up by private patients. In addition, the use of non-patient revenues to cover Medicaid deficits limits the hospitals' ability to use those revenues for care to the uninsured. Finally, it must be emphasized that these are aggregate figures and that some hospitals may have much greater difficulty in covering Medicaid and uncompensated care losses. For example, a municipal or county hospital might have a higher share of Medicaid or uninsured patients and might have few non-patient revenues or be required to turn those revenues over to general funds.

One other concept is important in assessing the financial impact of Medicaid on hospitals: that of variable cost. Hospitals, like any other business enterprise, have two kinds of costs: fixed and variable. Fixed costs are the costs a hospital incurs to remain in operation regardless of whether its beds are empty or full. A hospital must, for example, maintain certain minimum staffing levels regardless of how many patients it is treating on a given day. Variable costs are those that rise and fall depending on the number of patients the hospital is treating and the types of treatments they receive. For example, if the hospital is half full, it only needs to make half as many meals as would be required at full occupancy.

Ideally, the revenues from each individual patient will be sufficient to cover the variable cost associated with that patient and also a proportionate share of the hospital's fixed costs. However, if a hospital has an empty bed, it does better to admit a patient who will cover his or her own variable costs and make any contribution at all to fixed costs than to leave the bed empty and collect nothing. Because most hospitals have empty beds (occupancy in 1990 averaged 66 percent), they will not actually lose money by admitting a Medicaid patient so long as Medicaid pays the full variable costs for that patient. The Federal court ruling in the State of Washington's case rejected the contention that the requirements of the Boren amendment would be met if a State paid full variable cost. Still, States point out that underutilized hospitals are better off than they would be if Medicaid did not exist. In the hospitals' view, however, they would be smaller (and hence have lower fixed costs) if they did not have to accommodate Medicaid patients.

2. Nursing Facility Services

Until the enactment of OBRA 87, Medicaid law distinguished among three kinds of nursing facilities: skilled nursing facilities (SNFs), intermediate care facilities (ICFs), and intermediate care facilities for the mentally retarded (ICFs/MR). Services in SNFs were also covered by Medicare; the less intensive services provided by ICFs were not covered by Medicare but were covered under Medicaid in every State except Arizona (none of the territories covered ICF services). In addition, every State covers services in ICFs/MR.

Pre-1987 law required that States establish a "reasonable cost differential" between the State's average payment for a day of SNF care and the average payment for a day of ICF care. OBRA 87 eliminated the distinction between SNFs and ICFs, effective October 1, 1990, and created a single class of "nursing facility" services under both Medicaid and Medicare. This change reflected findings that there was no clear difference in the intensity of services provided by SNFs and ICFs or the types of patients they were treating. As a result, States now have a single payment system for all nursing facilities. (ICFs/MR are still a distinct category and may be paid on a different basis.)

The establishment of a single nursing facility category was part of a broader set of nursing facility reforms included in the OBRA 87, which provided stricter and more uniform standards for nursing facilities participating in Medicare and Medicaid. In addition to eliminating the SNF/ICF payment differential, the Act required that States adjust Medicaid payment rates to allow for the costs that would be incurred by facilities in meeting the new standards. (Facilities granted waivers of some of the standards might face a downward adjustment.) The adjustments were required to be reflected in the State plan by April 1, 1990.

a. Basic Methods

Table V-6 shows the basic nursing facility reimbursement methodologies used by States responding to a 1989 National Governors' Association (NGA) survey (43 States and the District of Columbia).[24] As in the case of hospital inpatient services, most States have shifted to PPSs for nursing facility services. Only three States (Massachusetts, Pennsylvania, and Tennessee) still paid entirely on a retrospective basis in 1989. Two others (Maine and New Hampshire) paid retrospectively for SNF services but had shifted to prospective payment for ICF services. (The NGA survey dates from before the elimination of the SNF/ICF distinction.) Five States used a combination of methods, paying prospectively for some components of a facility's costs and retrospectively for other components.[25]

---

[24]One additional State, Arizona, responded to parts of the survey, but has been omitted here because it purchases long-term care services on a capitated basis.

[25]The survey did not address reimbursement for ICF/MR services. A previous CRS analysis indicated that all but 8 States were paying prospectively for ICF/MR services by 1986. For ICF/MR services, the distinction between prospective and cost systems may not always be meaningful. Prospective rates are likely to be set at a level sufficient to meet the facilities' full anticipated costs, because most ICF/MR services are furnished in State facilities. If Medicaid reimbursement to these facilities is less than their full operating cost, the State will have achieved Medicaid savings only at the expense of another part of the State budget.

TABLE V-6. Medicaid Nursing Facility Payment Methods, 1989

	Basic method	Case mix	Individual or peer group rates	Cost center limits	Overall limits	Imputed occupancy rate
Alabama	Prospective		Individual	Yes	Yes	
Alaska	Prospective		Individual	Yes	Yes	
Arkansas	Prospective		Individual	Yes		85%
California	Prospective		Peer group	Yes		
Colorado	Combination		Individual	Yes	Yes	85%
Connecticut	Prospective		Individual	Yes	Yes	90%
Delaware	Prospective	Yes	Peer group	Yes		90%
District of Columbia	Prospective		Individual	Yes	Yes	85%
Florida	Prospective		Peer group	Yes		
Georgia	Prospective		Individual	Yes	NA	85%
Idaho	Combination		Individual	Yes	Yes	80%[a]
Illinois	Prospective	Yes	Individual	Yes		93%[b]
Indiana	Prospective		Peer group	Yes	Yes	80%
Iowa	Prospective		Individual		Yes	80%[c]
Kentucky	Prospective		Peer group	Yes	Yes	90%
Louisiana	Prospective		Peer group	Yes		
Maine	Retro. (SNF)	Yes	Individual	Yes		90%
Massachusetts	Retrospective		Peer group	Yes	Yes	96%
Michigan	Prospective		Individual		Yes	85%
Minnesota	Prospective		Peer group	Yes		96%[a]
Missouri	Prospective		Individual	Yes		90%[d]
Montana	Prospective		Peer group	Yes		90%
Nebraska	Combination	Yes	Peer group	Yes	Yes	85%
Nevada	Prospective		Individual	Yes		92%[a]
New Hampshire	Retro. (SNF)	Yes	Individual	Yes		85%
New Jersey	Prospective	Yes	Peer group	Yes		95%[e]
New Mexico	Prospective	Yes	Peer group	Yes	Yes	90%[f]
New York	Prospective		Peer group	Yes	Yes	90%
North Carolina	Prospective	Yes	Individual	Yes	Yes	
North Dakota	Prospective		Peer group	Yes		
Ohio	Combination		Peer group	Yes		85%[g]
Oklahoma	Prospective		Peer group			
Oregon	Combination	Yes	Individual	Yes		
Pennsylvania	Retrospective		Peer group	Yes	Yes	90%
Rhode Island	Prospective		Individual	Yes		98%

See notes at end of table.

TABLE V-6. Medicaid Nursing Facility Payment Methods, 1989--Continued

	Basic method	Case mix	Individual or peer group rates	Cost center limits	Overall limits	Imputed occupancy rate
South Carolina	Prospective	Yes	Peer group	Yes		98%
South Dakota	Prospective		Peer group	Yes	Yes	95%
Tennessee	Retrospective		Individual		Yes	80%[c]
Texas	Prospective		Peer group	Yes		85%[h]
Utah	Prospective		Individual		Yes	
Vermont	Prospective	Yes	Individual	Yes	Yes	90%
Virginia	Combination		Peer group	Yes	Yes	95%[i]
Wisconsin	Prospective		Peer group	Yes		85%
Wyoming	Prospective	Yes	Individual	Yes	Yes	90%[a]

[a]Only for property component.
[b]Only for capital component.
[c]ICF only.
[d]93 percent for capital costs.
[e]80 percent in first year of operation.
[f]Only for new construction.
[g]95 percent for cost of ownership.
[h]Only for facility and administrative costs.
[i]85 percent for facilities with 30 or fewer beds.

Source: National Governors' Association. Center for Policy Research. *Medicaid Payment for Nursing Facilities: Skilled Nursing Facilities and Intermediate Care Facilities (1986-1989)*. Washington, 1989.

Of the States using prospective payment, or a combination of retrospective and prospective methods, 21 established rates for each individual facility. Another 19 set rates for "peer groups" of facilities, classed according to such factors as location and number of beds. One State, Louisiana, used uniform Statewide rates for all SNFs and for two classes of ICFs. In general, the States use the historic costs for the individual facility or peer group as a base, update the cost with an inflation factor to establish a daily rate, and then reduce the rate if it exceeds one or more cost ceilings. (The States that pay on a retrospective cost basis use similar ceilings to cap allowable costs.) Ceilings may be based on a percentile of costs for a class of facilities, grouped by county, bed size, or ownership. Another approach is to use cost center ceilings. The costs of providing care are split into a number of components: administration, nursing, food, and so on. A separate cap is applied to each of these cost centers.

Cost ceilings may function implicitly as penalties for low occupancy. If a facility has the same fixed costs as others in its class but fewer patients, its per capita cost will exceed ceilings based on the average per capita cost for the class. A number of States have built explicit occupancy assumptions into their ceilings, setting cost limits in such a way as to penalize any facility that fails to maintain an "imputed" occupancy level, such as 85 percent or 90 percent. These penalties may apply only to capital-related costs (such as depreciation or interest), or only to new facilities; one State has lower occupancy expectations for smaller facilities.

Class averages may be used for other policy purposes as well. A number of States will share with a facility any difference between its actual costs and the ceiling for its class, as an incentive for efficiency. States may also modify rates directly to achieve policy goals. Illinois has developed a Quality Incentive Program (QUIP), which provides bonus payments to facilities meeting standards beyond the minimum. Some States have established disproportionate share adjustments, comparable to those for hospitals, to compensate facilities with a high number of Medicaid patients.

b. Case Mix Adjustments

Even before the SNF/ICF distinction was eliminated, some States had found that the two levels of care could not adequately reflect the full variation in cost and intensity of services required by different patients. Within the ICF level, for example, a bed-bound patient might require considerably more attention than an ambulatory one. If a State paid the same amount for both kinds of cases, facilities might have a financial incentive to refuse admission to "heavy care" patients. As a result, several States adopted case mix payment methodologies, under which reimbursement is partially dependent on the kinds of patients the nursing facility accepts.

In a case mix system, the State establishes classes of patients, according to their diagnosis, degree of disability, or service requirements, and sets different standard payment rates or payment adjustment factors for each class. The State may use a simple range, perhaps from "light care" to "heavy care." New York has experimented with 16 resource utilization groups (RUGs), which attempt to classify nursing facility patients by expected cost in the same way that DRGs classify hospital inpatients; a similar system is being tested in Texas.

As of 1989, 12 States were using some form of case mix payment. The establishment of a single class of nursing facilities is expected to encourage more States to develop payment systems that reflect variation in patient needs. HCFA has been funding evaluations of demonstrations of alternative case mix systems in Texas and Massachusetts.

In addition to modifying overall payments to reflect patient needs, a State may also provide enhanced reimbursement for specific types of services needed by certain patients. A bedridden patient may require periodic turning and repositioning to avoid bedsores; another patient may need tube feeding. The State may add a fixed amount to the standard daily rate for each day that a patient requires these services, or it may take the need for such services into account in measuring case mix.

c. Reserved Beds

Nursing facility patients will sometimes be away from the facility for a brief period, for a short-stay hospitalization or perhaps for a family visit. Where occupancy rates are high, the facility could conceivably admit another patient in this interval, leaving the absent patient unable to return. States may pay for leave days in order to ensure that a bed is reserved during a patient's absence. Rates may be reduced for these days, and a State may limit the number of reserve bed days it will pay in a year, either per patient or per facility.

d. Nursing Facility Reimbursement Levels

Table V-7 shows the Medicaid payment rates per day of patient care reported by the 45 States responding to the National Governors' Association survey. As was noted earlier, this survey dates from 1989, before the SNF/ICF distinction was abandoned. In addition, States were not yet required to adjust payments to reflect the cost of compliance with nursing home reforms. It should also be emphasized that States differ in their treatment of ancillary services, such as prescription drugs, received by nursing facility residents. Some States consider these services as part of nursing home care and include them in the per diem payment. Other States pay for the services separately; for example, payment for drugs would be made directly to the pharmacy that dispensed them, rather than to the nursing facility. For this reason, comparisons of different States' Medicaid nursing facility payment rates may not be meaningful.

TABLE V-7. Medicaid Per Diem Payment Rates for Nursing Facilities, 1989

	Skilled nursing facility (SNF)	Intermediate care facility (ICF)	Combined SNF/ICF rate
Alabama	$47.22	$35.54	
Alaska			$207.77
Arkansas	35.79	34.99	
California	60.26	44.22	
Colorado			54.30
Connecticut	83.86	64.18	
Delaware			65.21
District of Columbia	173.51	90.07	
Florida			61.14
Georgia	33.24	39.31	
Idaho			52.47
Illinois	49.69	39.73	
Indiana	63.70	51.08	
Iowa	83.55	36.89	
Kentucky	62.32	43.78	

See notes at end of table.

TABLE V-7. Medicaid Per Diem Payment Rates
for Nursing Facilities, 1989--Continued

	Skilled nursing facility (SNF)	Intermediate care facility (ICF)	Combined SNF/ICF rate
Louisiana	42.62	35.91	
Maine	83.07	58.33	
Massachusetts	90.94	58.76	
Michigan			50.78
Minnesota	68.31	50.90	
Missouri	46.95	44.06	
Montana			50.86
Nebraska	61.91	38.56	
Nevada	68.27	46.29	
New Hampshire	126.20	69.00	
New Jersey	73.70	67.31	
New Mexico	85.65	53.09	
New York	112.93	72.08	
North Carolina	61.40	46.33	
North Dakota	53.62	40.99	
Ohio	59.72	53.36	
Oklahoma	54.00	37.00	
Oregon	83.41	55.71	
Pennsylvania	76.36[a]	65.64[a]	
Rhode Island	75.11	65.00	
South Carolina			46.07[b]
South Dakota	42.17	33.40	
Tennessee	66.88	38.83	
Texas	49.16[c]	36.36[c]	
Utah	52.60	43.65	
Vermont			59.69
Virginia	70.59	51.78	
Wisconsin	57.27	46.24	
Wyoming			53.74

[a]Ceilings for private facilities in the largest urban areas.

[b]Shifted to separate rates for SNF and ICF in 1988; amount shown is the 1989 average of those rates.

[c]Texas changed to a case mix system in Apr. 1989. Rates shown are those used before that date.

NOTE: The following States did not respond to the National Governors' Association survey: Hawaii, Kansas, Maryland, Mississippi, Washington, and West Virginia. Arizona responded but did not furnish rate information.

Source: National Governors' Association. Center for Policy Research. *Medicaid Payment for Nursing Facilities: Skilled Nursing Facilities and Intermediate Care Facilities (1986-1989).* Washington, 1989.

There are no recent data on which to base a comparison between Medicaid rates and those paid by Medicare or paid directly by patients (other third-party payment for nursing facility services is still comparatively rare). The last comprehensive survey to address this issue was the 1985 National Nursing Home Survey (NNHS). At that time, Medicaid nursing home rates were generally lower than the rates charged to self-pay patients or to Medicare. Table V-8 shows the average basic per diem rates for nursing home care reported by survey respondents. The average Medicaid rate for SNF care was 80 percent of the average Medicare rate, and 82 percent of the average private pay rate. For ICF care, the Medicaid average was 82 percent of the private pay average.

TABLE V-8. Average Basic Per Diem Rates for Nursing Home Care, 1985

Payer	Skilled nursing facility	Intermediate care facility
Private payer	$61.01	$48.09
Medicare	62.02	a/
Medicaid	49.93	39.57

ªServices not covered.

Source: U.S. Dept. of Health and Human Services. National Center for Health Statistics. G. Strahan. Nursing Home Characteristics. Preliminary Data from the 1985 National Nursing Home Survey. Advance Data From Vital and Health Statistics No. 131. DHHS Pub. No. (PHS) 87-1250, Mar. 27,1987.

A comparison between national average private, Medicare, and Medicaid rates may be deceptive, because not all facilities participated in Medicaid. The facilities that did participate, and therefore could report a Medicaid rate, might have had lower private pay or Medicare rates than the average for their class. A better comparison, then, is between the Medicaid rate and other rates at each individual facility.

Tables V-9 and V-10 compare, by facility, 1985 Medicaid daily rates with the rates paid by Medicare for SNF services and by private payers for ICF services. The comparison is confined to ICFs whose private rate was from $45 to $49.99, and SNFs whose Medicare rate was from $55 to $59.99. These ranges were chosen because rates at these levels were those most commonly reported by facilities included in the NNHS. (It should be noted that the NNHS rate data are in $5 ranges. This means, for example, that a Medicaid rate reported as $50-$54.99 and a Medicare rate reported as $55-$59.99 might actually be as little as one cent or as much as $9.99 apart.)

TABLE V-9. Medicaid Per Diem Payment Rates, Intermediate Care Facilities with Private Per Diem Rate of $45 to $49.99, 1985

Basic Medicaid rate	Percent of facilities	Cumulative percent of facilities
Under $30	2.2	2.2
$30 to $34.99	21.1	23.3
$35 to $39.99	25.2	48.5
$40 to $44.99	29.1	77.6
$45 to $49.99	22.4	100.0

Source: Table prepared by the Congressional Research Service based on analysis of the National Nursing Home Survey, 1985.

TABLE V-10. Medicaid Per Diem Payment Rates, Skilled Nursing Facilities with Medicare Per Diem of $55 to $59.99, 1985

Basic Medicaid rate	Percent of facilities	Cumulative percent of facilities[a]
Under $30	1.7	1.7
$30 TO 39.99	11.2	12.9
$40 to $49.99	42.7	55.6
$50 to $54.99	14.4	70.0
$55 to $59.99	15.4	85.4
$60 to $64.99	7.2	92.6
$65 and over	7.4	100.0

[a]Omits Medicare facilities reporting no Medicaid rate.

Source: Table prepared by the Congressional Research Service based on analysis of the National Nursing Home Survey, 1985.

Among the ICFs whose private rate was $45 to $49.99, 52 percent reported a Medicaid rate of $40 or more, and 22 percent reported a rate in the same $45 to $49.99 range as their private rate. However, 23 percent of the ICFs reported a Medicaid rate of under $35 a day, at least $10 below their private rate.

Among the SNFs whose Medicare rate was $55 to $59.99, 12 percent reported a Medicaid rate below $40, and another 40 percent reported a rate below $50. Nearly 15 percent of the facilities reported a per diem Medicaid rate *higher* than the Medicare rate. This might occur in the States that include ancillary services (such as prescription drugs) in the Medicaid base rate; the comparable Medicare rate excludes these services.

Overall, the comparison suggests that Medicaid reimbursement in 1985 was more nearly equal to that of other payers at the ICF level and was generally lower than that of other payers at the SNF level. How Medicaid and other payment rates compare now that the SNF/ICF distinction has been eliminated is not yet known.

If Medicaid reimbursement rates are still generally lower than the rates charged to private payers (chiefly individuals), some degree of cost-shifting may occur. Because there are no data on nursing facility financial performance comparable to the hospital data discussed earlier, the extent to which private payers are subsidizing Medicaid beneficiaries cannot be determined. In addition, the situation may be complicated by the fact that many nursing home residents begin in private pay status and later become eligible for Medicaid.

As is discussed in *Appendix C, Medicaid, Long-Term Care, and the Elderly*, between 27 and 45 percent of Medicaid nursing home residents have "spent down"; that is, they qualify for Medicaid after they have used up their assets to pay for their care. If Medicaid payment rates were increased and private pay rates could therefore be reduced, residents beginning in private pay status might take longer to use up their assets and would therefore spend less of their total stay in Medicaid status. Medicaid would then be paying higher rates for fewer months of care, while private patients would pay lower rates for more months. The net effect, for the portion of the population that spends down, might be little or no change in the share of nursing facility costs paid by individuals and by Medicaid.

B. Physician and Outpatient Care

1. Physician Services

Medicaid payment rates for physicians are subject to the general requirement that payments be sufficient to attract enough providers to ensure that covered services will be as available to Medicaid beneficiaries as they are to the general population. OBRA 89 codified this rule and established specific reporting requirements with respect to payment rates for obstetric and pediatric services, to allow the Secretary to determine the adequacy of State payments for these services.

For services of physicians or other individual practitioners, Medicaid payment amounts are usually the lesser of the provider's actual charge for the service or a maximum allowable charge established by the State. Table V-11 shows the general approach used by each State in establishing maximum payments for physician services in 1989, as reported in a survey conducted by the Physician Payment Review Commission (PPRC) and the National Governors' Association (NGA). Two basic methods were in use: prevailing charge screens and fee schedules or relative value scales.

TABLE V-11. Medicaid Physician Payment Methodologies, 1989

State	Payment methodology	Fee schedule source and base year
Alabama	Fee Schedule	90 percent of 75th percentile of submitted charges, 1981
Alaska	Reasonable Charges	
Arizona	Negotiated Rate	
Arkansas	Fee Schedule	
California	Fee Schedule	1969 and 1974 California Relative Value Studies
Colorado	Fee Schedule	1976 Colorado Relative Value Study
Connecticut	Fee Schedule	Charges
Delaware	Fee Schedule	Charges
District of Columbia	Fee Schedule	Charges
Florida	Fee Schedule	
Georgia	Fee Schedule	Charges
Hawaii	Reasonable Charges	
Idaho	Fee Schedule	1974 California Relative Value Study
Illinois	Fee Schedule	Charges
Indiana	Reasonable Charges	
Iowa	Fee Schedule	Charges
Kansas	Fee Schedule	1974 California Relative Value Study
Kentucky	Reasonable Charges	
Louisiana	Fee Schedule	Charges
Maine	Fee Schedule	1974 California Relative Value Study
Maryland	Fee Schedule	1974 California Relative Value Study
Massachusetts	Fee Schedule	
Michigan	Fee Schedule	Michigan Relative Value Study, prevailing charges
Minnesota	Fee Schedule	Charges
Mississippi	Fee Schedule	1974 California Relative Value Study
Missouri	Fee Schedule	Charges
Montana	Fee Schedule	Charges
Nebraska	Fee Schedule	
Nevada	Fee Schedule	1974 California Relative Value Study
New Hampshire	Reasonable Charges	
New Jersey	Fee Schedule	Charges, 1973 New Jersey Blue Shield 500 Plan
New Mexico	Fee Schedule	1986 Colorado Relative Value Study
New York	Fee Schedule	1965 New York Medical Society Relative Value Study
North Carolina	Fee Schedule	Charges
North Dakota	Fee Schedule	Charges
Ohio	Fee Schedule	Charges
Oklahoma Medicaid	Fee Schedule	Lower of 75th percentile of Medicare and charges, 1986
Oregon	Fee Schedule	
Pennsylvania	Fee Schedule	Charges
Rhode Island	Fee Schedule	1967 Rhode Island Medical Society Negotiated Rates
South Carolina	Fee Schedule	1974 California Relative Value Study
South Dakota	Fee Schedule	Charges

TABLE V-11. Medicaid Physician Payment
Methodologies, 1989--Continued

State	Payment methodology	Fee schedule source and base year
Tennessee	Reasonable Charges	Percentage of usual, customary or prevailing charges
Texas	Reasonable Charges	
Utah	Fee Schedule	Utah Medical Association Relative Value Study
Vermont	Fee Schedule	1988 McGraw-Hill Relative Value Study
Virginia	Fee Schedule	15th percentile of charges
Washington	Fee Schedule	1974 California Relative Value Study
West Virginia	Fee Schedule	
Wisconsin	Fee Schedule	Charges
Wyoming	Reasonable Charges	

Source: National Governors' Association and Physician Payment Review Commission, 1990.

a. Prevailing Charge Screens

In eight States, maximum physician payments were determined through methods comparable to those used by Medicare in establishing reasonable charges for physician services. The Medicare reasonable charge for a specific service to a specific patient is the lowest of (a) the provider's actual charge for that service; (b) the provider's customary charge for comparable services; or (c) the "prevailing" charge in the area for comparable services.

For Medicare, the prevailing charge for an area is set at the 75th percentile of the customary charges established for all the providers in the area (because of rate of increase limits and other rules, the Medicare prevailing charge is in fact frequently lower than the 75th percentile). Some Medicaid systems use a different percentile, while others have dropped the prevailing charge "screen" and use the individual provider's customary charge as the maximum. In establishing customary or prevailing charges, States may use information developed by other payers, such as Medicare or Blue Shield, or may compile their own data.

As a result of changes made in OBRA 89, Medicare is phasing out the reasonable charge system for physician payments and shifting to a physician fee schedule based on a resource-based relative value system (see below). Medicaid policies are not directly affected by this change. However, State use of the prevailing charge method has declined sharply since 1986, when 19 States used prevailing charge screens for physician services.

b. *Fee Schedules and Relative Value Scales*

Forty-one States and the District of Columbia have developed fixed fee schedules, specifying a flat maximum payment amount for each type of service; the maximum may be unrelated to actual provider charges. Most Medicaid programs have developed these schedules on their own or through negotiation with provider groups. Fifteen States have used relative value scales (RVS), usually developed by an outside organization. In a relative value scale, each type of service is given a specific weight. A brief physician office visit might have a value of 3, an appendectomy a value of 150. The State then multiplies the different values by a single standard dollar amount. If a unit is valued at $5, the State will pay $15 for the brief office visit and $450 for the appendectomy. The effect is the same as under a fee schedule, except that the Medicaid agency has an external reference for its pricing decisions. Several standard RVS systems are available for States which choose this approach; the most familiar is the California Relative Value Studies for physician, laboratory, and x-ray services, used by nine States in 1989. Similar scales exist for other provider types, such as the Nevada scales for dental and ocular services. The Medicare program has developed its own "resource-based" relative value scale (RBRVS), which is being used in development of the new Medicare physician fee schedule.[26] The RBRVS is still being refined, but it might form a basis for some States' Medicaid fee schedules in the future.

A number of States have modified their physician reimbursement systems in order to encourage participation or increase access to care. Of particular concern in recent years has been access to obstetric and pediatric services. Even before the OBRA 89 provisions for reporting on these services, many States were moving to increase rates for pregnancy-related and early childhood care. The PPRC/NGA survey found that, while only 21 States had updated their overall physician payment rates in the 2 years ended April 1990, 11 more States had updated rates for maternity care, while 8 had done so for pediatric services. States have also provided enhanced reimbursement for primary care physicians and for ambulatory surgery.

c. *Physician Reimbursement Levels*

Medicaid payment rates for physician services vary widely among States. Table V-12 shows the range of reimbursement rates used by States in their 1989 fiscal years, as reported in the PPRC/NGA survey. There is greater variation in payment levels for some medical procedures than for others. The ratio of the highest to the lowest reported rate is 15 to 1 for comprehensive initial hospital visits, and 14.75 to 1 for intermediate emergency room visits. On the other hand, the highest rate for caesarean deliveries is 3.4 times the lowest.[27]

---

[26]The RBRVS measures the value of the resources (including physician work, practice expenses, and malpractice costs) that go into each medical procedure.

[27]PPRC suggests that variation in rates for pregnancy-related services has diminished as States have increased payments in order to improve access to

(continued...)

TABLE V-12. Range of Medicaid Fees by Service, State Fiscal Year 1989

	Minimum	Range: Median	Maximum
Comprehensive Office Visit, New Patient	$10	$44	$104
Limited Office Visit, Established Patient	10	17	39
Intermediate Office Visit, Established Patient	10	20	45
Intermediate Emergency Room Visit	8	25	118
Comprehensive Consultation, Initial	20	60	146
Psychotherapy, 45 to 50 minutes	18	42	86
Comprehensive Hospital Visit, Initial	10	51	150
Intermediate Hospital Visit, Subsequent	6	20	70
Total Obstetric Care, Vaginal Delivery	344	738	1316
Total Obstetric Care, Cesarean Delivery	453	903	1605
Vaginal Delivery	200	440	901
Cesarean Delivery	360	638	1231
Tonsillectomy & Adenoidectomy, under 12 years	60	164	475
Repair Inguinal Hernia, under 5 years	140	312	1016
Total Hysterectomy	166	614	1770
Cataract Removal	404	990	2915
Routine Electrocardiogram	10	23	55
Chest X-Ray, Two Views, Professional Component	5	10	21
Chest X-Ray, Two Views, Global Service	10	23	55
Endoscopy, Upper GI	80	205	411

NOTE: Total obstetric care generally includes prenatal services, delivery, and postpartum hospital and office visits.

Source: National Governors' Association and Physician Payment Review Commission, 1990.

[27](...continued)
obstetrical care. Physician Payment Review Commission. *Physician Payment Under Medicaid.* (PPRC Report No. 91-4) Washington, 1991. p. 26-7.

Comparison of States' physician payment rates is complicated by the fact there is no single unit of service (like a day of nursing home care) for which rates may be compared. Instead, States must set payments for a wide variety of services. One State may set higher payment rates for surgery, while another sets lower surgical fees but pays more for office visits, and so on. PPRC has attempted to overcome this problem by developing an index that bundles together payment rates for 18 different services that range from office visits to diagnostic tests to surgical procedures. This index provides some comparison of States with one another and also allows Medicaid rates to be compared with those payable under Medicare. Table V-13 shows the ratio of each State's rates for the bundle of services to the average for all States and then compares each State's rates to Medicare allowed charges and to estimated rates under the new Medicare fee schedule for the same bundle of services.

TABLE V-13. State Medicaid Physician Payment Rates
Relative to Medicaid Rates in Other States and to Medicare
Rates in the Same State, PPRC Bundle of 18 Services

	Ratio of Medicaid rates to:		
	Average of all States[a]	Medicare allowed charge[b]	Medicare fee schedule[c]
Alabama	1.07	0.80	0.73
Alaska	2.33	1.07	1.22
Arkansas	1.23	1.04	1.05
California	1.05	0.62	0.68
Colorado	0.78	0.62	0.57
Connecticut	1.01	0.64	0.62
Delaware	0.88	0.71	0.61
District of Columbia	0.97	0.57	0.58
Florida	1.35	0.73	0.78
Georgia	1.64	1.14	1.07
Hawaii	1.43	0.78	0.90
Idaho	0.89	0.82	0.74
Illinois	0.82	0.56	0.51
Indiana	1.55	1.18	1.05
Iowa	1.21	1.00	0.89
Kansas	0.86	0.69	0.66
Kentucky	0.62	0.51	0.49
Louisiana	0.88	0.64	0.58
Maine	0.67	0.59	0.52
Maryland	0.83	0.50	0.49
Massachusetts	1.30	0.89	0.86
Michigan	0.85	0.64	0.55
Minnesota	1.19	1.02	0.88
Mississippi	0.68	0.63	0.48
Missouri	0.61	0.52	0.46
Montana	0.98	0.81	0.77
Nebraska	1.20	1.03	0.95
Nevada	1.62	0.96	1.11
New Hampshire	0.69	0.61	0.52
New Jersey	0.50	0.34	0.32

See notes at end of table.

**TABLE V-13. State Medicaid Physician Payment Rates
Relative to Medicaid Rates in Other States and to Medicare
Rates in the Same State, PPRC Bundle of 18 Services--Continued**

	Ratio of Medicaid rates to:		
	Average of all States[a]	Medicare allowed charge[b]	Medicare fee schedule[c]
New Mexico	1.16	0.77	0.78
New York	0.53	0.28	0.26
North Carolina	1.07	0.88	0.81
North Dakota	1.01	0.83	0.69
Ohio	0.79	0.63	0.60
Oklahoma	1.18	0.86	0.83
Oregon	1.01	0.75	0.74
Pennsylvania	0.77	0.54	0.49
Rhode Island	0.68	0.48	0.49
South Carolina	0.92	0.82	0.70
South Dakota	0.87	0.77	0.71
Tennessee	1.05	0.88	0.82
Texas	1.20	0.82	0.81
Utah	0.99	0.83	0.74
Vermont	0.78	0.72	0.69
Virginia	0.81	0.74	0.65
Washington	0.86	0.66	0.64
West Virginia	0.61	0.40	0.36
Wisconsin	1.02	0.81	0.74

[a]Index of State's Medicaid payment rates for bundle of 18 services, relative to rates of other States, for State FY 1989.

[b]Index of State's FY 1989 Medicaid rates for bundle of 18 services, relative to Medicare allowed charges for the same 18 services.

[c]Index of State's Medicaid rates for bundle of 18 services, relative to estimated calendar year 1988 Medicare fee schedule rates for the same 18 services. (Fee schedule values used are based on a budget neutral conversion factor without a behavioral offset.)

Source: Physician Payment Review Commission. *Physician Payment Under Medicaid.* (PPRC Report No. 91-4). Washington, 1991.

While there is considerable variation among States in the index values computed by PPRC, the range for the full bundle of services is not as great as the range for individual services. Excluding Alaska, the highest-rate State (Georgia, with an index value of 1.64) pays 3.3 times as much as the lowest rate State (New Jersey, with a value of .50). This indicates that much of the variation in payments for particular procedures, as shown in table V-11, reflects different State decisions on the relative value of services, as well as different overall spending levels. PPRC investigated whether the overall variation in State payment levels could be explained by geographic differences in the costs of medical practice. However, correction for this factor did little to reduce the variation.

The last two columns in table V-13 compare maximum payable amounts under Medicaid in States' 1989 fiscal years to the actual amounts allowed by Medicare for comparable services in the same State, and to the amounts that would have been paid for those services in 1988 if the new Medicare physician payment system had been in effect. The average State's Medicaid rates were 73.7 percent of what would have been allowed under Medicare, and 69.8 percent of what would have been paid under the new Medicare system.[28]

There are several drawbacks to this comparison. First, Medicaid and Medicare patients may use different types of physicians. Medicaid patients may be more likely to visit pediatricians or obstetricians, while Medicare patients might see cardiologists. Second, there may be differences in the complexity of some of the services provided to Medicaid and Medicare patients. Finally, the rates are for slightly different time periods.

The gap between Medicaid physician payment rates and rates paid by private insurers is likely to be even greater. As PPRC notes, Medicare allowed charges tend to be lower than allowed charges under Blue Shield plans in the same area; the Medicare/Blue Shield ratio for 90 procedures was 79 percent in 1989.[29] As in the case of the Medicaid/Medicare comparison, there are some problems in comparing Medicare and Blue Shield allowed charges; service definitions and recordkeeping practices may vary, and the physicians submitting claims to the two programs may differ in a given State.

2. Hospital Outpatient Services

Medicaid regulations provide that aggregate payments for services in hospital outpatient departments or clinics may not exceed the amount that

---

[28]The Medicaid/Medicare ratio drops because the new Medicare system tends to increase payment rates for the services most commonly used under Medicaid. Note that the averages given here differ from those cited by PPRC, 64 and 62 percent respectively. PPRC used expenditure-weighted averages, giving greater weight to States with larger total Medicaid spending.

[29]Physician Payment Review Commission. *Fee Update and Medicare Volume Performance Standards for 1992.* (PPRC Report No. 91-3) Washington, 1991. p. 27.

would have been paid for comparable services under Medicare. (Medicare payments for many outpatient services, unlike those for most inpatient care, continue to be made on a reasonable cost basis. However, some services, including ambulatory surgery, dialysis, and diagnostic services, are now paid on a prospective or fee schedule basis.)

Table V-14 shows each State's basic Medicaid reimbursement methodology for outpatient hospital services, as reported in a 1989 survey by the Intergovernmental Health Policy Project. The survey found significant changes from the methodologies used in 1987, as reported in an earlier Congressional Research Service analysis. Only 10 States were still using retrospective cost reimbursement, compared to 23 in 1987. Twenty-nine States were using prospective payment systems, up from 9 in 1987. Another nine were using some form of fee schedule, while two (California and Hawaii) used negotiated rates. As in the case of inpatient services, States using prospective payment systems for outpatient care may base rates on a hospital's historic costs or those for a peer group; others use a budgeted system, under which rates are based on projections of probable utilization and hospital revenue requirements. Oklahoma sets basic outpatient clinic rates equal to 20 percent of the inpatient per diem rate established for the same hospital.

TABLE V-14. Basic Medicaid Hospital Outpatient Reimbursement Methodologies, January 1989

	Prospective	Retrospective	Fee schedule	Negotiated rates
Alabama			x	
Alaska		x		
Arkansas			x	
California				x
Colorado	x			
Connecticut		x		
Delaware	x			
District of Columbia		x		
Florida		x		
Georgia	x			
Hawaii				x
Idaho	x			
Illinois			x	
Indiana	x			
Iowa	x			
Kansas			x	
Kentucky	x			
Louisiana	x			
Maine	x			
Maryland		x		
Massachusetts		x		
Michigan	x			
Minnesota	x			
Mississippi	x			
Missouri	x			
Montana	x			
Nebraska	x			
Nevada			x	
New Hampshire	x			
New Jersey	x			
New Mexico	x			
New York			x	
North Carolina	x			
North Dakota	x			
Ohio	x			

**TABLE V-14. Basic Medicaid Hospital Outpatient
Reimbursement Methodologies, January 1989--Continued**

	Prospective	Retrospective	Fee schedule	Negotiated rates
Oklahoma		x		
Oregon	x			
Pennsylvania			x	
Rhode Island		x		
South Carolina			x	
South Dakota	x			
Tennessee	x			
Texas	x			
Utah	x			
Vermont	x			
Virginia	x			
Washington		x		
West Virginia			x	
Wisconsin		x		
Wyoming	x			
Total	29	10	9	2

Source: George Washington University. Intergovernmental Health Policy Project. *State Systems for Hospital Payment*. Washington, Apr. 1989.

Partly because of problems in obtaining access to physicians' services, many Medicaid beneficiaries have relied on hospital outpatient departments and emergency rooms as a primary source of care (see *Appendix H, Medicaid as Health Insurance: Measures of Performance* for a discussion of this problem). The cost for outpatient services may be considerably higher than the cost of identical services furnished in a physicians' office. Several States have reduced outpatient reimbursement to reflect the actual level of services provided. For example, Kansas limits payments for outpatient services to the amount that would be paid for the same service if rendered by a non-hospital provider. Other States pay reduced rates to emergency rooms for treatment of non-emergency cases.

As was noted earlier, available data do not permit separation of hospital inpatient and outpatient costs, and it is therefore not possible to assess independently the adequacy of Medicaid outpatient reimbursement. The AHA data reported earlier combine the two types of services, and some portion of the Medicaid shortfalls estimated by AHA may be attributable to outpatient care.

C. Prescription Drugs

Medicaid payment for a prescription drug furnished to a beneficiary on an outpatient basis has two components: an amount to cover the cost of the ingredients (the *acquisition cost*) and an amount to cover the pharmacy's costs to fill the prescription (the *dispensing fee*). Medicaid regulations establish upper limits on payment for acquisition costs, but do not limit dispensing fees; these must merely be "reasonable" (42 CFR 447.331). Two separate limits on acquisition costs are used, one for certain multiple source drugs--those for which therapeutic equivalents or "generic" versions are available from more than one manufacturer--and one for all other drugs. The limits are designed to encourage the substitution of lower cost generic equivalents for more costly brand name drugs.

OBRA 90 has established a system under which pharmaceutical manufacturers must grant rebates to State Medicaid programs for drugs dispensed and paid for on or after January 1, 1991. Under the new rebate requirements, States will in effect receive a volume discount in return for covering a manufacturer's drugs. The new rebate arrangements do not supersede the existing regulatory limits on Medicaid payments. During the period January 1, 1991 through December 31, 1994, the Secretary is prohibited from changing the regulatory formula for upper payment limits in a way that would result in a reduction in the limits. During the same period, States that were in compliance with the Federal rules may not reduce their own upper limits or dispensing fees.

The next section reviews the regulatory limits on reimbursement and summarizes State policies on acquisition costs and dispensing fees. The following section provides an overview of the new drug rebate program.

1. Pharmacy Reimbursement Methods

a. Multiple Source Drugs

For purposes of the upper payment limits, a "multiple source drug" is one that meets the following two requirements: (a) the drug is made available by at least three different suppliers, and (b) the Food and Drug Administration (FDA) has determined that at least three approved formulations of the drug are "therapeutically equivalent"--that is, contain identical doses of the active ingredient and have the same biological effects.[30] For each multiple source drug, HCFA establishes a price limit (known as the maximum allowable cost, or MAC) equal to 150 percent of the estimated wholesale cost of the least expensive therapeutic equivalent. The State's payments for such drugs during a given period may not exceed what would have been spent if the State had paid the price limit plus a reasonable dispensing fee.

---

[30]OBRA 90 overrides an existing requirement in regulations that *all* approved formulations of the drug be therapeutically equivalent.

The effect of this requirement is that, when a lower-cost "generic" equivalent exists for a brand-name drug, a pharmacy will be paid the generic price even if the brand-name drug is actually furnished. The pharmacy therefore has a financial incentive to substitute the generic equivalent for the brand-name drug. If the prescribing physician specifies that generic substitution is unacceptable (for example, by writing "dispense as written" or "no substitution" on the prescription), the HCFA price limits do not apply. The pharmacy must supply the brand-name drug and may be paid the full brand-name cost.

b. Other Drugs

For all other drugs (including multiple source drugs for which the prescribing physician has requested no substitution), statewide payments may not exceed the lesser of (a) the pharmacies' usual and customary charge to the general public and (b) the estimated acquisition cost (EAC) plus a dispensing fee. The EAC is the State's estimate of what providers are generally paying for a drug. Note that this limit applies only in the aggregate: a State may pay more for any particular drug so long as the total for all drugs does not exceed the aggregate limit. For most drugs, the ingredient cost is limited to the State's best estimate of what providers generally are paying for a drug.

Table V-15 shows the dispensing fee established by each State as well as the State's method of computing the ingredient cost or EAC. Most States base the EAC on average wholesale price (AWP), the price charged by wholesalers to retail pharmacies; in all but a few States, the AWP is reduced by a fixed percentage to reflect discounts available to retailers. A few States instead consider the wholesaler's acquisition cost (WAC), what the wholesaler paid for the drug, and then add a fixed percentage amount to reflect the wholesaler's markup. Two States (Delaware and Michigan) pay the actual acquisition cost (AAC), what a specific retailer actually paid for a drug; both States use charge screens to limit payment to a fixed percentage of AWP. Finally, New Jersey uses different ingredient cost estimates according to the size of the provider, on the assumption that high-volume pharmacies pay lower wholesale prices.

TABLE V-15. Basic Medicaid Reimbursement Policies for Prescription Drugs, July 1992

	Dispensing fee	Ingredient reimbursement basis
Alabama	$5.40	WAC + 9.2%
Alaska	3.45 - 11.46	AWP - 5%
Arkansas	4.51 + 10.3% of EAC	AWP - 10.5%
California	4.05	AWP - 5%
Colorado	4.08	Lesser of AWP - 10% or WAC + 18%
Connecticut	4.10[a]	AWP - 8%
Delaware	3.65	Lesser of AAC or AWP - 6%
District of Columbia	4.50	AWP - 10%
Florida	4.23	WAC + 7%
Georgia	4.41	AWP - 10%
Hawaii	4.67	AWP - 10.5%
Idaho	4.30	AWP
Illinois	Greater of 3.58 or 10% of cost	AWP - 10%
Indiana	4.00	AWP - 10%
Iowa	4.02 - 6.25[a]	AWP - 10%
Kansas	3.85 - 6.97	AWP - 10%
Kentucky	4.75	AWP - 10%
Louisiana	5.00	AWP - 10.5%
Maine	3.35	Lesser of EAC or AWP - 5%
Maryland	4.94 - 6.51	WAC + 10%
Massachusetts	4.06	WAC + 10%
Michigan	3.72	Lesser of AAC or AWP - 10%
Minnesota	4.10	AWP - 10%
Mississippi	5.16	AWP - 10%
Missouri	4.09	AWP - 10.43%
Montana	2.00 - 4.08	AWP - 10%
Nebraska	2.84 - 5.05	Lesser of WAC + 12.52% or AWP - 8.71%
Nevada	4.42	AWP - 10%

See notes at end of table.

TABLE V-15. Basic Medicaid Reimbursement
Policies for Prescription Drugs, July 1992--Continued

	Dispensing fee	Ingredient reimbursement basis
New Hampshire	$3.25 - 3.65[a]	AWP - 10%
New Jersey	3.73 - 4.07	Pharmacy-specific[b]
New Mexico	4.00	AWP - 10.5%
New York	2.60	AWP
North Carolina	5.60	AWP - 10%
North Dakota	4.25	AWP - 10%
Ohio	3.23	AWP - 7%
Oklahoma	5.10	AWP - 10.5%
Oregon	3.67 - 4.02	AWP - 11%
Pennsylvania	3.50	AWP
Rhode Island	3.40	AWP
South Carolina	4.05	AWP - 9.5%
South Dakota	4.75	AWP - 10.5%
Tennessee	3.91	AWP - 8%
Texas	[c]	AWP - 10.49%
Utah	3.90 - 4.40	AWP - 12%
Vermont	4.25	AWP - 10%
Virginia	4.40	AWP - 9%
Washington	3.45 - 4.38	AWP - 11%
West Virginia	2.75	AWP
Wisconsin	4.69	AWP - 10%
Wyoming	4.70	AWP - 11%

[a]Incentive fee added to pharmacy reimbursement for dispensing a lower cost product.

[b]Maximum reimbursement varies by pharmacy volume. Highest volume providers receive AWP-6 percent; lowest volume receive full AWP.

[c]Total payment equals (EAC + $4.55) divided by 0.970.

Abbreviations: AAC: actual acquisition cost. AWP: average wholesale price. EAC: estimated acquisition cost. WAC: wholesaler's acquisition cost. See text for definition of these terms.

NOTE: State Medicaid payments for certain multiple source drugs are subject to upper payment limits established by HCFA.

Source: National Pharmaceutical Council. *Pharmaceutical Benefits Under State Medical Assistance Programs*. Reston, VA. 1992.

Most States use a fixed dispensing fee per prescription for all pharmacies. Several States vary the fee according to pharmacy size or other factors. Arkansas, Illinois, and Texas vary the dispensing fee according to the cost of the drug, while Connecticut, Iowa, and New Hampshire pay a bonus when a pharmacy substitutes a lower cost drug (when the substitution is not mandatory). Several States will reduce the dispensing fee or pay no fee at all for drugs furnished directly by an institution or a physician.

The National Pharmaceutical Council estimates that Medicaid programs paid a national average of $19.30 per prescription in FY 1991.[31] Medicaid payment levels for prescription drugs appear to be very close to the prices paid by private insurers and individuals. One recent study by Schondelmeyer and Thomas estimates that the average retail prescription price in calendar year 1988 was $15.19, compared to $14.93 for Medicaid in FY 1988.[32] The difference, only 2 percent, might disappear if the same time periods were used; the Medicaid number reflects 3 months' less inflation than the retail number. (The comparison may not be exact if the types of drugs used by Medicaid beneficiaries differ from those furnished to other purchasers.)

Schondelmeyer and Thomas estimate that it cost the average chain pharmacy $6.39, in addition to ingredient cost, to fill prescriptions covered by insurance in 1989. (Prescriptions paid for by individuals cost less, because less paperwork is required.) This figure is well above the dispensing fees paid by most States. On the other hand, Medicaid programs may have been paying higher ingredient costs than some other payers.[33] Medicaid has not received discounts similar to those that some chain drug stores, hospitals, and HMOs or other managed care plans have been able to negotiate with drug manufacturers. Lower dispensing fees and higher ingredient costs may have offset one another to produce overall payments close to the national retail average. Much fuller data would be needed to determine whether this trade-off has in fact occurred. Still, concern that Medicaid was not receiving the price breaks offered to other high-volume purchasers led to the enactment of rebate requirements in OBRA 90.

2. Drug Rebate Requirements

OBRA 90 required that drug manufacturers, as a condition of coverage of their prescription drug products, agree to pay State Medicaid programs rebates for drugs dispensed and paid for on or after January 1, 1991. In return, States

---

[31]National Pharmaceutical Council. *Pharmaceutical Benefits Under State Medical Assistance Programs*. Virginia, 1991.

[32]Schondelmeyer, Stephen W., and Joseph Thomas III. Trends in Retail Prescription Expenditures. *Health Affairs*, v. 9, no. 3, fall 1990. p. 131-145.

[33]Schondelmeyer and Thomas note that "[c]omparison of prices paid by Medicaid with prices paid by other purchasers for similar drugs reveals that Medicaid usually pays the highest price in the market." However, the study does not provide supporting data for this assertion.

are required to cover under Medicaid all of the drugs marketed by that manufacturer (there are certain exceptions; see *Chapter V, Reimbursement*). Rebate requirements may also apply to a nonprescription item such as aspirin, if it is covered in a State's Medicaid plan. Rebate requirements do not apply to products dispensed as a part of a service provided in a hospital, physician's or dentist's office, or similar setting. Rebates will be computed each quarter on the basis of price information supplied by manufacturers to HCFA and utilization information furnished to the manufacturers by State Medicaid agencies.

Rebate requirements are being phased in during the period 1991 through 1993. In setting the amount of required rebates, the law distinguishes between two classes of drugs. The first includes single source drugs (generally, those still under patent) and "innovator" multiple source drugs (drugs originally marketed under a patent but for which generic competition now exists). The second class includes all other, "non-innovator" multiple source drugs (generics). Table V-16 shows the requirements applicable to the two different classes of drugs during the phase-in period.

a. Single Source and Innovator Multiple Source Drugs

For these drugs, manufacturers are required to pay State Medicaid programs a basic rebate for each covered drug, along with an additional rebate if drug product prices increase faster than inflation, as measured by the Consumer Price Index for all urban consumers (CPI-U).

Basic rebate amounts are determined by comparing the average manufacturer price (AMP) for a drug--the average price paid by wholesalers--to the "best price," the lowest price offered by the manufacturer in the same period to any wholesaler, retailer, nonprofit or public entity.[34] The basic rebate is the greater of a fixed percentage of the AMP or the difference between the AMP and the best price. Rebates are limited to 25 percent of the AMP in 1991 and 50 percent in 1992; no limits apply in later years.

The additional rebates are required for any individual drug whose price increases faster than the CPI in 1991 and 1992. Beginning in 1993, the rebates are required if the weighted average price for all of a given manufacturer's single source and innovator multiple source drugs rises faster than inflation. In determining the rebate, prices in effect on October 1, 1990, are used as a base; these are then compared with prices as of the month before the start of the period for which the rebate is to be issued.

Some manufacturers have reportedly responded to the requirement that they offer Medicaid their "best price" by raising the prices charged to other purchasers, such as hospitals and HMOs, instead of lowering the price to Medicaid. The Department of Veterans' Affairs (DVA), which has long enjoyed steep discounts on certain drugs, reported significant price increases in 1991 and has attributed these increases to the OBRA 90 best price requirement.

---

[34]Federal agency "depot" prices and prices paid under single-source contracts are not considered in determining the best price.

The Veterans Health Care Act of 1992 (P.L. 102-585) excludes from the determination of best price, effective October 1, 1992, the prices charged by manufacturers to DVA, the Department of Defense, the Public Health Service (PHS) and various PHS-funded health programs, and State (non-Medicaid) pharmacy assistance programs. (The exclusion of these prices from the "best price" potentially reduced Medicaid savings from the rebate program; to offset this, minimum rebates were increased to the percentages shown in table V-16.) The Act also provides, as a condition of Medicaid reimbursement for a manufacturer's drugs after January 1, 1993, that the manufacturer enter into an agreement with the Secretary to provide discounts and rebates to certain PHS-funded entities and public disproportionate share hospitals, as well as a new discount agreement with DVA.

b. Non-Innovator Multiple Source Drugs

For multiple source drugs, basic rebates are a fixed percentage of the AMP (10 percent in 1991 through 1993, and 11 percent beginning in 1994). Prices offered to other payers are not considered, nor is there any additional rebate for excess price increases.

TABLE V.16. Drug Rebate Requirements Under OBRA 90
(as amended by the Veterans Health Care Act of 1992)

	1991	1992	1993	1994	1995	1996 and later years
Single source and innovator multiple source drugs:						
Basic rebate	Greater of 12% of average manufacturer price (AMP) or difference between AMP and "best price."	Greater of 12% of AMP (15.7% after 10/1/92) or difference between AMP and "best price."	Greater of 15.7% of AMP or difference between AMP and "best price."	Greater of 15.4% of AMP or difference between AMP and "best price."	Greater of 15.2% of AMP or difference between AMP and "best price."	Greater of 15.1% of AMP or difference between AMP and "best price."
Maximum basic rebate	25%	50%	No limit.	No limit.	No limit.	No limit.
Additional rebate	Amount of price increase in excess of consumer price index (CPI) for specific drug between 10/1/90 and the month before the start of the quarter.	Amount of price increase in excess of CPI for specific drug between 10/1/90 and the month before the start of the quarter.	Amount of price increase in excess of CPI for specific drug between 10/1/90 and the month before the start of the quarter.	Weighted average increase in excess of CPI for all the manufacturer's single-source and innovator multiple source drugs between 10/1/90 and the month before the start of the quarter.	Same as 1994.	Same as 1994.
All other multiple source drugs:						
Rebate:	10%	10%	10%	11%	11%	11%

Source: Table prepared by the Congressional Research Service.

D. Other Services

The services described above account for over 82 percent of total Medicaid expenditures; remaining expenditures are distributed among a wide variety of providers and service types. The following discussion is limited to services for which special payment rules are established by Federal law.

1. Rural Health Clinics and Federally Qualified Health Centers

Payment to rural health clinics and federally qualified health centers (FQHCs)[35] must be equal to 100 percent of the facility's reasonable costs, subject to any reasonableness tests developed for the same services under Medicare rules (or, for Medicaid services not covered under Medicare, as would be allowed under principles similar to Medicare's).

2. Laboratories

Payment for a laboratory test performed by a physician, independent laboratory, or hospital (except tests for the hospital's own patients) may not exceed the amount that would be paid under Medicare rules for the same test. Medicare payment is based on regional fee schedules established by the Secretary for each type of test. (A previously scheduled shift to a national fee schedule was repealed by OBRA 89.)

3. Hospice Care

If the State elects to cover hospice services, it must follow Medicare reimbursement rules for hospices. Under Medicare rules, payment for each day of care furnished by the hospice is at fixed rates according to the nature of the care received by the patient: a day may be classed as routine home care, continuous home care, inpatient respite care, or general inpatient care. Average payments per patient are subject to an annual "cap amount" updated annually by the Secretary and applied on an aggregate basis. The cap for the year ended October 1, 1990, was $9787.

The aggregate number of inpatient care days provided by the hospice in any 12 month period may not exceed 20 percent of the total number of days of hospice care provided. (Medicaid inpatient days furnished to patients with AIDS are not counted towards this limit.) Under Medicaid, additional payment for room and board may be made for patients who receive hospice services while residing in a nursing facility or ICF/MR (this is not true under Medicare).

---

[35]Generally, a FQHC is a facility that is receiving Federal grant funding as a community or migrant health center or a health center for the homeless or that meets the eligibility requirements for such a grant.

364

4. Home and Community-Based Care

OBRA 90 established a new optional service under Medicaid, home and community-based care for functionally disabled elderly persons. See *Chapter VI, Alternate Delivery Options and Waiver Programs* for a discussion of the new services.) Payment rates for the care must be reasonable and adequate to meet the costs of providing the care efficiently, economically, and in conformity with laws and quality and safety requirements. However, payments over the course of a quarter for persons receiving the services may not exceed 50 percent of what would have been paid by Medicare to treat the same average number of patients in a nursing facility. (There are also annual limits on the national amount of Federal financial participation available for these services; see *Chapter VI, Alternate Delivery Options and Waiver Programs.*)

E. Volume Purchasing

States may arrange for "volume purchasing" of laboratory services (other than those provided by hospitals or rural health clinics) or medical devices, such as durable medical equipment or eyeglasses. One or more providers of the specified service may be selected by the State, through competitive bidding or other means, as the sole source of the items covered in an area or statewide. Some States will permit other providers to furnish the item or service, but only if they are prepared to meet the price of the approved source. The State must ensure that services remain accessible to beneficiaries. If the arrangement is for laboratory services, the laboratory must be State-licensed and/or meet other requirements established by the Secretary.

As of 1988, the following 16 States had some form of volume purchasing arrangement for optical services: Alabama, Arkansas, Florida, Georgia, Illinois, Maine, Massachusetts, Michigan, Minnesota, North Carolina, Ohio, Oregon, South Carolina, Vermont, Washington, and Wisconsin. Five States used volume purchasing for hearing aids: Alaska, Florida, Minnesota, South Carolina, and Texas. Minnesota, Vermont, and Washington had sole source contracts for oxygen; Minnesota also had a sole source for wheelchairs. Only Nevada had used volume purchasing for laboratory services.[36]

III. COORDINATION WITH OTHER PAYMENT SOURCES

Medicaid is the payer of last resort, secondary to any other insurance coverage a beneficiary may have or to any other third party who may be liable for medical payments or medical support on the beneficiary's behalf. In terms of dollar impact, the most important source of third party coverage for Medicaid beneficiaries is Medicare. Some beneficiaries may receive private health insurance through an employer or may be covered under the policy of another family member. The number of such beneficiaries is likely to increase as a result of OBRA 90 provisions requiring Medicaid payment of private insurance

---

[36]National Governors' Association. State Medicaid Program Information Center. *A Catalogue of State Medicaid Program Changes.* [1986-1988 editions] Washington, 1988-1989.

premiums for certain individuals. Other possible sources of third party payment include medical payments under automobile or other liability insurance or workers' compensation. Finally, an absent parent may be responsible for medical support payments.

A. Medicare

While coverage under Medicare Part A (hospital insurance) is automatic for persons meeting eligibility standards, coverage under Part B (supplemental medical insurance) requires payment of a monthly premium by the beneficiary.[37] Some persons not automatically eligible for Part A coverage may also obtain that coverage by paying a premium. In addition, Medicare beneficiaries are liable for cost-sharing, deductible and coinsurance payments for Medicare-covered services.

Since the beginning of the Medicaid program, States have been permitted to enter into an agreement with the Secretary under which Medicaid pays the Medicare Part B premium on behalf of Medicaid beneficiaries eligible for Part A coverage. (For certain beneficiaries eligible for Part A coverage only if they pay the Part A premium, Medicaid may pay this as well.) This arrangement is known as "buy-in." If a State pays the premium on behalf of a beneficiary, Medicare is responsible for payment for that beneficiary's services under its usual coverage and reimbursement rules. The Medicaid program then pays required beneficiary cost-sharing amounts.

1. Eligibility For Buy-In Coverage

By the mid-1980s, every State but Wyoming had entered into a buy-in agreement for at least some beneficiaries. Beneficiaries had to meet ordinary Medicaid eligibility standards. The Omnibus Budget Reconciliation Act of 1986 (OBRA 86, P.L. 99-509) allowed States, at their option, to provide Medicaid to aged and disabled persons who did not meet usual Medicaid standards but who met a higher income standard established by the State, up to 100 percent of the Federal poverty level, and whose resources did not exceed 200 percent of the limits for Supplemental Security Income (SSI) applicants. The State could provide this new group of beneficiaries with full Medicaid coverage, or it could choose to cover only the Medicare premiums and cost-sharing amounts.[38] Only three jurisdictions, the District of Columbia, Florida, and New Jersey, initially chose to cover the new group, known as *qualified Medicare beneficiaries* or *QMBs*.

---

[37]Medicare Part A, Hospital Insurance, covers inpatient hospital and skilled nursing facility care, hospice services, and some home health care. Part B, Supplemental Medical Insurance, includes physician, hospital outpatient, home health care, and a variety of ancillary services.

[38]States may also choose to make monthly payments to health maintenance organizations (HMOs) or similar entities that have contracted with HCFA to provide services to Medicare beneficiaries.

The Medicare Catastrophic Act of 1988 (P.L. 100-360) required all States to phase in coverage of QMBs with incomes up to 100 percent of the Federal poverty level and resources within 200 percent of the SSI limits. OBRA 90 accelerated this phase-in and phases in limited eligibility for beneficiaries with incomes up to 120 percent of the Federal poverty level by January 1, 1995. For those with incomes over 100 percent of poverty, States will be required to pay the Part B premium but not the Part A premium or any cost-sharing. Finally, States are required to pay the Part A premium, but not the Part B premium or cost-sharing, for "qualified disabled and working individuals." These are certain persons whose social security disability insurance benefits cease after they return to work but who are permitted to continue to receive Medicare by paying the Part A premium. (See *Chapter III, Eligibility* for a full discussion of the eligibility and transition rules.)

The requirements for coverage of QMBs supplement but do not supersede previous rules for Medicaid coverage of the aged and disabled. Many persons still qualify for Medicaid benefits under existing standards for the categorically or medically needy. At a State's option, a State may also continue to extend full Medicaid coverage to persons qualifying under the OBRA 86 option, instead of just paying Medicare premiums and cost-sharing. Thus a State could have three distinct classes of aged and disabled individuals qualifying for assistance. (See *Chapter III, Eligibility* for information on covered groups in each State.)

Although buy-in is now mandatory for QMBs, it remains optional for beneficiaries whose incomes exceed the poverty level but who qualify for benefits under standard Medicaid rules (chiefly persons in institutions). A State could choose not to pay the Medicare premiums for those beneficiaries and instead provide the usual benefits available under the State's Medicaid plan. However, States are given a financial incentive to obtain Part B coverage for all Medicaid beneficiaries who could qualify for it. If the State fails to buy in for a beneficiary and therefore covers as Medicaid, services that could have been covered by Medicare, it may not claim Federal matching for the resulting expenditures. (There is an exception for services furnished prior to the date of the beneficiary's Medicaid application and covered as a result of a retroactive grant of Medicaid eligibility).

Federal funding is available at the State's usual matching rate for Medicare premiums paid on behalf of categorically needy beneficiaries and QMBs. The State may also buy in for medically needy beneficiaries who are not QMBs (such as the over-poverty institutionalized persons mentioned above), but must pay the entire premium with State funds.

2. *Coverage and Payment Rules Under Buy-In*

In addition to having the Medicare premiums and cost-sharing amounts paid on their behalf, persons qualifying for Medicaid under standards other than the QMB rule may obtain services which are included in the State plan for Medicaid but which are not covered by Medicare, such as prescription drugs, dental care, or nursing facility care beyond the very limited Medicare coverage. In some States, on the other hand, the Medicaid plan may not include all the services covered by Medicare. For example, the State might not cover heart transplants, which Medicare covers. In this circumstance, the State may pay the Medicare deductible or coinsurance for those services, even though it would not pay for the service for other Medicaid beneficiaries.

Some States that use fee schedules to limit practitioner reimbursement may pay less than the full cost-sharing amount on Medicare claims. If, for example, the Medicare allowable charge for a particular service is $100, Medicare pays $80, leaving $20 to be paid as coinsurance. If the State's fee limit for the same service is $75, the State may conclude that the practitioner has already been paid in full. Other States will pay the full cost-sharing amounts determined by Medicare so long as these amounts are not themselves in excess of the State's fee limits. A Federal appeals court has recently overturned New York's policy of paying coinsurance only up to the limit of New York's Medicaid fee schedule.[39] The State may elect to pay the full cost-sharing amounts for QMBs even if it does not do so for other joint Medicare/Medicaid beneficiaries.

B. Group Health Plans and Other Third Party Liability

1. Enrollment in Group Health Plans

OBRA 90 requires States, effective January 1, 1991, to pay premiums and cost-sharing on behalf of beneficiaries eligible for enrollment in a group health plan when it is cost-effective to do so. For example, a beneficiary who is employed might be eligible for coverage under an employer health plan, but might be required to pay a monthly premium to join. Medicaid will pay that premium, as well as deductibles and coinsurance required under the plan, if the cost is less than the cost of the services that the employer plan will cover and that would otherwise have been paid directly by Medicaid. In some instances, it may be cost-effective for Medicaid to pay group health plan premiums on behalf of an individual who is not eligible, in order to enroll family members who are Medicaid beneficiaries. In these cases, Medicaid may pay premiums, but not cost-sharing, on behalf of the ineligible person.

The Secretary is required to develop guidelines for identifying cases in which enrollment of a beneficiary in a group health plan would be cost-effective. In such cases, beneficiaries (or their parents, in the children) are required to enroll in the plan as a condition of receiving Medicaid. Beneficiaries retain the right to Medicaid payment of any covered services not available under the group health plan. If, on the other hand, the plan includes services not ordinarily covered under Medicaid, the State is permitted to pay premiums and cost-sharing for those services. In addition, a State may at its option provide a minimum enrollment period of up to 6 months after the date of initial enrollment for a beneficiary enrolled under a group health plan. If the beneficiary loses Medicaid eligibility, the State may continue payments to the plan (but not other Medicaid benefits) until the end of that period.

---

[39]*New York City Health and Hospitals Corporation* v. *Perales*, 954 F2d 854 (1991).

Guidelines implementing the new provisions, including one suggested method for determining cost-effectiveness, were issued in April 1991; States were authorized to develop alternative methods of measuring cost-effectiveness. As of March 1992, only 27 States had filed State plan amendments implementing the new requirement. Of these, seven were using the cost-effectiveness methodology proposed by the Secretary.[40] Data on the number of persons enrolled under the OBRA 90 provision, and any resulting savings, are not yet available.

2. Other Third Party Liability

Applicants for Medicaid are required to disclose any insurance coverage or other potential third party payment source at the time of application or redetermination, and must assign to the State any right of recovery they may have. The State is required to have a system for pursuing third party claims; this system must be integrated with the State's Medicaid Management Information System (MMIS; see *Chapter VII, Administration*). States may act on the basis of the information furnished by beneficiaries or may identify potential payments by other means. For example, States must review cases of hospitalization resulting from accidental injury, on the possibility that a legal action is pending. States may also have agreements on data exchange with workers' compensation boards or State motor vehicle accident report files. Failure to maintain a third-party recovery system may subject the State to the penalties for failure to operate an approved MMIS; that is, reductions in Federal matching payments for administrative costs. The General Accounting Office (GAO) has reported that the MMIS penalties are not an adequate enforcement tool and has recommended that HCFA be given more direct authority to penalize States that do not comply with third-party recovery requirements.[41]

States must also have systems for collecting medical support payments from absent parents. Beneficiaries must cooperate in establishing paternity and obtaining medical support (this requirement may be waived for good cause, such as a possibility of reprisal). The Medicaid agency must have a cooperative agreement with the Title IV-D (child support enforcement) agency and other appropriate agencies. When subdivisions or other States assist in enforcement and collection action, the Medicaid agency must make an incentive payment to the other State or locality equal to 15 percent of the amount recovered; this payment comes entirely from the Federal share of the recovery.

A State may enforce third party responsibility (other than medical support payment) in either of two ways. Under the "cost avoidance" method, the State

---

[40]U.S. Dept. of Health and Human Services. Health Care Financing Administration. *Medicaid State Profile Data System: Characteristics of Medicaid State Programs*, v. 1, May 1992. Baltimore, 1992. p. 17-23.

[41]U.S. General Accounting Office. *Medicaid: HCFA Needs Authority to Enforce Third-Party Requirements on States*. Report to the Chairman, House Committee on Government Operations; (GAO/HRD-91-60), Apr. 1991. Washington, 1991.

denies reimbursement of claims for which potential third party liability is known to exist and instructs the provider to bill the responsible party. Under the "pay-and-chase" method, the State pays the claims and then seeks to collect from the responsible party on its own (unless the State concludes that the cost of collection is greater than the potential recovery). "Pay-and-chase" is mandatory for two kinds of claims: claims for prenatal or preventive pediatric care (including early and periodic screening, diagnostic and treatment (EPSDT) services) and claims involving late payment by a third party whose liability arises from a child support action. For all other kinds of claims, the statute permits the State to choose either approach. However, the Secretary has required by regulation that a State must use the cost avoidance method whenever possible unless it can demonstrate that its pay-and-chase system is equally cost-effective. All States have now shifted to a cost avoidance system as their basic method for enforcing third party liability. Some States continue to use pay-and-chase for certain services, usually prescription drugs.[42]

Some private health insurance policies have provisions which exclude coverage for any service which might be paid for by Medicaid. No Federal funding is available if a State pays for a service which would have been covered by the private policy but for such a provision. States have responded by prohibiting such provisions in the policies they regulate. However, GAO reports that problems have emerged with insurers beyond the reach of an individual State's regulation. These include out-of-State insurers and "self-insured" employer health plans.[43] Some of these plans may be denying payment for services obtained by Medicaid beneficiaries. Other insurers may refuse to recognize a beneficiary's assignment of recovery rights to the State. GAO has recommended a strengthening of Federal laws in these areas.[44]

One possible consequence of a cost avoidance system is that the provider will treat the beneficiary as a private patient and seek to collect from the beneficiary any difference between the amount received from the third party payer and the provider's usual charge. COBRA prohibits collection from the beneficiary if the third party payment is equal to the Medicaid rate for the service; if the payment is below the Medicaid rate, the provider may collect no more than the amount of any beneficiary cost-sharing permitted under the State plan. The State may recover triple the amount of the excess charge from any provider who violates this provision.

---

[42]Personal communication, Terry Derville, Medicaid Bureau, HCFA.

[43]Plans in which the employer assumes direct risk for the cost of health services used by employees, instead of buying a health insurance policy, are exempted from State regulation by the Employee Retirement Income Security Act of 1974 (ERISA).

[44]U.S. General Accounting Office. *Medicaid: Legislation Needed to Improve Collections from Private Insurers.* Report to the Chairman, Subcommittee on Health and the Environment, House Committee on Energy and Commerce; (GAO/HRD-91-25), Nov. 1990. Washington, 1990.

A second consequence of a cost avoidance system is that many claims are submitted directly by providers to the liable third parties; the State may never receive information about the services furnished or the amounts paid by the third parties. As a result there is no way of measuring the full impact of third party payments on Medicaid expenditures. HCFA reports that States' direct collections from third parties totalled $176 million in FY 1991. Estimates by States of the amounts saved through cost avoidance (not counting amounts paid by Medicare) totalled $1.2 billion in the same year.[45]

A State must generally limit Medicaid payment for deductibles and coinsurance imposed by a private insurer, so that the sum of the private insurance and Medicaid payments for a given service is no more than the usual Medicaid rate for the service. (This limitation is optional for Medicare cost-sharing, but mandatory for private insurance.) Under the new OBRA 90 program for enrollment of beneficiaries in group health plans, a State must pay all cost-sharing obligations for such beneficiaries.

C. Indian Health Service

The Indian Health Service (IHS) within the Department of Health and Human Services (DHHS) provides or purchases health services for certain groups of Native Americans and Alaska Natives. The IHS provides care in two different ways: directly through IHS facilities or tribally owned and operated facilities, and on a "contract care" basis through referral to off-reservation health care providers.

The IHS requires that alternative payment resources available to users of IHS services be exhausted before IHS will accept financial responsibility. Native Americans may qualify for Medicaid in the same way as any other population, by meeting categorical and financial standards. In the case of services provided in IHS facilities to Medicaid beneficiaries, IHS bills Medicaid directly. Federal matching funds for services in IHS facilities are available at 100 percent, rather than at the State's usual matching rate.[46] When services are furnished by a contract provider, the provider is expected to collect from any "alternative resource" available to the patient, including Medicaid, Medicare, or other health insurance, before seeking reimbursement from IHS. If Medicaid is the responsible payer, Federal funding is available at the State's usual matching rate; the State is liable for the remainder, as with any other Medicaid service.

---

[45]Unpublished report, HCFA. The report includes State by State breakdowns. These are not provided here because some States failed to report and States did not use uniform methods for estimating cost avoidance.

[46]The payment is not actually issued to the facility but is retained by the Secretary of Health and Human Services in a special fund for the purpose of improving IHS facilities. The Indian Health Care Amendments of 1988 (P.L. 100-713) established a demonstration project under which Medicaid payments would be made directly to certain tribally operated IHS facilities.

CHAPTER VI. ALTERNATE DELIVERY OPTIONS AND WAIVER PROGRAMS[1]

I. SUMMARY

Medicaid law provides a number of options for States wishing to use innovative methods for delivering or paying for Medicaid services. Since the earliest years of the Medicaid program, States have arranged for the enrollment of Medicaid beneficiaries under contracts with health maintenance organizations (HMOs) or comparable organizations. Omnibus Budget Reconciliation Act of 1981 (OBRA 81) established two new options, section 2175 (freedom-of-choice) and section 2176 (home and community-based services) waiver programs. Under these provisions, the Secretary may waive certain statutory requirements in order to allow States to develop cost-effective alternative methods of service delivery or reimbursement. The purpose of these provisions was to give States greater flexibility in managing their Medicaid programs.

In the case of the 2175 waiver option, also referred to as section 1915(b) waivers (after the section of Medicaid law in which the authority was established), the greater flexibility was intended to offset the temporary reductions in Federal Medicaid funding imposed by the same act. The section 2176 option, also referred to as section 1915(c) waivers, was intended to correct a perceived "institutional bias" in Medicaid services for the chronically ill by providing States an alternative of offering a broad range of home and community-based care to persons at risk of institutionalization. Two other home and community-based care waiver programs were subsequently established in Medicaid: one to allow States to serve elderly persons at risk of needing nursing home care and a second to allow them to provide services to certain children infected with the acquired immunodeficiency syndrome (AIDS) virus or who are drug dependent at birth. Most recently Omnibus Budget Reconciliation Act of 1990 (OBRA 90) established a new optional Medicaid benefit called home and community-based care for functionally disabled elderly persons.

Finally, States have periodically been granted waivers of Medicaid requirements in order to conduct demonstration projects. Some of these projects have been authorized by the Secretary under general statutory provisions allowing for tests of possible program improvements. Others have been specifically authorized by Federal legislation.

This chapter describes each of the five basic types of Medicaid alternate delivery options:

---

[1]This chapter was written by Mark Merlis and Richard Price.

- risk contracts with HMOs and comparable organizations known as prepaid health plans (PHPs);

- freedom-of-choice (section 1915(b)) waivers;

- home and community-based services waivers, including section 1915(c) waivers, 1915(d) waiver programs for the elderly, and 1915(e) waivers for "boarder babies" who are infected with the AIDS virus or who are drug dependent at birth;

- home and community-based care as an optional Medicaid benefit for functionally disabled elderly individuals;

- special demonstration projects authorized by the Secretary under general waiver authorities or specifically mandated by Congress.

II. RISK CONTRACTS

States may enter into risk contracts with HMOs or comparable entities. Under a risk contract, the organization agrees to make available a specified set of medical services to an individual beneficiary in return for a fixed periodic payment issued by the Medicaid program on the beneficiary's behalf. The payment, known as a premium or capitation payment, is usually issued monthly, at a rate based on a projection of costs for the services used by a typical patient. If the beneficiaries enrolled under the contract use more, or more costly, services than anticipated, the organization may suffer a loss. If the enrollees use fewer services than anticipated, the organization may realize a profit. The organization is therefore said to be "at risk" for the set of services covered by the contract.

The risk arrangement is intended to give the organization a financial incentive to furnish services more efficiently. The beneficiaries who are enrolled may obtain services covered under the contract only from providers affiliated with the organization, except in emergencies or for family planning services. As an incentive for participation, the State may arrange for an HMO to offer additional services not ordinarily covered by the Medicaid program, or the HMO may offer these services on its own. The State is not required to furnish the additional services to beneficiaries who are not enrolled under the risk contract.

The requirements governing risk contracts depend on the scope of services that the contractor has agreed to cover. A "comprehensive" contract is one in which the organization has agreed to accept risk for any three of the mandatory Medicaid services (see *Chapter IV, Services*), or for inpatient hospital care and any other mandatory service. Comprehensive contracts are subject to specific requirements set forth in section 1903(m) of the Social Security Act. A few States have entered into "partial capitation" arrangements, under which the organization contracts for a more limited scope of services. Such a contract might cover only physician and diagnostic services, or only dental care. No specific requirements for these contracts are included in Medicaid law, although they are subject to some regulatory requirements. Of the approximately 1.6

million Medicaid beneficiaries receiving services through risk contractors in June 1990, 92 percent were enrolled under comprehensive contracts (see *Appendix G, Managed Care* for enrollment by State). For this reason, the following discussion is confined to the requirements governing contracts subject to section 1903(m).

A State may enter into a 1903(m) comprehensive risk contract with two kinds of entities: HMOs and "PHPs."

An HMO may be federally qualified--determined by the Secretary to meet standards set forth in title XIII of the Public Health Service Act--or may be certified as eligible by the State.[2] A State-certified HMO must (a) be organized primarily for the purpose of providing health care services, (b) make the services it provides as accessible to enrollees as they are to nonenrolled beneficiaries, and (c) provide satisfactory assurances that beneficiaries will not become liable for the HMO's debts in the event that it becomes insolvent.

The PHPs include community, migrant, or Appalachian regional health centers which receive Federal grant funds and meet certain other conditions. Some entities which entered into a risk contract prior to 1970 may also be treated as PHPs.

No more than 75 percent of the enrollees of an HMO may be Medicaid or Medicare beneficiaries. This requirement may be waived for PHPs. It may be waived temporarily for publicly owned HMOs, HMOs with more than 25,000 enrollees that serve a designated "medically underserved" area and that previously participated in an approved demonstration project, or HMOs that have had a Medicaid contract for less than 3 years. Waivers for HMOs are permitted only if the HMO is making efforts to comply with the 75 percent limit, and (except for public HMOs) only if the Secretary determines that special circumstances warrant the exemption.[3]

Beneficiaries joining an HMO must ordinarily be permitted to disenroll at any time and return to ordinary Medicaid status; the withdrawal must take effect by the end of the month following the month in which disenrollment is

---

[2]Federally qualified HMOs are certified by HCFA as meeting certain financial, organizational, and quality standards. A qualified HMO is permitted to take advantage of the "dual choice" provisions of title XIII. An employer with more than 25 employees that is subject to the Fair Labor Standards Act and that provides health insurance benefits is required to offer an HMO option as an alternative to its standard health plan, if a federally qualified HMO is available in its area and asks to be included.

[3]Note that the 75 percent limit under Medicaid law is different from the rule for Medicare HMO contractors, which must generally have no more than 50 percent Medicaid or Medicare enrollees. Some HMOs contracting with Medicare are exempt from Medicare's 50 percent limit (these include contractors paid on a reasonable cost basis under section 1833 of the Social Security Act) but are subject to the higher limit under Medicaid.

requested. An exception to this rule is allowed for federally qualified HMOs, certain PHPs, and organizations with a risk contract under Medicare (but not for other State-certified HMOs). The State may restrict the enrollee's ability to disenroll from one of these organizations for a 5-month period, following a 1-month trial period. Disenrollment must be permitted at any time for cause; e.g., if the enrollee moves out of the area served by the HMO. The restriction may be renewed every 6 months, again with a 1-month period during which the beneficiary may disenroll without cause. For the same groups of organizations, with minor exceptions, the State may also provide for "guaranteed eligibility." For a period of up to 6 months from the date of initial enrollment, the State may continue premium payments to the HMO or PHP on behalf of an enrollee, even if the enrollee ceases to be eligible for Medicaid during that period.

The OBRA 90 added an additional option, available to any HMO, to address the problem of enrollees who lose Medicaid eligibility for a brief period and are later reinstated. A State may automatically reenroll such enrollees in the HMO once eligibility is regained, so long as the period of ineligibility is no more than 3 months.

Premium rates must be established on an actuarially sound basis. The Secretary has provided by regulation that rates may not exceed what has come to be known as the "fee-for-service equivalent." This is the amount which the State would have spent to provide the set of services covered by the HMO or PHP to an equivalent group of beneficiaries not enrolled in the organization and continuing to receive care on a fee-for-service basis. Conceptually, the fee-for-service equivalent is identical to the adjusted average per capita cost (AAPCC) used in calculating Medicare premium rates for HMOs. However, whereas Medicare premiums are fixed at 95 percent of the AAPCC, Medicaid payments may be at any level up to 100 percent of the fee-for-service equivalent; it is a ceiling rather than a basis for rate-setting. (No minimum or floor exists in Medicaid statute or regulation.) Some States do use the fee-for-service equivalent, or a percentage of this figure, as a premium rate. Others negotiate rates or set them on the basis of competitive bidding, while a few have developed more complex actuarial projection methodologies.[4]

Since 1986, Congress has added to the law a number of provisions intended to improve quality of care in prepaid programs or protect beneficiaries. States are now required to obtain an independent assessment of the quality of services furnished by contracting HMOs and PHPs, using either a utilization and quality control peer review organization (PRO) under contract to the Secretary or another independent accrediting body. In addition, States are prohibited from contracting with an organization which is managed or controlled by, or has a significant subcontractual relation with, individuals or entities potentially excludable from participation in Medicaid or Medicare (see *Chapter VII,*

---

[4]The OBRA 90 requires that, if an HMO contracts for the provision of services by a federally qualified health center (FQHC, such as a community or migrant health center), it must at the center's option pay for those services at the Medicaid fee-for-service rates for FQHCs. In turn, the State must adjust its capitation rates for the HMO to reflect this provision.

Administration for a discussion of the grounds for exclusion). Finally, States are now required to collect sufficient data on HMO enrollees' encounters with physicians to identify the physicians furnishing services to Medicaid beneficiaries.

The HMOs and PHPs that commit certain violations may also be subject to special monetary penalties or other sanctions, in addition to the general sanctions applicable to all Medicaid providers. Civil monetary penalties may be imposed on organizations that fail to furnish medically necessary services or, effective for contract years beginning in 1992, that make incentive payments to physicians in violation of rules governing such payments under Medicare.[5] Organizations may also be penalized for imposing illegal premiums on enrollees, discriminating in enrollment on the basis of health status, or supplying false information to the Secretary, the State, or any other individual or entity. (Details of the penalty provisions are included in the general discussion of civil monetary penalties in *Chapter VII, Administration.*)

In addition, the Secretary may deny Federal funding for Medicaid premiums paid on behalf of new enrollees joining the HMO after the date the Secretary notifies the HMO that it has committed a violation. The denial may continue until the Secretary is satisfied that the basis for the violation has been corrected and that the problems are not likely to recur.

III. FREEDOM-OF-CHOICE WAIVERS

A. Type of Freedom-of-Choice Waivers

Section 2175 of OBRA 81 added a new section 1915(b) to the Social Security Act, authorizing the Secretary to waive certain provisions of Medicaid law to allow States to develop innovative health care delivery or reimbursement systems. The section 1915(b) waiver program originally allowed for waivers of any provision of section 1902 of the Social Security Act, relating to basic requirements for State Medicaid plans, or section 1903(m),[6] relating to requirements for contracts with HMOs or PHPs, in order to allow a State to:

---

[5]Under the Medicare rules, added by OBRA 90, incentive plans must be reported to the Secretary, and no specific payment may be made to physicians as an inducement to withhold or limit services to specific enrollees. If physicians or physician groups are placed at serious risk for services than their own, the HMO must provide adequate stop-loss protection and must periodically survey enrollees to ensure that they have adequate access and are satisfied with the quality of services.

[6]The authority to waive section 1903(m), relating to requirements for HMOs and other risk contractors, was repealed by the Tax Equity and Fiscal Responsibility Act of 1982 (TEFRA 82, Public Law 97-248). See *Appendix G, Managed Care*, for a discussion of the reason for and impact of this change.

1. Implement a primary care case management program or specialty physician services arrangement which restricts the providers from whom a beneficiary may obtain covered services.

Under a primary care case management program, each participating beneficiary selects or is assigned to a single primary care provider. Except in an emergency, the beneficiary may obtain other services, such as specialty physician and hospital care, only with the authorization of the primary care provider. The aim of the program is to reduce the use of unnecessary services and provide better overall coordination of beneficiaries' care. Under a specialty physician services arrangement, beneficiaries could obtain specialty care only from a limited group of physicians selected by the State, perhaps on the basis of fee levels or cost-effective practice patterns (no State has implemented a program of this kind). Of the 35 section 1915(b) waiver programs operational or under development in January 1991, 30 involved case management.

2. Use a local agency as a "central broker" to assist beneficiaries in choosing among competing health care plans.

Under this option, a State may establish a limited number of alternative health plans in an area and require Medicaid beneficiaries to choose from among those plans. For example, the State might offer a choice among several HMOs or PHPs and a fee-for-service primary care case management program. Waivers for this purpose are ordinarily granted in conjunction with case management waivers. Five programs had both types of waivers in January 1991.

3. Share with beneficiaries, through the provision of additional services, savings resulting from the beneficiaries' use of cost-effective providers.

A beneficiary participating in a primary care case management program might, for example, receive expanded dental coverage or a waiver of required cost-sharing as an incentive to enroll. (Note that no waiver is required when additional services are made available to enrollees of an HMO or PHP.) Waivers for this purpose are also granted in conjunction with case management waivers. Six programs had both types of waivers in January 1991.

4. Restrict the providers from whom beneficiaries may receive services, except in emergencies, to those meeting reimbursement, quality, and utilization standards established by the State.

A State may use this option to establish a selective contracting program, such as the California and Illinois (until 1991) systems of competitive negotiations for inpatient hospital services described in *Chapter V, Reimbursement*. Other States have combined selective contracting with primary care case management programs to establish coordinated care systems. Nine States restrict providers in the context of a case management program, while five have waivers for restriction of providers alone. Of those five, three involve hospital contracting, one is for transportation services, and one is for pharmaceuticals. Omnibus Budget Reconciliation Act of 1989 (OBRA 89, Public

Law 101-239) provided that a State with a selective contracting system must still comply with Medicaid requirements for additional payments for hospitals serving a disproportionate share of low-income patients, and OBRA 90 provided that payments under a selective contracting system are subject to requirements for timely claims payment.

Table VI-1 shows the types of programs for which section 1915(b) waiver proposals--including those withdrawn, disapproved, or never implemented--have been submitted to the Secretary from 1981 through January 1991. Of the 120 requests, 59 were approved. Most approved waiver proposals have related to primary care case management and other "managed care" programs. Table VI-2 shows the current status of those proposals that were actually implemented, while table VI-3 shows the States with operational programs in January 1991 (including approved programs not yet fully implemented), along with the nature of the waivers for those programs. Of the 35 programs, 30 were managed care programs; details of these programs are provided in *Appendix G, Managed Care*. The other six projects included the selective contracting programs cited above and a Utah program for capitation payments to mental health providers.

TABLE VI-1. Waiver Requests Under Section 1915(b), 1981 to 1991

	1981	1982	1983	1984	1985	1986	1987	1988	1989	1990	1991	Total
Managed care												
Approved	3	12	6	3	4	4	3	2	5	3		45
Disapproved						2			1			3
Withdrawn		4	3	1	2	2	2	2				16
Pending					1	1		1	1	4	1	9
Selective contracting												
Approved		4	1	2	1			3	1			12
Disapproved												0
Withdrawn		1	4	2	3	2	1					13
Pending				1	1	2	1					5
Waive 1903(m) rules												
Approved	1	1										2
Disapproved												0
Withdrawn		1										1
Pending												0
Nonresponsive[a]												
Disapproved	5	2	1									8
Withdrawn	1	3	1			1						6
Total requests	10	28	16	9	12	14	7	8	8	7	1	120

[a]Requests labeled as "nonresponsive" were for purposes other than those specified in section 1915(b) or required waivers of provisions of law for which waivers were not authorized by that section. Among these were proposals to impose new copayment requirements on beneficiaries or to waive eligibility rules.

Source: Table prepared by the Congressional Research Service based on analysis of unpublished Health Care Financing Administration (HCFA) reports. Data reflect applications filed and State or HCFA actions taken as of Jan. 31, 1991.

TABLE VI-2. Status of Approved Section 1915(b) Waivers, January 1991

Type of waiver	Still in initial waiver period	Operating under approved renewal	Terminated or expired	Total
Managed care	11	19	15	45
Selective contracting	3	3	6	12
Waive 1903(m) rules	0	0	2	2
Total	14	22	23	59

Source: Table prepared by the Congressional Research Service based on analysis of unpublished HCFA reports.

TABLE VI-3. Location and Type of Operational Section 1915(b) Waiver Programs, January 1991

	Case management	Locality as central broker	Share savings	Restrict providers
Alabama: Case management, pregnant women	x		x	x
California:				
Selective contracting, hospital services				
Primary care case management	x			x
San Mateo organized health system	x			x
Santa Barbara health initiative	x			x
Colorado: Primary care case management	x			
Florida: Primary care case management	x			
Illinois: Illinois competitive access and reimbursement equity program (Note: this program was eliminated later in 1991)				x
Iowa: Medicaid patient access to health	x			
Kansas: Kansas primary care network	x			

See notes at end of table.

TABLE VI-3. Location and Type of Operational Section 1915(b) Waiver Programs, January 1991--Continued

	Case management	Locality as central broker	Share savings	Restrict providers
Kentucky: KENPAC	x			
Louisiana: Selective contracting, medical transportation				x
Maryland:				
Diabetes managed care	x		x	
Maryland access to care	x			
Michigan:				
Primary care physician sponsor program	x			
Capitated ambulatory program	x			
Physician sponsors for SSI population	x			
Minnesota: Case management for chemical and substance abuse	x			x
Missouri: Missouri Medicaid managed health care plan	x	x		

See notes at end of table.

TABLE VI-3. Location and Type of Operational Section 1915(b) Waiver Programs, January 1991--Continued

	Case management	Locality as central broker	Share savings	Restrict providers
New Mexico: Primary care network	x			
New York:				
PCMP.-Erie County	x			
Erie County physician case management	x	x		
North Carolina:				
Primary care case management	x			
Ohio: Dayton area health plan	x	x		
Oregon:				
Capitated physician case management	x			x
Selective contracting--pharmaceuticals				x
Pennsylvania: HealthPass	x		x	x
South Carolina:				
High risk channeling project	x		x	x
Mental health case management	x			

See notes at end of table.

TABLE VI-3. Location and Type of Operational Section 1915(b) Waiver Programs, January 1991--Continued

	Case management	Locality as central broker	Share savings	Restrict providers
Tennessee: Primary care case management	x			
Utah:				
Choice of health care delivery system	x	x		
Mental health capitation	x	x	x	x
Washington:				
KPS capitation plan	x			
Selective hospital contracting				x
Wisconsin:				
HMO primary care case management	x		x	x
Total	30	5	6	14
Number of programs:	35			
Number of States with programs:	24			

Source: Table prepared by the Congressional Research Service based on analysis of unpublished HCFA reports.

B. Statutes Waived and Application Process

There are three statutory provisions for which section 1915(b) waivers have most frequently been granted. The first is *freedom-of-choice*, the requirement that beneficiaries be able to obtain covered services from any qualified provider willing to accept Medicaid reimbursement. Waiver of this requirement has, for example, permitted States to mandate beneficiary enrollment in case management systems. (As with HMO contracts, the beneficiary's right to select a provider of family planning services may not be restricted, nor can a program exclude the services of "FQHCs"; see *Chapter IV, Services* for a discussion of these providers.) Waiver of this rule is so common a feature of section 1915(b) programs that they are often spoken of generically as "freedom-of-choice waivers." The other two statutory provisions often waived are *comparability* and *statewideness*, the requirements that the scope of covered services be the same for all categorically needy beneficiaries and that the Medicaid program operate uniformly throughout the State. Waiver of these requirements has allowed States to target section 1915(b) programs to particular groups of beneficiaries, such as AFDC recipients in a particular county.

In requesting a 1915(b) waiver, the State must demonstrate that its proposed program will be cost-effective and must provide assurances that the restrictions established by the waiver will not impair beneficiaries' access to medically necessary services of adequate quality. Waivers are deemed granted unless the Secretary denies the request or asks for additional information within 90 days. The maximum period for which waivers may be granted is 2 years, but waivers may be renewed after a reapplication process.

IV. HOME AND COMMUNITY-BASED SERVICES WAIVERS

Medicaid law contains other waiver authorities that are intended to allow States to offer community-based long-term care services to persons who would otherwise require nursing home care or other forms of institutional care. Community-based long-term care services include homemaker/home health aide services, personal care assistance, adult day care, and other noninstitutional services needed by persons who have lost some capacity for self-care because of a chronic illness or condition.

The first of these waiver authorities to be enacted was the Medicaid Home and Community-Based Services Program, often referred to as the "2176 waiver program," after the section of OBRA 81 which authorized it. This program is also called the 1915(c) waiver program, for the section of Medicaid law in which it is authorized. Under 1915(c) waivers, States provide a broad range of home and community-based services to elderly, mentally retarded, and other disabled and chronically ill persons.

A second waiver program for home and community-based services was established by Omnibus Budget Reconciliation Act of 1987 (OBRA 87, Public Law 100-203) to address concerns of some States that the 1915(c) authority constrained their ability to provide services to a growing elderly population at risk of needing nursing home care. To respond to these concerns, Congress established a new waiver authority, referred to as the 1915(d) waiver program. With a 1915(d) waiver, States may serve only elderly persons at risk of requiring nursing home care.

Congress established the original 1915(c) waiver program in response to general concern about the lack of Federal funding for home and community-based care. The waiver program was also intended to respond to specific concerns that Medicaid provided far greater support for nursing home care than for home and community-based care. Prior to 1981, many of the nonskilled personal care and supportive services needed by chronically impaired persons to remain in the community were simply not covered under Medicaid. These services, however, are typically covered as part of Medicaid's nursing home benefit.

Policymakers had also observed that Medicaid actually created financial incentives for persons to use nursing home care rather than community care. In certain instances, the program's financial eligibility rules had allowed persons to become eligible for Medicaid coverage of institutional care under standards that were more liberal than those used for community-based care.[7]

In establishing the waiver programs, Congress did not, however, authorize States to provide home and community-based care as mandatory or optional services for which Federal Medicaid matching funds are available without prior approval. Instead, both the 1915(c) and 1915(d) waiver authorities require States to make special application to the Secretary of the Department of Health and Human Services (DHHS) for each of the specific programs under which they propose to provide home and community-based care. The programs must be reviewed and approved by the Secretary before covered services become eligible for Federal matching payments.

---

[7]One of the barriers to eligibility for persons needing home and community-based care had been Medicaid's deeming rules. An individual is eligible for Supplemental Security Income (SSI) payments, and therefore, automatic Medicaid eligibility, if his or her resources and income are below established limits. In making this determination, the total income and resources of the applicant's spouse, or applicant's parent in the case of a child under 18, are automatically considered available, or "deemed," to the individual. However, the "deeming" provisions only apply to individuals living in the same household as their spouse or parents. Under SSI deeming rules, an institutionalized individual is no longer considered to be living in the same household as his/her spouse or parents after the first full month of institutionalization. Therefore, after the first month, only the institutionalized individual's own income and resources are considered for purposes of eligibility.

In addition, Medicaid has permitted States to use a higher income eligibility standard for persons needing nursing home care than for persons living in the community. States may cover under their Medicaid programs persons needing nursing home care, so long as their monthly income does not exceed 300 percent of SSI (in 1992, $1,266). The "300 percent rule" is discussed in greater detail in *Chapter III, Eligibility.*

The need for special review and approval for waiver programs grew out of concern about the costs of expanding Federal support for home and community-based care. Federal long-term care demonstrations have generally shown that expanded community-based services result in new costs that are not offset by reductions in nursing home spending. In addition, policymakers have been concerned about the potential demand for community-based care, especially given the lack of financing for these services. For these reasons, 1915(c) and 1915(d) waiver authorities contain specific limitations in spending for covered services, and States must demonstrate to the Secretary in their applications that spending for home and community-based care will not exceed levels specified in law and regulations.

To assist States in developing programs that would meet the law's spending tests, both the 1915(c) and 1915(d) authorities provide States greater flexibility in offering home and community-based care than they have for all other Medicaid covered services. This flexibility is provided through waivers of certain requirements that otherwise apply to States' Medicaid plans and the services they cover. Specifically, the Secretary is allowed to waive the Medicaid "statewideness" requirement, so that States may cover home and community-based care in only a portion of the State, rather than in all geographic jurisdictions. The Secretary may also waive the requirement that covered services be comparable in amount, duration, and scope for persons in particular eligibility groups. As a result, States may limit coverage of home and community-based care to certain State-defined individuals. Finally, the 1915(c) and 1915(d) programs allow States to waive the financial eligibility standards that apply to persons living in the community and to use for these individuals the more liberal financial standards they may use for persons needing institutional care.[8]

Because of administrative burdens involved in making special applications under the 1915(c) and 1915(d) waiver programs and meeting budget neutrality tests, Congress recently established under OBRA 90 a new optional Medicaid benefit called home and community-based care for the elderly. As an optional service, States no longer will need to demonstrate that home and community-based care programs will be budget neutral. This optional service, however, is different from all other services in that it is subject to a cap on Federal outlays-- a total of $580 million for 5 years. This new authority is described in greater detail below.

---

[8]This may include (depending on the State plan), but is not limited to, individuals who would be eligible for Medicaid in an institution because income from a spouse or parents is not deemed available to them, and individuals who would be eligible under the 300 percent rule. Many States are using these more liberal standards for their waiver populations. See Lipson, Linda and Susan Laudicina. *State Home and Community-Based Services for the Aged Under Medicaid: Waiver Programs, Optional Services Under the Medicaid State Plan, and OBRA 1990 Provisions for a New Optional Benefit.* American Association of Retired Persons, Apr. 1991. p. 10.

A. 1915(c) Waivers

Under the 1915(c) waiver authority, States with approved applications may provide home and community-based care to persons who, without these services, would require institutional care that would be covered by Medicaid. In the first years after enactment, States provided services to elderly, disabled, and chronically mentally ill persons at risk of needing nursing home care and to persons with mental retardation and developmental disabilities who required intermediate care facilities for the mentally retarded (ICFs/MR) care. Subsequent amendments to the authority have allowed States to include persons needing hospital care and those with specific illnesses and conditions. As a result, States are now also serving chronically ill and disabled children and persons with AIDS.

In establishing the waiver program, Congress sought to prevent or postpone institutionalization of persons who could be served in the community. To that end, 1915(c) waivers permit States to cover services that go beyond the medical and medically-related benefits that have been the principal focus of Medicaid law. With approved waiver programs, States are authorized to cover a wide variety of nonmedical, social, and supportive services that have been shown to be critical in allowing persons to remain in the community. These include case management,[9] homemaker/home health aide services, personal care, adult day health, habilitation services,[10] respite care,[11] and other services requested by the State and approved by the Secretary. For the chronically mentally ill, the waiver program also authorizes day treatment or other partial hospitalization, psychosocial rehabilitation services, and clinic services (whether or not furnished in a facility). The law prohibits coverage of room and board for targeted populations.[12]

With the waiver of Medicaid statewideness and comparability requirements permitted under 1915(c), States have flexibility to define the geographic areas and the target populations they wish to serve. In addition, for covered persons,

---

[9]Case management is commonly understood to be a system under which responsibility for developing a care plan for an impaired or disabled individual, locating and coordinating services specified in the care plan, and monitoring services over time rests with a designated person or organization.

[10]Habilitation services are designed to assist persons with mental retardation and developmental disabilities in acquiring, retaining, and improving the self-help, socialization, and adaptive skills necessary to reside successfully in community-based settings.

[11]Respite care provides relief to the primary caregiver of a chronically ill or disabled individual. Respite services may be provided either in the home or a facility, so as to allow the absence of the caregiver for a period of time.

[12]The OBRA 90, however, permitted payment of rent and food of an unrelated personal caregiver who is residing in the same household with an individual eligible to receive waiver services.

they may provide any one or combination of services authorized in law and may provide these in amounts they determine necessary.

States are, however, constrained by a budget neutrality test in defining the populations and services they wish to cover. The law requires that States demonstrate to the Secretary that estimated average per capita expenditures for persons receiving waiver services will not exceed expenditures that would have been incurred for these individuals in the absence of the waiver.

In implementing this provision, the Health Care Financing Administration (HCFA) developed a formula that States must use to demonstrate that their programs will meet the statutory budget neutrality test. The formula requires, among other things, that States estimate the number of persons who would be served in Medicaid-certified nursing home beds and other institutions participating in the program, in the absence of a waiver. This estimate must include all current Medicaid certified beds by type of facility, all additional beds that would be built and certified during the life of the waiver, and all beds closed as a direct result of the waivers.

The HCFA has used this estimate of bed supply as a ceiling on the number of persons who may be served under the waiver. This policy has presented problems particularly for those States that have attempted to control Medicaid spending for nursing home care by limiting construction of new nursing home beds or by actually closing beds in such facilities as ICFs/MR. Because they have fewer beds with which to serve persons at risk of institutionalization, these States can serve fewer people under the waiver. States that have a greater supply of nursing home beds because they have not limited their growth would be allowed to serve larger numbers of persons under the waiver.

Congress attempted to address this problem in two ways. First, it created a new 1915(d) waiver program for the elderly that is not dependent on a State's supply of nursing home beds. Second, it changed the budget neutrality test for programs designed to serve the mentally retarded and developmentally disabled. OBRA 87 provided a less restrictive budget neutrality test for individuals with developmental disabilities who are residents of ordinary nursing facilities but who require the level of care provided by an ICF/MR. The amendment allows States to compare waiver costs to the costs that would have been incurred if the participants had been in an ICF/MR. In addition, an amendment in OBRA 90 allows States to compare projected costs under the waiver to costs that are incurred for ICF/MR care, even if the ICF/MR has been terminated from Medicaid participation, so that residents of these facilities may be deinstitutionalized and served in the community.

In addition to assurances that their waiver programs will be budget neutral, States must demonstrate to the Secretary that they will be able to evaluate and determine potential waiver participants' need for institutional care. They must provide assurance they will take necessary safeguards to protect the health and welfare of persons receiving waiver services. Individuals determined to be eligible for community-based services must be given a choice between waiver services and institutional care. Waiver programs are approved for an initial period of 3 years and may be extended for additional 5-year terms.

B. Model Waivers

In 1982, HCFA established a variation of "regular" 1915(c) waivers called "model" waivers. HCFA created this separate category of model waivers to deal with an eligibility problem faced by certain disabled persons, many of whom are children.

If a child lives at home, the parents' financial resources are deemed to be available for the child's medical care. If the same child is institutionalized, after the first month away from home, only the child's own financial resources are deemed to be available for the child's care. The child may then qualify for Medicaid. Because of these "deeming" rules, some children who could have been cared for at home might remain in institutions because, if they were to return home, they would lose Medicaid benefits. The same rules apply to married couples, with the resources of the noneligible spouse deemed available for the other spouse who requires nursing home level of care.

A model waiver allows a State to waive the deeming rules and pay for services that will allow disabled children and adults to be served in the community. Model waivers follow the requirements of regular waivers but the application requires less information. Limited to smaller populations, these waivers are given priority in the review process and are usually approved more quickly than regular waivers. Originally HCFA limited the number of persons who could be served under model waivers to 50, but an amendment to section 1915(c) prohibits HCFA from imposing a limit of fewer than 200 persons.[13]

C. Current State 1915(c) Waiver Activity

1. Target Populations and Numbers of Persons Served

Table VI-4 summarizes the number and type of regular and model 1915(c) waivers States had in operation as of December 2, 1991. At that time, almost all States (with the exception of Alaska, Arizona, and the District of Columbia) were using the 1915(c) waiver authority to provide community-based services to populations at risk of institutionalization. States had a total of 167 waivers--

---

[13]The TEFRA 82 also allows States to extend Medicaid coverage to certain disabled children under 18 who are living at home and who would be eligible for Medicaid if institutionalized. The State must determine that (1) the child requires the level of care provided in an institution; (2) it is appropriate to provide care outside the facility; and (3) the cost of care at home is no more than institutional care. If a State elects this option, however, it must grant eligibility to all children who meet these criteria, rather than to a limited number as under the model waivers. See *Chapter III, Eligibility* for additional details.

129 regular waivers and 38 model waivers--in operation at the end of 1991. In FY 1991, 1915(c) waivers served more than 185,000 persons.[14]

Table VI-5 shows that most States with regular waivers served the aged/disabled[15] and the mentally retarded/developmentally disabled. In December 1991, 40 States operated 53 waiver programs serving the aged and disabled, and 46 States operated 61 programs for the mentally retarded and developmentally disabled. (One State operated a program serving both of these groups.) Thirteen States served persons with AIDS under the waiver authority. Only one State served the chronically mentally ill.

A similar analysis of State model waiver activity, contained in table VI-6, shows that 13 States were using this variation to serve disabled children and children with AIDS. States also used the model waiver to serve the aged/disabled (11 States) and the mentally retarded/developmentally disabled (7 States).

As shown in figure VI-2, regular and model waivers served approximately 135,000 aged/disabled persons in FY 1991, or 73 percent of total persons served; 40,000 mentally retarded/developmentally disabled persons, or 21 percent of the total; 6,200 persons with AIDS, or 3.4 percent of the total; and 976 chronically ill and disabled children, or 0.5 percent of the total.[16]

[14]Unpublished HCFA data based on analysis of HCFA Form 372s that States must annually submit to report on numbers of persons served, services used, and costs of services. HCFA uses this form to evaluate the budget neutrality of each waiver program. The total reflects data from 47 States that operated 138 regular and model waivers at that time.

[15]In almost all cases, HCFA's summary information about aged/disabled waivers does not indicate the age of the disabled being served. In only a few cases where States have established waivers that serve the physically disabled under 65 or disabled children is it possible to make inferences about the age of waiver participants.

[16]Unpublished HCFA data based on analysis of HCFA Form 372s. The totals reflect data from 47 States that operated 138 regular and model waivers in FY 1991. These totals do not include an additional 3,800 persons who in 1991 were participants in waiver programs serving at least two different population groups, e.g., the aged/disabled and the mentally retarded/developmentally disabled. For these waivers, a breakdown of the number of participants in each group was not available.

**TABLE VI-4. 1915(c) Regular and Model Waivers,
by State and Target Population, December 2, 1991**

	Regular waivers		Model waivers	
	Population	Total	Population	Total
Alabama	1 A/D		1 A/D	
	1 MR/DD	2	1 C/D	2
Alaska	None	0	None	0
Arizona	None	0	None	0
Arkansas	1 A/D			
	1 MR/DD	2	None	0
California	2 A/D			
	1 P/D			
	1 AIDS			
	1 MR/DD	5	1 A/D	1
Colorado	1 A/D			
	1 MR/DD			
	1 DD			
	1 AIDS	4	1 C/D	1
Connecticut	1 A/D			
	1 MR/DD			
	1 DD	3	1 MR/DD and D	1
Delaware	1 A/D			
	1 MR/DD	2	1 AIDS	1
Dist. of Columbia	None	0	None	0
Florida	2 A/D			
	1 MR/DD			
	1 AIDS	4	1 D	1
Georgia	1 A/D			
	1 MR/DD	2	1 C/D	1
Hawaii	2 A/D			
	1 MR/DD			
	1 AIDS	4	None	0
Idaho	1 A/D and MR/DD	1	None	0

See notes at end of table.

TABLE VI-4. 1915(c) Regular and Model Waivers,
by State and Target Population, December 2, 1991--Continued

	Regular waivers		Model waivers	
	Population	Total	Population	Total
Illinois	1 D 1 A 1 MR/DD 1 AIDS	4	1 C/D and AIDS	1
Indiana	1 A/D	1	1 DD	1
Iowa	2 MR 1 AIDS	3	1 A/D, C/D, MR/DD 1 A/D	2
Kansas	1 A/D 1 MR/DD	2	1 D 1 C/D	2
Kentucky	1 A/D 1 MR/DD	2	1 C/D 1 D	2
Louisiana	1 A/D 1 MR/DD	2	None	0
Maine	1 A 1 P/D 1 MR/DD	3	None	0
Maryland	2 MR/DD	2	1 C/D	1
Massachusetts	1 A/D 1 MR/DD	2	None	0
Michigan	1 MR/DD	1	1 MR/DD	1
Minnesota	1 A 1 P/D 2 MR/DD	4	1 D	1
Mississippi	1 A/D	1	None	0
Missouri	2 A/D 2 MR/DD 1 AIDS	5	None	0
Montana	1 A 1 A/D 1 MR/DD	3	None	0

See notes at end of table.

TABLE VI-4. 1915(c) Regular and Model Waivers,
by State and Target Population, December 2, 1991--Continued

	Regular waivers		Model waivers	
	Population	Total	Population	Total
Nebraska	1 A/D 1 MR/DD	2	1 MR/DD	1
Nevada	1 A/D • 1 MR/DD	2	1 P/D	1
New Hampshire	1 A/D 1 MR/DD	2	None	0
New Jersey	1 A/D 1 MR/DD 1 AIDS	3	3 B and D	3
New Mexico	1 A/D 1 D 1 MR/DD 1 AIDS	4	None	0
New York	1 A/D 1 MR/DD	2	1 C/DD 2 C/D	3
North Carolina	1 A/D 1 MR/DD	2	1 C/B, C/D, and C/AIDS	1
North Dakota	1 A/D 1 MR/DD	2	None	0
Ohio	1 A 1 D 1 C/D 1 AIDS 2 MR/DD	6	2 MR/DD	2
Oklahoma	2 MR	2	None	0
Oregon	1 B and D 1 MR/DD	2	None	0
Pennsylvania	1 MR/DD 2 MR 1 AIDS	4	1 C/D	1

See notes at end of table.

TABLE VI-4. 1915(c) Regular and Model Waivers,
by State and Target Population, December 2, 1991--Continued

	Regular waivers		Model waivers	
	Population	Total	Population	Total
Rhode Island	2 A/D 1 MR/DD	3	1 P/D 1 C/D	2
South Carolina	1 A/D 1 AIDS 1 MR	3	1 C/D	1
South Dakota	1 A 1 MR/DD	2	None	0
Tennessee	1 A/D 1 MR/DD	2	1 MR/DD	1
Texas	1 C/D 1 MR/DD 2 MR	4	None	0
Utah	1 MR/DD	1	None	0
Vermont	1 A/D 2 MR/DD 1 MI	4	None	0
Virginia	1 A/D 2 MR/DD	3	1 D 1 AIDS	2
Washington	1 A/D 1 MR/DD 1 MR 1 AIDS	4	1 B and D	1
West Virginia	1 A/D 1 MR/DD	2	None	0
Wisconsin	1 A/D 2 DD	3	None	0
Wyoming	1 DD	1	None	0
TOTAL		129		38

KEY:

A/D	includes aged/disabled persons.
A	includes aged persons.

**TABLE VI-4. 1915(c) Regular and Model Waivers,
by State and Target Population, December 2, 1991--Continued**

KEY (continued):

P/D	includes physically disabled persons.
C/D	includes disabled children.
C/DD	includes developmentally disabled children.
B and D	includes blind and disabled persons.
D	includes disabled persons.
MR/DD	includes mentally retarded and/or developmentally disabled persons.
MR	includes mentally retarded persons.
DD	includes developmentally disabled persons.
MI	includes mentally ill persons
AIDS	includes persons diagnosed with acquired immunodeficiency syndrome (AIDS), AIDS-related complex, or human immunodeficiency virus (HIV) infection.

Source: Table prepared by the Congressional Research Service based on analysis of unpublished HCFA reports.

TABLE VI-5. 1915(c) Regular Waivers by Target Population, December 2, 1991

Population	Number of programs	Number of States[a]
Aged/disabled(A/D); Aged (A); Physically disabled (P/D); Disabled children (C/D); Blind and disabled (B and D); and Disabled (D)	53	40
Mentally retarded/developmentally disabled (MR/DD); Mentally retarded (MR); and Developmentally disabled (DD)	61	46
Mentally ill (MI)	1	1
Acquired immunodeficiency syndrome (AIDS)[b]	13	13
Aged/disabled and mentally retarded/ developmentally disabled (A/D and MR/DD)	1	1
States with no waivers[c]	NA	3
TOTAL	129	

[a]A State can have more than one waiver program for a target population.

[b]Includes persons diagnosed with AIDS, AIDS-related complex (ARC), or HIV infection.

[c]Includes the District of Columbia.

NOTE: NA = Not applicable.

Source: Table prepared by the Congressional Research Service based on analysis of unpublished HCFA reports.

TABLE VI-6. 1915(c) Model Waivers by Target Population, December 2, 1991

Population	Number of programs	Number of States[a]
Aged/disabled (A/D); Physically disabled (P/D); Blind and disabled (B and D); and Disabled (D)	14	11
Disabled children (C/D)	11	10
Mentally retarded/developmentally disabled (MR/DD); Developmentally disabled (DD); Developmentally disabled children (C/DD); and Mentally retarded/developmentally disabled and disabled (MR/DD and D)	8	7
Acquired immunodeficiency syndrome (AIDS)[b]; Blind children, disabled children, and children with AIDS (C/B, C/D, and C/AIDS); Disabled children and AIDS (C/D and AIDS)	4	4
Aged/disabled, disabled children, and mentally retarded/developmentally disabled (A/D, C/D, and MR/DD)	1	1
States with no waivers[c]	NA	24
TOTAL	38	

[a]A State can have more than one waiver program for a target population.

[b]Includes persons diagnosed with AIDS, AIDS-related complex (ARC), or HIV infection.

[c]Includes the District of Columbia.

NOTE: NA = Not applicable.

Source: Table prepared by the Congressional Research Service based on analysis of unpublished HCFA reports.

398

2. Services Covered

Table VI-7 presents information about the range of services States cover under their regular waiver programs. For their aged/disabled waivers, States covered with almost equal frequency case management, homemaker services, adult day care, and respite. Personal care was also covered in a number of programs. All of these services contain a strong social service component that Federal demonstrations and State programs have found to be important in allowing persons needing long-term care to remain in their homes. States also frequently exercised their option to provide "other" services approved by the Secretary. These often included minor home modifications and transportation.

The mix of covered services is somewhat different in waivers for the mentally retarded and developmentally disabled. States most frequently covered habilitation services, followed by respite and case management. Habilitation services assist the mentally retarded and developmentally disabled in acquiring and improving self-help skills that are necessary to reside successfully in the community. Not nearly as many mentally retarded/developmentally disabled waiver programs covered homemaker services as aged/disabled waivers did. This may be the result of persons with mental retardation and developmental disabilities being able to do light household tasks themselves or having caregivers available to do these tasks for them. The aged/disabled waivers, on the other hand, may be serving persons who are more physically disabled and/or more likely to be living alone. States also covered a wide variety of "other" services, including transportation and minor home modifications.

For the 13 regular waiver programs serving persons with AIDS, States most frequently covered the same range of social services that they used to serve the aged/disabled. However, 11 of the 13 programs also included skilled nursing care among "other" covered services, reflecting the medical needs of persons with AIDS.

TABLE VI-7. 1915(c) Waiver Services, by Regular Waiver Programs and Populations Served, December 2, 1991

	A/D, A, PD, C/D, B&D, and D[a]	MR/DD, MR, and DD[b]	MI[c]	AIDS[d]	A/D and MR/DD[e]
Case management	40	37	1	9	0
Homemaker	38	16	0	8	0
Home health aide	13	6	0	5	0
Personal care	27	24	0	9	1
Adult day	38	14	1	7	0
Habilitation	5	58	1	1	0
Respite	42	52	1	5	0
Miscellaneous:					
Minor home modification	19	28	0	4	0
Transportation	19	24	0	5	0
Home-delivered meals	15	4	0	5	0
Nursing[f]	13	16	0	11	0
Other[g]	43	45	0	12	0

[a]Includes aged/disabled (A/D), aged (A), physically disabled (PD), disabled children (C/D), blind and disabled (B and D), and disabled (D).

[b]Includes mentally retarded/developmentally disabled (MR/DD), mentally retarded (MR), and developmentally disabled (DD).

[c]Includes mentally ill (MI).

[d]Includes persons diagnosed with AIDS, AIDS-related complex (ARC), or HIV infection.

[e]Includes aged/disabled and mentally retarded/developmentally disabled (A/D and MR/DD).

[f]Includes skilled nursing and/or private duty nursing.

[g]Includes family therapy, in-home support services, psycho-social counseling, emergency response systems, nonmedical transportation, nutritional assessment, medical supplies, prevocational services, supported employment, client support services, child supervision, assistive devices, substance abuse treatment, or any other service approved by HCFA.

Source: Table prepared by the Congressional Research Service based on analysis of unpublished HCFA reports.

3. Spending for 1915(c) Waivers

Spending for 1915(c) waiver services has grown dramatically since the enactment of the authority in 1981. Figure VI-1 and table VI-8 indicate that Federal and State spending increased from $3.8 million in FY 1982 to $1.7 billion in FY 1991.[17]

Table VI-8 also shows that programs serving the mentally retarded/developmentally disabled accounted for the largest share of total waiver spending--65 percent in FY 1991. Programs serving the aged/disabled accounted for 31 percent of total spending. When combined waiver programs serving both the aged/disabled and mentally retarded/developmentally disabled are included in the total, these two groups accounted for almost 98 percent of total waiver spending in FY 1991.

Figure VI-2 illustrates how different the relative *spending* shares for aged/disabled waivers and mentally retarded/developmentally disabled waivers are from the shares these population groups represent of total *persons served*. The aged/disabled represented 73 percent of all persons served in 1991, but accounted for only 31 percent of total spending. The mentally retarded/developmentally disabled accounted for 21 percent of total waiver participants, but 65 percent of total spending. More intensive service needs of the mentally retarded and developmentally disabled, resulting in higher average costs of waiver services for this population, may explain this disparity.[18]

While spending for disabled children and persons with AIDS has been increasing both in dollars and as a percent of the total, these two groups account for only a small portion of total spending. Spending for the chronically mentally ill has always been a small portion of total waiver spending; as noted above, in December 1991 only one State operated a waiver program for the chronically mentally ill.

---

[17]Spending data are from HCFA's Form 64 that reflect waiver expenditures by date of payment and not date of service. A State may have a waiver program in operation, but may not yet have claimed Federal matching payments for the program. The Form 64 total, therefore, may not reflect all waiver activity and may even include waivers that have expired.

[18]U.S. Dept. of Health and Human Services. Health Care Financing Administration. Office of Research and Demonstrations. *Medicaid 2176 Home and Community-Based Care Waivers: 1982-1989.* Prepared by Nancy A. Miller. Unpublished paper presented at the 1990 American Public Health Association annual meeting. p. 8. Analysis of 1987 data showed average waiver costs for the mentally retarded and developmentally disabled to be almost twice as high as those for the aged/disabled--$10,574 for persons with mental retardation and developmental disabilities compared to $5,363 for persons who were aged or disabled.

FIGURE VI-1. Federal and State Medicaid Home and Community-Based Waiver Program Expenditures, FY 1982-1991

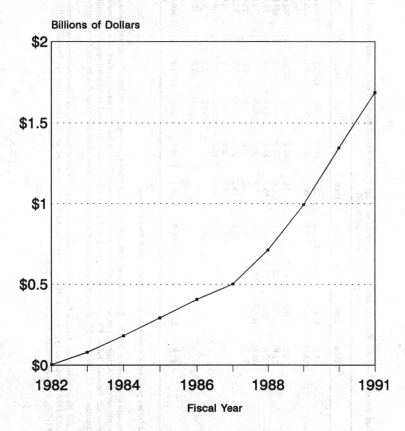

Source: Congressional Research Service analysis of HCFA Form 64 for fiscal years 1990-1991; and Nancy Miller, *Medicaid 2176 Home and Community Based Care Waivers: 1982-89*, paper presented at the 1990 American Public Health Association annual meeting.

TABLE VI-8. 1915(c) Waiver Program Federal and State Expenditures by Target Population: Fiscal Years 1982 to 1991
(expenditures in millions)

Target group	1982	1983	1984	1985	1986	1987	1988	1989	||	1990	1991
Aged and disabled (AD)	$0.6	$19.5	$66.7	$118.3	$162.1	$180.0	$258.9	$338.7	||	$433.4	$524.4
Percent of yearly total[a]	(15.8)	(24.3)	(36.6)	(40.5)	(39.9)	(35.9)	(36.4)	(34.1)	||	(32.2)	(31.1)
Mentally retarded/ developmentally disabled (MR/DD)	1.2	9.8	47.7	105.3	207.0	286.2	427.1	627.6	||	869.0	1,099.7
	(31.6)	(12.2)	(26.2)	(36.1)	(51.0)	(57.0)	(60.0)	(63.1)	||	(64.5)	(65.2)
Both AD and MR/DD	2.0	51.0	67.9	66.6	33.8	30.3	17.9	13.0	||	19.9	23.0
	(52.6)	(63.5)	(37.2)	(22.8)	(8.3)	(6.0)	(2.5)	(1.3)	||	(1.5)	(1.4)
Disabled children			0.1	0.7	1.0	2.9	5.5	10.0	||	16.6	28.4
			(0.1)	(0.2)	(0.2)	(0.6)	(0.8)	(1.0)	||	(1.2)	(1.7)
Chronically mentally ill				1.1	2.2	2.6	1.6	1.8	||	2.0	2.1
				(0.4)	(0.5)	(0.5)	(0.2)	(0.2)	||	(0.1)	(0.1)
Persons with AIDs							0.9	2.8	||	5.4	10.2
							(0.1)	(0.3)	||	(0.4)	(0.6)
TOTAL	$3.8	$80.3	$182.4	$292.0	$406.1	$502.0	$711.9	$993.9	||	$1,346.3	$1,687.9

[a]Numbers in parentheses equal target population's percentage share of a given year's totals.

NOTE: All expenditure amounts are in millions of dollars. Expenditures include Federal and State spending. FY 1982 to FY 1989 estimates are based on Nancy Miller's American Public Health Association (APHA) meeting paper. FY 1990 estimates are based on Federal spending data supplied on a waiver-by-waiver basis and the Federal matching assistance percentage for each State. FY 1991 estimates are based on total computable (Federal and State) spending amounts for each waiver as reported on HCFA Form 64. Estimates for FY 1990 and FY 1991 are not strictly comparable to those for earlier years due to the accounting methods used.

Source: U.S. Dept. of Health and Human Services. Health Care Financing Administration. Office of Research and Demonstrations. *Medicaid 2176 Home and Community Based Care Waivers: 1982-1989.* Prepared by Nancy A. Miller. Unpublished paper presented at the 1990 American Public Health Association annual meeting. Table based on analysis of HCFA Form 64 and HCFA Form 372 data.

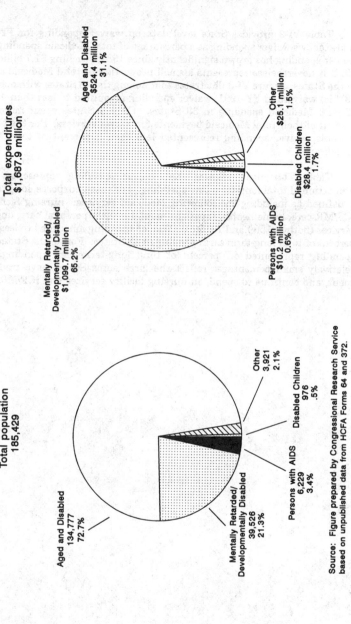

FIGURE VI-2. Relative Size of Populations Served and Spending for Home and Community-Based Care Waiver Programs, FY 1991

Total population
185,429

Aged and Disabled
134,777
72.7%

Mentally Retarded/
Developmentally Disabled
39,526
21.3%

Persons with AIDS
6,229
3.4%

Disabled Children
976
.5%

Other
3,921
2.1%

Total expenditures
$1,687.9 million

Aged and Disabled
$524.4 million
31.1%

Mentally Retarded/
Developmentally Disabled
$1,099.7 million
65.2%

Other
$25.1 million
1.5%

Disabled Children
$28.4 million
1.7%

Persons with AIDS
$10.2 million
0.6%

Source: Figure prepared by Congressional Research Service based on unpublished data from HCFA Forms 64 and 372.

Table VI-9 provides State level data on waiver spending for FY 1991.[19] It also shows waiver spending as a percentage of total Medicaid spending. While waiver spending has grown significantly since 1981, reaching $1.7 billion in FY 1991, it nevertheless represents a small proportion of total Medicaid spending in the States. Figure VI-3 illustrates that among the 48 States with operational 1915(c) waivers in FY 1991, waiver spending amounted to less than 4 percent of total Medicaid spending in 33 States. Only 5 States spent more than 7 percent of their total Medicaid payments for waiver services. For the Nation as a whole, waiver spending represented less than 2 percent of total Medicaid spending.

Table VI-9 also indicates that waiver spending represents a small proportion of total long-term care spending. For these purposes, long-term care is defined as including the following Medicaid services: nursing facility care, ICF/MR care, home health, inpatient mental health, personal care, and waiver services (both 1915(c) and 1915(d)). Waiver spending amounted to less than 10 percent of total long-term care spending in 35 States. For all the States, waiver spending represented 4.7 percent of total long-term care spending. These relatively small percentages reflect the large sums States have traditionally spent, and continue to spend, on nursing facility services and ICF/MR care.

---

[19]Oregon's total includes spending for both 1915(c) and 1915(d) waiver programs. Oregon is the only State with a 1915(d) program for the elderly.

TABLE VI-9. 1915(c) Waiver Expenditures for FY 1991, by State,
and Waiver Expenditures as a Percent of Long-Term Care Spending
and Total Medicaid Payments
(expenditures in thousands)

State	Federal expenditures	State expenditures	Total expenditures	Waivers as a % of long-term care expenditures	Waivers as a % of total Medicaid payments
Alabama	$27,162	$10,165	$37,327	10.4%	3.5%
Alaska	0	0	0	0.0%	0.0%
Arizona	0	0	0	0.0%	0.0%
Arkansas	1,698	562	2,261	0.7%	0.3%
California	45,387	45,387	90,775	4.8%	1.1%
Colorado	32,509	17,342	49,851	15.4%	6.7%
Connecticut	44,220	44,220	88,440	8.6%	5.8%
Delaware	3,916	3,916	7,832	8.6%	4.2%
District of Columbia	0	0	0	0.0%	0.0%
Florida	16,200	13,542	29,742	2.9%	0.9%
Georgia	20,899	13,172	34,071	5.5%	1.7%
Hawaii	4,074	3,451	7,525	7.3%	3.0%
Idaho	4,124	1,475	5,599	5.6%	2.7%
Illinois	32,134	32,134	64,267	5.7%	2.6%
Indiana	339	226	565	0.1%	0.0%
Iowa	930	542	1,472	0.4%	0.2%
Kansas	8,417	6,259	14,676	4.3%	2.4%
Kentucky	19,403	7,191	26,594	6.3%	1.8%
Louisiana	785	269	1,054	0.2%	0.1%
Maine	12,214	7,023	19,237	6.5%	3.3%
Maryland	19,715	19,715	39,430	8.1%	2.7%
Massachusetts	52,712	52,712	105,424	5.9%	2.3%
Michigan	32,418	27,248	59,667	5.7%	1.8%
Minnesota	44,979	39,204	84,183	7.9%	4.9%
Mississippi	1,040	261	1,301	0.5%	0.2%
Missouri	24,047	16,152	40,199	7.7%	2.4%
Montana	9,521	3,752	13,273	12.9%	5.6%
Nebraska	14,834	8,845	23,679	11.5%	5.9%
Nevada	$1,840	$1,840	$3,679	5.7%	2.0%

See notes at end of table.

TABLE VI-9. 1915(c) Waiver Expenditures for FY 1991, by State, and Waiver Expenditures as a Percent of Long-Term Care Spending and Total Medicaid Payments--Continued
(expenditures in thousands)

State	Federal expenditures	State expenditures	Total expenditures	Waivers as a % of long-term care expenditures	Waivers as a % of total Medicaid payments
New Hampshire	21,938	21,938	43,877	20.9%	11.3%
New Jersey	73,635	73,635	147,269	10.5%	5.1%
New Mexico	11,271	4,089	15,360	11.1%	4.1%
New York	6,110	6,110	12,219	0.2%	0.1%
North Carolina	22,780	11,424	34,204	4.2%	1.7%
North Dakota	13,040	5,234	18,274	12.8%	8.0%
Ohio	11,122	7,475	18,597	1.1%	0.5%
Oklahoma	8,238	3,590	11,827	2.9%	1.4%
Oregon	56,044	32,289	88,333	26.7%	13.4%
Pennsylvania	67,161	51,407	118,568	6.2%	2.9%
Rhode Island	11,892	10,237	22,130	8.4%	3.4%
South Carolina	22,772	8,549	31,321	7.9%	2.4%
South Dakota	10,336	4,082	14,418	13.3%	7.1%
Tennessee	6,308	2,891	9,199	1.8%	0.5%
Texas	8,836	5,144	13,980	0.9%	0.3%
Utah	15,736	5,276	21,012	17.5%	6.1%
Vermont	9,246	5,674	14,921	16.6%	7.6%
Virginia	16,274	16,274	32,549	5.8%	2.6%
Washington	47,804	40,379	88,182	13.5%	5.8%
West Virginia	14,996	4,479	19,476	8.0%	3.2%
Wisconsin	34,938	23,663	58,602	6.5%	3.4%
Wyoming	1,003	469	1,472	4.4%	1.6%
U.S. Total	966,997	720,913	1,687,910	4.7%	1.9%

NOTE: All spending amounts are in thousands. Total long-term care payments represent payments for nursing facilities, personal care, home and community-based care, intermediate care for the mentally retarded, home health, and inpatient mental health services. Total Medicaid payments represent Federal and State expenditures for medical assistance payments and exclude any administrative spending.

Source: Table prepared by the Congressional Research Service based on analysis of HCFA Form 64 data for FY 1991.

FIGURE VI-3. Waiver Spending as a Percent of Total Medicaid Spending, by State, FY 1991

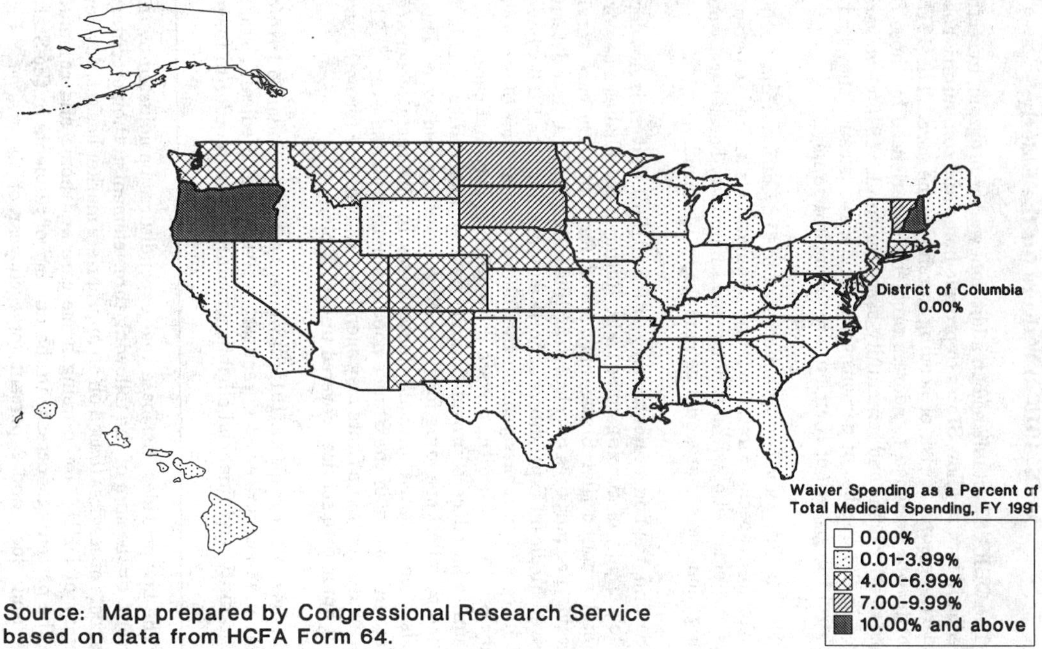

District of Columbia
0.00%

Waiver Spending as a Percent of Total Medicaid Spending, FY 1991

0.00%
0.01-3.99%
4.00-6.99%
7.00-9.99%
10.00% and above

Source: Map prepared by Congressional Research Service based on data from HCFA Form 64.

D. 1915(d) Waivers for the Elderly

The OBRA 87 established an additional waiver program, in section 1915(d) of Medicaid law, to allow States to provide home and community-based services to elderly persons at risk of needing nursing home care. The 1915(d) waiver authority was designed to address problems experienced by those States that wished to offer home and community-based care under 1915(c) waivers, but were limited in the number of persons they could serve because they had attempted to control the growth of their nursing home bed supply.

The 1915(d) waiver program created in 1987 differs from 1915(c) waivers in two major respects. First, the target population is limited to persons 65 years of age and older who, without home and community-based care, would require nursing home care that would be paid for by Medicaid.

Second, the budget neutrality test for 1915(d) waivers is not dependent on a State's supply of nursing home beds. Rather it establishes a cap or ceiling on the total amount that States may spend for long-term care services under Medicaid. For purposes of calculating this ceiling, HCFA first determines from approved Medicaid expenditure reports submitted by the States how much the State has spent in a base year on the following categories of services: nursing facility care, home health, private duty nursing, personal care, and home and community-based care provided under waiver authorities. This amount is adjusted to reflect spending for those 65 years of age and over. This base year total is then updated annually for changes in the costs of services and for changes in the size of the State's population aged 65 and over.[20] This amount is the maximum that a State may spend in a waiver year for both nursing home and all home care services covered under its plan.

In most other respects, 1915(d) waivers are very similar to 1915(c) waivers. States are authorized to request waivers of Medicaid statewideness, comparability, and financial eligibility requirements in order to target services

---

[20]The law provides that base year expenditures be adjusted by *the lesser of* 7 percent, or the sum of the following three elements: the percentage increase in the costs of services (based on an appropriate market basket, developed by the Secretary of DHHS, for nursing home care and home and community-based care), the percentage increase in the number of residents in the State 65 years of age and older, and 2 percent for each year of the waiver. Prior to the publication of interim final regulations on June 30, 1992, HCFA had been using the Medicare skilled nursing facility input price index to adjust for increases in the cost of nursing home services. For home and community-based care, it had been using the Medicare home health agency input price index. The law requires that after the publication of final regulations for the 1915(d) waiver program, HCFA must adjust base year expenditures by *the greater of* 7 percent or the sum of the items enumerated above. In the final regulations, HCFA indicated that it will continue to use the Medicare skilled nursing facility inflator to adjust for increases in nursing facility costs and the Medicare home health agency inflator for increases in costs of home and community-based services.

on persons whom they believe they can serve cost-effectively. With approved programs, States may provide case management, homemaker/home health aide services, personal care, adult day health services, respite care, and other medical and social services that can contribute to the health and well-being of individuals and their ability to reside in the community. They must provide assurances that they will take necessary safeguards to protect the health and welfare of persons receiving services. Waiver programs are approved for an initial period of 3 years and may be extended for additional 5-year terms.

Only one State, Oregon, is operating a 1915(d) waiver program. It is also the only State that has applied for approval of a program. Other States may be reluctant to apply for a 1915(d) waiver because their capacity to redirect spending from nursing home care is limited by a growing supply of beds and/or increasing costs of these services. In addition, they may be constrained by limited spending for home and community-based care in a base year.

E. Home and Community-Based Care as an Optional Medicaid Benefit for Functionally Disabled Elderly Individuals

Since the implementation of the 1915(c) waiver program, States have expressed concern with the budget neutrality test and the lengthy and burdensome application process HCFA has required for approval of programs. In response to these problems, Congress included in OBRA 90 another alternative that States may choose for covering home and community-based care under their Medicaid plans. Effective July 1, 1991, OBRA 90 established a new optional Medicaid benefit called home and community-based care for functionally disabled elderly persons. Under this option, States are not required to demonstrate budget neutrality as they are under 1915(c) and 1915(d) waivers. Nor are they limited in the number of people they may serve by their nursing home bed supply. Federal matching payments for this optional benefit, however, are capped at specific amounts for each fiscal year.

Persons eligible for coverage under this optional benefit must be functionally disabled individuals age 65 or over who are eligible for Medicaid in the community because they have low income and resources, or, if they live in a State with a medically needy program, because they have incurred large medical expenses that deplete their income and resources. Generally, States are *not* permitted to apply to persons served under this optional benefit the more liberal financial standards that they may use for persons served under 1915(c) and 1915(d) waivers (unless they decide to discontinue their waiver programs and serve waiver participants under the new optional benefit).[21]

---

[21]The law also permits Texas, which has provided personal care services to functionally disabled persons under a special demonstration project authority, to extend home and community-based services to aged and disabled persons who meet the program's functional disability test. In addition, the State may use its "300 percent rule" for financial eligibility standards for persons receiving home and community-based care as an optional service.

The optional benefit requires that eligible persons be functionally disabled. This is different from the 1915(c) and 1915(d) waiver standard that requires persons to be at risk of needing institutional care that Medicaid would cover. The new home and community-based care optional benefit defines functionally disabled persons as individuals who are unable to perform without substantial human assistance at least two of three specified activities of daily living (toileting, transferring, and eating). Alternatively, they could also include persons who have a primary or secondary diagnosis of Alzheimer's disease and (a) who are unable to perform without substantial human assistance (including verbal reminding or physical cuing) or supervision at least two of five activities of daily living (bathing, dressing, toileting, transferring, and eating); or (b) who are cognitively impaired so as to require substantial human supervision because the person engages in inappropriate behaviors that pose serious health or safety hazards to himself or herself or others.

Services that States may cover under the optional benefit include homemaker/home health aide services; chore services; personal care; nursing care; respite care; training for family members in managing the individual; adult day care; day treatment or other partial hospitalization, psychosocial rehabilitation services, and clinic services for persons with chronic mental illness; and other services approved by the Secretary.

Under the optional benefit, States are required to conduct a comprehensive assessment of potentially eligible individuals to determine whether they meet the functional disability criteria of law. For those persons determined to be eligible, the assessment is then used by a case manager to develop a care plan that specifies the amount, duration, and scope of services needed by the individual.

The Secretary is required to establish minimum quality standards for providers of home and community-based care and for settings in which services are provided. States are then responsible for certifying the compliance of providers and community-care settings with these requirements. These detailed specifications are different from the general provision in 1915(c) and 1915(d) waiver authorities that requires only that States provide assurances to the Secretary that they will take necessary safeguards (including establishing adequate standards for providers) to protect the health and welfare of persons receiving services.

Federal matching payments for optional home and community-based care benefits are capped at $40 million for FY 1991; $70 million for FY 1992; $130 million for FY 1993; $160 million for FY 1994; and $180 million for FY 1995. In making allocations to the States, the Secretary is required to take into account the number of persons age 65 and older in a State in relation to the number of individuals age 65 and over nationally (considering to the maximum extent possible, the number of elderly persons who are low-income). In addition, Federal matching payments to each participating State in any calendar quarter may not exceed 50 percent of the aggregate amount that would have been spent to provide Medicare skilled nursing facility services to persons receiving home and community-based care under the optional benefit.[22] To the extent that a State electing the optional benefit fails to maintain levels of nonfederal expenditures for home and community-based care for functionally disabled elderly individuals (excluding 1915(c) waiver services and Medicaid home health and personal care), its Federal matching payments will be reduced by the amount it no longer spends.

States submitting Medicaid plan amendments to provide home and community-based care as an optional Medicaid benefit must define the election period during which they will offer these services. An election period must be 4 or more calendar quarters. For the duration of its election period, a State must provide services to eligible individuals, regardless of the availability of Federal matching payments. States are permitted to limit eligibility for services based on reasonable classifications, such as age, degree of functional disability, and need for services. They are not required to provide services on a statewide basis.

As of July 1992, only two States, Texas and Rhode Island, had Medicaid plan amendments approved to provide home and community-based care as an optional service.

F. 1915(e) Waivers for "Boarder Babies"

The Medicare Catastrophic Coverage Act of 1988 (Public Law 100-360) established another home and community-based care waiver program targeted at "boarder babies," children who are infected with the acquired immunodeficiency syndrome (AIDS) virus or who are drug dependent at birth and who may remain in hospitals indefinitely because of problems in finding an alternative placement. This waiver program, established in section 1915(e) of Medicaid law, allows States to provide services to such children, as well as to any children with AIDS, who (i) are under age 5, (ii) are receiving or are expected to receive federally funded adoption or foster care assistance, and (iii) would be likely, in the absence of waivered services, to require the level of care provided by a hospital or nursing facility. Services that States may cover under this waiver program include nursing care, physicians' services, respite care, prescription drugs, medical devices and supplies, transportation, and any other service requested by the State and approved by the Secretary.

As with other home and community-based services waivers, the State is required to provide assurances that the health and safety of waiver participants will be protected, that there will be financial accountability for program funds, and that the projected per capita cost of the program will not exceed the costs that the Medicaid program would have incurred for the same individuals in the absence of a waiver. States may request waivers of Medicaid statewideness and

---

[22]The law specifically provides that Federal payments may not exceed 50 percent of the product of the following: (1) the average number of individuals receiving home and community-based care in the quarter, (2) the average per diem rate of payment for Medicare skilled nursing facility services in that State for the quarter, and (3) the number of days in a quarter.

comparability requirements. Waiver programs may be granted for an initial term of 3 years, and are renewable for 5-year periods unless the Secretary determines that the required assurances have not been met. The Secretary cannot refuse to grant a waiver or waiver renewal to a State meeting the statutory requirements; any denial is subject to appeal.

No State has ever applied for a waiver under the 1915(e) option. Some States have used regular and model 1915(c) waivers to provide services for children who are infected with the AIDS virus or who are drug dependent at birth. Several of these programs are targeted specifically at children in foster care. States may have decided to use the 1915(c) waiver authority to cover these children, in the event that the natural parents decide to resume custody of their children. In that case, the children would no longer be eligible for foster assistance and could not be covered under a 1915(e) waiver.

G. Comparison of Major Features of State Options for Covering Home and Community-Based Care

Table VI-10 summarizes the major features of options States may use to cover home and community-based care under their Medicaid plans.

TABLE VI-10. Comparison of Major Features of State Options for Covering Home and Community-Based Care Under Their Medicaid Plans

Feature	1915(c) regular waivers	1915(c) model waivers	1915(d) Waivers	Optional home and community-based care	1915(e) waivers
Target populations covered	Persons who would otherwise require institutional care that would be covered by Medicaid.	Up to 200 persons who would otherwise require institutional care that would be covered by Medicaid, and especially those who require deeming rules to be waived in order to be served in the community.	Elderly persons 65 years of age and older who would otherwise require nursing home care that would be covered by Medicaid.	Elderly persons 65 years of age and older who would be eligible for Medicaid in the community and who are functionally disabled, defined as including those who are unable to perform without human assistance at least two of three specified activities of daily living and certain persons with Alzheimer's disease.	Children under age 5, who are infected with AIDS or who are drug dependent at birth, and who are eligible for adoption or foster care assistance, and who would otherwise require institutional care that would be covered by Medicaid.

See note at end of table.

TABLE VI-10. Comparison of Major Features of State Options for Covering Home and Community-Based Care Under Their Medicaid Plans—Continued

Feature	1915(c) regulars waivers	1915(c) model waivers	1915(d) waivers	Optional home and community-based care	1915(e) waivers
Covered services	Case management; homemaker/home health aide; personal care; adult day health; habilitation services; respite care; day treatment or other partial hospitalization psychosocial rehabilitation, and clinic services for the chronically mentally ill; and other services approved by the Secretary.	Same as for 1915(c) regular waivers.	Case management, homemaker/home health aide, personal care, adult day health, respite care, and other medical and social services that can contribute to the health and well-being of individuals and their ability to reside in the community.	Case management; homemaker/home health aide; chore services; personal care; nursing care; respite care; training for family members in managing the individual; adult day care; day treatment or other partial hospitalization, psychosocial rehabilitation services and clinic services for persons with chronic mental illness; and other services approved by the Secretary.	Nursing care, respite care, physicians' services, prescribed drugs, medical devices and supplies, transportation services, and other services approved by the Secretary.

See note at end of table.

TABLE VI-10. Comparison of Major Features of State Options for Covering Home and Community-Based Care Under Their Medicaid Plans--Continued

Feature	1915(c) regulars waivers	1915(c) model waivers	1915(d) waivers	Optional home and community-based care	1915(e) waivers
Spending limits	Average per capita expenditures for persons receiving waiver services can not exceed expenditures that would have been incurred for these individuals in the absence of the waiver. For this budget neutrality test, States must estimate the number of Medicaid-certified nursing home beds and beds in other institutions participating in the program that could serve waiver participants.	Same as for 1915(c) regular waivers.	Total long-term care spending (defined as including nursing facility care, home health, private duty nursing, personal care, and home and community-based care provided under waiver authorities) can not exceed the amount spent for these services in a base year, adjusted for changes in the costs of services and for changes in the size of the State's population aged 65 and over.	Total Federal matching payments for optional home and community-based care are capped at $40 million for FY 1991; $70 million for FY 1992; $130 million for FY 1993; $160 million for FY 1994; and $180 million for FY 1995. In making allocations to the States, the Secretary must take into account the State's relative share of persons age 65 and older (considering to the maximum extent possible, the number of elderly persons who are low-income). In addition, Federal matching payments to a State are capped at 50 percent of the amount that would have been spent to provide Medicare nursing home services to covered persons.	Average per capita expenditures for persons receiving waiver services can not exceed expenditures that would have been incurred for these individuals in the absence of the waiver.

See note at end of table.

TABLE VI-10. Comparison of Major Features of State Options for Covering Home and Community-Based Care Under Their Medicaid Plans—Continued

Feature	1915(c) regulars waivers	1915(c) model waivers	1915(d) waivers	Optional home and community-based care	1915(e) waivers
Medicaid requirements authorized to be waived	Statewideness and comparability requirements and income and resource rules that apply to persons receiving services in the community.	Same as for 1915(c) regular waivers.	Same as for 1915(c) regular waivers.	Statewideness requirements.	Statewideness and comparability requirements.
Duration of waiver programs	An initial term of 3 years, renewable for 5-year periods.	Same as for 1915(c) regular waivers.	Same as for 1915(c) regular waivers.	States must define the election period during which they will offer the option. An election period must be four or more quarters.	Same as for 1915(c) regular waivers.
Quality of care requirements	States must assure Secretary that they will take necessary safeguards to protect the health and welfare of beneficiaries.	Same as for 1915(c) regular waivers.	Same as for 1915(c) regular waivers.	Secretary is required to establish minimum quality standards for providers of services and settings in which services are provided. States must certify compliance of providers and settings with these requirements.	Same as for 1915(c) regular waivers.

See note at end of table.

TABLE VI-10. Comparison of Major Features of State Options for Covering Home and
Community-Based Care Under Their Medicaid Plans--Continued

Feature	1915(c) regulars waivers	1915(c) model waivers	1915(d) waivers	Optional home and community-based care	1915(e) waivers
Numbers of States and approved waiver programs	As of December 2, 1991, 48 States operated 129 programs.	As of December 2, 1991, 27 States operated 38 programs.	As of July 1, 1992, one State, Oregon, had an approved program.	As of July 1, 1992, two States, Texas and Rhode Island had approved State plan amendments to provide optional services.	As of July 1, 1992, no States had ever applied to operate a program.

Source: Table prepared by the Congressional Research Service.

V. OTHER WAIVER AUTHORITIES

Several statutes give the Secretary a broad authority to waive statutory requirements for Medicaid and other programs in order to conduct demonstration projects. For Medicaid purposes, the most important of these in recent years has been section 1115(a) of the Social Security Act, which allows waiver of any provision of Medicaid law for demonstrations "likely to assist in promoting the objectives" of the program. A State may be exempted from compliance with usual requirements or may receive Federal financial participation for expenditures not ordinarily eligible for Federal matching.[23] (There are restrictions on the use of demonstration waiver authorities to impose cost-sharing requirements on beneficiaries beyond those ordinarily permitted by law.)

Demonstration waivers differ from the other waiver programs described above in several respects. They are granted for research purposes, to test a program improvement or investigate an issue of interest to HCFA. Projects must usually include a formal research or experimental methodology and provide for an independent evaluation. Most projects run for a limited period, no more than 3 or 4 years, and are usually not renewable. Finally, the number and subject matter of the demonstrations are generally at the discretion of the Secretary.[24] A State does not qualify for a demonstration waiver, as it does for the 1915(b) and 1915(c) waivers, simply by meeting certain established conditions.

Projects conducted under the various demonstration authorities have played a major role in the development of Medicaid policy. Some past projects include early experiments with prospective payment for inpatient services and the first primary care case management programs.

More recently, the entire medical assistance program for AFDC and SSI recipients in Arizona has been operated as an 1115(a) demonstration, known as the Arizona Health Care Cost Containment System (AHCCCS). In place of the usual open-ended Federal matching funds for service expenditures, AHCCCS receives a Federal per capita payment for each eligible beneficiary. Most beneficiaries are required to join an HMO contracting with AHCCCS. Initially, long-term care services were excluded, as were mental health services for the chronically mentally ill. The omission of these services, normally mandatory under Medicaid, is one key reason that Arizona's program has not legally amounted to a Medicaid program (another is the use of a fixed per capita Federal payment in place of matching funds).

---

[23]Other demonstration project authorities, rarely used for Medicaid projects, appear in section 402 of the Social Security Amendments of 1967 (Public Law 90-248) and section 222 of the Social Security Amendments of 1972 (Public Law 92-603).

[24]There is no specific limit on total expenditures for demonstration projects under the 1115(a) authority. Projects are funded through the general Medicaid appropriation, rather than through a distinct research appropriation.

Under a newer component of the AHCCCS demonstration, known as the Arizona Long-Term Care System (ALTCS), counties and private contractors are furnishing long-term care on a prepaid basis to elderly and physically disabled and developmentally disabled populations with Federal financial participation. ALTCS covers the continuum of long-term care services, from nursing home care to home and community-based care. Arizona negotiates rates for covered services with contractors and pays them a single amount to cover both nursing home care and home and community-based care. Home and community-based care for the elderly and physically disabled is subject to a cap. Persons receiving this care can not exceed 25 percent of a contractor's caseload in FY 1992, and 30 percent in FY 1993. No limit is placed on home and community-based care for the developmentally disabled. Mental health services are still omitted from AHCCCS. (See *Appendix G, Managed Care* for a fuller discussion of the AHCCCS program.)

Table VI-11 lists the section 1115(a) demonstration projects in operation as of October 1991.[25]

---

[25]For a full summary of research and demonstration projects in progress see U.S. Dept. of Health and Human Services. Health Care Financing Administration. Office of Research and Demonstrations. *Status Report: Research and Demonstrations in Health Care Financing.* HCFA Pub. No. 03323, Mar. 1992. Baltimore, 1992.

TABLE VI-11. Active Section 1115 Projects, October 1991

State	Project name
COMMUNITY-BASED CARE:	
California	Capitation Reimbursement for Comprehensive Long-Term Care (On Lok) SCAN Health Plan (S/HMO)
Massachusetts	The Program of All-Inclusive Care for the Elderly
New York	The Program of All-Inclusive Care for the Elderly
Oregon	The Program of All-Inclusive Care for the Elderly
South Carolina	The Program of All-Inclusive Care for the Elderly
Wisconsin	The Program of All-Inclusive Care for the Elderly
Colorado	The Program of All-Inclusive Care for the Elderly
Texas	The Program of All-Inclusive Care for the Elderly
Minnesota	Ebenezer Society and Group Health Plan (S/HMO)
New Jersey	New Jersey Respite Care Pilot Program
New York	Elder-Care (S/HMO)
INSTITUTIONAL CARE:	
Texas	Texas Nursing Home Case Mix Demonstration
Maine	Maine Long-Term Care Case Mix Demonstration Project
South Dakota	South Dakota Long-Term Care Case Mix Demonstration Project
Kansas	Kansas Long-Term Care Case Mix Demonstration Project
Mississippi	Mississippi Long-Term Care Case Mix Demonstration Project
New York	New York Long-Term Care Case Mix Demonstration Project
CAPITATION:	
Arizona	Arizona Health Care Cost Containment System (AHCCCS)
Maryland	Program for Prepaid Managed Health Care
Minnesota	Medicaid Voucher Demonstration
New York	Health Care Plus

TABLE VI-11. Active Section 1115 Projects, October 1991--Continued

State	Project Name

WELFARE REFORM (incidental Medicaid components):

New Jersey . . . . Realizing Economic Achievement (REACH)
Wisconsin . . . . Wisconsin Welfare Reform Demonstration
Washington . . . . Family Independence Program

ACCESS TO CARE:

Michigan . . . . Medicaid Extension of Eligibility to Pregnant Women and Children
Florida . . . . Medicaid Extension of Eligibility to Pregnant Women and Children
Maine . . . . Medicaid Extension of Eligibility to Pregnant Women and Children
Maryland . . . . Improving Access to Care for Pregnant Substance Abusers
Washington . . . . Improving Access to Care for Pregnant Substance Abusers
Maine . . . . Improving Access to Care for Pregnant Substance Abusers
New York . . . . Improving Access to Care for Pregnant Substance Abusers
South Carolina . . . . Improving Access to Care for Pregnant Substance Abusers
Maine . . . . Medicaid Extension of Eligibility to Certain Low-Income Families
South Carolina . . . . Medicaid Extension of Eligibility to Certain Low-Income Families
Washington . . . . Medicaid Extension of Eligibility to Certain Low-Income Families

Source: Unpublished list obtained from HCFA.

Finally, Congress has periodically mandated specific demonstration projects or special waivers in legislation. The following is a listing of the Medicaid or joint Medicare-Medicaid projects for which mandates have been enacted since 1984. Some of these projects are direct congressional initiatives. Others were initiated by the Secretary under 1115(a) or other authorities but were terminated or scheduled to expire; in these cases the congressional mandate was for an extension of the existing project.

One project that began with demonstration waivers provided by HCFA and was subsequently continued with congressionally mandated waivers is the On Lok program in San Francisco. On Lok uses the HMO model to provide all acute care and long-term care services needed by a frail elderly population at risk of nursing home placement. It covers the costs of all these services in return for fixed monthly payments from Medicare and Medicaid. On Lok received its first waivers from HCFA in 1977. Congress mandated continued waivers for On Lok in the Social Security Amendments of 1983 (Public Law 98-21) and again in Consolidated Omnibus Budget Reconciliation Act (COBRA); the COBRA extension continues indefinitely unless On Lok ceases to comply with the conditions of its waivers.

Omnibus Budget Reconciliation Act of 1986 (OBRA 86, Public Law 99-509) mandated waivers for up to 10 projects intended to replicate the On Lok program in other areas, in an initiative known as the Program for All-inclusive Care for the Elderly (PACE); OBRA 90 increased the number to 15. As of July 1992, waivers had been granted for 8 PACE sites in New York City, Rochester, Boston, Milwaukee, Portland, Oregon, El Paso, Columbia, South Carolina, and Denver. Projects are also under development in Chicago, Oakland, Sacramento, and Honolulu. The Secretary is authorized to continue the waivers for these projects beyond their first 3 years of operation if they comply with the conditions of their original waivers.

Deficit Reduction Act of 1984, Public Law 98-369

- Social health maintenance organizations (S/HMOs), which provide a continuum of health and social services to the elderly on a prepaid, capitated basis. (Extension)

[Continuing Appropriations, FY 1986], Public Law 99-190

- Municipal Health Services programs, which provide primary care in community-based facilities linked to municipal hospitals in 4 cities. (Extension)

Consolidated Omnibus Budget Reconciliation Act of 1985 (COBRA 85, Public Law 99-272)

- The On Lok program in San Francisco, which provides health and social services on a prepaid basis to the frail elderly at risk of institutionalization. (Extension)

- Access: Medicare (Monroe County, New York), which assesses the long-term care needs of Medicare-Medicaid beneficiaries and provides ongoing case management. (Extension)

- Oregon's capitated ambulatory plans, which furnish physician and related services, but not inpatient care, on a prepaid basis. (Extension)

- Texas' system of care for the elderly, which promotes community services in place of nursing home care. (Extension)

- Wisconsin's Medicaid HMO program, which mandates HMO enrollment for beneficiaries in Madison and Milwaukee. (Extension)

Omnibus Budget Reconciliation Act of 1986, (OBRA 86, Public Law 99-509)

- Chronically mentally ill demonstration programs in several cities, which integrate medical care with housing and social services. (New program)

- Frail elderly demonstration projects, which would replicate the On Lok program in other cities. (New program)

- Massachusetts' Case Managed Medical Care program, which provides close medical monitoring of nursing home patients to reduce the need for inpatient hospital stays or outpatient visits. (Extension)

- New Jersey's respite care pilot project, which provides support services for family caregivers to prevent institutionalization of the elderly or disabled. (New program)

Omnibus Budget Reconciliation Act of 1987, (OBRA 87, Public Law 100-203)

- New York's prenatal/maternity/newborn care pilot program, which would provide an alternative to conventional Medicaid coverage for pregnant women and newborns. (New program)

- AHCCCS, which the State operates as an alternative to a Medicaid program. (Extension)

- OBRA 87 also authorizes waivers of certain Medicaid requirements to facilitate Washington State's Family Independence Project, an employment and training program for AFDC recipients.

Medicare Catastrophic Coverage Act of 1988, Public Law 100-360

- Texas' system of care for the elderly, which promotes community services in place of nursing home care. (Extension)

Omnibus Budget Reconciliation Act of 1989, (OBRA 89, Public Law 101-239)

- Demonstration projects to study the effect of allowing States to extend Medicaid to pregnant women and children not otherwise qualified to receive Medicaid benefits.

- Texas' system of care for the elderly, which promotes community services in place of nursing home care. (Extension)

Omnibus Budget Reconciliation Act of 1990, (OBRA 90, Public Law 101-508)

- Demonstration projects to study the effect of allowing States to extend Medicaid coverage to certain low-income families not otherwise qualified to receive Medicaid benefits.

- Demonstration project to provide Medicaid coverage for human immunodeficiency virus (HIV)-positive individuals.

- Frail elderly demonstration projects, which would replicate the On Lok program. (Expansion)

- New Jersey's respite care pilot project, which provides support services for family caregivers to prevent institutionalization of the elderly or disabled. (Extension)

Public Law 102-276, Waiver for Dayton Area Health Plan

- Waiver of requirement limiting the maximum number of Medicare and Medicaid beneficiaries enrolled in the HMO.

Public Law 102-317, Waiver for Tennessee Primary Care Network

- Waiver of requirement limiting the maximum number of Medicare and Medicaid beneficiaries enrolled in plan. (Extension)

CHAPTER VII. ADMINISTRATION[1] [2]

I. INTRODUCTION

The Medicaid program is administered by State agencies under the general oversight of the Health Care Financing Administration (HCFA), Department of Health and Human Services (DHHS). States must designate a single administrative agency for program operations. The basic responsibilities of these agencies include: eligibility determination; provider certification; claims processing; review and inspection of facilities providing care, as well as the maintenance of the program's integrity and administration. This chapter provides an overview of Federal and State administrative activities.

II. FEDERAL ADMINISTRATION

The Medicaid program is administered by the States within broad Federal guidelines. Federal administration is assigned by law to DHHS. The Secretary of DHHS has delegated authority to HCFA which also administers the Federal Medicare program. In March 1990, a separate Medicaid Bureau was established within HCFA in order to provide greater visibility for the program. (Figure VII-1 presents the organizational chart for the Medicaid Bureau.) The mission statement for this new entity outlines its major functions as follows:

- directing the planning, coordination, and implementation of the Medicaid program;

- ensuring the development of effective relationships between HCFA and other governmental jurisdictions;

- providing direction for HCFA in the area of intergovernmental affairs, including advising the Administrator on all policy and program matters which affect other HCFA and other governmental units;

- planning and overseeing Medicaid quality control financial management systems and national budgets for States;

---

[1]This chapter was written by Jennifer O'Sullivan, Mark Merlis, and Richard Price.

[2]The major sources for information in this chapter are Federal laws and regulations and personal communications from HCFA.

(425)

- developing requirements, standards, procedures, guidelines and methodologies pertaining to the review and evaluation of State agencies' automated systems;

- developing, operating, and managing a program for performance evaluation of State agencies and fiscal agents; and

- coordinating (in cooperation with the Office of General Counsel) litigation affecting Medicaid and conducting Medicaid hearings not within the jurisdiction of another entity.[3]

[3]*Federal Register*, v. 55, no. 49, Mar. 13, 1990. p. 9364.

FIGURE VII-1. Medicaid Bureau, HCFA

as of April 30, 1991

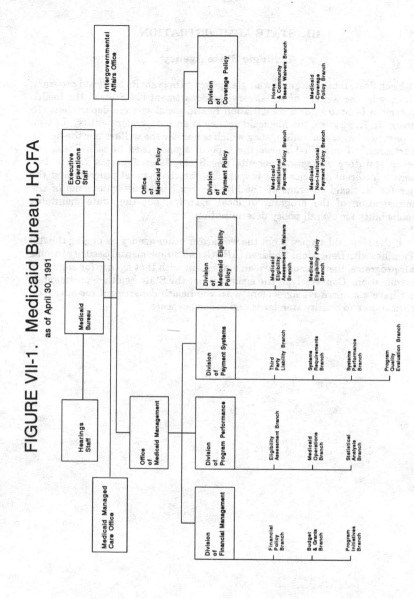

Source: Figure prepared by the Congressional Research Service.

III. STATE ADMINISTRATION

A. Single State Agency

Each State must designate a single agency to operate its Medicaid program. This may be the welfare or social services department (24 States), the health department (4 States), or a combination health/social services department (15 States). In five States, the Medicaid agency is an independent entity. In two, it is part of a larger umbrella agency which is neither the welfare nor the health department.[4] Table VII-1 shows the type of agency used in each State. (A specific statutory exemption permits one State, Massachusetts, to use two separate Medicaid agencies--one responsible for the general program and the other for Medicaid coverage of the blind.) Six States delegate some of the administration of the program to local agencies, but the State maintains responsibility for overall policy determination.

If the Medicaid agency is not the welfare or other agency managing the Aid to Families with Dependent Children (AFDC) and Supplemental Security Income (SSI) programs, then it must have an agreement with that agency for eligibility determination. Conversely, if the agency is not the State health department, it must have a cooperative agreement with the health department for advice on certification and quality standards and other purposes.

---

[4]When the Medicaid program is only one of many programs operated by the State agency, the State must have an approved cost allocation plan to ensure that Federal funds for administrative costs are claimed only for Medicaid-related functions.

TABLE VII-1. Medicaid Administration,
December 31, 1990

State	Medicaid agency
Alabama	Medicaid
Alaska	Health/Social Services
Arkansas	Social Services
California	Health*
Colorado	Social Services
Connecticut	Social Services
Delaware	Health-Social Services
District of Columbia	Health-Social Services
Florida	Health-Social Services
Georgia	Medicaid
Hawaii	Social Services
Idaho	Health-Social Services
Illinois	Social Services
Indiana	Social Services
Iowa	Social Services
Kansas	Social Services
Kentucky	Medicaid
Louisiana	Health-Social Services
Maine	Health-Social Services
Maryland	Health
Massachusetts	Social Services
Blind only	Commission for the Blind
Michigan	Social Services
Minnesota	Social Services*
Mississippi	Medicaid
Missouri	Social Services
Montana	Social Services
Nebraska	Social Services
Nevada	Health-Social Services
New Hampshire	Health-Social Services
New Jersey	Umbrella
New Mexico	Social Services
New York	Social Services*
North Carolina	Health-Social Services*

See notes at end of table.

TABLE VII-1. Medicaid Administration, December 31, 1990--Continued

State	Medicaid agency
North Dakota	Social Services*
Ohio	Social Services*
Oklahoma	Social Services
Oregon	Health-Social Services
Pennsylvania	Social Services
Rhode Island	Social Services
South Carolina	Umbrella
South Dakota	Social Services
Tennessee	Health
Texas	Social Services
Utah	Health
Vermont	Social Services
Virginia	Medicaid
Washington	Health-Social Services
West Virginia	Health-Social Services
Wisconsin	Health-Social Services
Wyoming	Health-Social Services

*Some administration (other than eligibility) delegated to counties.

Source: HCFA, personal communication, Apr. 1991.

The Medicaid agency must have agreements with the agencies administering the maternal and child health block grant and the State's vocational rehabilitation programs, to ensure maximum use of resources. It is also required to coordinate its activities with the State's operation of the Special Supplemental Food Program for Women, Infants, and Children (WIC). There are other State agencies or programs that provide services to populations served by Medicaid and with which the Medicaid agency's functions potentially overlap, such as mental retardation and mental health agencies, and offices on aging. Although many Medicaid agencies coordinate their activities with these other programs, coordination is not required and may not always occur.

Personnel of the Medicaid agency must be employed under a merit system; those responsible for expenditure of substantial funds are subject to Federal conflict of interest provisions relating to activities of current and former employees. The agency must have a program to train and employ beneficiaries and other low-income persons in what the statute terms "subprofessional" jobs and to use volunteers. The State agency is not subject to Federal contracting or procurement rules.

Medicaid regulations require that each State establish a Medicaid advisory committee, including provider and beneficiary representatives, to review and make recommendations on Medicaid policy.

B. State Plan

Each State's Medicaid program is operated in accordance with a State plan for medical assistance which describes the State's basic eligibility, coverage, reimbursement, and administrative policies. Many of the basic provisions in Medicaid law take the form of requirements for the content of State plans; the State plan thus constitutes the fundamental control mechanism for the program. The State plan must be amended periodically to reflect changes in Federal law or regulations or material changes in State law or policy. HCFA ordinarily notifies States when an amendment is needed because of a change in Federal rules.

The HCFA regional offices have the authority to approve State plan amendments with the exception of reimbursement changes which must be approved by the HCFA central office. A State plan amendment is deemed approved unless the Secretary denies it within 90 days after its submission. A denial of a State plan amendment is subject to administrative appeal within DHHS and to review by Federal courts. The effective date of a plan amendment is no earlier than the first day of the calendar quarter in which the change was submitted.

C. Basic Program Operations

A Medicaid program pays claims for medically necessary covered services rendered by qualified providers to eligible beneficiaries. This basic program description defines the chief functions performed by the single State agency.

- It must determine which individuals are eligible to receive services.

- It must determine which providers are qualified to furnish those services.

- It must have a system for processing claims.

- It must maintain program control mechanisms, both to monitor its own performance and to ensure that the services it purchases are medically necessary and appropriate for the specific beneficiary receiving them.

- It must have systems for detecting fraud against the program or abuse of program benefits.

Subsequent sections of this chapter provide an overview of State performance of these basic functions.

D. Compliance and Disallowance Actions

The HCFA may use several mechanisms to ensure State compliance with Federal requirements. These include compliance and disallowance actions.

1. Compliance Actions

Under a compliance action, HCFA could withhold Federal funds, in whole or in part, if it makes a determination that the State plan no longer complies with Federal requirements or that in the administration of the plan there is failure to comply substantially with any of the requirements. Such a finding could not be made until the State had been given notice and an opportunity for a hearing. Hearings are not called until a reasonable effort has been made to resolve the issues through conferences and discussions.

The compliance process is actually a multi-stage and lengthy process which is used by HCFA to encourage States to meet Federal requirements. The first stage involves an informal notice to the State; if the State does not demonstrate, within a reasonable time period, that it is making a good faith effort to achieve compliance, it is put on the compliance report by the regional office. Subsequent stages involve a conference between the Medicaid Bureau Director and the director or other official of the State agency. This may be followed by a recommendation by the Bureau Director to the HCFA Administrator for an administrative hearing. Actions may be dropped at any point along the path if the State shows that it has made a good faith effort to come into compliance.

The pace of the process is deliberately slow to allow States plenty of opportunity to come into compliance. Termination of a State's Federal financial participation for all of its program, or that portion of its program found not in compliance, would be the end result of the compliance process. However, no State has ever had any money withheld as part of this process. A number of States have, however, been put on the compliance report. For the October 1, 1989-March 31, 1991 period, 106 compliance issues were reported. Close to one-half of the issues related to payments for services and nearly one-third involved eligibility issues. The remainder related to a variety of Federal requirements.[5]

2. Disallowance Actions

The method generally chosen to address noncompliance with Federal requirements is the disallowance action under which HCFA retrospectively disallows Federal matching for State expenditures for failure to meet Federal requirements.[6] The State may request payment of disputed Federal matching

---

[5]HCFA, Personal communication, July 1991.

[6]One of the responsibilities of the DHHS Inspector General is to conduct audits of State expenditures; this may lead to disallowance recommendations.

funds pending the outcome of an appeal before the DHHS Departmental Appeals Board (DAB). If the State loses or withdraws its appeal, it is then liable for interest at a rate equal to the average of the bond equivalent of the weekly 90-day Treasury bill auction rates during the period the appeal was pending.

For the period May 1979-March 1991, the DAB had made decisions with respect to disallowed Medicaid expenditures totalling $2.2 billion. Of this total, $1.5 billion represented decisions for HCFA (including interest) and $0.7 billion for the States. Total disallowances pending at the DAB as of March 31, 1991, were $243 million; 21 States were involved in pending cases.

IV. ELIGIBILITY DETERMINATIONS

A. Agencies Used

Many Medicaid beneficiaries qualify automatically as a result of their eligibility for cash assistance. Determination of Medicaid eligibility for persons receiving AFDC must be performed by the same agency that determines AFDC eligibility. States have three options in determining Medicaid eligibility for persons receiving SSI.

• In a State where SSI beneficiaries are automatically eligible for Medicaid, section 1634 of the Social Security Act allows the State to contract with the Social Security Administration (SSA) to perform Medicaid determinations for those beneficiaries. Social Security may also determine eligibility for the aged, blind, or disabled medically needy in SSI-related categories if the State's standards for these groups are essentially the same as those for SSI. States that choose to contract with SSA for these Medicaid determinations are sometimes called "1634 States." The State must pay SSA 50 percent of the costs attributable to Medicaid certification activities.

• A State may instead choose to conduct its own, separate Medicaid determinations, even though SSI beneficiaries are automatically eligible and the State could have contracted with SSA.

• A State that uses more restrictive standards for Medicaid eligibility than for SSI (so-called "209(b) States"; see *Chapter III, Eligibility*) must conduct its own Medicaid determinations.

Table VII-2 shows the option elected by each State.

For categories of beneficiaries other than AFDC and SSI (and the SSI-related medically needy in some States), Medicaid eligibility determination is a distinct process conducted by the Medicaid agency. Because the State must offer the opportunity to apply for benefits on a statewide basis, applications are generally taken at local welfare or social services offices. The Medicaid agency may have its own workers in those offices or may contract to have determinations done by social services workers. In some States, applications may also be taken by on-site eligibility workers at hospitals or other facilities.

These workers may be employed by the facilities themselves, although the actual determination of eligibility must be conducted by State or county workers.

Eligibility determinations for "qualified Medicare beneficiaries" ("QMBs", see *Chapter III, Eligibility*) is also conducted by the Medicaid agency. SSA does not conduct eligibility determinations for this population group, though it is making efforts to expand its QMB public awareness activities. DHHS has indicated that social security offices have insufficient resources to perform the eligibility determination process. In addition, State Medicaid offices are better able to determine if a QMB applicant is also entitled to full Medicaid benefits.

TABLE VII-2. SSI Eligibility Determination, December 31, 1990

State	SSI determination
Alabama	1634
Alaska	State
Arkansas	1634
California	1634
Colorado	1634
Connecticut	209(b)
Delaware	1634
District of Columbia	1634
Florida	1634
Georgia	1634
Hawaii	209(b)
Idaho	State
Illinois	209(b)
Indiana	209(b)
Iowa	1634
Kansas	State
Kentucky	1634
Louisiana	1634

See notes at end of table.

**TABLE VII-2. SSI Eligibility Determination,
December 31, 1990--Continued**

State	SSI determination
Maine	1634
Maryland	1634
Massachusetts	1634
Michigan	1634
Minnesota	209(b)
Mississippi	1634
Missouri	209(b)
Montana	1634
Nebraska	209(b)
Nevada	State
New Hampshire	209(b)
New Jersey	1634
New Mexico	1634
New York	1634
North Carolina	209(b)
North Dakota	209(b)
Ohio	209(b)
Oklahoma	209(b)
Oregon	State
Pennsylvania	1634
Rhode Island	1634
South Carolina	1634
South Dakota	1634
Tennessee	1634
Texas	1634
Utah	1634
Vermont	1634
Virginia	209(b)
Washington	1634
West Virginia	1634
Wisconsin	1634
Wyoming	1634

Source: HCFA, personal communication, Apr. 1991.

B. Application Process

Anyone must be permitted to complete an application. Persons who are potentially eligible in more than one category must be allowed to choose the category under which their application will be considered. (This requirement is meaningful in States which offer greater benefits to the categorically needy than to the medically needy.) States are required to complete the eligibility determination process and furnish assistance to eligible persons with "reasonable promptness." This has been defined in regulations as 90 days from the date of application for applicants claiming disability and 45 days for all other applicants. (As discussed in *Chapter III, Eligibility* may be granted retroactively for up to 3 months before the date of application.)

The State must verify the information furnished on applications, largely through data exchange with other agencies. Each State is required to have an income and eligibility verification system for Medicaid and several other programs: AFDC, Unemployment Compensation, Food Stamps, and SSI. The State agencies responsible for these programs exchange benefit information, and can also obtain wage and income data from the SSA and the Internal Revenue Service. To facilitate these cross-checks, every applicant is now required to furnish a Social Security number; however, if the applicant has never opened a Social Security account, benefits may not be delayed while the applicant is obtaining a number. The State must also have a system for direct collection of wage information from all employers (this requirement may be waived if the State has an adequate alternative). The information obtained through the verification system is used, not only to establish the applicant's eligibility, but also to assist in the collection of any child support payments due to the applicant.

For applicants who are not United States citizens, the State must also verify immigration status (assistance to illegal aliens may be furnished only for emergency care); 100 percent Federal funding is available for this activity. (See *Chapter III, Eligibility* for a discussion of eligibility for aliens, refugees, and illegal aliens.)

Establishment of eligibility for Medicaid is not permanent. The State must conduct periodic redetermination of eligibility and must also take action between redeterminations if it learns of changes in a beneficiary's circumstances. The Secretary has established by regulation that redetermination must occur at least every 12 months; longer intervals are permissible for blind or disabled beneficiaries. Redetermination intervals for recipients of AFDC and SSI are set by the regulations for those programs; the interval is 6 months for AFDC and varies for different groups of SSI beneficiaries.

Applicants who are denied eligibility must be given notice and an opportunity for a fair hearing. If the beneficiary is terminated because of a redetermination, the beneficiary must be given advance notice of the action; if an appeal is made on a timely basis, the State is required to continue benefits pending the outcome of the appeal, unless the sole issue in the appeal is one of Federal or State law or policy (as opposed, for example, to some fact about the particular beneficiary). If the State's position is sustained by the fair hearing decision, the State may recover from the beneficiary payments resulting from the eligibility extension.

C. Streamlined Eligibility for Pregnant Women and Children

States are employing a number of mechanisms to streamline the eligibility process for pregnant women and children. Some of these mechanisms, such as dropping assets tests, involve liberalizing eligibility requirements; these are discussed in *Chapter III, Eligibility*. Other mechanisms involve simplifying the application process. Examples of this approach include using the presumptive eligibility option and shortening application forms.

The Omnibus Budget Reconciliation Act of 1986 (OBRA 86, Public Law 99-509) gave States the option to establish "presumptive eligibility" for low-income pregnant women. The purpose of the provision is to ensure that prenatal care is not delayed because a woman does not have a Medicaid card during the time it takes for a State to process an ordinary Medicaid application. Certain providers of care may make an interim determination, on the basis of preliminary information, that a pregnant woman seeking treatment may be financially eligible for Medicaid benefits. Providers permitted to make this determination include individual practitioners, clinics participating in a number of federally funded health-related programs or in a State perinatal care program, and Indian Health Service facilities. The provider must notify the Medicaid agency of the presumptive eligibility determination within 5 days, and must inform the woman that she is required to make a formal application for Medicaid by the last day of the month following the month in which the determination of presumptive eligibility was made.

Once the provider has established tentative eligibility, the woman may receive ambulatory prenatal care. If the woman fails to apply for Medicaid, her presumptive eligibility ends the last day of the month after the month she is determined presumptively eligible. If she applies for Medicaid, her presumptive eligibility period continues until the day on which the State makes a final eligibility determination. Even if the State should ultimately determine that the woman is not eligible, payment could still be made to the provider for services rendered during the presumptive eligibility period.

The National Governors' Association (NGA) reports that as of January 1, 1992, 26 States had implemented the presumptive eligibility option. (See table VII-3.)

As of July 1, 1991, States are required to provide for receipt and initial processing of applications by pregnant women and poverty-related children at locations other than welfare offices. Many States had already initiated such efforts. NGA reports that as of January 1, 1991, 24 States were giving pregnant women and children the opportunity to apply for Medicaid at the sites where they receive health care. While there was great variation in how States structured these "outstationing" efforts, the majority used social service eligibility workers placed in hospitals and public health clinics. A growing number of States were training clinical and administrative staff at the health care sites. As noted earlier, these personnel cannot process applications; however, they can initiate the application and assist women in completing the form.

The NGA also reported that 33 States had shortened the Medicaid application form for pregnant women and children. Fourteen States had instituted an expedited eligibility process. In these States, applications made on behalf of pregnant women are given priority and decisions regarding eligibility are made within a predetermined amount of time ranging from 5 to 10 days.

TABLE VII-3. State Strategies to Streamline Medicaid Eligibility for Pregnant Women and Children, January 1992

State	Presumptive eligibility	Outstationing eligibility workers[a]	Shortened application[b]	Expedited eligibility
Alabama		Yes	Yes	Yes
Alaska				Yes
Arizona				Yes
Arkansas	Yes	Yes	Yes	
California		Yes		
Colorado	Yes		Yes	
Connecticut	Yes			
Delaware		Yes	Yes	
District of Columbia	Yes			
Florida	Yes	Yes	Yes	
Georgia		Yes	Yes	Yes
Hawaii	Yes		Yes	
Idaho	Yes		Yes	
Illinois	Yes		Yes	
Indiana			Yes	
Iowa	Yes	Yes	Yes[c]	
Kansas				Yes
Kentucky		Yes	Yes	
Louisiana	Yes	Yes	Yes	
Maine	Yes			
Maryland	Yes	Yes[d]	Yes	
Massachusetts	Yes		Yes	
Michigan		Yes[d]	Yes	

See notes at end of table.

TABLE VII-3. State Strategies to Streamline Medicaid Eligibility for Pregnant Women and Children, January 1992--Continued

State	Presumptive eligibility	Outstationing eligibility workers[a]	Shortened application[b]	Expedited eligibility
Minnesota			Yes	Yes
Mississippi		Yes	Yes	
Missouri	Yes	Yes	Yes	
Montana	Yes			
Nebraska	Yes			
Nevada				
New Hampshire		Yes		
New Jersey	Yes		Yes	
New Mexico	Yes	Yes[d]	Yes	
New York	Yes			
North Carolina	Yes	Yes	Yes	Yes
North Dakota				
Ohio		Yes[d]	Yes	Yes
Oklahoma	Yes			
Oregon			Yes	Yes
Pennsylvania	Yes			
Rhode Island				
South Carolina		Yes	Yes	
South Dakota			Yes	
Tennessee	Yes	Yes	Yes	
Texas	Yes	Yes	Yes	
Utah	Yes	Yes		
Vermont		Yes[d]	Yes	Yes
Virginia		Yes	Yes	Yes
Washington			Yes	Yes
West Virginia		Yes	Yes	Yes
Wisconsin	Yes		Yes	Yes
Wyoming				
Total States	26	24	33	14

[a]Information current as of January 1991.
[b]In some States (e.g., New York) applicants are instructed to eliminate parts of the standard form in lieu of a shortened form. This information may not be reflected in the table.
[c]State plans to implement strategy in the future.
[d]Instead of placing eligibility workers at health care site, these States are training provider staff in these settings to administer Medicaid applications to potentially-eligible clients.
Source: National Governors' Association, 1992.

V. CLAIMS PROCESSING

Most Medicaid payments must be issued directly to the provider furnishing the service, not to the beneficiary.[7] Providers are prohibited from using "factors." Factors are collection agents to whom providers sell their accounts receivable or who are reimbursed on the basis of the amounts recovered. Providers may use collection agents who are paid on a fixed fee basis or may assign their billing rights to their employer or to the facility in which they practice.

States are required to pay 90 percent of "clean" claims from practitioners within 30 days, and 99 percent within 90 days. A clean claim is one which has been correctly completed and which has all the information required for payment, such as a valid beneficiary number and a full description of the services rendered. The prompt payment requirement may be waived by the Secretary for good cause. In general, this requirement applies only to practitioner claims. However, States are also required to meet the timely payment requirements for providers paid under selective contracting arrangements under a freedom-of-choice waiver.

Before issuing payment, the State must subtract from the amount due to the provider certain amounts which the State or Federal Government is entitled to recover. These include prior overpayments under either Medicare or Medicaid, amounts due from the provider under Internal Revenue Service or other garnishment proceedings, and overcharges subject to recovery under the third party liability rules described in *Chapter V, Reimbursement*. The State's claim for Federal financial participation must be adjusted to reflect these recoveries. In the case of Medicaid overpayments, the Secretary may reduce funding to the State after 60 days even if the State has not actually recovered the funds (unless circumstances, such as a provider's bankruptcy, make recovery impossible).

Many States use outside fiscal agents to process claims. The agent may be used for all claim types or only for specific services, such as pharmacy. Table VII-4 shows the States using fiscal agents and the services for which the agent is used. The fiscal agent may be a local organization, such as a Blue Cross/Blue Shield plan; there are also several national firms which sell claims processing services to States. In States that use fiscal agents it is common for the agent to operate the State's Medicaid Management Information System or MMIS (see discussion below).

---

[7]Federal Medicaid law provides that beneficiaries who are not receiving cash assistance may be reimbursed directly for services furnished by physicians or dentists. It is not known whether any State actually uses this option.

TABLE VII-4. Medicaid Claims Processing Status as of April 1991

State	Type of claim				
	Inpatient hospital	Physician services	Dental services	Prescription drugs	Long-term care facilities
Alabama	F	F	F	F	F
Alaska	F	F	F	F	F
Arkansas	HS	HS	HS	HS	HS
Arizona	F	F	H	HS	HS
California	F	F	F	F	F
Colorado	F	F	F	F	F
Connecticut	F	F	F	F	F
Delaware	F	F	F	F	F
District of Columbia	F	F	F	F	F
Florida	F	F	F	F	F
Georgia	F	F	F	F	F
Hawaii	F	F	F	F	F
Idaho	F	F	F	F	F
Illinois	S	S	S	S	S

See notes at end of table.

TABLE VII-4. Medicaid Claims Processing Status as of April 1991–Continued

State	Type of claim				
	Inpatient hospital	Physician services	Dental services	Prescription drugs	Long-term care facilities
Indiana	H	H	H	H	F
Iowa	F	F	F	F	F
Kansas	F	F	F	F	F
Kentucky	F	F	F	F	F
Louisiana	F	F	F	F	F
Maine	S	S	S	S	S
Maryland	S	S	S	S	S
Massachusetts	F	F	F	F	F
Michigan	S	S	S	S	S
Minnesota	S	S	S	S	S
Mississippi	F	F	F	F	F
Missouri	F	F	F	F	F
Montana	F	F	F	F	F
Nebraska	S	S	S	S	S
Nevada	FS	FS	FS	FS	FS

See notes at end of table.

TABLE VII-4. Medicaid Claims Processing Status as of April 1991–Continued

State	Inpatient hospital	Physician services	Dental services	Prescription drugs	Long-term care facilities
New Hampshire	F	F	F	F	F
New Jersey	F	F	F	F	F
New Mexico	F	F	F	F	F
New York	F	F	F	F	F
North Carolina	F	F	F	F	F
North Dakota	S	S	S	S	S
Ohio	S	S	S	S	S
Oklahoma	F	F	F	F	F
Oregon	S	S	S	S	S
Pennsylvania	S	S	S	S	S
Rhode Island	S	S	S	S	S
South Carolina	S	S	S	S	S
South Dakota	S	S	S	F	S
Tennessee	F	F	F	F	F
Texas	H	H	S	S	S

See notes at end of table.

TABLE VII-4. Medicaid Claims Processing Status as of April 1991–Continued

State	Type of claim				
	Inpatient hospital	Physician services	Dental services	Prescription drugs	Long-term care facilities
Utah	S	S	S	S	S
Vermont	F	F	F	F	F
Virginia	F	F	F	F	F
Washington	FS	FS	FS	FS	FS
West Virginia	F	F	F	F	F
Wisconsin	F	F	F	F	F
Wyoming	F	F	F	F	F

KEY: F–Fiscal agent processes claims
S–State agency processes claims
FS–Both State and fiscal agent processes claims
H–Health insuring organization processes claims
HS–Health insuring organization and State agency process claims

Source: HCFA, personal communication, Apr. 1991.

Three States have entered into arrangements under which the fiscal agent assumes direct financial responsibility for payment of services. The State issues a fixed monthly payment to the agent, known as a "health insuring organization" or HIO, for each eligible beneficiary. The HIO uses the funds to reimburse providers, and may retain some of the savings--or suffer a loss--if amounts paid to providers differ from the total payment received from the State. These arrangements are not the same as the State contracts with health maintenance organizations (HMOs) or prepaid health plans described in *Chapter VI, Alternate Delivery Options and Waiver Programs*. Although the HIO is paid a fixed amount and is at risk for costs in excess of that amount, it does not directly provide or arrange care, and beneficiaries are not required to use a specific group of providers affiliated with the organization. The HIO pays for services rendered by any qualified Medicaid provider. It may control costs through preauthorization systems or intensified claims review, but does not generally engage in the activities known as "managed care" (see *Appendix G, Managed Care*). In Texas and Indiana, an HIO arrangement is used for all beneficiaries in the State. In California, an HIO serves beneficiaries eligible for dental services.[8]

VI. PROVIDER CERTIFICATION

States must have standards and procedures for determining the eligibility of providers of services to participate in the program. Federal law is specific about the standards and certification procedures for institutional providers, such as hospitals and nursing facilities. For certain other kinds of providers, such as physicians and pharmacies, States follow their own laws on licensure and monitoring.

The Omnibus Budget Reconciliation Act of 1987 (OBRA 87) established a new set of standards for nursing facilities participating in Medicare or Medicaid, a new system for monitoring compliance with those standards, and a new set of sanctions for noncompliant facilities. These provisions are discussed separately in subsection VIII below.

A. Standard Setting Authority

Medicare law provides for the use of the State health agency or other appropriate State agency to determine compliance by institutional providers with Medicare standards. This same agency must be designated for the purpose of establishing and maintaining health standards for institutional providers under Medicaid. A State authority or authorities must also be designated for establishing standards, other than those relating to health, for such institutions.

Standards for facilities include those relating to professional supervision and staffing levels, State licensure where applicable, utilization review (UR) programs, and management and budgetary practices.

---

[8]In recent years, some States have entered into contracts with another kind of organization, also known as an HIO, which more closely resembles a HMOs. These very different arrangements are described in *Appendix G, Managed Care*.

B. Survey Agency

A survey agency determines for the State whether institutions and agencies meet the requirements for participation in Medicaid. This is either the State standard setting authority or another agency responsible for licensing health institutions. The Secretary may validate the determinations if he or she has cause to question their adequacy. (This is known as a "look-behind" survey.) On that basis, the Secretary may make independent and binding determinations concerning the extent to which individual institutions and agencies meet the participation requirements.

The survey agency staff must be the same staff as that used for making determinations under Medicare. For hospital certification, both Medicare and Medicaid may rely on the findings of one of two organizations (the Joint Commission on the Accreditation of Health Care Organizations or the American Osteopathic Association, whichever is appropriate) for determining whether an institution meets the majority of program requirements.

Intermediate care facilities for the mentally retarded (ICFs/MR) are not covered by Medicare. The Medicaid agency thus deals directly with the survey agency for these providers.[9]

Facilities must be inspected and recertified every 12 months. The State Medicaid agency is required to have a procedure for disclosing the pertinent findings from surveys made by the survey agency to determine if an entity meets the requirements for Medicaid participation.

The law includes additional provisions for specific types of providers and suppliers. It specifies that facilities certified as qualified rural health clinics under Medicare are deemed to meet certification standards under Medicaid. The law also requires that any laboratory services paid for by Medicaid must be provided by a laboratory meeting Medicare requirements.

The OBRA 90 authorized surveys for a new provider type--home and community-based care settings. The Secretary is required to establish minimum quality standards for providers of these services and for settings where the services are provided. The States are responsible for surveying and certifying the compliance of providers and community care settings with the statutory requirements, subject to validation by the Secretary.

---

[9]In some instances, the Medicaid agency and the State survey agency are within the same department. In addition, some of the facilities reviewed by the survey agency, such as public hospitals and ICFs/MR, may be State-operated.

C. Remedial and Enforcement Action

A State may terminate the certification of a facility found no longer to meet substantially the requirements for participation. Alternatively, if the deficiencies do not immediately jeopardize the health and safety of patients, the provider may be granted a reasonable period of time to achieve compliance if it submits an acceptable correction plan.

In the case of an ICF/MR, the State may, after notice to the facility and the public, deny Medicaid payment to any new patients admitted after a notice of noncompliance. Reimbursement may be continued for existing patients. The State may not make any decision with respect to a facility until it is given a reasonable opportunity to correct its deficiencies and reasonable notice and opportunity for a hearing.

After a payment denial decision has been made, the ICF/MR is given a limited period to correct the problems. Certification must be terminated if the facility is still not in substantial compliance, or is found not to have made a good faith effort to achieve compliance, by the end of the 11th month following the initial finding of noncompliance.[10]

D. Noninstitutional Providers

States generally follow their own procedures for certifying physicians and other health care practitioners and certain other noninstitutional providers such as pharmacies. Ordinarily, the State agency relies on the findings of the applicable governing body or board.

The OBRA 90 specified that, effective January 1, 1992, Federal matching payments may not be made for physicians' services provided to children or pregnant women unless the physician: is certified in family practice or in pediatrics or obstetrics, whichever is appropriate, by the appropriate specialty board; is employed by or affiliated with a federally qualified health center; holds admitting privileges in a hospital participating in Medicaid; is a member of the National Health Service Corps; documents a current, formal, consultation and

---

[10]The COBRA provided a temporary choice between correction or reduction plans for an ICF/MR in cases where the Secretary found deficiencies which were substantial, but did not impose an immediate threat to residents. A State could submit a plan for correction for all observed deficiencies, including a timetable for rectifying all staffing and physical plant problems within 6 months. Alternatively it could submit a 3-year plan for reduction of the total patient load at the facility to the point at which it would be possible to bring the facility into compliance for its remaining patients by closing deficient parts of the facility or improving staff-patient ratios. Reduction would be accomplished by shifting patients to home and community-based treatment. The option became effective April 7, 1986, and expired January 1, 1990. A limited number of facilities availed themselves of this option. Nationwide, eight facilities used correction plans and three facilities used the reduction plan (though one of these was terminated by Medicaid anyway).

referral arrangement with a board-certified pediatrician or family practitioner or obstetrician; or has been certified by the Secretary as qualified to provide services to pregnant women or children. OBRA 90 included additional provisions directed at the quality of physicians' services. It required the use of unique physician identifiers on all claims; maintenance of encounter data by HMOs; maintenance of a list of physicians participating in Medicaid (together with their identifier numbers), and prohibition on the issuance of unique identifiers for foreign medical graduates who have not passed the Foreign Medical Graduate Examination in the Medical Sciences (FMGEMS) or Education Commission for Foreign Medical Graduates (ECFMG). It also required States to report to the Secretary on any negative action or findings by State licensing authorities or other entities reviewing the services provided.

For several years, there were concerns that some providers who lost their licenses or faced other disciplinary action could take up practice in other States or continue to practice as employees of hospitals or other entities. The Medicare and Medicaid Patient and Program Protection Act of 1987 (Public Law 100-93) requires States to report to the Secretary any adverse action by a licensing authority, including revocation or suspension of a license, reprimand, censure, or probation. The State must also report cases in which a provider surrenders a license voluntarily or leaves the State while an adverse action is pending. The Secretary may then disseminate this information to agencies administering Federal health programs (including Medicare intermediaries and carriers); other States' licensing agencies, health agencies and Medicaid fraud units; hospitals or other providers that might consider the practitioner for employment or staff appointment; and other parties, such as peer review organizations (PROs), the United States Attorney General and other law enforcement officials, and the General Accounting Office. The Secretary is required to maintain confidentiality, except for the disclosures authorized by law.

VII. PROGRAM CONTROLS

A Medicaid agency must engage in a variety of activities to ensure that the program is properly administered:

- It must monitor its own administrative performance, subject to Federal oversight, through a quality control system.

- It must collect information on program utilization and expenditures and complete reports required by the Secretary. In most States, these functions must be performed by a federally certified MMIS.

- It must have systems for reviewing the adequacy and appropriateness of services furnished to beneficiaries.

A. Medicaid Quality Control

Medicaid, like other federally funded, State administered programs, has quality control systems, under which each State monitors aspects of its own administrative performance. The chief focus for Medicaid Eligibility Quality Control (MEQC) is the identification of eligibility errors that may result in improper Federal payments.

The law provides for two types of penalties--retrospective and prospective-- for States which have error rates exceeding certain tolerances. States which are notified of potential disallowances generally appeal the determination. Congressional actions have required recalculations of error rates for certain time periods. As of September 1991, the Department was in the process of reissuing revised error rates to the States. No final action had been taken on appeals.

States select monthly samples of cases for review, which may involve conducting field interviews with beneficiaries and obtaining information from other sources. A portion of the State sample is re-reviewed directly by HCFA. HCFA may review an entire sample of its own if a State has failed to comply with review requirements. Sample error rates are assumed to reflect statewide error rates.

The Federal and State findings are combined to yield an official State eligibility payment error rate which may be used for disallowance purposes. Simply stated, the error rate is the ratio of Medicaid dollars spent erroneously to the total Medicaid dollars spent in the sample. If a State's fiscal year error rate is greater than 3 percent, then Federal payments for Medicaid services may be reduced by a percentage equal to the excess error rate. For example, if a State's error rate during a year is 3.5 percent, its excess error rate is .5 percent, and Federal payments for services during that year will be reduced accordingly. This reduction excludes payments for SSI beneficiaries in States where Social Security determines SSI eligibility. Also technical errors, such as failure to obtain an applicant's Social Security number, are not counted if the errors did not result in erroneous payments. Reductions are made for errors that result in erroneous excess payments; penalties are not imposed for determinations that incorrectly deny coverage or for delays in making eligibility determinations.

States may request a waiver of disallowances resulting from their annual payment error rates by showing that a good faith effort was made to reduce the error rate. If the waiver is not granted, it may be appealed through the DHHS administrative hearing process. In every case, except three small disallowances in FY 1983, the State has appealed the disallowances where waivers were not granted. States may opt to retain the funds in dispute, and will owe interest on these monies if the disallowances are sustained.

Payment reductions may occur in another way. Congress mandated that HCFA project future error rates on a quarterly basis. This is accomplished using the lower of the latest annual or 6-month error rate to estimate future rates. This estimate is compared to the 3 percent tolerance level and is used to reduce the State's quarterly Federal grant by the amount exceeding that level.

States are given an opportunity to rebut the projections based on erroneous data. When final fiscal year error rates become available, any overestimates are returned to the States.

A number of recent actions by Congress have affected the MEQC system. First, COBRA provided for a study of the methodologies used in the AFDC-QC and MEQC systems. DHHS and National Academy of Sciences reports were submitted to Congress in 1988. The Academy study suggested that the quality control system was too narrowly focused on eligibility errors. The DHHS report found that the system is performing a necessary function; it recommended that more emphasis be added to protecting persons inappropriately denied payments.

The law established a moratorium on AFDC-QC penalties pending completion of the study, but did not apply the same moratorium to MEQC penalties. OBRA 87 did provide for a moratorium on MEQC penalties, but did not prohibit subsequent collection of penalties for State errors occurring during the moratorium period. HCFA has reinstituted the processes for identifying and assessing penalties.

The Medicare Catastrophic Coverage Act of 1988 (Public Law 100-360) modified, retroactive to 1982, provisions that required States' methodologies for determining eligibility for medically needy beneficiaries to conform to the methodology for determining eligibility for the related categorically needy group (i.e., SSI for the aged, blind, and disabled, and AFDC for families with children). Prior to this change, the law required that the methodologies be the "same;" now the medically needy methodology must simply be "no more restrictive" than the categorically needy methodology. A significant portion of the eligibility errors counted against States from 1982 on have related to the rules affected by this change. HCFA is in the process of reassessing errors and recomputing error rates for these years to resume the disallowance process.

The President's FY 1993 Budget Request indicated that HCFA planned to collect prior period disallowances in FY 1992 and subsequent fiscal years. It expected that $2.8 million would be collected in FY 1992 and $11.6 million in FY 1993. Further, prospective withholdings for FY 1992 and subsequent fiscal years were projected at $11 million annually.

The Omnibus Budget Reconciliation Act of 1990 (OBRA 90) contains two maternal and infant health provisions affecting the MEQC program. The first provision requires that the Department submit a report to Congress by July 1991 on the extent of quality control errors for maternal and infant health cases. The second provision requires that no MEQC eligibility errors be cited for these cases until at least 1 year from the report submittal date. The report had not been submitted as of September 1992.

B. Medicaid Management Information System (MMIS)

In the early 1970s, HCFA's predecessor agency (the Social and Rehabilitation Service) began development of a model data processing system for State Medicaid agencies, the MMIS. The model MMIS included basic systems for maintaining information on beneficiaries and providers and for processing claims. In addition it included systems intended to improve program management, including a system for generating budgetary and statistical reports and a Surveillance and Utilization Review subsystem (S/URS) to help identify abusive or fraudulent practices by beneficiaries and providers. The Social Security Amendments of 1972 (Public Law 92-603) provided that States could receive 90 percent Federal financial participation in the costs of developing an MMIS or comparable system, and 75 percent funding for ongoing operations of the system.

The Mental Health Systems Act of 1980 (Public Law 96-398) required all States to have a MMIS meeting Federal standards by September 30, 1982 (later changed to 1985), or face reductions in Federal financial participation in program administrative costs. Exceptions were permitted for States with a population of less than 1,000,000 and with total Medicaid expenditures of less than $100 million in FY 1976, as well as for territories. As of January 1991, only one state--Rhode Island--was exempt from the requirement to have an operational MMIS. All the other States either had passed their initial MMIS certification review or had an initial MMIS under development.

Continued State compliance with the MMIS requirements is monitored by HCFA through a process called Systems Performance Review, or SPR. SPR considers, not only the performance of the computer system itself, but also the extent to which States use the system in program management. A State which fails the annual SPR will be subjected to financial penalties.

C. Review of Appropriateness and Quality of Care

Medicaid law and regulations include detailed provisions relating to the quality and appropriateness of care rendered to Medicaid beneficiaries. Both States and institutions are required to meet specific procedural requirements. This section includes a discussion of requirements applicable for inpatient services provided by hospitals, mental hospitals, and ICFs/MR. (For a discussion of provisions applicable to nursing facilities, see section VIII below.)

Required State activities include development of a UR plan and provision for external reviews known as inspection of care. Activities conducted by the facilities themselves include initial and periodic recertification of each patient's need for care, development of plans for the care of each patient, and operation of an approved UR program.

1. State Plan

The State health or other appropriate medical agency is required to establish a plan, consistent with HCFA regulations, for review by appropriate health personnel of the appropriateness and quality of care furnished to Medicaid beneficiaries in order to provide guidance to the State Medicaid agency in administering the State plan.

The law also requires States to provide methods and procedures (including but not limited to the use of UR plans) necessary to: (1) safeguard against unnecessary utilization of care and services; (2) assure that payments are consistent with efficiency, equality and economy of care; and (3) assure that payment is sufficient to enlist enough providers so that care and services are available to the Medicaid population to the same extent they are available to the general population in the same geographic area. Each hospital, mental hospital, and ICF/MR admission is to be reviewed or screened by impartial professional personnel. Information obtained from the reviews and screenings, together with other data concerning necessity for admissions and continued stays, is to be used to construct samples of admissions that can disclose patterns of inappropriate admissions or utilization.

2. Certification and Plans of Care

A physician must certify the patient's need for the level of care furnished by the institution at the time of admission, or at the time the patient qualifies for Medicaid benefits, if this occurs after admission. For care in psychiatric facilities, the initial certification must be reviewed by the Medicaid agency and must include a social and psychiatric evaluation.

The need for institutional care must be periodically recertified by a physician, at intervals which vary according to the type of facility. For hospital and mental hospital inpatient care, recertification is required every 60 days. For ICF/MR services, recertification must be scheduled at the following intervals from the date of admission: 60 days, 180 days, 12 months, 18 months, 24 months, and every 12 months thereafter.

In addition to certifying the need for institutional services, the attending physician must develop a written plan of care for each patient. The plan must specify the treatment and other services to be furnished to the patient and include plans for continuing care and, if appropriate, for discharge. The plan of care must be reviewed by the physician--or in some cases a multidisciplinary team--at specified intervals.

3. Institutional Utilization Review (UR)

Each institution is required to have a plan for ongoing internal UR, including periodic assessments of the care required by each patient and general reviews, known as medical care evaluation studies, to identify patterns of care and problem areas and to recommend changes. (The general studies are not required at ICFs/MR.)

These activities are carried on by a UR committee at each institution, generally made up of the facility's own attending physicians and outside professionals. For facilities which are also Medicare providers, the UR plans and committees must be the same as those used for Medicare. This requirement may be waived if the State shows that it has an equally effective system of its own.

The UR committee must periodically reassess each patient's need to continue receiving care from the facility. These assessments are distinct from the physician recertifications; the physician certifying the need for continued care may not participate in the independent assessment of the UR committee, and the intervals between reviews are different. For hospital inpatient services, the periods between reassessments vary according to established norms for different patient conditions. In mental hospitals, the first review is due 30 days after admission. For ICFs/MR, the first review is due within 6 months. The deadlines for reassessment may be waived for facilities in rural areas, where it may not be possible to convene the UR committee often enough to meet the deadlines.

4. Inspection of Care

The Medicaid agency is required to conduct annual on-site inspections of care at every mental hospital and ICF/MR in the State. A professional review team is required to conduct a medical review of every beneficiary who has received 90 or more days of care in a mental hospital, or 60 or more days of care in an ICF/MR, to assure that services are adequate and to determine whether alternatives to institutional care are appropriate.

5. Penalties

A State may face financial penalties for failure to have effective utilization control program. To avoid a penalty a State must make a satisfactory showing that it has met the following requirements for each beneficiary: (1) certification and recertification of the need for inpatient care; (2) establishment of a plan of care; (3) a continuous program of review of long stays in institutional settings (60 days in a hospital or ICF/MR; 90 days in an institution for mental diseases); and (4) a regular program of medical review and required annual on-site inspections.

Federal funding for all services at a level of care during a quarter may be reduced by an amount equal to one-third times a noncompliance ratio. This ratio is the number of beneficiaries who received services in facilities not meeting these requirements divided by the total number of beneficiaries receiving services in facilities in which a satisfactory showing is required.

A State is considered to be in compliance with the on-site inspection requirement if it is in compliance for 98 percent of all facilities, and for all facilities with 200 or more beds. A facility is deemed to be noncompliant if a single beneficiary at the facility has not been reviewed by the end of the quarter 1 year after the previous review.

Penalties do not apply if the State contracts with a utilization and quality control PRO to perform Medicaid reviews. These are entities used by the Secretary to conduct Medicare reviews. In FY 1990, 34 States, the District of Columbia and Puerto Rico had contracts with PROs to review Medicaid services.

VIII. REQUIREMENTS FOR NURSING FACILITIES

The OBRA 87 comprehensively revised the statutory authority that applies to nursing homes participating in Medicaid. This revision, often referred to as nursing home reform, responded to general congressional concern about the quality of nursing home care paid for by the Medicaid and Medicare programs, as well as findings and recommendations of a 1986 Institute of Medicine (IOM) report. In its review of nursing home care and Federal regulation of these providers, the IOM had found the quality of care provided by many nursing homes to be unsatisfactory.[11] It recommended that more effective government regulation, including a stronger Federal role, would substantially improve the quality of life of nursing home residents.

The nursing home reform law eliminated the Medicaid program's previous distinction between skilled nursing facilities and intermediate care facilities. It established a single category of nursing home provider (called "nursing facility" (NF)) and a single nursing home benefit. The revised law established a separate set of requirements for NFs for each of the three major areas of Federal regulation discussed above for other providers of services under the Medicaid program: (1) requirements that must be met in order to participate in the program; (2) the survey and certification process that States must use for determining whether nursing homes comply with these requirements; and (3) sanctions and enforcement actions that the States and HCFA may impose against noncompliant nursing homes.

A. Requirements for Nursing Facilities

Effective October 1, 1990, OBRA 87 established in Medicaid law detailed requirements for providing care that NFs must comply with in order to participate and receive reimbursement under the program. These requirements address such issues as the scope of services a NF must provide, levels of staffing in the facility and the qualifications of staff (including special requirements for the training and competency evaluation of nurse aides), residents' rights, and the physical environment of the facility, among others. NFs must also conduct and periodically update a comprehensive assessment of each resident's functional capacity.

This combination of detailed requirements and resident assessments is intended to focus requirements on actual facility performance in meeting residents' needs, rather than on the capacity of the facility to provide appropriate services. Regulations implementing many of the requirements of

---

[11]Institute of Medicine. *Improving the Quality of Care in Nursing Homes.* Washington, National Academy Press, 1986. p. 21.

the revised law became effective October 1, 1990. Today, the new requirements apply to 15,175 nursing homes participating in Medicaid as NFs.[12]

The law also prohibits NFs from admitting any individual who is mentally ill or mentally retarded unless the State mental health authority or State mental retardation authority, respectively, has determined that the individual requires the level of services provided by the facility. These requirements originated out of concern that many mentally ill and mentally retarded persons were inappropriately placed in nursing homes where they would not receive the care and, particularly, the active treatment services needed for their conditions.[13]

B. Survey and Certification Process for Nursing Facilities

The OBRA 87 established a new process for surveying NFs to determine their compliance with the standards for participation. Under the new law, States are responsible for surveying and certifying the compliance of NFs with these requirements.[14]

The revised law provides for two different surveys for certification. State survey officials must use an unannounced *standard survey* to inspect every NF participating in Medicaid. NFs found in the standard survey to be providing substandard care must be reexamined through an *extended survey*. This two-tiered process is intended to focus survey resources on deficient facilities. HCFA

---

[12]Data provided by the HCFA for facilities participating as of August 13, 1991. On that date, 6,193 facilities were participating solely under the Medicaid program as NFs and another 8,982 facilities were participating as both NFs under Medicaid and SNFs under Medicare. The 1985 National Nursing Home Survey estimated the total number of nursing homes in the country, including those not participating in Medicaid, to be 19,100 in 1985. The American Health Care Association, an association representing for-profit nursing homes, estimates that this number may have grown by 10 percent between 1985 and the present.

[13]A 1987 General Accounting Office (GAO) report, *Medicaid: Addressing the Needs of Mentally Retarded Nursing Home Residents*, found that the active treatment needs of mentally retarded residents of nursing homes in three States had generally not been identified and met. States used placements in nursing homes in order to reduce overcrowding in large State-operated intermediate care facilities for the mentally retarded (ICFs/MR). In addition, States had a financial incentive to place the mentally retarded in nursing homes rather than in ICFs/MR, since the costs for ICF/MR care are generally much higher than the costs for nursing home care. These higher costs are attributable, in part, to the costs of active treatment which must be provided in ICFs/MR. States also had an incentive to place the mentally ill in Medicaid-certified nursing homes where the Federal Government would share in the cost of their care. Medicaid cannot participate in the cost of care provided in mental hospitals to persons aged 22-64.

[14]The Secretary of DHHS is responsible for surveying and certifying the compliance of State-owned NFs with these requirements.

began using the general methodology required by law through instructions to the States that became effective October 1, 1990.

Each facility's standard survey must be conducted not later than 15 months after the date of the previous standard survey. The average interval between standard surveys in a State cannot exceed 12 months. In addition to a review of whether facilities are meeting the general requirements for participation, standard surveys must include, for a case-mix stratified sample of residents, a review of the quality of care furnished by the facility, a review of written plans of residents' care and assessments, and the facility's compliance with requirements pertaining to residents' rights. These requirements are intended to assure that the survey process be resident-centered and outcome-oriented, and not be limited to observations of the facility, its policies, and procedures.

A standard survey (or an abbreviated standard survey) may also be conducted within 2 months of any change of ownership, administration, or management of a NF, or a change in its director of nursing, in order to determine whether the change has resulted in any decline in the quality of care furnished by the facility.

Each NF found under a standard survey to have provided substandard care must be subject to an extended survey. This survey must be conducted immediately after the standard survey and must identify the policies and procedures that resulted in substandard care. The extended survey must also determine compliance with every requirement for participation in Medicaid, and must include a review of staffing, in-service training, and an expanded sample of residents' assessments. At the discretion of the State or Secretary, any other facility, besides those found to be providing substandard care, can be subject to an extended survey (or a partial extended survey).

Federal matching rates for State costs of survey and certification activities are 90 percent for FY 1991, and will be 85 percent for FY 1992, 80 percent for FY 1993, and 75 percent for FY 1994 and for fiscal years thereafter. For FY 1991, HCFA estimates that the Federal share of survey costs of NFs will be $96,270,900.[15]

Under the new requirements, the Secretary of DHHS must also conduct onsite validation or "look-behind" surveys of at least 5 percent of the facilities surveyed by the State each year in order to determine the adequacy of State survey activities. If after these validation surveys the Secretary finds State performance to be inadequate, the Secretary must reduce matching payments to the State for survey and certification activities. This reduction must be equal to 33 percent of the ratio of the total number of residents in noncompliant facilities to the total number of residents in facilities surveyed by the Secretary in validation surveys.

---

[15]This includes Medicaid's share of the costs of surveying nursing homes participating in both Medicaid and Medicare as well as the costs of surveying facilities participating in Medicaid only.

C. Remedial and Enforcement Action

Prior to the enactment of nursing home reform law, HCFA and the States had limited sanction authority with which to deal with nursing homes found in the survey and certification process to be deficient in meeting the requirements for participation. OBRA 87 revised and expanded the sanctions that States and the Secretary may impose against noncompliant facilities. States were required to amend their Medicaid plans to include the law's new sanctions by October 1, 1989. On October 1, 1990, the expanded authority began to be applied to the new standards NFs must meet.

In general, the sanctioning process of the new law distinguishes between nursing homes with deficiencies which do and do not immediately jeopardize the health or safety of residents. If the State finds after a survey that a facility is not in compliance with the requirements for participation, and that its deficiencies immediately jeopardize the health or safety of its residents, the State must either (1) take immediate action to remove the jeopardy and correct the deficiencies through the appointment of temporary management, or (2) terminate the facility's participation in Medicaid. In addition, the State may impose other specified remedies that include denial of payment for new admissions; civil money penalties; or, in the case of an emergency, closing of the facility or transfer of residents, or both. Similar authority is provided to the Secretary.

If the State finds that a facility is not in compliance and that its deficiencies do not immediately jeopardize the health or safety of its residents, then the State may terminate the facility's participation in Medicaid and/or invoke other sanctions.[16] These include denial of payment for new admissions; civil money penalties for each day of noncompliance; temporary management selected by the State; and, in the case of an emergency, closing of the facility or transfer of residents, or both. Similar authority is provided to the Secretary. The revised law also specifies procedures to be followed where the State and Secretary do not agree on findings of noncompliance.

If a facility has not complied with the law's requirements within 3 months after a finding of noncompliance, the State must deny payment for new admissions. For facilities found on three consecutive standard surveys to have provided substandard care, States must deny payment for new admissions and monitor the facility until it has demonstrated that it is in compliance and will

---

[16]These new intermediate sanctions were intended to address a concern that, if the only penalty available for a violation is termination, deficiencies not serious enough to warrant termination might not be addressed. This problem was pointed out by the General Accounting Office in a 1987 report. U.S. General Accounting Office. *Medicare and Medicaid: Stronger Enforcement of Nursing Home Requirements Needed.* GAO/HRD-87-113, July 1987. Washington, 1987.

remain in compliance.[17] In the case of facilities that are taking steps to eliminate deficiencies according to a plan of correction submitted by the State and approved by the Secretary, the Secretary may continue Federal matching payments for not longer than 6 months.

In addition to establishing new sanction authority for noncompliance, OBRA 87 also authorized States to establish a program to reward, through public recognition or incentive payments, or both, NFs that provide the highest quality care to residents who are Medicaid beneficiaries. These incentive awards are eligible for Federal matching payments at the 50 percent rate.

The HCFA has not yet established a system for collecting information on the full range of sanctions that may be imposed against deficient NFs. It does, however, collect information on nursing homes terminated under Medicaid and/or Medicare. As of September 1991, 35 nursing homes had been terminated from participation in one or both of these programs since October 1, 1990; three nursing homes had payment denied for new admissions in one or both of these programs.

IX. PROGRAM INTEGRITY

Program integrity activities are those intended to detect, investigate, and sanction fraud against or abuse of the Medicaid program by providers or beneficiaries. Fraud consists of obtaining payments or other benefits to which the provider or beneficiary is not entitled, through misrepresentation or withholding of relevant information. Abuse of the program consists of activities which are not fraudulent but which are inconsistent with sound fiscal, business, or medical practices and which result in inappropriate expenditures of program funds. A physician who submits a claim for an operation that was never performed has committed fraud; if the operation was actually performed but was clearly unnecessary, the provider has committed abuse. Similarly, a beneficiary who is certified as eligible for Medicaid because he or she knowingly failed to report all income has committed fraud. A beneficiary who visits multiple physicians in order to obtain duplicate prescriptions for a single drug has committed abuse.

---

[17]The GAO report cited above noted that, under the previous rules, a facility could correct a deficiency temporarily, be found compliant in a recertification review, and then resume the violation. So long as it corrected the problem again each time it was uncovered, the facility could continue participating indefinitely.

A. General Requirements

1. Identification and Investigation

Each State is required to establish methods for identifying and investigating cases of potential fraud and abuse. A State may rely on the S/URS of the MMIS, which processes data on paid claims and selects exceptional providers or beneficiaries according to criteria established by the State. Cases may also be developed through other means, such as financial audits of cost-reimbursed providers, information obtained during the Medicaid quality control process, referrals from licensing and other agencies, or direct calls from the public.

States are required to develop methods of investigation that ascertain the facts without violating due process or the rights of individuals. Further they must have procedures for referring suspected cases to law enforcement officials. The State must report to HCFA the number of fraud and abuse cases warranting a "preliminary investigation" and the number of such complaints warranting a full investigation.

All cases of suspected provider fraud must be referred to the State Medicaid fraud control unit if the State has such an entity. Upon referral from the unit, the State Medicaid agency must initiate available administrative and judicial action to recover improper payments from providers.

Cases of apparent abuse are generally handled within the Medicaid agency. The agency may take steps to reeducate the provider or beneficiary involved or may impose one of the sanctions described below.

The State is also required to have in effect a system for reporting and providing access to information for use by the Secretary and other officials concerning licensing revocations and other sanctions taken against providers and practitioners by State licensing authorities.

2. State Medicaid Fraud Control Units

The Medicare-Medicaid Anti-Fraud and Abuse Amendments (Public Law 95-142, 1977) provided special Federal funding for State Medicaid fraud control units (MFCUs). A MFCU must be independent of the State agency operating the Medicaid program. It must be part of the State Attorney General's office or coordinate with that office, and must either have statewide prosecutorial authority or the ability to refer to local prosecutors. The MFCU investigates State law fraud violations (Federal violations are prosecuted by United States Attorneys), and also reviews and prosecutes cases involving neglect or abuse of beneficiaries in nursing homes and other facilities.

Federal matching is available at 90 percent for the first 3 years of an MFCU's operations and at 75 percent thereafter. However, funding is limited to the higher of $125,000 or one quarter of 1 percent of total State and Federal Medicaid expenditures for the State.

In a State without a MFCU, the Medicaid agency must maintain its own fraud investigation capacity and refer cases of suspected fraud to appropriate State or Federal law enforcement agencies.

3. Federal Activities

Federal agencies may act on their own to pursue Medicaid fraud or abuse cases. The Secretary of DHHS, acting through the Office of the Inspector General, may investigate cases of provider fraud or abuse and may impose civil monetary penalties or exclusion from program participation (see below). U.S. Attorneys may prosecute criminal and civil cases of fraud against the Medicaid program.

B. Sanctions

Four basic kinds of sanctions may be used against providers and beneficiaries found to have violated program requirements, depending on the nature and severity of the offense. Individual providers and beneficiaries, or the owners or managers of institutional providers, may be subject to criminal prosecution. They may be liable for civil monetary penalties. They may be excluded from program participation, temporarily or permanently. Finally, a temporary restriction on the use of Medicaid services, known as "lock-in," may be imposed on beneficiaries found to have used services inappropriately.

Note that the sanctions described in this section are distinct from the sanctions, described earlier, for an institutional provider's failure to comply with quality standards.

1. Criminal Penalties

The following Medicaid-related violations are crimes under Federal law:

- Knowingly and willfully making a false statement in an application for, or for use in determining the right to, a Medicaid payment or benefit.

- Having knowledge of a change affecting the right or continued right to a benefit and failing to disclose such knowledge with an intent to defraud.

- Applying for a benefit on behalf of another and then converting the benefit to one's own use.

- Claiming payment for a service by an unlicensed physician.

- Paying or receiving kickbacks or other remuneration (with exceptions for legitimate discounts or purchasing agent arrangements) for referrals for services or in return for purchasing, leasing, or otherwise obtaining covered items and services.

- Making a false statement to obtain certification as a hospital, NF, or home health agency.

- Charging a beneficiary for a service reimbursed by Medicaid, except for any allowable cost-sharing amounts.

- "Supplementation," i.e., soliciting contributions from beneficiaries or their relatives as a condition for admission or continued stay in an institutional facility.

Some of these violations, such as making false statements in application for benefits, may be committed by either a beneficiary or provider; others are applicable to providers alone. A violation by a provider is a felony, punishable by imprisonment for up to 5 years and a fine of up to $25,000. Violations by beneficiaries or third parties are misdemeanors, punishable by imprisonment for up to 1 year and a fine of up to $10,000. When a beneficiary is convicted of a Medicaid-related offense, the State may exclude the beneficiary from Medicaid eligibility for up to 1 year. Other family members may not be excluded if otherwise eligible.

State laws may also provide for criminal penalties for fraudulent practices. States may have specific laws relating to Medicaid fraud or may rely on general statutes covering fraud or false pretenses. Some States have also adopted legislation providing criminal penalties for abuse of NF residents.

2. Civil Monetary Penalties

The Secretary may, under procedures agreed to by the U.S. Attorney General and subject to judicial review, impose civil monetary penalties on Medicaid providers up to the following limits (the list excludes violations applicable only under Medicare):

- $2,000 for each item or service not provided as claimed, fraudulently claimed, provided by an unlicensed or otherwise unqualified physician, or furnished by a provider excluded from the program, plus an assessment of up to twice the amount claimed.

- $2,000 for each instance in which a provider charges a beneficiary an amount greater than permitted under the provider's agreement with the Medicaid agency or under any provision of Medicaid rules, plus an assessment of up to twice the amount claimed.

- $2,000 for each instance in which a hospital or rural primary care hospital knowingly makes a payment to a physician as an inducement to limit services. A physician knowingly accepting such payment is also subject to a $2,000 fine.

- $25,000 for each instance in which an HMO or similar organization fails to provide medically necessary care to an enrollee, if the failure has adversely affected, or has a substantial likelihood of affecting, the enrollee.

- Up to $25,000 for each instance in which the Secretary determines that an HMO has imposed premiums on enrollees in excess of the premiums permitted under Medicaid law, plus double the amount of the overcharges. The overcharges must be deducted from any such penalties and refunded to the enrollees.

- Up to $100,000 for each instance in which the Secretary determines that an HMO has expelled or refused to re-enroll beneficiaries on the basis of health status or need for health services, or has engaged in practices that could reasonably be expected to deny or discourage enrollment of beneficiaries likely to have a substantial need for services. The HMO may also be penalized an additional $15,000 for each individual not enrolled as a result of these practices.

- Up to $100,000 for each instance in which the Secretary determines that an HMO has misrepresented or falsified information furnished to the Secretary or the State and up to $25,000 for such actions with respect to any other individual or entity.

- Up to $25,000 for each determination that an HMO has failed to comply with the Medicare requirements relating to physician incentive plan arrangements.

- $2,000 for any case in which an individual notifies a NF in advance of a standard scheduled survey. (As noted above, these surveys are supposed to be unannounced.)

- $1,000 for certifying, or $5,000 for causing to be certified, a false statement in the assessment of a NF resident's functional capacity.

Again, individual States may have their own provisions for imposition of civil penalties. State law or regulations must provide for civil penalties for noncompliant nursing homes unless the State can demonstrate to the Secretary that it has equally effective alternative remedies.

3. Exclusion From Participation

a. Federal Requirements

A State may exclude a provider from Medicaid participation on its own initiative or in response to action by the Secretary. The law specifies certain actions which must result in exclusion from Medicare and certain actions which may result in exclusion from that program. If the Secretary excludes a provider from participation in Medicare, the State must exclude the provider from the Medicaid program. The Medicaid exclusion must last at least as long as the Medicare exclusion; the State may at its discretion provide for a longer exclusion period.

A mandatory exclusion must last at least 5 years except that the Secretary may waive the exclusion, upon request of a State, in the case of a sole community provider or sole source of essential specialized services in the community. Such a waiver may not be granted where the provider has been convicted of patient abuse or neglect. In the case of permissive exclusions, waivers may be granted upon request of a State. Exclusion is generally effective immediately upon notice to a provider, but may be delayed for 30 days for patients receiving institutional, home health, or hospice services, if there is no immediate danger to their health and welfare.

The Secretary **must** exclude from Medicare (and hence the State must exclude from Medicaid) any provider who has been: (1) convicted of a crime involving the delivery of Medicare services or services under Medicaid or any other State health care program, or (2) convicted of a criminal offense involving patient abuse or neglect.

The Secretary **may** exclude a provider, after notice and an opportunity for a hearing, for any of the following:

- Federal or State conviction of fraud, embezzlement, theft, other financial misconduct;

- Federal or State conviction relating to obstruction of an investigation;

- Federal or State conviction relating to controlled substances.

- Revocation or suspension of a provider's license for reasons of professional competence or performance or financial integrity, or voluntary surrender of that license while a formal disciplinary proceeding was pending.

- Exclusion or suspension from any Federal or State health program for reasons bearing on the provider's professional competence or performance or financial integrity. (The Secretary may thus exclude a provider from Medicare after one State excludes the provider from Medicaid; the exclusion then becomes binding on all other States' Medicaid programs.)

- Overcharging or providing excessive services or services that fail to meet professionally recognized standards under Medicare, Medicaid, or any other State health program. Failure, in the case of an HMO or a provider under a section 2175 case management program (see *Chapter VI, Alternate Delivery Options and Waiver Programs*) to provide necessary services, if the failure adversely affects or has a substantial likelihood of affecting the health of beneficiaries.

- Determination by the Secretary that a provider has committed any of the acts for which criminal or civil monetary penalties could be imposed, as described above.

- In the case of an institutional provider, control or management by an individual who has been excluded from program participation, subjected to civil monetary penalties, or convicted of certain crimes.

- Failure to make required disclosures relating to ownership, management or control of the provider by sanctioned individuals, or relationships between the provider and its subcontractors and suppliers.

- Failure to supply information requested by the Secretary or State agency on ownership and business transactions of subcontractors and suppliers;

- Failure to supply information needed to verify amounts payable by Medicare or a State health program;

- Failure to grant immediate access to Federal and State auditors, reviewers, or investigators.

- In the case of a hospital, failure to take corrective action after a finding that the hospital has provided inappropriate services under Medicare;

- Default on health education loan or scholarship obligations.

b. State Requirements

States are required to maintain their own administrative procedures for excluding providers from Medicaid. They must report any such action to the Inspector General, DHHS, and must also report any criminal convictions. In addition, States must obtain information on ownership and management from all providers, and may act on their own to exclude a provider with an excludable owner or manager or which fails to make full disclosure. If the provider is an HMO or similar organization, exclusion on this basis is mandatory.

4. Sanctions Imposed

For FY 1990, the Office of Investigations of the Office of the Inspector General reported 16 criminal convictions and $1.2 million in fines, recoveries, and savings related to Medicaid. It also reported $1.9 million in civil monetary penalties. A total of 824 providers were excluded from Medicare and Medicaid during the period.[18]

Additional actions were reported by the MFCUs. MFCUs operated in 39 States in FY 1990 and received a total of $51 million in Federal matching funds. For that year, the MFCUs reported 729 convictions and $37.3 million in fines, restitutions, and overpayments collected. Additionally, 326 civil monetary

---

[18]Communications with officials of the Office of Inspector General, DHHS, Aug. and Sept. 1991.

penalties were imposed and $6.5 million in penalties were assessed. (A small portion of the penalty dollars may overlap those reported for the Office of Investigations above.) Further, 321 persons were excluded from Medicaid for health care provider violations.[19]

5. Lock-In

A form of sanction known as "lock-in" is available for cases in which a beneficiary is determined to have made inappropriate or excessive use of services.[20]   The State is permitted, after notice to the beneficiary and an opportunity for a hearing, to restrict the providers from whom the beneficiary may obtain care. Typically, the State will require the beneficiary to choose a single primary care physician. Except in emergencies, the beneficiary may obtain care from other providers only with the primary care physician's authorization.[21]   In some States an effort is made to counsel beneficiaries and give them an opportunity to modify their own behavior before lock-in is imposed.

---

[19]Ibid.

[20]A parallel sanction for providers, known as "lock-out," was eliminated by the Medicare and Medicaid Patient and Program Protection Act of 1987 (P.L. 100-93). The lock-out provision gave the States the option of temporarily suspending a provider who furnished unnecessary services. It has been replaced by a provision authorizing the exclusion of such a provider from program participation; see above.

[21]The arrangement may somewhat resemble the primary care case management programs described in *Appendix G, Managed Care*. Those programs, however, generally apply to entire populations rather than scattered individuals and are permitted only under a section 2175 waiver of Medicaid requirements approved by the Secretary.

CHAPTER VIII. FINANCING[1]

SUMMARY

Medicaid services and associated administrative costs are jointly financed by the Federal Government and the States. State governments administer the program, determining who is eligible, what medical services are to be reimbursed, and what amount and methods should be used in reimbursing health service providers. These program policies follow general Federal guidelines. The Federal Government, in turn, provides grants in aid to the States. These grants pay a share of the program's costs. From a Federal budget perspective, Medicaid is viewed as an entitlement program. Entitlement programs provide benefits to all people or jurisdictions who are eligible and receive benefits. Spending levels for entitlements are determined not by the annual appropriation process, but, by the number of persons who participate in the program, and program benefit levels. Under the Budget Enforcement Act of 1990 (title XIII of OBRA 90, P.L. 101-508), Medicaid spending falls into the "pay-as-you-go" category with other entitlement programs. The budget law requires that for FYs 1991 through 1995 any legislation affecting these programs should be deficit neutral as a group. That is, as a group, any legislative changes to these "pay-as-you-go" programs should not increase the size of the Federal deficit.

The Federal Government uses general funds to share in the cost of Medicaid services through grants to the States. The Federal share of a State's payments for services is known as the Federal medical assistance percentage (FMAP). FMAPs are calculated annually based on a formula designed to provide a higher percentage of Federal matching payments to States with lower per capita incomes. The Federal share of administrative costs is 50 percent, though higher rates are applicable for specific items. Overall, the Federal share of Medicaid payments is 57 percent. Figure VIII-1 shows the Federal and State shares of medical assistance payments and administrative costs in FY 1991. Table VIII-1 provides State-by-State detail for these payments.

Participating States are responsible for the nonfederal share of Medicaid payments. For many State budgets, Medicaid expenditures represent one of the fastest growing items. Some States require local governments to share a part of the cost of Medicaid. Some States have been using provider contributions or provider specific taxes as a source of the State's share of Medicaid expenditures. These provider donations or taxes are treated as part of a State's share of payments and matched with Federal payments. Controversy has surrounded the use of these revenue sources. In the fall of 1991 legislation was enacted that clarifies the use of voluntary donations and provider specific taxes by States.

---

[1]This chapter was written by Richard Rimkunas, Melvina Ford, and Dawn Nuschler.

FIGURE VIII-1.
Federal and State Share of Total
Medicaid Spending, FY 1991

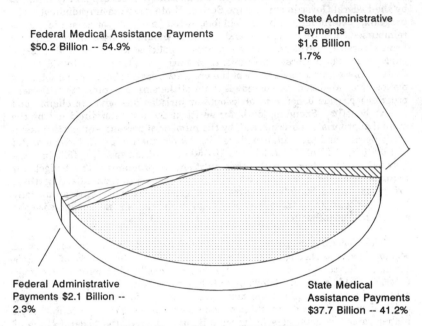

Federal Medical Assistance Payments
$50.2 Billion -- 54.9%

State Administrative
Payments
$1.6 Billion
1.7%

Federal Administrative
Payments $2.1 Billion --
2.3%

State Medical
Assistance Payments
$37.7 Billion -- 41.2%

Total Spending = $91.5 Billion

Source: Figure prepared by Congressional Research Service based on State-reported spending information for FY 1991.

TABLE VIII-1. Medicaid Payments for Medical Assistance and Administration, as Reported by the States, FY 1991
(in thousands of dollars)

State	Medical assistance payments			Administrative payments			Total payments		
	Federal	State	Total	Federal	State	Total	Federal	State	Total
Alabama	777,846	290,359	1,068,204	19,784	14,451	34,235	797,630	304,810	1,102,439
Alaska	94,218	83,385	177,603	7,755	5,035	12,789	101,973	88,420	190,392
Arizona	482,865	287,730	770,595	44,074	37,614	81,688	526,939	325,344	852,282
Arkansas	545,884	180,361	726,245	15,426	11,549	26,975	561,310	191,910	753,220
California	4,242,957	4,197,073	8,440,030	306,627	252,728	559,355	4,549,584	4,449,801	8,999,384
Colorado	401,109	342,843	743,952	20,477	13,686	34,163	421,586	356,529	778,115
Connecticut	725,535	721,334	1,446,869	32,295	26,588	58,883	757,830	747,922	1,505,752
Delaware	92,269	91,475	183,744	6,489	3,891	10,380	98,758	95,366	194,124
Distr. of Columbia	242,647	241,316	483,963	12,660	9,334	21,994	255,307	250,650	505,956
Florida	1,771,192	1,475,394	3,246,587	74,918	59,882	134,800	1,846,110	1,535,277	3,381,387
Georgia	1,189,396	741,747	1,931,144	60,525	42,636	103,160	1,249,921	784,383	2,034,304
Hawaii	139,962	117,750	257,711	8,438	6,862	15,300	148,400	124,612	273,011
Idaho	153,378	54,437	207,815	9,493	6,103	15,597	162,871	60,540	223,411
Illinois	1,224,720	1,215,678	2,440,398	85,516	65,582	151,098	1,310,236	1,281,261	2,591,497
Indiana	1,109,835	642,349	1,752,185	22,009	19,855	41,864	1,131,844	662,205	1,794,049
Iowa	494,229	283,350	777,580	18,287	14,083	32,371	512,517	297,434	809,950
Kansas	389,504	290,325	679,829	16,580	9,819	26,399	406,084	300,144	706,228
Kentucky	1,056,105	390,006	1,446,111	23,852	17,128	40,980	1,079,957	407,134	1,487,091
Louisiana	1,485,616	508,976	1,994,592	23,305	17,442	40,747	1,508,921	526,418	2,035,339
Maine	366,559	209,857	576,416	12,778	9,871	22,649	379,337	219,728	599,065

See notes at end of table.

TABLE VIII-1. Medicaid Payments for Medical Assistance and Administration, as Reported by the States, FY 1991--Continued

(in thousands of dollars)

State	Medical assistance payments			Administrative payments			Total payments		
	Federal	State	Total	Federal	State	Total	Federal	State	Total
Maryland	728,575	723,956	1,452,531	44,132	34,574	78,706	772,707	758,530	1,531,237
Massachusetts	2,230,320	2,222,987	4,453,307	50,827	40,432	91,260	2,281,147	2,263,419	4,544,566
Michigan	1,826,144	1,533,840	3,359,984	62,232	47,674	109,906	1,888,376	1,581,514	3,469,891
Minnesota	897,637	777,860	1,675,497	49,884	42,312	92,196	947,521	820,172	1,767,693
Mississippi	645,644	161,235	806,880	17,062	12,470	29,531	662,706	173,705	836,411
Missouri	988,920	661,080	1,650,000	26,342	22,079	48,421	1,015,262	683,159	1,698,421
Montana	170,990	64,402	235,392	7,702	4,961	12,663	178,692	69,363	248,056
Nebraska	251,630	148,334	399,965	12,786	8,533	21,319	264,416	156,868	421,283
Nevada	93,357	92,310	185,667	6,931	5,932	12,863	100,288	98,242	198,530
New Hampshire	195,163	193,972	389,135	6,768	4,517	11,285	201,931	198,489	400,420
New Jersey	1,458,114	1,433,199	2,891,313	69,587	54,416	124,003	1,527,701	1,487,614	3,015,316
New Mexico	277,234	97,442	374,676	8,995	7,051	16,046	286,229	104,493	390,722
New York	7,584,007	7,538,571	15,122,578	227,456	170,164	397,620	7,811,463	7,708,736	15,520,199
North Carolina	1,351,444	673,309	2,024,753	44,750	39,058	83,807	1,396,194	712,367	2,108,561
North Dakota	156,256	65,496	221,752	5,626	4,621	10,246	161,881	70,117	231,998
Ohio	2,254,975	1,498,788	3,753,763	66,869	57,183	124,052	2,321,844	1,555,971	3,877,815
Oklahoma	592,322	254,501	846,823	38,924	32,049	70,974	631,247	286,550	917,796
Oregon	423,323	241,855	665,178	47,077	36,111	83,189	470,400	277,967	748,367
Pennsylvania	2,408,590	1,830,291	4,238,882	86,692	76,097	162,789	2,495,282	1,906,388	4,401,670
Rhode Island	340,974	292,909	633,883	5,939	5,589	11,528	346,913	298,498	645,411

See notes at end of table.

TABLE VIII-1. Medicaid Payments for Medical Assistance and Administration, as Reported by the States, FY 1991--Continued

(in thousands of dollars)

State	Medical assistance payments			Administrative payments			Total payments		
	Federal	State	Total	Federal	State	Total	Federal	State	Total
South Carolina	900,009	338,158	1,238,166	27,820	21,451	49,271	927,829	359,608	1,287,437
South Dakota	143,884	54,201	198,085	3,244	2,275	5,520	147,128	56,476	203,604
Tennessee	1,270,533	581,791	1,852,323	28,958	19,948	48,907	1,299,491	601,739	1,901,230
Texas	2,564,957	1,456,895	4,021,853	118,060	89,032	207,092	2,683,018	1,545,927	4,228,945
Utah	260,039	86,797	346,836	15,000	10,743	25,743	275,039	97,540	372,579
Vermont	123,233	74,742	197,975	8,225	5,701	13,926	131,458	80,443	211,901
Virginia	639,417	631,238	1,270,655	31,627	23,107	54,734	671,044	654,345	1,325,389
Washington	819,608	685,379	1,504,987	54,032	45,260	99,291	873,640	730,639	1,604,279
West Virginia	445,084	131,614	576,698	10,388	7,581	17,969	455,473	139,195	594,667
Wisconsin	1,033,968	695,327	1,729,295	34,955	26,503	61,457	1,068,923	721,829	1,790,752
Wyoming	63,894	29,270	93,164	3,860	2,317	6,177	67,753	31,587	99,341
American Samoa[a]									
Guam	1,555	1,547	3,102	283	256	539	1,838	1,803	3,642
No. Mariana	392	392	784	68	68	136	460	460	920
Puerto Rico	51,716	51,716	103,432	3,747	3,747	7,495	55,463	55,463	110,927
Virgin Islands	1,145	1,145	2,290	294	287	580	1,439	1,432	2,870
U.S. Total	50,180,885	37,692,292	87,873,177	2,048,429	1,608,240	3,656,668	52,229,313	39,300,552	91,529,845

[a]American Samoa did not provide estimates for medical assistance payments or administrative payments.

Source: Table prepared by the Congressional Research Service based on State reported data from the *Quarterly Medical Statement of Expenditures for the Medical Assistance Program*, HCFA Form 64, Mar. 1992.

I. MEDICAID SPENDING

A. Medicaid as a Federal Entitlement Program

Medicaid is the largest federally supported program targeted at individuals with low incomes.[2] Administered by the States within broad Federal guidelines, the program is jointly financed by Federal and State governments. The Federal Government provides grants for the cost of Medicaid services by means of a variable matching formula designed to give more Federal funding to the poorest States. Medicaid spending results from statutory entitlements. Each participating State administers the program through a single agency in accordance with a State plan. The State's plan defines its eligibility, coverage, reimbursement, and administrative policies based on Federal requirements. In addition to the mandatory eligibility and service groups, the Federal Government also allows for Federal matching payments for optional eligibility groups and services. States have the choice to incorporate these optional services and eligibility groups into their State plan. Individuals who meet the mandatory or covered optional eligibility requirements are entitled to have States pay for covered services provided to them; participating States are entitled to receive matching payments from the Federal Government to cover the Federal share of outlays for these services. The size of the Federal payment is determined by the size of State spending and a matching formula and there is no dollar limit on the size of this Federal payment to the State. Individual States determine the method and amount of reimbursement to the providers of covered services.

B. The Size of Federal Medicaid Spending

In FY 1991, total Medicaid spending reached more than $91 billion, more than double the amount spent in FY 1983. Of the amount spent in FY 1991, the Federal share was $52.5 billion, 11 percent of the Department of Health and Human Services (HHS) budget and 4 percent of total Federal spending in that year. Figure VIII-2 shows Federal Medicaid spending as a percent of total Federal outlays, 1980 to 1991 and projected spending as a percent of projected Federal outlays, 1991 to 1997.

On a program by program basis, Medicaid represents one of the largest Federal spending categories. Only Social Security ($269 billion in FY 1991) and Medicare ($104 billion in FY 1991) represent larger Federal social welfare program spending categories.[3] Unlike Medicare and Social Security which

---

[2] Not all poor persons are eligible for Medicaid, nor are all Medicaid enrollees poor. See *Chapter III, Eligibility* for specific eligibility requirements for Medicaid. It should also be noted that while Medicaid is the largest federally supported needs-tested program, other programs such as Social Security and Medicare also provide benefits to individuals with low income.

[3] Social welfare spending includes spending for such programs as: Social Security, Federal employees' civilian and military retirement, Medicare, (continued...)

provide benefits to individuals without regard to income, Medicaid beneficiaries must meet a test of low income and resources. By far the largest Federal spending category among these means tested programs is Medicaid. Figure VIII-3 compares FY 1991 Medicaid expenditures with Federal outlays for other major programs for low-income persons.

Medicaid is the largest Federal grant-in-aid program to State and local governments. Medicaid has grown from 15.3 percent of total grant-in-aid to States in 1980 to 34.6 percent in FY 1991. Grant-in-aid programs represent spending by the Federal Government to help finance State and local government services and income transfers. There is tremendous variety in the scope, structure and purpose of these grants. The grants represent income to State and local governments for entitlement programs that provide payments to individuals like Medicaid, and Aid to Families with Dependent Children (AFDC); grants like urban development grants, urban mass transit grants, education grants and many more. In FY 1991, these grants-in-aid to States totalled more than $152 billion. Table VIII-2 traces Federal grant-in-aid spending for Medicaid as a share of all Federal grants-in-aid to State and local governments from FY 1966 through FY 1991.[4]

---

³(...continued)
unemployment compensation, cash and noncash welfare programs, education programs, job training, social services, and veterans' benefits.

⁴For an in-depth history of the role of Medicaid as a Federal grant-in-aid program see Miller, Victor. *Medicaid Financing Mechanisms and Federal Limits: A State Perspective.* [In] Medicaid Provider Tax and Donation Issues, by Health Policy Alternatives, Inc., Washington, D.C., July 1992.

TABLE VIII-2. Federal Medicaid Outlays as a Share of Federal Grants to States and Local Governments, 1966 to 1991

Fiscal year	Federal Medicaid outlays (in millions)	Total grants to State and local governments (in millions)	Medicaid as a percent of total
1966	$ 770	$ 12,887	6.0%
1967	1,173	15,233	7.7
1968	1,806	18,551	9.7
1969	2,285	20,164	11.3
1970	2,727	24,065	11.3
1971	3,362	28,099	12.0
1972	4,601	34,375	13.4
1973	4,600	41,847	11.0
1974	5,818	43,857	13.3
1975	6,840	49,791	13.7
1976	8,568	59,094	14.5
1977	9,876	68,415	14.4
1978	10,680	77,889	13.7
1979	12,407	82,858	15.0
1980	13,957	91,451	15.3
1981	16,833	94,762	17.8
1982	17,391	88,195	19.7
1983	18,985	92,495	20.5
1984	20,061	97,577	20.6
1985	22,655	105,897	21.4
1986	24,995	112,379	22.2
1987	27,435	108,446	25.3
1988	30,462	115,382	26.4
1989	34,604	121,976	28.4
1990	41,103	135,377	30.4
1991	52,533	152,017	34.6

Source: Table prepared by the Congressional Research Service based on data from the Budget of the United States Government, Fiscal Year 1993 Supplement. Feb. 1992.

FIGURE VIII-2.
Federal Medicaid Spending as a Percent of
Total Federal Outlays, FY 1980-FY 1991

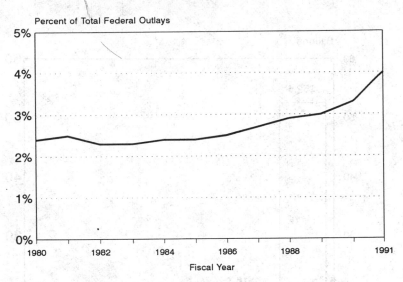

Source: Figure prepared by Congressional Research Service based on data obtained from OMB.

Projected Federal Medicaid Spending as a Percent of
Total Federal Outlays, FY 1991-FY 1997

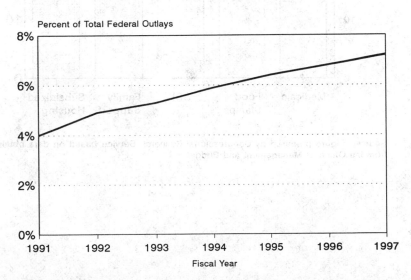

NOTE: Projected spending is based on CBO baseline estimates in August 1992. These estimates will be revised.
Source: Figure prepared by Congressional Research Service based on data from CBO.

FIGURE VIII-3.
Federal Outlays for Selected Programs for Low-Income Persons, FY 1991

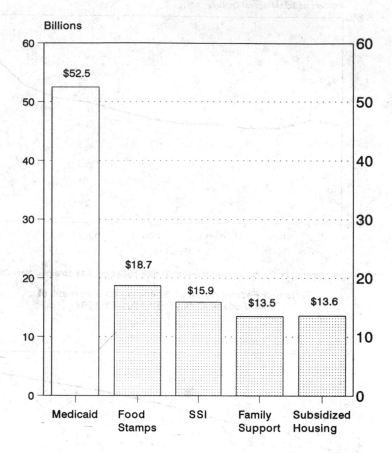

Source: Figure prepared by Congressional Research Service based on data obtained from the Office of Management and Budget.

II. FINANCING MEDICAID

A. Medicaid and the Congressional Budget Process

Medicaid is a permanently authorized entitlement program under which States pay for covered services provided to beneficiaries. Because it is an entitlement program, its spending is determined by the number of people receiving services, the number of services they receive, and the size of the reimbursement for these services. Though permanently authorized, Congress could change the entitlement at any time. The legal budget authority for Medicaid (i.e., the ability to enter into spending agreements with the State) is provided through annual appropriation acts.

The congressional budget process is generally governed by the Budget Impoundment and Control Act of 1974, and the Balanced Budget and Emergency Deficit Control Act of 1985 (known as Gramm-Rudman-Hollings). These laws were most recently amended by the Budget Enforcement Act (BEA) of 1990.[5] Prior to the BEA, much of the budget debate focused on reducing the size of the Federal deficit. Each year, Congress faced the task of achieving the savings necessary to meet a deficit target and avert an automatic sequester of budget funds. The BEA changed the focus of congressional budgeting from meeting the Gramm-Rudman-Hollings fixed deficit targets to constraining any legislation that would breach the budget agreement reached between the Bush Administration and the Congress at the end of the 101st Congress.[6] Generally, the Congress is not required to come up with new spending reductions each year. Instead, the BEA amended the budget process acts to ensure that the agreed upon savings in the fall 1990 agreement come to pass.

The BEA divides the Federal budget into three main parts: (1) entitlements and other mandatory spending programs and revenues; (2) Social Security; and (3) discretionary spending. Medicaid is an entitlement, and subject to the BEA's *pay-as-you-go* rules. The BEA requires that the sum of entitlement and revenue legislation enacted in a congressional session be at least deficit neutral, unless the President and Congress both declare that the legislation meets an "emergency." If entitlement increases and any offsetting revenues are not deficit neutral and no emergency exists, a sequester, or across the board cut in spending will be applied to all nonexempt entitlement programs. Some programs are exempt from the sequestration, Medicaid is one of these programs. Under the BEA, discretionary programs are subject to fixed budget authority and outlay caps. Appropriations responding to an "emergency" declared by both the President and Congress are exempt from these caps. The President and Congress could also suspend BEA enforcement because of war or recession.

---

[5] Title XIII of the Omnibus Budget Reconciliation Act of 1990, P.L. 101-508.

[6] The BEA retained the Gramm-Rudman-Hollings "maximum deficit amounts," but provided that these amounts be adjusted each year for changes in economic and technical assumptions.

1. Budget Resolution

The Budget Impoundment and Control Act, as amended, requires Congress to annually adopt a concurrent resolution, outlining a fiscal policy plan for the upcoming year and 5 subsequent years. As a concurrent resolution adopted by the House and Senate, the budget resolution does not require the President's signature nor does it have the force of law.

The budget resolution includes recommended levels of total budget revenues, budget authority, and budget outlays. It also allocates recommended budget authority and budget outlays by function. Medicaid is categorized in function 550 (Health), and its budget authority and outlays are included in the function total shown in the budget resolution.

Budget resolutions do not in themselves change Federal spending or amend Federal programs. However, the resolution's spending levels often assume specific policy changes. These changes may include changes in the services covered by the program, or the type of individuals eligible.

The Budget Act includes two methods of enforcing the budget resolution's plan. It requires that the resolution's recommended budget authority and outlay levels be allocated among the appropriations and authorizing committees of each house.[7] In addition, in the House the committee allocations include a report of entitlement authority, with such authority for Medicaid included in the House Energy and Commerce Committee's allocation of entitlement authority.

These allocations are in turn enforced through rules of congressional procedure. The Budget Act provides for a *point of order* against any legislation that would cause a violation of these allocations. That is, when the estimated effect of legislation increases the program's outlay so that the committee's allocation is exceeded, a member may object to the consideration of the legislation on the grounds that it violates the Budget Act. In the House, an entitlement program's allocation may be exceeded as long as the legislation provides for offsetting revenues or spending cuts.

The Budget Act's second method of enforcing the budget resolution is *reconciliation*. The Act provides that a budget resolution may include instructions to congressional committees to change laws within their jurisdiction to conform spending levels with those recommended in the resolution. Like the budget resolution's other allocations, reconciliation instructions provide the committees with an aggregate amount of spending or revenue changes. These instructions do not recommend specific program changes. The committees report back legislation to the budget committees, which then report the entire reconciliation package to the floor of each house.

Reconciliation instructions have generally been used to instruct committees with jurisdiction over entitlement programs to change entitlement eligibility or

---

[7]For FY 1991 to FY 1995, these allocations are made in accordance with section 602 of the Budget Act.

benefit rules to cut spending to the level recommended in the budget resolution. Some Medicaid program expansions have been packaged with cuts to other entitlement programs in reconciliation bills, other expansions have been packaged with offsetting Medicaid cuts.[8]

2. The Authorization Process

Medicaid is permanently authorized in title XIX of the Social Security Act and thus does not require periodic renewal by Congress. However, because Medicaid is an entitlement, the eligibility and benefit rules of its authorizing law affect its spending. Generally, Congress must amend title XIX's eligibility and covered services requirements to influence its spending. Thus, title XIX has been frequently amended. In the 1980s, these amendments frequently were made in reconciliation bills. Both the Office of Management and Budget (OMB) and the Congressional Budget Office (CBO) make estimates of the effect of legislated changes on the Federal budget.[9]

3. The Appropriation Process

Though Medicaid is a permanently authorized entitlement, its law provides no automatic mechanism for providing budget authority. Budget authority is the legal authority to enter into spending commitments. Therefore, Medicaid's budget authority must be annually provided in appropriation acts. This budget authority provides the legal spending authority to cover spending mandated by Medicaid's authorizing law.

The appropriation bills specify a fixed amount of "grants to the States" for the fiscal year, with the amount to remain available until expended. In general, appropriation bills also provide spending authority for "such sums as may be necessary" beginning in the last quarter of a fiscal year to cover unanticipated costs. They also provide budget authority for the first quarter of the subsequent fiscal year.

4. Enforcement

If the pay-as-you go requirement is violated in a congressional session, the BEA provides that a *sequester* take place on nonexempt entitlements. Sequestration is the automatic cancellation of budgetary resources to eliminate a breach of the pay-as-you go requirement.

Medicaid legislation could cause a sequestration, if an eligibility or benefit expansion were not offset by increased revenues or spending cuts. However, Medicaid along with a number of other programs targeted at low-income persons is exempted from sequestration in the event of a breach in the pay-as-you-go

---

[8]See *Chapter IX, Recent Legislative History* for a discussion of program changes.

[9]See *Chapter IX, Recent Legislative History* for details on these changes, and CBO estimates of changes in Federal spending levels.

requirement. Any breach of the entitlement targets would result in the sequestration of the nonexempt entitlement programs. Most of the cuts of such a sequester would fall on Medicare.

It should be noted that increased entitlement spending that results from provisions in current law can not cause a sequestration under the pay-as-you-go requirement. For example, Medicaid spending increases that come as a result of an economic downturn triggering increases in State Medicaid rolls would not cause a sequester on the nonexempt entitlement programs.

B. Determining the Size of the Federal Share of Medicaid Spending

1. Payments to States for Covered Services

In the States and the District of Columbia, the Federal share of payment for Medicaid services is paid to a State according to a formula that is set in statute. The Federal share of a State's expenditures for medical assistance is called the Federal medical assistance percentage (FMAP). The statutory formula for determining the FMAP follows:

$$FMAP = 100 \; percent \; minus \; State \; share$$

$$State \; share = \frac{State \; per \; capita \; income^2}{U.S. \; per \; capita \; income^2} \times .45$$

The formula is designed to provide a higher Federal matching percentage to States with lower relative per capita income, and a lower Federal matching percentage to States with higher per capita income. Under this formula, if a State's per capita income is equal to the national average, the Federal share would equal 55 percent. The law establishes a minimum FMAP of 50 percent and a maximum of 83 percent.

Wilbur Cohen, the undersecretary of the Department of Health, Education and Welfare at the time of the enactment of Medicaid, has noted that the Medicaid formula was appropriate for three reasons.[10] First, relying on a

---

[10]See Weiss, Richard. *Regional Disparities in Federal Medicaid Assistance.* Northeast-Midwest Research Institute, Nov. 28, 1977; and U.S. Library of Congress. Congressional Research Service. *Analysis of Federal-State Cost Sharing in the Aid to Families with Dependent Children Program.* CRS Report for Congress No. 82-62 EPW, by Vee Burke. Much of the analytical description of the Medicaid formula in this section is based on this earlier CRS report.

formula for Federal matching percentages would mean that States could not easily manipulate it for their own gains. Second, the formula relied on data that was periodically published and could be estimated with reasonable accuracy. Finally, the use of per capita income was used as a proxy for tax capacity, it was thought that the income measure bore a "reasonable relevance" to the underlying concept of a State's capacity to pay for these medical services. That is, it was thought that a State's per capita income is a rough indicator of the economic well being of residents in a State. States with a higher per capita income are likely to have a higher standard of living, while States with a lower per capita income are likely to have a lower standard of living. Generally, this lower standard of living may mean that there is a potentially greater demand for Medicaid services in the State and that the State may not have the fiscal capabilities to pay for them. As a result, it was thought that States with lower per capita incomes should receive larger Federal matching payments.

In 1983 the U.S. General Accounting Office (GAO) released a report that concluded:[11]

> the [Medicaid] formula is not as equitable to States as it could be. This is because per capita income--a key formula factor--does not adequately reflect the greater tax burden of States with a high proportion of needy and because it is not the best available measure of States' ability to finance Medicaid from State revenue sources."

In a more recent report, the GAO again concluded that a more equitable distribution of funds would be produced by replacing per capita income in the formula with two other factors: total taxable resources, and people in poverty. The GAO reports that these factors provide better measures of a State's ability to fund Medicaid services, and the need for services.[12] It was also noted that incorporating these changes in the funding formula, while still maintaining some form of budget neutrality resulted in a sizable redistribution of Federal Medicaid funds. Under varying assumptions, the GAO formula would result in about half the States gaining Federal funds, and about half the States losing Federal funds.

Figure VIII-4 provides a graphical picture of the relationship between a State's per capita income and the possible Federal matching rate for FY 1992. This figure depicts the possible matching percentages for all States over a range of income levels. The matching percentage that a State actually receives depends on its individual per capita income. Two features of the graph should be noted. First, for all States with a per capita income in excess of 1.05 times the national average, about $17,400 for the FY 1992 FMAPs, the Federal matching percentage equals 50 percent. If the statute defining the formula did

---

[11]U.S. General Accounting Office. *Changing Medicaid Formula Can Improve Distribution of Funds to States.* GAO/GGD-83-27, Mar. 9, 1983.

[12]See U.S. General Accounting Office. *Medicaid: Alternative for Improving the Distribution of Funds.* Fact sheet for the Honorable Dale Bumpers. GAO/HRD-91-66FS. May 20, 1991.

not contain a minimum matching percentage, these States would receive a lower matching rate (denoted by the dotted curved line on the figure). Likewise, if any State's per capita income was less than 61.4 percent of the national average, about $10,200 for the FY 1992 FMAPs, it could receive no more than the maximum Federal matching percentage of 83 percent. For the FY 92 FMAPs, no State has a per capita income so low that it receives this maximum Federal matching percentage. Second, the use of squared per capita income in the formula results in its non linear shape. Moving from lower to higher per capita income, the formula slope becomes increasingly steeper. This means that the Federal matching rate declines more rapidly with each dollar of income. For example, for FY 1992, a $1,000 increase in per capita income from $11,000 to $12,000, results in a decline of 3.8 percentage points in the Federal matching percentage. This can be compared to a decline of 5.4 percentage points when per capita income increases from $16,000 to $17,000.

FIGURE VIII-4.
Federal Medical Assistance Percentage
by State's Per-Capita Income, FY 1992

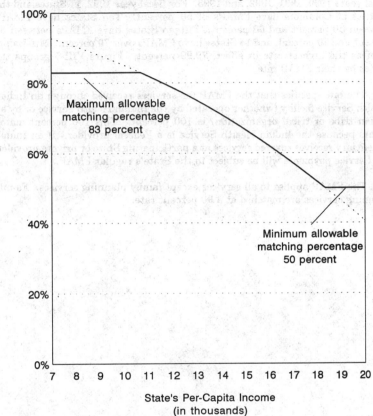

Federal Medical Assistance Percentage

Maximum allowable
matching percentage
83 percent

Minimum allowable
matching percentage
50 percent

State's Per-Capita Income
(in thousands)

Source: Figure prepared by Congressional Research Service.

The Social Security Act requires the Secretary of HHS to promulgate the FMAP between October 1 and November 1 of each year. This FMAP is in effect for the 1-year period beginning the following October. Thus, the FMAP for fiscal year 1993, the year beginning October 1992, was promulgated in 1991. The percentages are based on the average per capita income of each State and the U.S. for the three most recent calendar years for which data are available from the Department of Commerce. Table VIII-3 shows the FMAP by State for fiscal years 1990, 1991, 1992, and 1993. For fiscal year 1992, 11 States and the District of Columbia have FMAPs of 50 percent. Ten States have FMAPs between 50 percent and 60 percent. Fifteen States have FMAPs between 60 percent and 70 percent, and 14 States have FMAPs over 70 percent. Mississippi receives the highest rate in effect, 79.99 percent. Figure VIII-5 groups the States by their FMAP rate.

The law specifies that the FMAP for services received through an Indian Health Service facility (whether operated by the Indian Health Service or by an Indian tribe or tribal organization) is 100 percent. This 100 percent match occurs because the Indian Health Service is a Federal provider. If an Indian beneficiary receives covered services at a participating State or private provider, the Service payments will be subject to the State's regular FMAP.

The FMAP applies to all services except family planning services. Family planning services are matched at a 90 percent rate.

TABLE VIII-3. Federal Medical Assistance Percentages,
Fiscal Years 1990 to 1993

State	FY 1990	FY 1991	FY 1992	FY 1993
Alabama	73.21	72.73	72.93	71.45
Alaska	50.00	50.00	50.00	50.00
Arizona	60.99	61.72	62.61	65.89
Arkansas	74.58	75.12	75.66	74.41
California	50.00	50.00	50.00	50.00
Colorado	52.11	53.59	54.79	54.42
Connecticut	50.00	50.00	50.00	50.00
Delaware	50.00	50.00	50.00	50.00
District of Columbia	50.00	50.00	50.00	50.00
Florida	54.70	54.46	54.69	55.03
Georgia	62.09	61.34	61.78	62.08
Hawaii	50.00	50.00	50.00	50.00
Idaho	73.32	73.65	73.24	71.20
Illinois	50.00	50.00	50.00	50.00
Indiana	63.76	63.24	63.85	63.21
Iowa	62.52	63.41	65.04	62.74
Kansas	56.07	57.35	59.23	58.18
Kentucky	72.95	72.96	72.82	71.69
Louisiana	73.12	74.48	75.44	73.71
Maine	65.20	63.49	62.40	61.81
Maryland	50.00	50.00	50.00	50.00
Massachusetts	50.00	50.00	50.00	50.00
Michigan	54.54	54.17	55.41	55.84
Minnesota	52.74	53.43	54.43	54.93
Mississippi	80.18	79.93	79.99	79.01
Missouri	59.18	59.82	60.84	60.26
Montana	71.35	71.73	71.70	70.92
Nebraska	61.12	62.71	64.50	61.32
Nevada	50.00	50.00	50.00	52.28
New Hampshire	50.00	50.00	50.00	50.00
New Jersey	50.00	50.00	50.00	50.00
New Mexico	72.25	73.38	74.33	73.85
New York	50.00	50.00	50.00	50.00
North Carolina	67.46	66.60	66.52	65.92
North Dakota	67.52	70.00	72.75	72.21
Ohio	59.57	59.93	60.63	60.25
Oklahoma	68.29	69.65	70.74	69.67
Oregon	62.95	63.50	63.55	62.39
Pennsylvania	58.86	56.64	56.84	55.48
Rhode Island	55.15	53.74	53.29	53.64

**TABLE VIII-3. Federal Medical Assistance Percentages,
Fiscal Years 1990 to 1993--Continued**

State	FY 1990	FY 1991	FY 1992	FY 1993
South Carolina	73.07	72.58	72.66	71.28
South Dakota	70.90	71.69	72.59	70.27
Tennessee	69.64	68.57	68.41	67.57
Texas	61.23	63.53	64.18	64.44
Utah	74.70	74.89	75.11	75.29
Vermont	62.77	61.97	61.37	59.88
Virginia	50.00	50.00	50.00	50.00
Washington	53.88	54.21	54.98	55.02
West Virginia	76.61	77.00	77.68	76.29
Wisconsin	59.28	59.62	60.38	60.42
Wyoming	65.95	68.14	69.10	67.11
American Samoa	50.00	50.00	50.00	50.00
Guam	50.00	50.00	50.00	50.00
Northern Mariana	50.00	50.00	50.00	50.00
Puerto Rico	50.00	50.00	50.00	50.00
Virgin Islands	50.00	50.00	50.00	50.00

Source: Table prepared by the Congressional Research Service based on data obtained from the Health Care Financing Administration.

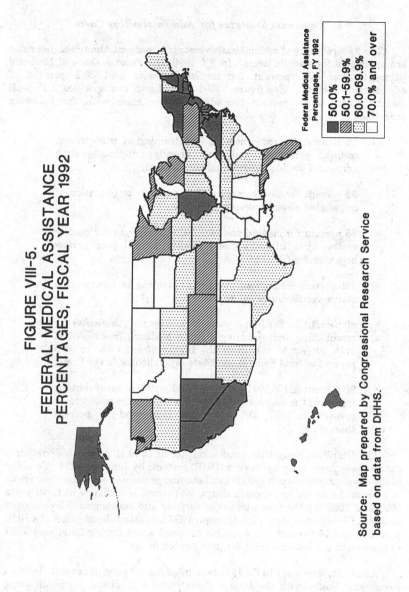

FIGURE VIII-5.
FEDERAL MEDICAL ASSISTANCE
PERCENTAGES, FISCAL YEAR 1992

Federal Medical Assistance
Percentages, FY 1992

50.0%
50.1-59.9%
60.0-69.9%
70.0% and over

Source: Map prepared by Congressional Research Service
based on data from DHHS.

2. Payments to States for Administrative Costs

The Federal share of administrative costs is 50 percent, though higher rates are applicable for specific items. In FY 1990, the Federal share of Medicaid payments was 57.1 percent for medical services and 56.8 percent of administrative costs. (See figure VIII-1.) Medicaid law specifies a Federal matching rate of 50 percent for administrative costs with the following exceptions:

- 75 percent for compensation and training of professional medical personnel, and staff directly supporting such personnel used in program administration;

- 90 percent for development and 75 percent for operation of automated claims processing systems;

- 75 percent for medical and utilization review, or for quality review by a utilization and quality control peer review organization (PRO);

- 100 percent for implementing and operating an immigration status verification system; and

- 90 percent for the first 3 years, and 75 percent thereafter for establishing and operating a State Medicaid fraud control unit, subject to a limit of the higher of $125,000 or .025 percent of total Federal and State expenditures in the State;

- 90 percent in FY 1991 for survey and certification of nursing facilities; the matching rate for this activity decreases to 85 percent in 1992, 80 percent in 1993, and 75 percent thereafter.

The Omnibus Budget Reconciliation Act of 1990 (P.L. 101-508) requires States to establish drug use review (DUR) systems by January 1993. To assist in the development of such systems and encourage the use of electronic systems to process claims for prescription drugs, 90 percent is available in fiscal years 1991 and 1992 for the procurement of services and equipment; 75 percent is available for calendar years 1991 through 1993 for statewide adoption of a DUR program; and 75 percent was available for sums spent during fiscal year 1991 to implement a rebate program for prescription drugs.

Administrative costs in FY 1991 accounted for 4.0 percent of total Medicaid payments. States with the largest share of total Medicaid payments going toward administrative costs include: Oregon, Arizona, Utah, Idaho, and Utah. States with the lowest share of total Medicaid payments going toward administrative costs include: New York, Indiana, Massachusetts, Louisiana, and Rhode Island. Administrative payments as a percent of total payments in each State are presented in table VIII-4.

489

TABLE VIII-4. Administrative Payments as a Percent of Total
Computable Medicaid Payments, Fiscal Year 1991

State	Administrative payment as a percent of total Medicaid payments
Alabama	3.1%
Alaska	6.7
Arizona	9.6
Arkansas	3.6
California	6.2
Colorado	4.4
Connecticut	3.9
Delaware	5.3
District of Columbia	4.3
Florida	4.0
Georgia	5.1
Hawaii	5.6
Idaho	7.0
Illinois	5.8
Indiana	2.3
Iowa	4.0
Kansas	3.7
Kentucky	2.8
Louisiana	2.0
Maine	3.8
Maryland	5.1
Mass Total	2.0
Michigan	3.2
Minnesota	5.2
Mississippi	3.5
Missouri	2.9
Montana	5.1
Nebraska	5.1

TABLE VIII-4. Administrative Payments as a Percent of Total
Computable Medicaid Payments, Fiscal Year 1991--Continued

State	Administrative payment as a percent of total Medicaid payments
Nevada	6.5%
New Hampshire	2.8
New Jersey	4.1
New Mexico	4.1
New York	2.6
North Carolina	4.0
North Dakota	4.4
Ohio	3.2
Oklahoma	7.7
Oregon	11.1
Pennsylvania	3.7
Rhode Island	1.8
South Carolina	3.8
South Dakota	2.7
Tennessee	2.6
Texas	4.9
Utah	6.9
Vermont	6.6
Virginia	4.1
Washington	6.2
West Virginia	3.0
Wisconsin	3.4
Wyoming	6.2
U.S. Total	4.0

NOTE: Estimates are based on payment information supplied to the Health
Care Financing Administration by the States.

Source: Table prepared by the Congressional Research Service based on data
contained on HCFA Form 64.

3. *Payments to the Outlying Areas*

For Puerto Rico and other Outlying Areas, the Social Security Act sets the matching rate at 50 percent for services and administrative costs with a maximum annual dollar limit on the amount each area can receive. The dollar limits in effect since FY 1990 are shown in table VIII-5.

TABLE VIII-5. Maximum Annual Payments to Outlying Areas

Outlying area	Maximum payment
American Samoa	$ 1,450,000
Guam	2,500,000
Northern Mariana Islands	750,000
Puerto Rico	79,000,000
Virgin Islands	2,600,000

If the dollar limit is reached, these areas have the choice of suspending Medicaid services or paying for them with nonfederal funds. Consequently, some Outlying Areas contribute more than 50 percent of the costs of their Medicaid programs.

C. State Funding for Medicaid

1. *The Size of State Medicaid Spending*[13]

In 1990, Medicaid accounted for more than 12 percent of total State spending, second only to the 23 percent of State funds spent on elementary and secondary education. Not only does Medicaid represent a large share of State spending, it also is a growing share. In 1987, Medicaid represented 10 percent of State spending. By 1991, it is estimated to represent almost 14 percent. Figure VIII-6 provides total State spending by selected service categories for State's fiscal year 1990.

---

[13]This discussion of Medicaid and State spending is based on data collected by the National Association of State Budget Officers (NASBO) in a survey of States. The NASBO survey provides detailed information on State spending by fund source (State general funds, other State funds, Federal funds, bond funds, and total funds) as well as spending category (Medicaid, education, cash assistance programs, etc.). It should be noted that estimates of the share of total spending by States on Medicaid includes any Federal grant-in-aid. The survey collects information on State spending and revenue and excludes funds from local sources. It should be remembered in any State by State comparison that some States require local funding. These local funds are not reflected in these estimates.

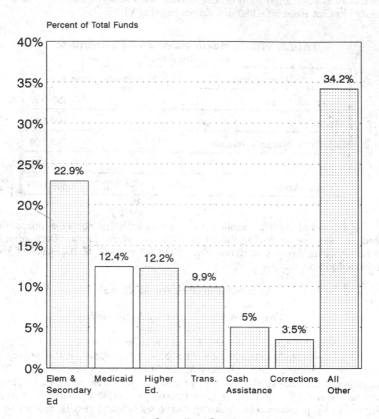

FIGURE VIII-6.
Share of State and Federal Funds Spent on
Selected Spending Categories, 1990

NOTE: Funds include Federal grants-in-aid and State spending.
Source: Figure prepared by Congressional Research Service based on National Association of State Budget Officers Survey of States, 1991.

It is important to note, however, that Medicaid spending as reported by many States includes Federal matching funds as well as State funds. Medicaid is the largest Federal grant program in State budgets, accounting for 35 percent of all Federal grant-in-aid received by States in FY 1991. Any analysis of State Medicaid spending as a share of total State expenditures has to take Medicaid's share of Federal grants to the States into account.

For the 49 States reporting on the most recent National Association of Budget Officers (NASBO) survey, Medicaid expenditures equalled 6.8 percent of the State's nonfederal spending in 1990.[14] For that year, NASBO data show that the nonfederal funds that States spent on Medicaid ranged from 2.0 percent (Wyoming) to 10.9 percent (Rhode Island) of total State spending. The States with the largest share of nonfederal funds being spent on Medicaid include: Rhode Island, New Hampshire, New York, Michigan, and Minnesota. The States with the lowest share of nonfederal funds being spent on Medicaid include: Wyoming, New Mexico, Alaska, South Carolina, and Delaware. Table VIII-6 provides the State by State percentages for FY 1988 through FY 1991.

As can be seen in table VIII-6, Medicaid has consumed a larger proportion of spending in most States since 1988. Of the 49 States providing information to NASBO, 39 States are spending a larger share of State funds on Medicaid in FY 1990 than in FY 1988. Those States experiencing the most rapid increase in the share of State funds going towards Medicaid include: West Virginia, Alabama, Alaska and South Carolina.

---

[14]Excluding any local funds.

TABLE VIII-6. State Medicaid Spending as a Share of State Funds, State Fiscal Years 1988 to 1990 and Projected State Fiscal Year 1991

State	FY 1988	FY 1989	FY 1990	FY 1991[a]
Alabama	3.3%	3.9	6.2%	7.6%
Alaska	1.7	1.9	2.8	3.6
Arizona	5.0	6.0	6.2	7.1
Arkansas	3.9	4.4	4.6	4.6
California	7.0	6.9	7.2	7.5
Colorado	6.2	6.3	7.2	8.2
Connecticut	5.1	5.3	5.5	7.0
Delaware	2.9	3.0	3.3	3.9
Florida	4.7	5.2	5.6	6.3
Georgia	6.1	6.2	5.9	7.9
Hawaii	3.8	3.8	3.3	2.9
Idaho	3.2	3.1	3.4	4.0
Illinois	6.4	7.9	7.9	8.2
Indiana	6.4	6.6	8.1	9.0
Iowa	3.9	3.8	4.4	4.8
Kansas	5.4	5.4	5.1	5.9
Kentucky	3.7	4.1	4.3	4.3
Louisiana	5.6	6.5	5.9	6.4
Maine	6.7	6.9	6.5	6.5
Maryland	6.6	6.8	6.7	6.9
Massachusetts	6.4	6.6	9.7	9.2
Michigan	6.3	6.0	9.3	8.2
Minnesota	7.8	8.0	8.3	8.7
Mississippi	3.6	3.5	4.6	4.6
Missouri	4.4	5.0	5.3	7.4
Montana	4.4	4.0	3.7	3.4
Nebraska	5.2	5.3	4.5	4.1
New Hampshire	8.5	9.2	10.2	11.8
New Jersey	7.4	7.5	8.6	9.6
New Mexico	2.6	3.0	2.5	3.0
New York	9.7	9.5	9.6	11.1
North Carolina	3.8	4.2	4.8	5.1
North Dakota	5.3	5.5	5.2	6.5
Ohio	6.2	6.1	7.0	7.9
Oklahoma	6.0	5.7	5.0	4.9

See notes at end of table.

TABLE VIII-6. State Medicaid Spending as a Share of State Funds, State Fiscal Years 1988 to 1990 and Projected State Fiscal Year 1991--Continued

State	FY 1988	FY 1989	FY 1990	FY 1991[a]
Oregon	2.2	2.2	3.3	4.3
Pennsylvania	7.8	8.2	8.1	10.9
Rhode Island	9.6	9.2	10.9	12.6
South Carolina	2.0	2.7	3.1	5.0
South Dakota	5.3	6.4	6.3	6.1
Tennessee	7.0	6.4	7.8	9.1
Texas	6.4	6.9	6.6	7.8
Utah	2.7	2.8	2.8	3.0
Vermont	4.7	4.8	6.6	8.5
Virginia	4.1	4.6	4.7	5.8
Washington	5.6	5.5	6.0	6.0
West Virginia	2.1	3.0	4.0	3.8
Wisconsin	6.2	6.3	6.9	6.9
Wyoming	1.3	2.3	2.0	1.7
49 State Total[b]	6.1	6.3	6.8	7.5

[a]State FY 1991 figures are based on estimates of expected State spending. These figures are likely to change with additional information.

[b]Total is based on the 49 States providing information to the National Association of Budget Officers survey in 1991. Data was not obtained for Nevada or the District of Columbia.

NOTE: Estimates are based on total State funds and State funds spent on Medicaid. These spending amounts exclude any Federal matching grants or any revenues obtained from local governments. It should also be noted that these estimates are based on responses to a NASBO survey and are likely to differ from information from other sources.

Source: Based on a State survey of expenditures conducted by the National Association of State Budget Officers, 1991.

2. Local Funding as a Share of State Medicaid Payments

The nonfederal portion of State Medicaid payments can be financed entirely through State funds. Alternatively, States may require local governments to share in financing program costs. However, States must assure that the lack of adequate funds from local sources will not result in diminished services in the State. States themselves are required to provide at least 40 percent of the nonfederal share of Medicaid expenditures. As of September 1991, 14 States required local funding of at least some portion of medical assistance payments. (See table VIII-7.) In addition, to these local financing formulas some States will allow other public entities to share in Medicaid financing. For instance, hospital districts in Texas transfer funds to the State which are used in the calculation of the State's nonfederal share of Medicaid. Table VIII-9 notes States where these intergovernmental transfers occur.

TABLE VIII-7. County Funding Formulas for Medicaid Vendor Payments as of September 1991

Arizona	Under Arizona's Health Care Cost Containment System, counties pay 100 percent of the nonfederal share of long term care for the elderly and physically disabled, and fund a variable portion of acute care services.
Florida	Counties pay $55 per month for each nursing home resident, and 100 percent of the nonfederal share for the 13th through 45th inpatient hospital days.
Iowa	Counties pay 100 percent of the nonfederal share of ICF/MR and MH/MR/DD home and community-based waivers for persons normally served by ICFs/MR; and 50 percent of the nonfederal share of certain mental health "enhancements" (i.e., title XIX case management, partial hospitalization, and day treatment for the chronically mentally ill, mentally retarded and developmentally disabled).
Minnesota	Counties pay 100 percent of the nonfederal share of Medicaid administrative expenses related to client services except for the child health plan where the share varies. Counties also loan funds to the State, without interest, for a portion of the State's benefit payments for the first 6 months of each fiscal year.
Montana	Counties pay 18 percent of the nonfederal share of the eligibility personnel costs.
New Hampshire	Counties pay 61.5 percent of the nonfederal share of intermediate nursing care services, except for ICFs/MR.
New York	Counties pay 20 percent of the nonfederal share of long term care; and 50 percent of the nonfederal share of all other services.

**TABLE VIII-7. County Funding Formulas for Medicaid Vendor
Payments as of September 1991--Continued**

North Carolina . . . . Counties pay 15 percent of the nonfederal share of
services, and 100 percent of the nonfederal share of
administrative expenses.

North Dakota . . . . Counties pay 15 percent of nonfederal share except
for: ICF/MR, clinic services, and waivered home and
community-based services for mentally retarded,
aged, and disabled recipients. In the 1989-90
biennium, the county share averaged 9.8 percent of
the nonfederal share of all services.

Ohio . . . . Counties pay 10 percent of the nonfederal share of
of Medicaid eligibility costs.

Pennsylvania . . . . Counties pay 10 percent of the nonfederal share for
county nursing homes plus $3 per invoice.

South Dakota . . . . Counties pay $60 per month for each ICF/MR
resident; and $200 per month for each mental
health resident in State inpatient facilities.

Utah . . . . For mental health, counties must provide a match
equal to 20 percent of the amount paid by the State,
which is equivalent to 16.7 percent of the
nonfederal share.

Wisconsin . . . . Counties pay the nonfederal share for certain
mental health programs (i.e., community support
program services and targeted case management),
but up to 90 percent of the county match may be
offset by funding provided by the State through
payments to counties under the State's "community
aid for human services."

NOTE: While the State of Colorado does not require counties to provide
funds for Medicaid vendor payments, counties in the State pay 40 percent of the
nonfederal share of administrative costs related to eligibility.

Source: Table prepared by the National Association of Counties (NACo)
based on information from State associations of county officials and State
Medicaid offices.

D. Provider Donations and Tax Programs and State Funding[15]

Rising Medicaid costs have placed increasing strains on State budgets. In order to alleviate this increased fiscal stress and implement mandatory or optional expansions of coverage and reimbursement, without altering the types of covered services, number of beneficiaries or reallocating State general funds, some States have used funds donated by health care providers, and taxes paid by these providers to draw greater Federal matching payments. States receive donations from Medicaid providers or levy taxes specifically on Medicaid providers (e.g., a tax on each day of hospital care or each hospital bed). In turn, these provider generated revenues have been treated as part of the State's share of spending for covered services and have been matched with Federal dollars. Increased revenues from these sources are used by States to extend eligibility, expand benefits to those eligible, increase reimbursements to providers, and help alleviate the fiscal pressures that indigent care places on health care providers and the States.[16]

In 1991, a controversy erupted over these provider donations and taxes. Concerns over the provider-generated revenue stemmed from the specific nature of the taxes and donations and how they are related to Medicaid reimbursement. If a State receives a donation or imposes a specific tax on Medicaid providers, it could use the provider-generated funds to claim Federal matching payments, then repay the taxes or donations to the Medicaid provider along with the Federal funds without having spent State revenues (i.e., raising any new State revenues).

An example will clarify how the donation/provider-specific tax process worked. Table VIII-8 assumes that a State has a matching rate of 60 percent, approximately equal to the 57 percent average Federal share. In this hypothetical example the State receives a hospital donation equal to $40; the State pays the hospital $100 and receives $60 in Federal matching funds. The State's share is $40 or zero after crediting the hospital donation.

---

[15]This section of the chapter is based on: U.S. Library of Congress. Congressional Research Service. *Medicaid: Provider Donations and Provider-Specific Taxes.* CRS Report for Congress No. 91-722 EPW, by Mark Merlis. Washington, 1991.

[16]See Miller, Victor. *Medicaid Financing Mechanisms and Federal Limits: A State Perspective.* [In] Medicaid Provider Tax and Donation Issues, by Health Policy Alternatives, Inc., July 1992.

TABLE VIII-8. Effect of a Hypothetical State Provider
Donation Program on State Medicaid Spending

(State with a Federal matching assistance percentage = 60 percent)

Hospital donation	$ 40
Total Medicaid payment to hospital	100
Amount of payment allowed by HCFA	100
Computed Federal share of payment	60
State share of payment (total Medicaid payment--Federal share)	40
Net cost to State (State share less donation)	0

NOTE: This is a hypothetical example. The size of the net cost to the State and Federal Government as well as the provider's net payment are influenced by three factors: the State's Federal matching assistance percentage, the payment level and the size of the provider donation.

The controversy over provider donations and provider specific taxes was further complicated with some States using intergovernmental transfers as a source of Medicaid funding. These transfers represent funds from local entities (e.g., county governments or local hospital districts) transferred to the State. When the transferred funds are treated as part of Medicaid, the funds can be matched with Federal dollars. When the source of the transferred funds was also a Medicaid provider, such as a public hospital, the intergovernmental transfer could be viewed as another mechanism to limit State Medicaid cost sharing. However, it should be noted that these intergovernmental transfers may differ from donations and provider-specific taxes in that they can act as a "new" source of State revenues. The transfer can represent local taxes transferred to the State for the support of Medicaid.

By FY 1991 many States began to use these revenue sources. In February of 1992, States reported that provider-specific taxes, provider donations, and intergovernmental transfers resulted in FY 1991 revenue totals of more than $3.2 billion.[17] In FY 1992, the combined effect of these revenue sources were expected to amount to more than $10.5 billion. For some States these revenues amounted to a sizable share of their Federal Medicaid grant. For instance, revenue from provider voluntary donations and intergovernmental transfers in Alabama were expected to equal 70 percent of the State's FY 1992 Federal matching dollars. New Hampshire's projections equalled about 67 percent of their Federal grant, Tennessee's projections equalled about 48 percent.

---

[17]Ibid., detailed State by State table. The estimates presented in this discussion are based on unaudited State reports to HCFA. The data should be viewed as preliminary and subject to change.

1. A Short History of the Controversy Surrounding Donated Funds and Provider Specific Taxes

Until 1985, Federal Medicaid rules permitted the use of donated funds for the costs of training State administrative personnel (former 42 CFR 432.60), but did not explicitly allow the use of donations for any other purpose. According to the Health Care Financing Administration (HCFA), the use of donations for purposes other than training was not allowed because a "'kickback' situation could result from private donations made by a proprietary organization, such as a long-term care facility or data processing company, in return for Medicaid business."[18]

However, in 1985, HCFA had concluded that the likelihood of abuse was small and that private donations could be used to finance the State share of any Medicaid service or administrative spending. A new regulation (42 CFR 433.45(b)) established two conditions for the use of donated funds:

- the funds had to be transferred to the Medicaid agency and be under its administrative control; and

- the funds could not revert to the donor unless the donor was a nonprofit organization and the Medicaid agency decided on its own to use the donor's facility.

In 1986 and 1987, West Virginia and Tennessee developed programs under which donations made to the State by hospitals were used to finance part of the State's share of Medicaid spending. After initial HCFA approval, Federal matching funds were later denied to the States. However, upon appeal these denials of matching funds were overturned.

In 1988, HCFA indicated that it would issue new regulations limiting the use of donations as the State share of Medicaid funds. But before HCFA could issue new rules, Congress intervened. The Technical and Miscellaneous Revenue Act of 1988 (P.L. 100-647), enacted in 1988, included a provision prohibiting the Secretary from issuing final rules that would change the treatment of voluntary contributions or provider-specific taxes before May 1, 1989. The prohibition on the issuance of a final rule on provider donations was extended to December 1990 with the passage of OBRA 89, and then to December 1991 with the passage of OBRA 90. OBRA 90 also permanently prohibited the Secretary from interfering with the use of provider specific taxes except in certain cases.[19]

---

[18]50 *Federal Register* 46657, Nov. 12, 1985.

[19]In particular, section 1903(i)(10) of the act states that Federal matching payments shall not be made: "with respect to any amount expended for medical assistance for care or services furnished by a hospital, nursing facility, or intermediate care facility for the mentally retarded to reimburse the hospital or facility for the costs attributable to taxes imposed by the State sole[l]y with respect to hospitals or facilities."

In September 1991, HCFA published interim final rules scheduled to be effective January 1, 1992. Under this rule, revenues derived from donations and from provider specific taxes on hospitals, nursing homes, or intermediate care facilities for the mentally retarded would be deducted from a State's expenditures for Medicaid before the Federal share of the State's Medicaid expenditures was calculated. The status of intergovernmental transfers was, in the view of the States, ambiguous under the interim final rule. Some States felt the interim rule allowed the Administration too much discretion in the treatment of these transfers.

The Administration was concerned that the use of donations and taxes effectively reduced a State's share of Medicaid spending. In testimony before the House Subcommittee on Health and the Environment, Gail Wilensky, then the administrator of the Health Care Financing Administration stated:

> State donation and tax programs present a complex issue, but it is clear that they have the potential to undermine a basic premise of the Medicaid program--that funding be shared through a Federal match of State monies. In a matching program, those responsible for expenditure decisions and the direct fiscal management of the program must have a reasonable stake in program costs. This shared responsibility works to shape their decision-making to contain costs. The requirement for a State share of payment has always acted as a restraint on the otherwise open-ended Medicaid program.

> Without a limit on evolving State donation and tax programs, we will move quickly toward a system of *fourth party payment* where the Federal Government, not the patient, the provider, or the manager of the program is at risk for the cost of services. State provider tax and donation programs threaten to alter fundamentally the intended funding relationship between Federal and State government.[20]

The Administration's perspective was based on the idea that a connection existed between the size of the donation or tax revenue that the State received from the provider and the amount the provider received in the form of a Medicaid payment. In contrast, the States argued that provider donation and tax systems in many States were thoroughly considered and fell within the realm of the statute at the time of this debate. Donations and taxes were a legitimate and viable revenue source from the States' perspective. Furthermore, the primary reliance on donation or provider specific taxes was as a revenue measure to help in supporting higher reimbursement rates for providers. This in turn would promote access to the health care system. For example, the

---

[20]U.S. Congress. House. Committee on Energy and Commerce. Subcommittee on Health and the Environment. *State Financing of Medicaid*. Statement of Honorable Gail R. Wilensky, Ph.D., Administrator. Health Care Financing Administration. Hearing, Serial No. 102-79, Sept. 30 and Oct. 16, 1991. Washington, GPO, 1991. p. 277. (Hereafter cited as Wilensky, *State Financing of Medicaid*)

Alabama State Medicaid Agency Commissioner noted before the House Subcommittee on Health and the Environment:

> With voluntary contributions, Alabama has been able to meet Federal mandates and enhance services for children, pregnant women and mothers. With provider specific taxes, the work begun in 1988 can continue and services can be further enhanced. Should Alabama lose its ability to use provider specific taxes as a part of the State's share for Federal matching funds, the Medicaid program will collapse. In fact, the loss of provider specific taxes and the Federal matching funds they generate will be catastrophic for the entire health care delivery system in the State. Alabama will regress to the "dark ages" of health care. Children and pregnant women will lose access to the medical services they need, the infant mortality rate will go up again, and the elderly will lose eligibility for care in a nursing home.[21]

The Administration provided some concrete examples of why they felt the use of donations undermined a State's fiscal responsibilities for the program. In explaining how the donation program worked in the State of Pennsylvania Dr. Wilensky noted:

> What they [Pennsylvania] did was 170 hospitals got together, formed a foundation borrowed some $365 million from a lending institution. They donated that money to the State treasury. The Federal match for Pennsylvania is such that the State got $380 million to match the $365 million they put up. The $365 million that was put up by this group of 170 hospitals went back to the 170 hospitals as increased disproportionate share payments, so they were made completely whole including the cost of actually borrowing the money.
>
> The $380 million that the Feds put in, the only new money in the system, went to some 260 hospitals in the State in order to fulfill their court settlement to increase rates to hospitals . . . .[22]

The Administration argued that provider-specific taxes violated an important quality of a tax. A provider-specific tax linked back to some selective reimbursement was argued not to be redistributive in nature. Rather than a broad based revenue mechanism, it was argued that a small number of providers were being taxed only to be directly reimbursed with Federal matching funds. No "new" State funds were involved, and no redistribution was occurring. If a State used a broad-based tax, rather than a provider specific tax, some providers who would have to pay the tax would not receive any Medicaid reimbursement. A broad-based tax would redistribute Federal matching dollars and **State** revenues to providers within the State.

---

[21]U.S. Congress. House. Committee on Energy and Commerce. Subcommittee on Health and the Environment. Statement of Carol A. Herrmann, Commissioner, Alabama State Medicaid Agency. p. 89.

[22]Wilensky, *State Financing of Medicaid*, p. 296.

Central to the Administration's example is the State's reliance on the Medicaid program's disproportionate share payments. Disproportionate share payments are supplemental payments to State specified hospitals that serve a disproportionate share of low-income patients with special needs. In 1987, the Congress defined minimum criteria to be used by States in designating hospitals for this supplemental payment. But, States could use more liberal definitions. No cap was placed on the size of the supplemental payments, and the payment methodology could be developed by the States as long as similar types of hospitals were treated equally. The flexibility given to States in designating disproportionate share hospitals as well as the States' ability to designate reimbursement methodologies allowed for these payments to be an important avenue for increased reimbursements.

If a State can **selectively** raise reimbursement rates it has a mechanism that can hold providers "harmless" from the effect of their donations or Medicaid taxes. Disproportionate share payments provide a source for this selectivity. The rather dramatic increase in disproportionate share payments and the increase in the number of States that use donation and provider tax revenues have placed focus on the connection between these revenue and reimbursement sources. Based on data compiled by the HCFA, in the spring of 1992, of the 11 States relying on acute care hospital donations, 10 States used the proceeds from those donations for disproportionate share payments.[23] At least 18 States levied provider-specific taxes on acute care hospitals. Sixteen of these States used the proceeds from these taxes for disproportionate share payments.[24] It should be noted that while States indicate that disproportionate share payments are financed through these approaches, this association between donation/taxes and these payments does not completely explain the rather rapid increase in disproportionate share payments.

Table VIII-9 provides a compilation of the revenue sources used by States in May 1992. Twenty-two States used some form of provider specific taxes as revenue in 1992. Most of these States (18) levied a tax on hospitals, in 12 States nursing homes paid provider-specific taxes. Provider donations were a source of State revenues in 15 States. Seventeen States relied on intergovernmental transfers as a source of funds for the Medicaid program.

---

[23]Health Care Financing Administration. *Medicaid State Profile Data System: Characteristics of Medicaid State Programs.* National Comparison, v. 1, HCFA Publication No. 02178, May 1992. Tables 5-1 and 5-2.

[24]Ibid., table 5-1.

TABLE VIII-9. Provider Specific Funding Devices Used by States, May 1992

State	Provider specific taxes						Donations	Intergovernmental transfers
	Hospitals	Physicians	Nursing homes	Mental health facilities	Pharmacy	Other		
Alabama[a]								
Alaska								
Arizona								
Arkansas	Yes	Yes	Yes	Yes	Yes			
California							Details not available	Counties, hospitals[b]
Colorado	Pending		Pending				Hospitals	Hospitals
Connecticut[a]								
Delaware[a]								
District of Columbia[a]								
Florida	Yes					Yes	Other	
Georgia							Hospitals	
Hawaii								
Idaho								

See notes at end of table.

TABLE VIII-9. Provider Specific Funding Devices Used by States, May 1992--Continued

State	Provider specific taxes						Donations	Intergovernmental transfers
	Hospitals	Physicians	Nursing homes	Mental health facilities	Pharmacy	Other		
Illinois	Yes		Yes	Yes				Pending
Indiana	Yes			Yes				County[c]
Iowa	Pending	Pending	Pending		Pending	Pending		Hospitals (pending)
Kansas								Community mental health, community developmental disability and local health/education agencies
Kentucky	Yes	Yes	Yes		Yes	Yes		
Louisiana							Hospitals	
Maine[a]								
Maryland		Yes	Yes		Yes	Yes		
Massachusetts	Yes							Public hospitals[d]
Michigan							Hospitals	Pending

See notes at end of table.

TABLE VIII-9. Provider Specific Funding Devices Used by States, May 1992--Continued

| State | Provider specific taxes | | | | | | Donations | Intergovernmental transfers |
	Hospitals	Physicians	Nursing homes	Mental health facilities	Pharmacy	Other		
Minnesota	Yes		Yes			Yes		
Mississippi	Yes	Yes	Yes	Yes	Yes	Yes	Hospitals	Hospitals
Missouri							Hospitals, nursing homes	
Montana			Yes					
Nebraska								
Nevada	Yes							Counties[e]
New Hampshire	Yes							
New Jersey[d]								
New Mexico								Hospitals, counties[f]
New York	Yes		Yes	Yes				
North Carolina							Hospitals, nursing homes	

See notes at end of table.

TABLE VIII-9. Provider Specific Funding Devices Used by States, May 1992--Continued

State	Provider specific taxes						Donations	Intergovernmental transfers
	Hospitals	Physicians	Nursing homes	Mental health facilities	Pharmacy	Other		
North Dakota								
Ohio	Yes							
Oklahoma								Details not available
Oregon[a]								
Pennsylvania							Hospitals, nursing homes	
Rhode Island								
South Carolina	Details on taxes not available						Details not available	ICF mental health services
South Dakota								
Tennessee[a]								
Texas	Yes						Hospitals	Hospitals[g]

See notes at end of table.

TABLE VIII-9. Provider Specific Funding Devices Used by States, May 1992--Continued

State	Provider specific taxes						Donations	Intergovernmental transfers
	Hospitals	Physicians	Nursing homes	Mental health facilities	Pharmacy	Other		
Utah							Hospitals[h]	[h]
Vermont	Yes		Yes			Yes		
Virginia								
Washington	Yes						Hospitals, mental health facilities	Hospitals[i]
West Virginia		Yes				Yes		Mental health facilities, others
Wisconsin			Yes				Hospitals, others (pending)	Hospitals, nursing homes, others[j]
Wyoming								
Total number of States using revenue source	18	6	12	5	5	8	15	17

See notes at end of table.

TABLE VIII-9. Provider Specific Funding Devices Used by States, May 1992.--Continued

[a]State did not respond to survey, see note below for additional information.

[b]Counties, local hospitals, and University of California teaching hospitals that license disproportionate share payments make transfers to State.

[c]Marion County will transfer funds beginning in FY 1993 to the State.

[d]Transfer from City of Boston.

[e]Joint State-local program for SSI recipients. Counties provide SSI funds from $714 per recipient to 300 percent of SSI maximum.

[f]Counties make voluntary contributions to county-supported Medicaid fund.

[g]Disproportionate share hospitals use local funds from public hospital districts and State-owned teaching hospitals.

[h]The University of Utah Hospital provides donations to the State. Since the hospital is considered a State agency, this donation can be considered an intergovernmental transfer.

[i]Two State teaching hospitals participate in intergovernmental disproportionate share hospital program with the Department of Social and Health Services. In addition, 43 rural hospitals receive disproportionate share monies from the same program.

[j]Counties, cities, towns or villages can elect to provide funds for case management, community support programs, community supported living, hospital and nursing home programs.

TABLE VIII-9. Provider Specific Funding Devices Used by States, May 1992--Continued

NOTE: Eight States and the District of Columbia did not respond to this survey. Based on information provided to the Health Care Financing Administration in February of 1992, some additional information is available:

Alabama--Relied on (or intends to use) provider-specific taxes and intergovernmental transfers in FY 1992 and FY 1993.
Connecticut--No specified funding device was noted.
Delaware--Intends to use provider-specific taxes in FY 1993.
District of Columbia--Intends to use provider-specific taxes in FY 1993.
Maine--Relied on (or intends to use) provider-specific taxes and intergovernmental transfers in FY 1992 and FY 1993.
New Jersey--No specified funding devices.
Oregon--No specified funding devices.
Tennessee--Relied on (or intends to use) provider specific taxes in FY 1992 and FY 1993.

Additional information for these States was not available. States not specifying funding devices may still rely on these devices.

Source: Table prepared by the Congressional Research Service based on information contained in the National Conference of State Legislatures' *1992 Survey of State Medicaid Provider Assessment Changes.*

2. Medicaid Voluntary Contribution and Provider-Specific Tax Amendments of 1991

After much debate, the controversy was reconciled primarily through negotiations between the National Governors' Association and the Administration.[25] The result of this negotiation is found in the Medicaid Voluntary Contribution and Provider-Specific Tax Amendments of 1991 (P.L. 102-234). The act deals with this issue by:

• defining acceptable State taxing authorities;

• defining what a bona fide donation is;

• setting a cap on revenues from provider-specific taxes and donations; and

• limiting disproportionate share payments.

In addition, the law explicitly eliminates the issuance of any interim final regulations on intergovernmental transfers. Furthermore, the law nullified the October 1991 interim regulations. Through the use of transition rules, the law allowed States time to convert their existing provider-specific tax and donation programs to acceptable revenue programs. These transition rules allowed States to continue to use these revenue devices after January 1, 1992, the cutoff date that would be in effect under the regulations.

Generally, the voluntary contribution and provider specific tax amendments prohibit the use of Federal funds to match revenues obtained from provider specific taxes or voluntary donations unless these revenue sources meet the definition of a broad-based health care related tax or a bona fide donation. The elimination of these matching payments would be effective as of January 1, 1992, except if a State already had a donation program in place by September 30, 1991 and the program is in effect in fiscal year 1992 or a tax program enacted by November 22, 1991. For States with tax or donation programs already in place, Federal matching payments for revenues under the current tax or donation plans would continue until the following dates:

• for States with a fiscal year beginning on or before July 1-October 1, 1992;

• for States with a fiscal year beginning after July 1-January 1, 1993; and

• for States who did not have regular legislative session in 1992, or 1993 (i.e., States with biennial legislatures), or if a

---

[25]A detailed description of the debate associated with this bill can be found in Health Policy Alternatives, Inc. *Medicaid Provider Tax and Donation Issues: The Federal Debate.*

State enacted a provider-specific tax on November 4, 1991-July 1, 1993.

a. Defining a Health Care Related Tax

The Medicaid voluntary contribution and provider-specific tax amendments specified that States could use broad-based health care related taxes as a revenue source for the Medicaid program. These taxes should apply uniformly within a class of providers. Classes of providers include:

- inpatient hospital services;

- outpatient hospital services;

- nursing facility services;

- intermediate care facility for the mentally retarded services (ICF/MR);

- physician services;

- home health care services;

- outpatient prescription drugs;

- services provided through health maintenance organizations;

- and other service groups defined through regulation.[26]

The law covers taxes that are related to health care items or services, or under general tax provisions (e.g., a sales tax) if the tax treats health care items or services differently. Taxes are considered relating to health care items or services if at least 85 percent of the burden falls on health care providers.

Qualifying taxes include taxes based on: 1) the revenues or receipts of a provider; and 2) a licensing fee or similar tax. These taxes must be levied uniformly. This means that in the case of taxes on revenues and receipts the tax is the same for all providers of the services. In the case of licensing fees or similar taxes based on the number of licensed hospital beds, the tax should be the same for each bed for every provider. Taxes on revenues must apply to all revenues related to services subject to the tax, except that Medicaid and/or Medicare revenues may be excluded. If a local government imposes the tax, the tax must apply to all providers within the local jurisdiction. Taxes are not considered uniform if the State provides for exclusions, deductions, or credits to providers in an attempt to return to the provider all or a portion of the tax paid or the State employs a hold harmless provision.

---

[26]As of Oct. 1992, Federal regulations specifying additional classes were not issued.

A hold harmless provision occurs if: 1) any Medicaid reimbursement to the provider paying a tax varies based on the amount of the tax; 2) any State or local government payment, outside of a Medicaid reimbursement, varies based on the health-care related tax; or 3) any State or local government payment, offset, or waiver has the intention of guaranteeing that the provider will not face an increased tax. Public providers can be excluded from a tax. If a provider specific tax does not meet these criteria, the State can seek a waiver from the Secretary. Two conditions must be met for a waiver to apply: 1) the net effect of the tax and associated expenditures is redistributive in nature; and 2) the amount of the tax is not directly associated with Medicaid payments. The law specifies that rural and sole-community providers can be exempted from a tax under a waiver.

b. Defining a Bona Fide Donation

A bona fide donation is any donation that does not have a direct or in-direct relationship with Medicaid payments to that provider, to a class of providers, or to a related entity.[27] The Secretary HHS will determine what donations are considered "bona fide" donations. Any donations made by a hospital, clinic, or similar entity for the direct cost of persons placed at the site to determine Medicaid eligibility and to provide outreach services for the program are also acceptable donations. However, donations associated with eligibility determination and outreach activities can not exceed 10 percent of administrative spending in the State in Federal FY 1993 and subsequent years.

c. Setting a Limit on the Use of Donations and Taxes as a Revenue Source

In addition to defining what are acceptable types of taxes and donations, the voluntary contribution and tax amendment sets limits on the use of these revenue sources. For January 1, 1992 through FY 1993 the sum of revenues from all donations and provider taxes may not exceed:

- 25 percent of the nonfederal share of Medicaid spending; or

- the percent of nonfederal Medicaid spending that donations and taxes collected in State FY 1992 represent.[28]

In addition, from January 1 1992 through September 30, 1995 collections from broad-based taxes may not exceed these limits.

---

[27]A related entity includes: an organization, association, or partnership form by or on behalf of the health care providers; a person with ownership or a controlling interest in the provider; a employee, spouse, child or someone who has a similar close relationship to the provider.

[28]In States where a health-care related tax or donation is in effect for only part of the year, or the rate or base changed during the year, the Secretary will base the limit on a projected figure for that State.

d. Limiting Disproportionate Share Payments to Hospitals

The other major focus of the 1991 amendments was to set an upper limit on the payments to disproportionate share hospitals. Effective January 1, 1992, national aggregate DSH payment adjustments during each fiscal year are limited to 12 percent of total Medicaid spending for that year. Individual States' payments in January through September 1992 are generally limited to those made under methodologies in effect by the end of FY 1991. For FY 1993 and subsequent fiscal years, each State will have its own DSH limit. "High DSH" States, those whose payments are already above the 12 percent limit, will be allowed to increase their payments by no more than the projected growth in their overall Medicaid spending. Other "non-high DSH" States will be allowed larger increases, so long as aggregate national payments do not exceed the national cap. If projected DSH payments for a year under States' current rules are less than 12 percent of total projected Medicaid spending, the difference will constitute a pool of funds that may be divided among the non-high DSH States. Each State will receive the lesser of (a) a share of the pool proportionate to the State's share of all Medicaid spending by non-high DSH States or (b) the amount that would raise the State's allowable payment adjustments to 12 percent of its Medicaid spending.

The Act allows an exception to the DSH limits beginning January 1, 1996, but only if Congress has taken certain action by that date. States would not be subject to the limits if they designated as DSHs only hospitals that have above-average Medicaid or low-income utilization rates, account for at least 1 percent of all Medicaid days in the State, or meet other criteria established by the Secretary. However, this alternative would become available only if Congress enacts legislation limiting DSH payments in the States that elect the option.

Chapter V, Reimbursement provides State DSH allocations for FY 1993.

CHAPTER IX. RECENT LEGISLATIVE HISTORY[1]

I. SUMMARY

The Medicaid program was established by the Social Security Amendments of 1965, (P.L.89-97). Prior to 1980, amendments to this program were generally incorporated in legislation amending the Social Security Act. Beginning in 1980, budget reconciliation bills have been the major legislative vehicle for program changes. The intent of these reconciliation bills has been to provide for reductions in Federal spending across government programs. However, many of these bills provided for slight increases in Medicaid outlays; these were primarily attributable to expansions in the eligible population. In addition to reconciliation bills, several other laws also included modifications to the Medicaid program.

Taken together, these measures have resulted in a number of changes in the nature of the Medicaid program since 1980. Perhaps the most significant change is the severing of the automatic link between cash assistance and Medicaid eligibility and the resultant expansion in the population groups served by the program. Other changes included providing States increased flexibility in the design and administration of their programs, strengthening the quality of care requirements for nursing facility services, providing for savings on prescription drug expenditures, and expanding the list of covered Medicaid services.

Beginning in 1984, Congress began expanding the protection available to low-income pregnant women and children. Initially, the focus was on expanding coverage for individuals meeting the income and resources requirements for cash assistance, but not actually receiving a cash assistance payment. Subsequently, the Congress enacted legislation expanding first the optional, and then the required coverage for other low-income pregnant women and children. States are now required to cover all pregnant women with incomes below 133 1/3 percent of the Federal poverty line. They are required to cover all children born after September 30, 1983 who meet State-established eligibility standards. They are also required to cover all children under age 6 with incomes below 133 1/3 percent of the Federal poverty line. Beginning July 1, 1991 they are required to cover all children under age 19 born after September 30, 1983 with incomes below 100 percent of the Federal poverty line. Thus, all poor children under age 19 will be covered by the year 2002. All Medicaid-eligible children, including new coverage groups as they become eligible, are entitled to all medically necessary services needed to treat conditions uncovered during early and periodic screening, diagnostic, and treatment (EPSDT) services.

---

[1]This chapter was written by Jennifer O'Sullivan.

Expansions in Medicaid coverage have not been restricted to pregnant women and children. Recent legislation has extended assistance to low-income elderly and disabled persons who are also eligible for Medicare. States are now required to pay Medicare cost-sharing charges for all such persons with incomes below 100 percent of the Federal poverty line.

A second important theme of legislation enacted in recent years was the increased flexibility given States in the design and administration of their programs. In 1981, both in response to rapidly escalating program costs and to an Administration proposal to cap Federal Medicaid expenditures, the Congress approved temporary reductions in Federal Medicaid payments. However, of greater long-term significance for the program were the increased flexibilities authorized under the freedom-of-choice and home and community-based services waiver authorities. (See discussion below). This flexibility has been cited as a factor in encouraging States to explore alternative health services delivery approaches. The legislation also continued the process begun in 1980 of allowing States increased flexibility in determining reimbursement rates for institutional services.

Another important concern of the Congress has been the quality of care received by program beneficiaries. This concern was exemplified in the passage of nursing home reform legislation in 1987 and subsequent amendments to that legislation. Beginning in 1990, all nursing facilities participating in Medicaid were required to meet a single set of quality standards. A new process was established for State and Federal monitoring of nursing facility compliance with the new requirements.

Finally, a major theme of the 1990 reconciliation bill was the effort to stem Federal and State expenditures for prescription drugs. Under the new legislation, drug manufacturers are required, as a condition of Federal matching, to enter into, and comply with, an agreement to provide each State periodic rebates on the manufacturer's products purchased for Medicaid beneficiaries in the State.

Also included in Omnibus Budget Reconciliation Act of 1990 (OBRA 90, P.L. 101-508) was Title XIII, the Budget Enforcement Act (BEA) of 1990, which has important implications for any future legislative changes. BEA established new budget enforcement rules. Under these rules, Federal spending is divided into the following categories: direct (entitlement) spending, three discretionary spending categories (international, defense, and domestic) and social security. Medicaid is in the direct spending category. Direct spending programs are subject to "pay as you go" rules for the FY 1991-FY 1995 period. Any legislation that would increase the direct spending category must be offset by spending reductions or financed by increased revenues. Other factors that influence Medicaid spending, such as an economic downturn or changes in State eligibility rules, are not affected by BEA.

This chapter reviews the major legislative changes which have been enacted over the 1980-1992 period. These changes were incorporated in nine reconciliation bills and several other measures:

- Public Law 96-499, Omnibus Reconciliation Act of 1980 (technically ORA 80, generally referred to as OBRA 80),

- Public Law 97-35, Omnibus Budget Reconciliation Act of 1981 (OBRA 81),

- Public Law 97-248, Tax Equity and Fiscal Responsibility Act of 1982 (TEFRA),

- Public Law 98-369, Deficit Reduction Act of 1984 (DEFRA),

- Public Law 99-272, Consolidated Omnibus Budget Reconciliation Act of 1985 (COBRA),

- Public Law 99-509, Omnibus Budget Reconciliation Act of 1986 (OBRA 86),

- Public Law 100-93, Medicare and Medicaid Patient and Program Protection Act of 1987,

- Public Law 100-203, Omnibus Budget Reconciliation Act of 1987 (OBRA 87),

- Public Law 100-360, Medicare Catastrophic Coverage Act of 1988 (MCCA),

- Public Law 100-485, Family Support Act of 1988 (FSA),

- Public Law 100-647, Technical and Miscellaneous Revenue Act of 1988 (TAMRA),

- Public Law 101-234, Medicare Catastrophic Coverage Repeal Act of 1989,[2]

- Public Law 101-239, Omnibus Budget Reconciliation Act of 1989 (OBRA 89),

- Public Law 101-508, Omnibus Budget Reconciliation Act of 1990 (OBRA 90),

- Public Law 102-234, Medicaid Voluntary Contribution and Provider - Specific Tax Amendments of 1991,

---

[2] This legislation did not repeal the Medicaid expansions authorized under MCCA.

- Public Law 102-276, waiver for Dayton Area Health Plan,

- Public Law 102-317, waiver for Tennessee Primary Care Network, and

- Public Law 102-585, Veterans Health Care Act of 1992.

The following highlights the major changes incorporated in these laws. More details are contained in the following sections of these chapters. For the location of specific provisions in the Medicaid statute, see the index to the Medicaid statute in the addendum.

A. Eligibility Expansions

Coverage of pregnant women, infants and young children. Beginning with DEFRA, legislation expanded requirements with respect to coverage of pregnant women and children who had a linkage with the cash assistance programs. States are now required to cover all pregnant women meeting the States' income and resources requirements, whether or not they are receiving cash assistance. They are also required to cover all children born after September 30, 1983, who meet such income and resources requirements, though this requirement is effectively superseded by the requirements pertaining to poverty-related coverage.

Beginning in 1987, States were permitted to significantly expand their programs to provide coverage for low-income pregnant women and children who did not have a direct link to the cash assistance system. Subsequent legislation identified those groups for whom States were required to extend protection. Effective April 1, 1990, States were required to cover all pregnant women and children under age 6 with incomes below 133 1/3 percent of the Federal poverty line. Effective July 1, 1991, States are required to extend coverage to all children under age 19, born after September 30, 1983, with incomes below the Federal poverty line.

Coverage of elderly and disabled poor. Beginning in 1987, States were permitted to provide Medicaid coverage to elderly and disabled persons with incomes above the cash assistance standard but below the Federal poverty line. Alternatively they could cover just the Medicare cost-sharing charges for this population group.

The MCCA required States to phase-in, generally over 4 years, coverage of Medicare cost-sharing charges for all elderly and disabled persons below the Federal poverty line. OBRA 90 accelerated implementation of this provision; by January 1, 1991, most States were required to provide this coverage for elderly and disabled Medicare beneficiaries who have incomes below the poverty line and who meet the assets test. In addition, OBRA 90 required States, beginning in 1993, to cover Medicare Part B premiums (but no other Medicare cost-sharing charges) for persons with incomes below 110 percent of poverty and assets below a specified level; beginning in 1995, the income limitation for this group is raised to 120 percent of poverty.

Coverage of Working Disabled Persons. OBRA 86 required States to continue Medicaid coverage for disabled persons with severe impairments who lose their eligibility for cash assistance because of their earnings from work.

OBRA 89 required States to pay Medicare Part A premiums for certain low-income working disabled persons not otherwise eligible for Medicaid.

1. Eligibility Modifications for Nursing Facility Population

* *Deterring Financial Gaming In Order to Qualify for Nursing Home Benefits.* Beginning in 1982, legislation was enacted to prevent persons with substantial assets from gaining eligibility for Medicaid prior to spending excess assets on medical care. TEFRA strengthened existing provisions relating to liens and to treatment of resources transferred for less than fair market value. COBRA added potential payments from Medicaid qualifying trusts to the list of income and resources available to an individual and therefore considered in determining eligibility. MCCA established a national transfer of assets policy.

* *Prevention of Spousal Impoverishment.* MCCA included provisions intended to protect a portion of a couple's income and resources, but only up to specified maximums, for the needs of the spouse of an institutionalized individual.

2. Expansion in the Types of Services Offered Under State Medicaid Programs

The OBRA 80 required States to cover nurse midwife services. Subsequent legislation expanded the list of mandated services to include nurse practitioner services, federally qualified health center services, and personal care services. During the 1980-1990 period, the list of optional services was also expanded. Services States may offer include hospice care, targeted case management and home respiratory care for ventilator dependent persons.

The OBRA 90 added a provision requiring drug manufacturers, as a condition of Federal matching, to enter into rebate agreements with the Secretary. States are prohibited from using formularies to deny coverage for a drug of a manufacturer that has entered into a rebate agreement.

The OBRA 90 established two capped entitlement programs within Medicaid. The first permits States to provide home and community-based services to functionally disabled persons otherwise eligible for Medicaid. The second permits States to provide community-supported living arrangements services to persons with mental retardation or related conditions.

3. Modified Rules for Establishing Payment Rates

Increased Flexibility for States in Establishing Payment Rates

- *Payments to Skilled Nursing and Intermediate Care Facilities (SNF/ICF).* Prior to enactment of OBRA 80, States were required to pay for SNF and ICF services on a "reasonable cost" basis. OBRA 80 repealed this requirement. It required States to reimburse such facilities at rates that are reasonable and adequate to meet the cost which must be incurred by efficiently and economically operated facilities in order to provide care in conformity with applicable State and Federal laws, regulations, and quality and safety standards.

The OBRA 87 eliminated, effective October 1, 1990, the distinction between SNFs and ICFs and at the same time eliminated the requirement that States pay less for ICF than for SNF services. States are also required to adjust their payment rates to reflect the costs facilities incur in implementing the 1987 reforms.

- *Payments to Hospitals.* OBRA 81 eliminated the requirement that States pay for hospital services on a reasonable cost basis; it gave States increased flexibility to develop their payment rates, comparable to that authorized for SNFs and ICFs under OBRA 80. At the same time States were required to take into account the situation of hospitals serving a disproportionate number of low-income patients. This "disproportionate share" provision was strengthened several times in subsequent legislation.

Requiring Manufacturers to Offer Rebates for Prescription Drugs. OBRA 90 substantially reformed Medicaid reimbursement for outpatient prescription drugs in all States. It denied Federal matching funds for all of a manufacturer's products in any State unless the manufacturer enters into, and complies with, an agreement to provide each State periodic rebates on the manufacturer's products purchased for Medicaid beneficiaries in the State. OBRA 90 included the manufacturer's "best price" in the calculation of the rebate. The Veterans Health Care Act of 1992 excluded from the determination of best price, effective October 1, 1992, the prices charged by manufacturers to the Department of Veterans' Affairs (DVA), the Department of Defense, the Public Health Service (PHS) and various PHS-funded health programs, and State (non-Medicaid) pharmacy assistance programs.

4. Increased Flexibility in Delivery of Services

"Freedom-of-Choice Waiver". OBRA 81 authorized the Secretary to waive certain State plan requirements to enable a State to restrict the provider from or through whom the individual could obtain nonemergency services.

Home and Community-Based Services Waivers. OBRA 81 authorized the Secretary to waive Federal requirements to enable a State to provide home and community-based services (other than room and board) to individuals who would otherwise require SNF or ICF services which would be paid by Medicaid. Services which could be provided under these waivers included certain supportive services not normally covered by Medicaid. Subsequent amendments to the original waiver authority generally addressed issues raised by implementing regulations and/or administration of the program by Health Care Financing Administration (HCFA).

"1915(d) Waiver". OBRA 87 established a separate waiver authority that allowed States, on a budget neutral basis, to provide a mix of home and community-based and institutional services to the elderly at risk of nursing home care.

5. Nursing Home Reform

The OBRA 87 contained major nursing home revisions for both Medicaid and Medicare. Beginning October 1, 1990, all nursing facilities participating in Medicaid have to meet a single set of quality standards pertaining to the provision of services, residents' rights, and administration. The law also established a new process for State and Federal monitoring of nursing facility compliance with the new Medicaid requirements. OBRA 89 and OBRA 90 contained technical amendments addressing implementation issues arising after enactment of OBRA 87.

6. Limits on Voluntary Contributions and Provider-Specific Taxes

Beginning in 1986, States developed programs to use funds donated by health care providers or taxes paid by these providers to draw greater Federal matching payments. The Congress delayed the Secretary's authority to regulate in this area several times over the 1988-1990 period.

The Medicaid Voluntary Contribution and Provider-Specific Tax Amendments of 1991 prohibited the use of most provider donations or provider taxes that are not "broad-based" (such as taxes imposed solely on Medicaid revenues) although States using such revenues at the time were permitted to phase them out in 1992 and 1993. Total revenues from donations and taxes (whether or not broad-based) are limited to 25 percent of the State's share of Medicaid, again with exceptions for States that were relying more heavily on these revenues. The Act also limited aggregate spending for disproportionate share hospital payment adjustments.

7. Expansion of Penalty, Enforcement, and Intermediate Sanction Remedies

The OBRA 81 authorized the Secretary to impose civil monetary penalties for fraudulent Medicaid and Medicare claims; these were in addition to the criminal penalties already included in the law. OBRA 86 expanded the actions for which such penalties could be imposed. Public Law 100-93 expanded the anti-fraud provisions in the law and clarified the criminal and civil penalty provisions.

The OBRA 87 expanded the remedies available to both the Secretary and the States for the purposes of deterring and sanctioning noncompliance by institutional long-term facilities with Medicaid requirements. The Secretary's new remedies were effective January 1, 1988, with respect to existing requirements for SNFs and ICFs; they were to apply with respect to compliance by nursing facilities with the new requirements when those took effect October 1, 1990. States were required to have the new remedies in place no later than October 1, 1989. The law detailed intermediate remedies (including the imposition of civil monetary penalties) that could be taken if a facility's deficiencies did not immediately jeopardize the health or safety of residents.

This chapter provides a further background on the legislative history of Medicaid since 1980. The discussion is divided into eight parts: eligibility, services, reimbursement, alternative delivery systems, administration, financing, long-term care, and anti-fraud measures. The final section of this chapter outlines the cost estimates made at the time of enactment of the 1981-1990 reconciliation bills and related legislation.

II. ELIGIBILITY

The major eligibility changes incorporated in recent legislation have been first, the expansions in required and optional coverage of low-income pregnant women and children, and second, the expansions in coverage for the low-income elderly and disabled. Recent legislation also included several other modifications to Medicaid eligibility provisions including expanding eligibility for families with a linkage to the Aid to Families With Dependent Children (AFDC) program, giving States more flexibility in designing their medically needy programs, requiring them to cover the working disabled who lose cash assistance, and establishing coverage rules for persons with access to private health insurance. Eligibility modifications for the nursing facility population included strengthening requirements in order to deter financial gaming on the part of those seeking to qualify for nursing home benefits, and protecting a portion of a couple's income and resources for the maintenance needs of the noninstitutionalized spouse.

A. Coverage for Persons With AFDC Linkage

1. Required Coverage for Pregnant Women and Children Meeting AFDC Income and Resources Requirements but Not Otherwise Receiving AFDC or Medicaid

The OBRA 81 included certain limitations on AFDC coverage which had the effect of limiting required Medicaid coverage. It limited AFDC eligibility to children under age 18, or at State option under 19, but only if the child was a full-time student in a secondary or technical school and could reasonably be expected to complete the program before reaching age 19. The law further provided that States could limit Medicaid coverage to any person under age 19 who met the definition of dependent child under AFDC. At State option, States could extend Medicaid to all persons between the ages of 18 and 20 or any reasonable classification of such persons. OBRA 81 also prohibited States from making AFDC cash payments to a pregnant woman on the basis of her unborn child until the sixth month of pregnancy. However, States were permitted to extend Medicaid eligibility to these women from the time pregnancy had been medically verified.

Beginning with DEFRA, major changes occurred in Federal policies relating to the coverage of pregnant women and children. These changes can be divided into two groups--first, those relating to coverage of persons meeting AFDC income and resources requirements but not otherwise eligible for Medicaid, and second, those relating to coverage of persons with incomes above the State AFDC level. (See item B below for discussion of this second group).

The DEFRA required States to cover certain pregnant women and children even though they were not actually receiving cash assistance. DEFRA required States to provide coverage to the following groups of persons meeting State AFDC income and resources requirements:

• First time pregnant women from medical verification of pregnancy;

• Pregnant women in two-parent families where the principal breadwinner was unemployed, from the medical verification of pregnancy; and

• Children born after September 30, 1983, up to age 5.

The DEFRA also provided that a child born to a woman eligible for and receiving Medicaid at the time of birth was deemed eligible for 1 year as long as the woman remained eligible.

The COBRA expanded these provisions by requiring States to provide Medicaid coverage to pregnant women in two-parent families that met AFDC income and resources standards even where the principal breadwinner was not unemployed. COBRA also specified that States were not required to extend comparable benefits to other beneficiaries when they provide additional services related to pregnancy to all pregnant women. States were required to provide post-partum coverage to eligible pregnant women until the end of the 60 day period beginning on the last day of their pregnancy.

The OBRA 87 further expanded the required coverage of children meeting the income and resources requirements of the State's Medicaid plan. A State was required to extend Medicaid coverage to all such children under age 7 (or at State option under age 8) born after September 30, 1983.

The OBRA 90 required States to continue eligibility through the 60 day post-partum period to pregnant women who would otherwise lose eligibility due to a change in income. Further, States were required to extend eligibility for a year for an infant born to a Medicaid eligible woman so long as the infant remained in the woman's household and the woman would remain Medicaid eligible if still pregnant.

2. Expanded Coverage for Families

a. Transitional Medicaid Coverage for Working Poor Families

The FSA expanded the Medicaid protection available to families who leave cash assistance due to earnings. Prior law had required States to provide Medicaid coverage for 4 additional months to families who lost AFDC due to earnings. It also provided for a 9 month Medicaid extension, which could be extended for an additional 6 months for families that lost AFDC because they no longer qualified for one of the AFDC time limited monthly income disregards. FSA established new requirements effective for the period April 1, 1990-September 30, 1998. States were required to provide 6 months of extended coverage to each family that received assistance in at least 3 of the 6 months preceding the month the family lost assistance due to either increased employment hours or income of the caretaker relative or a family member's loss of one of the time-limited AFDC monthly income disregards. States were required to provide full Medicaid coverage or alternatively provide "wrap around coverage." Under this option, States could pay the family's expenses for premiums, deductibles, and coinsurance for any health care coverage offered by the employer of the caretaker relative (with direct coverage available for any services not offered by the third party plan).

The FSA further provided that families covered during the entire first 6-month extension period, and earning below 185 percent of the poverty line, would qualify for a second 6 month extension period. During this period States were given a number of options. They could offer regular Medicaid benefits or limit coverage to acute care services. They could provide wrap around coverage. They could also offer to enroll families in alternative coverage such as an employer or state employee plan, a state uninsured plan, or an Health Maintenance Organization (HMO). The Act further permitted States to impose premiums for the second 6-month extension period if the family's income exceeded the poverty line. Premiums were limited to 3 percent of the family's average gross monthly earnings. TAMRA clarified that the premium could not exceed 3 percent of the family's average gross monthly earnings less the average monthly costs for child care necessary to accommodate the caretaker relative's employment.

b. Coverage of Families With Unemployed Parents

The FSA required all States, effective October 1, 1990, to extend cash assistance benefits to two-parent families where the principal earner was unemployed. States that had such a program as of September 26, 1988, were required to continue operating such programs. Other States were permitted to limit cash assistance coverage to 6 months in any 12 month period. However, the Act required all States to provide full Medicaid coverage to all family members even in months where cash assistance was not paid due to a State-established time limit. FSA specified that this requirement was effective through September 30, 1998.

B. **Expansions in Coverage for Low-Income Pregnant Women, Infants, and Children**

Beginning in 1986, legislation was enacted which significantly expanded the numbers of low-income pregnant women, infants and children eligible for Medicaid. Initially, this expanded coverage was optional with the States. More recently, many of the expansions became mandatory.

The OBRA 86 created a new *optional* categorically needy group composed of pregnant women, infants up to age 1, and on an incremental basis, children up to age 5 with family incomes below a State established level. States could choose an income level between the AFDC level and 100 percent of the Federal poverty line. Imposition of resource standards was optional with the States. The provision was effective April 1, 1987 for pregnant women and infants. Beginning in FY 1988, States could increase the age level by one in each fiscal year until all children under age 5 were included. States could not elect to cover one age group unless all younger age groups were covered.

The OBRA 87 included provisions which allowed States to expand the scope of coverage under this provision. It permitted States to accelerate coverage of children under age 5 whose income was below the poverty line. Effective July 1, 1988, States could cover children under age 2, 3, 4, or 5 (as selected by the State) who were born after September 30, 1983. Effective October 1, 1988, States could expand coverage to children under age 8 born after September 30, 1983. States would thus be able to cover all such children by FY 1991.

The OBRA 87 also permitted States, effective July 1, 1988 to increase the State-established income level for pregnant women and infants (up to age 1) with incomes up to 185 percent of the Federal poverty level. States could impose a premium for such coverage. The amount of the premium could not exceed 10 percent of the amount by which the family's income (less child care expenses) exceeded 150 percent of the poverty line for a comparable sized family.

Beginning in 1988, legislation was enacted which mandated coverage for certain pregnant women and infants whose coverage was previously optional with the States. MCCA required States to phase-in coverage of pregnant women and infants with incomes below 100 percent of the poverty line. Effective July 1, 1989, States were required to cover such persons with incomes at or below 75 percent of poverty and effective July 1, 1990, States were required to cover those with incomes below 100 percent of poverty.

The OBRA 89 required States, effective April 1, 1990, to extend Medicaid coverage to all pregnant women and children up to age six with family incomes below 133 1/3 percent of the Federal poverty level.

The OBRA 89 further required the Secretary to conduct demonstration projects in several States for the purposes of developing innovative programs to extend health insurance coverage to uninsured pregnant women and their children under age 20 and of encouraging workers to obtain health insurance for themselves and their children. Federal financial participation was limited to $10 million in each of the fiscal years 1990, 1991, and 1992.

The OBRA 90 required States, effective July 1, 1991, to provide Medicaid coverage to all children under age 19 born after September 30, 1983 in families with incomes at or below 100 percent of the Federal poverty level. Thus, all poor children under age 19 would be covered by the year 2002.

The OBRA 90 provided for demonstration projects in up to four States to test the effect of eliminating categorical Medicaid eligibility requirements for individuals with family incomes below 150 percent of the Federal poverty level.

C. Coverage of Elderly and Disabled Poor

The OBRA 86 also created a new optional categorically needy coverage group composed of the aged and disabled with family incomes up to a State-established level that did not exceed 100 percent of the Federal poverty line. A State choosing this option would have to offer the benefit package available to other categorically needy persons. As an alternative, States could cover just the Medicare cost-sharing charges for this population group. (This is sometimes referred to as buy-in coverage). In either case, States would be required to use the Supplemental Security Income (SSI) resource standards, except that if it had a medically needy program with higher standards it could use the higher standards for the new group. A State electing expanded coverage of the aged and disabled would be required to cover some newly eligible pregnant women and infants (as described in item B above). States could begin offering expanded coverage under this provision effective July 1, 1987.

Beginning in 1988, legislation was enacted which required States to phase-in buy-in coverage for poor Medicare beneficiaries with incomes below the poverty line. Specifically, MCCA required States to pay Medicare premiums, deductibles and coinsurance for elderly and disabled individuals whose incomes were at or below the poverty line and whose non-exempt resources were at or below twice the resource standard used under the SSI program. Persons receiving benefits under this provision became known as qualified Medicare beneficiaries or QMBs. In all but five States the income standard would be phased-in over 4 years with coverage extended as follows:

- January 1989--persons with incomes at or below 85 percent of poverty;

- January 1, 1990--persons with incomes at or below 90 percent of poverty;

- January 1, 1991--persons with incomes at or below 95 percent of poverty; and

- January 1, 1992--all persons with incomes below 100 percent of poverty.

In the five States using Medicaid income criteria more restrictive than SSI, the threshold would be set at 80 percent of poverty on January 1, 1989, increasing 5 percentage points each year.

The TAMRA deleted the provision limiting QMB coverage to persons otherwise ineligible for Medicaid. OBRA 89 clarified that the provision applied in "209(b)" States.

The OBRA 90 accelerated the implementation of the MCCA provision. The income standard was increased to 100 percent of poverty effective January 1, 1991; in the five States using more restrictive criteria than SSI, the standard was raised to 95 percent on January 1, 1991 and 100 percent on January 1, 1992. OBRA 90 also required States to cover Medicare Part B premiums (but no other Medicare cost-sharing charges) for certain low-income Medicare beneficiaries with assets at or below twice the SSI level. These are persons with incomes below 110 percent of poverty in 1993 and 1994 and below 120 percent of poverty in 1995 and thereafter.

The MCCA had also provided, beginning January 1, 1991, Medicare catastrophic prescription drug coverage, subject to specified deductible and coinsurance charges. MCCA required State Medicaid programs, on the same phase-in schedule applicable to other benefits, to pay the additional deductibles and coinsurance amounts for Medicare beneficiaries. The law gave States the option of meeting the prescription drug deductible requirement by either covering incurred drug charges below the Medicare deductible or providing the same drug coverage as the State offered to its Medicaid beneficiaries. P.L.101-234 repealed both the provision providing for Medicare catastrophic prescription drug coverage and the related Medicaid provision.

D. Coverage of the Disabled

1. Medicaid Coverage of Home Care for Certain Disabled Children

The TEFRA allowed States to extend Medicaid coverage to certain disabled children under age 18 who were living at home and would be eligible for SSI (and therefore Medicaid) if they were institutionalized. The State was required to determine that the (a) the child required the level of care provided in an institution; (b) it was appropriate to provide such care outside the facility; and (c) the cost of the care at home was no more than institutional care.

2. Working Disabled

The OBRA 86 required States to continue Medicaid coverage for disabled persons with severe impairments who lost their eligibility for cash assistance because of earnings from work. A "qualified severely impaired individual" was one who: (a) was under 65; (b) in the month preceding the first month this provision applied, received cash assistance benefits or special benefits under Section 1619 of the Social Security Act; and (c) received Medicaid benefits. Further such individual: (a) had to continue to be blind or have a disabling physical or mental impairment; (b) had to meet, except for earnings, all other requirements for SSI eligibility; and (c) would have been seriously inhibited from continuing work in the absence of Medicaid coverage; and (d) did not have earnings that would be sufficient to provide a reasonable equivalent of the Medicaid, SSI or publicly funded attendant care benefits that would be available if he did not work. This provision paralleled the section in Public Law 99-643, the SSI Improvement Amendments of 1986 which revised and extended on a permanent basis the authority contained in Section 1619 of the Social Security Act.

The OBRA 89 required States, effective July 1, 1990, to pay Medicare Part A premiums for certain working disabled persons not otherwise eligible for Medicaid. These were individuals with incomes below 200 percent of the poverty level and resources less than twice the maximum allowable under the SSI program. States were permitted to charge a premium for persons whose incomes were above 150 percent of the poverty level. The premium was to be set based on a sliding scale from zero percent (at 150 percent of poverty) to 100 percent (at 200 percent of poverty).

3. HIV Infected Persons

The OBRA 90 directed the Secretary to establish demonstration projects in two States for the purpose of providing coverage for a broad range of services, in addition to the standard Medicaid benefit package, to individuals who are infected with the HIV virus and whose income and resources do not exceed levels set by the State for Medicaid beneficiaries.

E. Coverage of Other Persons

1. Homeless

Homelessness does not automatically qualify an individual for Medicaid. However, OBRA 86 clarified that if an individual was otherwise qualified, States or localities could not impose any residence requirement which excluded from Medicaid an individual who resided in the State, regardless of whether the residence was maintained permanently or at a fixed address.

2. Aliens

The OBRA 86 specified that Federal matching payments were not available for State expenditures for aliens who were not lawfully admitted for permanent residence or permanently residing in the U.S. under color of law (e.g., certain aliens admitted pursuant to the discretionary authority of the Attorney General). An exception was made for services provided to an individual who was otherwise eligible for Medicaid and had an emergency medical condition, including emergency labor and delivery.

The Immigration Reform and Control Act of 1986 (Public Law 99-603) provided that aliens who lived in the country continuously since January 1, 1982 could apply for legalization. If their status was adjusted to lawful temporary resident (LTR) status they were immediately eligible for Medicaid (provided they met the appropriate financial and categorical criteria) only if the following conditions were met. They had to be under 18, a Cuban-Haitian entrant, or aged, blind, or disabled as defined under the SSI program. A LTR alien, meeting the appropriate financial and categorical requirements but not falling into one of these groups, was only eligible for emergency services or services for pregnant women. These persons could be eligible for the full range of Medicaid benefits beginning 5 years after they were granted LTR status.

F. Coverage of and Services for the Medically Needy

1. Expanded Flexibility for States

The OBRA 81 modified existing law pertaining to conditions a State had to meet if it chose to offer coverage to its medically needy population. It repealed the requirements that: (1) coverage had to be provided to all medically needy groups (i.e., aged, blind, disabled, and members of families with dependent children); (2) services for all medically needy groups had to be comparable in amount, duration, and scope; (3) States had to offer a minimum set of services to this population group; and (4) States had to offer a mix of institutional and noninstitutional care and services. OBRA 81 placed the following requirements on State medically needy programs. If a State provided medically needy coverage for any population group, it had to provide ambulatory services for children and prenatal and delivery services for pregnant women. If a State provided institutional services for any medically needy group, it was also required to provide ambulatory services for this population. Further, if a State provided medically needy coverage for persons in intermediate care facilities for the mentally retarded (ICFs/MR), it had to offer to all covered medically needy groups a minimum set of services, as required under prior law.

2. Medicaid Moratorium

The TEFRA amended the Medicaid statute to clarify that Congress did not intend to change the policies governing income and resources standards and methodologies for determining eligibility of the medically needy from those in effect prior to OBRA 81. The TEFRA provision specified that the methodology to be used in determining income and resource eligibility for the medically needy was to be the same as that used under the relevant cash assistance program. The DEFRA conference report stated that a strict interpretation of this provision led to unintended consequences. DEFRA therefore established a moratorium period during which the Secretary was directed not to take any compliance, disallowance penalty or other regulatory action against a State because a State in determining eligibility for noncash Medicaid eligibles was using an income or resource standard or methodology that was less restrictive than the applicable cash assistance standard or methodology. The Secretary was directed to report to Congress within 12 months of enactment on the impact on States and beneficiaries of applying income and resources standards and methodologies under the cash assistance programs to noncash eligibles. The moratorium was to run until 18 months after submission of the report.

The MCCA clarified that the moratorium applied to any State Medicaid plan change submitted to the Secretary either before or after enactment of DEFRA whether or not approved, disapproved, acted on or not acted on. The law further provided that noncash eligibles included noncash categorically needy recipients. It also specified that during the moratorium period an institutionalized person could sell his home in the same manner that applied at the beginning of the moratorium.

The MCCA provided, retroactive to October 1, 1982, that States had the flexibility to establish income and resource methodologies under medically needy, optional categorically needy, and under the "209(b)" option that were less restrictive, i.e., more generous, than those applied in the corresponding cash program. This provision has been used by States to cover individuals whose resources and/or income would not otherwise allow them to be covered.

3. Income Level

The OBRA 89 prohibited the Secretary from issuing final regulations to reduce medically needy income levels for single individuals before December 31,1990. OBRA 90 permitted States which already did so to continue to base their medically needy income limit for a family of one on the AFDC maximum payment for a family of two.

4. Spenddown

The OBRA 90 permitted States to allow individuals to establish medically needy eligibility by making monthly premium payments to the States.

G. Provisions Affecting Eligibility for Nursing Home Benefits

1. Modifications in Lien and Transfer of Assets Provisions

The TEFRA modified prior law provisions pertaining to liens and transfer of assets. TEFRA permitted States to impose liens on real property of institutionalized Medicaid beneficiaries who the State determined, after notice and opportunity for a hearing, were reasonably likely to remain in a nursing home for the remainder of their lives. States were not permitted to impose a lien on the home of a beneficiary if the spouse, child under 21, disabled child, or sibling with an equity interest was residing in the home. The lien dissolved if the individual was discharged from the institution and returned home.

The TEFRA specified that a State could not foreclose on a lien until the beneficiary voluntarily sold his property or until after his death. Foreclosure actions could not be taken until after the death of the surviving spouse and/or any children who were blind or disabled; protection was offered for additional family members where the lien had been imposed on the individual's home.

The TEFRA also expanded existing transfer of assets provisions. It permitted States, subject to certain exceptions, to deny Medicaid eligibility for 24 months to institutionalized persons who, within 24 months prior to application for Medicaid, disposed of their homes for less than fair market value even though such disposal would not have made them ineligible for SSI. States could deny eligibility for a longer period if the uncompensated value was greater than the cost of 24 months of care. They were required to set a shorter period if the uncompensated value was less than the value of 24 months of care.

The MCCA provided, effective with respect to transfers occurring on or after July 1, 1988, that States were required to determine, at the time of application for Medicaid benefits, whether an institutionalized individual had disposed of resources for less than fair market value within the preceding 30 months. Where such a disposal occurred, States were required to delay Medicaid eligibility for the number of months equal the quotient of the uncompensated value of the transferred assets divided by the cost of nursing home care. MCCA further repealed existing SSI transfer-of-assets provisions with respect to cash assistance benefits; the new Medicaid rules were to be applied in considering an individual's eligibility for Medicaid if and when such individual entered a medical institution or nursing facility.

The FSA provided that the determination of whether a disposal of resources had occurred was to be made at the point the individual became institutionalized if the individual was Medicaid eligible; otherwise the determination was to be made at the point of application.

The OBRA 89 provided that the transfer prohibitions also applied to the spouse of the institutionalized individual.

2. Treatment of Potential Payments from Medicaid Qualifying Trusts

The COBRA added potential payments from "Medicaid qualifying trusts" to the list of income and resources available to an individual and therefore considered in determining eligibility. A qualifying trust was defined as one which had been established (other than by a will) by an individual under which the individual could be the beneficiary of part or all of the payments from the trust and the distribution of such payments was determined by one or more trustees who were permitted to exercise any discretion with respect to the amount distributed to the individual. Distributions were to be considered available to the individual whether or not they were actually made.

The OBRA 86 clarified that the COBRA provision relating to the treatment of income from certain trusts did not apply to such trusts if they were established before April 7, 1986, solely for the benefit of residents of ICFs/MR.

3. Personal Needs Allowance

The OBRA 87 raised the monthly personal needs allowance for nursing home residents from $25 to $30.

4. Protection of Income and Resources of Couple for Maintenance Needs of Community Spouse

The MCCA included provisions intended to protect against so-called spousal impoverishment. The law provided that after an institutionalized individual had established eligibility for Medicaid, the State would be required to allow the community spouse to receive a certain portion of the institutionalized spouse's income. The amount had to be sufficient to raise the community spouse's monthly income to at least: 122 percent of the poverty level for a couple, effective September 30, 1989; 133 percent of such level, effective July 1, 1991, and 150 percent of such level, effective July 1, 1992. The monthly protected income could not exceed $1,500 (as adjusted after 1989 for inflation), except where a higher level was determined necessary by a fair hearing or court order.

The MCCA also included provisions relating to protection of resources. Effective September 30, 1989, States were required, in making eligibility determinations for institutionalized persons, to total all nonexempt resources held by either the community spouse or the institutionalized spouse and divide them equally. States would be required to protect a minimum of $12,000 for the community spouse; they could raise the minimum to $60,000. The community spouse's share could not exceed $60,000, except where a higher amount was provided under a fair hearing or court order. These income levels are indexed for inflation in subsequent years.

Both OBRA 89 and OBRA 90 contained technical modifications to the spousal impoverishment provisions. OBRA 90 clarified that State community property laws applied to redeterminations of eligibility but not post-eligibility of income. Further, it specified that computation of the spousal share would occur only once at the beginning of the first continuous period of institutionalization.

5. Beginning Date of Optional Coverage for Individuals in Medical Institutions

The COBRA clarified that Medicaid payment could begin at the beginning of any 30 consecutive day period of institutionalization in the case of institutionalized persons for whom a State applied a special income standard.

H. Coverage of Persons With Access to Private Health Insurance

1. Medicaid Payment of Premiums and Cost-Sharing for Enrollment Under Group Health Plans

The OBRA 90 required States to purchase group health insurance coverage for Medicaid beneficiaries where cost effective as defined by the Secretary. States would be required to pay the requisite premiums and cost-sharing charges for services otherwise covered under Medicaid and to furnish "wrap around" coverage to insure that beneficiaries had the full scope of Medicaid benefits. The provision was effective January 1, 1991.

2. Medicaid Payment of Premiums for COBRA Continuation Coverage

The COBRA, as amended, requires an employer with 20 or more employees to provide his or her employees and their families the option of continued coverage under the employer's group health plan in the case of certain designated events. Such events include lay offs or death of or divorce from the covered worker. Coverage is extended for 18 or 36 months depending on the nature of the event. The employer is not required to pay for the coverage. OBRA 90 permitted Medicaid coverage of premiums for COBRA continuation coverage offered by employers with 75 or more employees. This coverage could be extended to individuals with incomes at or below 100 percent of poverty and resources at or below twice the SSI level. The coverage could only be provided where the State determined that anticipated Medicaid savings would exceed premium costs.

III. SERVICES

Legislation enacted over the 1980-1990 period expanded the list of mandated services to include nurse midwife services, nurse practitioner services, federally qualified health center services, and personal care services. The list of optional services was also expanded. Services States may offer include hospice care, targeted case management and home respiratory care for ventilator dependent persons.

The OBRA 90 established two programs within Medicaid that cap Federal matching payments for FY 1991-FY 1995. The first permits States to provide home and community-based services to functionally disabled persons otherwise eligible for Medicaid. The second permits States to provide community-supported living arrangements services to persons with mental retardation or related conditions.

A. Mandated Services

1. Nurse Midwife Services

The OBRA 80 required States to provide coverage for services furnished by a nurse midwife that he or she is legally authorized to perform whether or not he or she is under the supervision of, or associated with a physician or other health care provider.

2. Federally Qualified Health Center Services

The OBRA 89 mandated coverage of certain services which had previously been optional with the States. Under the mandate, States were required to cover ambulatory services provided by federally qualified health centers (FQHCs). These centers were defined as community health centers, migrant health centers, or health care for the homeless programs. Also included were clinics that met the standards of these programs but were not actually receiving grant funds. States were required to pay these centers 100 percent of their reasonable costs for providing covered services. OBRA 90 included, within the definition of FQHCs an outpatient health program or facility operated by a tribe or tribal organization under the Indian Self-Determination Act.

3. Nurse Practitioner Services

The OBRA 89 required States, effective July 1, 1990, to cover services of certified pediatric nurse practitioners and certified family nurse practitioners practicing within the scope of State law. Services were to be covered regardless of whether or not the individual was under the supervision of, or associated with, a physician.

4. Personal Care Services

The OBRA 90 expanded the definition of home health services to include coverage of personal care services, effective FY 1995. Such services were defined as those which are prescribed by a physician, provided by a qualified provider who is not a family member, supervised by a registered nurse and furnished in a home or other location which is not a hospital or nursing facility.

B. Optional Services

1. Hospice Benefits

The COBRA allowed States to cover hospice care as an optional service for terminally ill individuals who elected to receive hospice care and waived their eligibility for certain other benefits. The definitions of hospice care and hospice program were the same as those used under Medicare, except States could define the length of coverage.

The OBRA 87 provided that for Medicaid services only, a hospice could exclude inpatient care provided to acquired immune deficiency syndrome (AIDS) patients from the law's 20 percent inpatient day limit.

2. Case Management

The COBRA added targeted case management services to the list of covered Medicaid services and allowed States to cover such services without regard to the statewideness or comparability requirements. OBRA 86 provided that States were allowed to limit the provision of services to individuals with AIDS or with AIDS-related conditions, or with either. A State could also limit the provision of case management services to persons with chronic mental illness. OBRA 87 permitted States to limit case managers available for persons with developmental disabilities or chronic mental illness in order to assure that case managers were capable of ensuring that such persons received needed services.

The TAMRA specified that a State could not refuse to approve a State plan amendment or deny State payment for case management services on the basis that either State law required State provision of such services or that the State is or was paying for such services from nonfederal funds.

3. Technology-Dependent Persons

The COBRA required the Secretary to establish a task force concerning alternatives to institutional care for technology dependent children. The task force was required to report to the Secretary and the Congress within 2 years of enactment.

The OBRA 86 permitted States to provide optional coverage of respiratory care services in the home for individuals who: (a) were medically dependent on a ventilator for life support at least 6 hours a day; (b) were so dependent at least 30 days as inpatients; (c) had adequate social support services at home; (d) wished to be cared for at home; and (e) in the absence of such care would require respiratory care on an inpatient basis for which Medicaid would pay.

4. Optional Home and Community-Based Services for the Frail Elderly

The OBRA 90 established a new program within Medicaid to permit States to provide home and community-based services to functionally disabled elderly persons otherwise eligible for Medicaid. A functionally disabled person was defined as a person who is (a) unable to perform two of out of three of the following activities of daily living: toiletting, transferring, or eating; or (b) has a primary or secondary diagnosis of Alzheimer's disease and is unable to perform at least two of the five activities of daily living. The law specified that services covered under the option were to be furnished in accordance with a community plan of care developed by a case manager. Covered services included homemaker/home health aide services, chore services, personal care services, nursing care services, respite care services, training for family members, and adult day care. The law required the Secretary to establish minimum quality standards for providers and for settings where services are provided. Federal expenditures under this provision were capped at $580 million over the FY 1991-FY 1995 period. Money was to be allocated by the Secretary to States electing this option. In making the allocations, the Secretary was directed to take into account the number of aged persons in the State

5. Community-Supported Living Arrangements

The OBRA 90 established a new program within Medicaid to permit States to provide community-supported living arrangement services to persons with mental retardation or related conditions. Services covered under the provision were personal assistance, training and rehabilitation, emergency assistance, assistive technology, adaptive equipment, support services and other services specified by the Secretary (excluding room and board and the cost of prevocational, vocational and supported employment). Eligible individuals were persons living with a family or legal guardian in their own home in which no more than three other persons receiving such services resided. Between two and eight States could elect this option. OBRA 90 required States electing the option to maintain existing spending levels for such services and to establish and maintain a quality assurance program. Federal expenditures were capped at $100 million over the FY 1991-FY 1995 period.

C. Requirements for Services

1. Organ Transplants

The COBRA prohibited Federal matching for organ transplant procedures unless: (1) the State plan provided written standards for coverage; and (2) the standards provided that similarly situated individuals were treated alike and any restrictions placed on providers who could provide the care were consistent with access to high quality care.

The OBRA 87 clarified that if a State covered organ transplants, such services had to be sufficient in amount, duration, and scope to achieve their purpose.

2. Early and Periodic Screening, Diagnostic, and Treatment Services

The OBRA 89 established a statutory definition for required early and periodic screening, diagnostic, and treatment (EPSDT) services. Under the definition, States were required to provide screening, vision, dental, and hearing services. They were required to provide necessary health care, diagnostic services, treatment and other services to correct physical or mental defects found, regardless of whether the follow-up services were generally covered under the State's Medicaid plan. The Secretary was required to establish annual participation goals (beginning by July 1, 1990). States were required to report annually to the Secretary on the number of children who were provided services, referred for treatment, or receiving dental services. Further, States were required to report results in meeting annual participation goals.

3. Day Habilitation Services

The OBRA 89 prohibited the Secretary from denying Federal funding for day habilitation services for the mentally retarded until final regulations were issued. The prohibition applied to services provided under a State plan amendment approved on or before June 30, 1989.

4. Rehabilitation Services

The OBRA 90 codified the existing regulatory definition of rehabilitation services. Such services were defined as those that are provided in a facility, home or other setting for the maximum reduction of physical or mental disability and restoration of the individual to the best possible functional level.

5. Physicians' Services

The OBRA 90 included several provisions relating to the quality of physicians' services. It required the Secretary to establish a unique identifier for each physician providing Medicaid services which would be used on all claims submitted for physicians services by July 1, 1991. It also established, effective January 1, 1992, minimum qualifications, other than State licensure, which physicians must meet in order to receive payment for services provided to Medicaid eligible children or pregnant women.

D. Cost-sharing

The TEFRA modified prior cost-sharing requirements by permitting States to impose cost-sharing charges for all persons for all services with certain exceptions. States were prohibited from imposing such charges on services provided to children under age 18, services related to pregnancy, services provided to inpatients of SNFs and ICFs (subsequently changed to nursing facilities and ICFs/MR), family planning or emergency services, and categorically needy HMO enrolles. TEFRA specified that if a State imposed cost-sharing charges on other Medicaid beneficiaries they had to be nominal in amount. The Secretary could waive the nominality requirement in the case of nonemergency services in emergency rooms where the State had established, to the satisfaction of the Secretary, that alternative sources of nonemergency services were actually available and accessible. The Secretary could approve other waivers of cost-sharing requirements only for 2 years and only if certain specified conditions were met.

IV. REIMBURSEMENT

Prior to 1990, the major reimbursement changes related to calculation of payment rates for institutional services. Several laws addressed the calculation of rates for hospitals serving a disproportionate number of low-income patients.

The OBRA 90 substantially reformed Medicaid reimbursement for outpatient prescription drugs in all States. It denied Federal matching funds for all of a manufacturer's products in any State unless the manufacturer enters into, and complied with, an agreement to provide each State periodic rebates on the manufacturer's products purchased for Medicaid beneficiaries in the State.

A. Reimbursement of Hospitals

Prior to enactment of OBRA 81, States were required to reimburse hospitals on a reasonable cost basis as then defined under Medicare unless they had approval to use an alternative payment method. OBRA 81 required instead that State payments for inpatient hospital services be reasonable and adequate to meet the costs which must be incurred by efficiently and economically operated facilities in order to meet State and Federal laws, regulations, and quality and safety standards. The law required States, in developing their payment rates to take into account the situation of hospitals serving a disproportionate number of low-income patients. Further, the payment rates were to be sufficient to assure that Medicaid patients had reasonable access (taking into account geographic location and reasonable travel time) to services of adequate quality.

The COBRA required the Secretary to submit a report to Congress by October 1, 1986 which (1) described the methodology used by States to take into account the situation of hospitals serving a disproportionate number of low-income patients; and (2) identified the hospitals that received a disproportionate share adjustment and specified the proportion of low-income and Medicaid patients at such hospitals.

The OBRA 86 provided that nothing in the Medicaid law was to be construed as authorizing the Secretary to limit the amount of payment adjustments that could be made under a State Medicaid plan with respect to hospitals serving a disproportionate number of low-income patients with special needs.

The OBRA 87 implemented the requirement that States take into account the situation of hospitals serving a disproportionate number of low-income patients with special needs. It required States, by July 1, 1988, to submit a Medicaid plan amendment that defined disproportionate share hospitals and provided for an appropriate increase in the payment rate for inpatient services provided by these hospitals. A hospital would be deemed a disproportionate share hospital if: (a) its Medicaid inpatient utilization rate was in excess of one standard deviation above the mean rate for the State; or (b) it had a low-income utilization rate of 25 percent. Payment adjustments would be phased in over a 3 year period.

The MCCA provided that States which imposed durational limits on Medicaid payments for inpatient hospital services had to establish exceptions to such limits in the case of medically necessary inpatient services received by an infant (up to age 1) in a disproportionate share hospital. The law further provided that if a State paid for inpatient hospital services on a prospective basis, it must provide for an outlier share adjustment for disproportionate share hospitals providing medically necessary inpatient services for infants.

The OBRA 90 prohibited States from limiting the duration of coverage or denying outlier payments in reimbursing for hospital services provided to Medicaid-eligible children up to age 6 in disproportionate share hospitals and infants in all hospitals.

The OBRA 90 further required inclusion of Medicaid nursery, psychiatric, and administrative days for purposes of determining eligibility for and amount of disproportionate share payments.

The OBRA 90 provided that a State could use a formula resulting in different payments to different types of disproportionate share hospitals. Payments were to be reasonably related to costs, volume, or services provided to Medicaid or low-income patients served by that type of hospital.

The Medicaid Voluntary Contribution and Provider-Specific Tax Amendments of 1991 limited national aggregate spending for disproportionate share payment adjustments to 12 percent of total Medicaid program spending, roughly the level projected for FY 1992. States with payments already exceeding 12 percent could not increase those payments; other States could do so, subject to the national cap.

B. Reimbursement of Skilled Nursing and Intermediate Care Facilities

Prior to the enactment of OBRA 80, States were required to pay SNFs and ICFs on a reasonable cost-related basis in accordance with methods and standards developed by the State on the basis of cost-finding methods approved and verified by the Secretary. OBRA 80 required instead that States reimburse such facilities at rates that are reasonable and adequate to meet the cost which must be incurred by efficiently and economically operated facilities in order to provide care in conformity with applicable State and Federal laws, regulations, and quality and safety standards.

The OBRA 87 contained major nursing home reform provisions for both Medicare and Medicaid. Effective October 1, 1990, the existing distinction between SNFs and ICFs was eliminated as was the requirement that States pay less for ICF services than for SNF services.

The OBRA 87 specified that nursing facility rates must be sufficient to take into account the costs of complying with the new nursing facility requirements. OBRA 90 clarified that these costs include the costs of services required to attain or maintain the highest practicable physical, mental, and psychosocial well-being of each Medicaid-eligible resident.

C. Flexibility in Setting Payment Rates for Hospitals Furnishing Long-Term Care Services

The DEFRA modified the requirements pertaining to establishment of payment rates for small rural hospitals furnishing long-term care services by permitting States to use the special payment rates or alternatively the same criteria generally applicable for payment of long-term care services.

D. Payment for Hospice Services

The OBRA 86 clarified rules for payment with respect to an individual, who was eligible for both Medicare and Medicaid, resided in a SNF or ICF, was having Medicaid payments made on his/her behalf for such institutional services, elected Medicare hospice coverage, and resided in a State which did not cover hospice services under Medicaid. The SNF or ICF and the hospice must have entered into a written agreement under which the program took full responsibility for the professional management of the individual's hospice care and the facility agreed to provide room and board. In such circumstances, the State was directed to pay the Hospice program an amount equal to the amounts allocated under Medicaid for room and board in a SNF or ICF, plus applicable coinsurance amounts.

The OBRA 89 specified that States providing hospice services to terminally ill nursing facility residents were required to include in the payment to the hospice an additional amount equal to at least 95 percent of the rate that would have been paid by the State to the facility for the beneficiary.

E. Payment for Obstetrical and Pediatric Services

The OBRA 89 codified the existing regulatory requirement that payments for services must be sufficient to enlist enough providers so that care and services are available to Medicaid beneficiaries at least to the same extent that they are available to the general population in the area.

The OBRA 89 further required each State to submit by April 1, of each year State plan amendments specifying payment rates for noninstitutional obstetrical and pediatric care.

F. Outpatient Prescription Drugs

The OBRA 90 made significant changes in the way Medicaid reimburses for outpatient prescription drugs, effective January 1, 1991. The law barred Federal matching funds for outpatient prescription drugs unless the manufacturer had entered into and had in effect a rebate agreement. The law required rebates to be calculated on a drug-by-drug basis for 3 years after which rebates would be calculated on an aggregate basis. States were required to cover all rebated drugs of manufacturers entering into rebate agreements. However, States could exclude specified categories of drugs from coverage. States were also permitted to subject any covered drug to prior authorization provided its procedures provided for response within 24 hours of a request and provided for dispensing of at least a 72-hour supply in an emergency situation.

The law required manufacturers to enter into an agreement with the Secretary on behalf of the States, except that the Secretary could authorize the State to enter directly into an agreement with the manufacturer. Agreements existing at the time of enactment could be considered to be in compliance provided there was a minimum rebate of 10 percent. OBRA 90 specified how rebates were to be calculated. It specified that there would be a basic rebate and an additional rebate for single source and innovator multiple source drugs (brand name drugs). The basic rebate would equal the number of dosage units dispensed times the greater of: (1) the difference between the average manufacturer price (AMP) and 87.5 percent of such price (85 percent beginning in 1993) for the quarter, or (2) the difference between the AMP and the manufacturers best price. The basic rebate was capped at 25 percent in 1991 and 50 percent in 1992. The additional rebate would be calculated to recover any increases in the AMP exceeding general inflation increases after October 1, 1990.

The OBRA 90 specified that the amount of the rebate for other drugs (generic and over the counter) was equal to the number of dosage units times 10 percent of the AMP for the first 3 years and 11 percent thereafter.

The OBRA 90 further barred Federal matching funds for outpatient prescription drugs after January 1, 1993 unless a State had in place a drug utilization review program which complied with minimum standards for prospective review, retrospective review, and educational outreach. The program would assess drug use data against predetermined standards and take remedial action as necessary.

Some manufacturers reportedly responded to the requirement that they offer Medicaid their "best price" by raising the prices charged to other purchasers, such as hospitals and HMOs, instead of lowering the price to Medicaid. The DVA, which long enjoyed steep discounts on certain drugs, reported significant price increases in 1991. The Veterans Health Care Act of 1992 excluded from the determination of best price, effective October 1, 1992, the prices charged by manufacturers to the DVA, the Department of Defense, the PHS and various PHS-funded health programs, and State (non-Medicaid) pharmacy assistance programs. The Act also provided, as a condition of Medicaid reimbursement for a manufacturer's drugs after January 1, 1993, that the manufacturer enter into an agreement with the Secretary to provide discounts and rebates to certain PHS-funded entities and public disproportionate share hospitals, as well as enter into a new discount agreement with DVA.

G. Revaluation of Assets

The DEFRA specified that Medicare payments to providers could not be increased to reflect higher capital costs that resulted solely from the sale of a facility. Capital costs to the new owner were to be the lesser of the historical cost (less depreciation) or the acquisition cost. Medicaid payments were subject to similar limits. COBRA amended the Medicaid provision to allow a State's aggregate cost payments to SNFs and ICFs to reflect increases in valuation due to their change in ownership, subject to certain limits.

H. Payment for Physicians' Services

The OBRA 81 removed the prior law requirement that payment for physicians' and certain other services could not exceed the reasonable charge levels as defined under Medicare.

The OBRA 90 permitted a physician to bill for services provided on a temporary basis to his or her patients by another physician.

I. Treatment of Educationally-Related Services

The MCCA specified that Federal matching funds were available for the cost of services furnished in connection with the Education of the Handicapped Act (provided the services were covered under a State's Medicaid program). Services which could be covered under Medicaid were either those furnished to a handicapped child pursuant to a child's individual education program established under the Act or services furnished to a handicapped infant or toddler which were included in the child's individualized family service plan adopted pursuant to that Act.

V. ALTERNATIVE DELIVERY SYSTEMS

The OBRA 81 included several provisions designed to give States increased flexibility in the design and implementation of their Medicaid plans. The most significant of these were two waiver authorities: the freedom-of-choice waiver and the home and community-based services waiver. OBRA 87 established a separate waiver authority that allowed States, on a budget neutral basis, to provide a mix of home and community-based and institutional services to the elderly at risk of nursing home care.

During the 1981-1990 period the Congress also approved a number of waivers for individual States to test various alternative delivery approaches.

A. Inapplicability of Freedom-of-Choice and Other State Plan Requirements

The OBRA 81 authorized the Secretary to waive certain State plan requirements as might be necessary to achieve certain program purposes. These so-called "2175 waivers" were to enable a State to:

(1) implement a case management system or specialty physicians' services arrangement which restricted the provider from or through whom individuals could obtain primary care services (other than under emergency circumstances), so long as the restriction did not substantially impair access to services of adequate quality;

(2) allow a locality to act as a central broker in assisting individuals in selecting among competing health care plans;

(3) share with eligibles any cost savings (through provision of additional services) resulting from the use by the eligible of more cost-effective medical care; and

(4) restrict the provider from or through whom an individual could obtain services (other than in emergency circumstances) to providers or practitioners who complied with State plan reimbursement, quality, efficiency, and utilization standards, so long as the restriction did not discriminate among classes of providers on grounds unrelated to their demonstrated effectiveness and efficiency in providing those services.

The TEFRA deleted the authority of the Secretary, under the "2175 waiver provision", to waive the requirements for HMOs and other prepaid entities contracting on a risk basis to provide Medicaid services.

The OBRA 90 required States to meet the same prompt payment standards for practitioners under a selective contracting waiver as they were required to meet for other health care practitioners.

B. Waivers to Provide Home and Community-Based Services

The OBRA 81 authorized the Secretary to waive Federal requirements to enable a State to provide home and community-based services (other than room and board), pursuant to a written plan of care, to individuals who would otherwise require SNF or ICF services which would be reimbursed by Medicaid. Services which could be provided under these "2176 waivers" (in addition to those otherwise authorized under Medicaid) included case management, homemaker/home health aide and personal care services; adult day health; habilitation services; respite care; and other services requested by the State and approved by the Secretary. The Secretary could not approve a "2176 waiver" unless the State provided the following assurances:

- Necessary safeguards were taken to protect the health and welfare of individuals receiving services and to assure financial accountability for expended funds;

- The State would provide an evaluation of the individual's need for SNF or ICF care;

- Individuals determined likely to require SNF or ICF care would be informed of the feasible alternatives available at their choice under the waiver;

- The average per capita expenditure for individuals provided services under the waiver would not exceed the average per capita amount which would have been expended for such individuals if the waivers had not been in effect;

- The State would annually provide information to the Secretary on the impact of the waiver on the type and amount of medical assistance provided and on the health and welfare of recipients.

Amendments to the original 2176 waiver authority generally addressed issues raised by implementing regulations and/or administration of the program by HCFA. The following were the major COBRA modifications:

- The law clarified that the estimated per capita expenditure amount for medical services in any fiscal year could not exceed 100 percent of the average per capita expenditure that the State reasonably estimated would have been incurred in that year if the waiver had not been approved. The Secretary was prohibited from requiring that actual total expenditures under a 2176 waiver could not exceed the approved estimates for these services. The Secretary was prohibited from denying Federal matching payments under the waiver on the grounds that a State failed to limit actual total expenditures to the approved estimates. Further, States were allowed, in estimating average per capita expenditures for physically disabled individuals in SNFs and ICFs to use only expenditures associated with this group of patients.

- States could establish, for individuals receiving wavered services in the community, higher maintenance needs allowances than the maximum amounts specified in regulations in effect on July 1, 1985.

- The Secretary was required, upon the request of a State, to extend for a minimum of 1 year and a maximum of 5 years any 2176 waiver that expired on or after September 30, 1985 and before September 30, 1986. The Secretary was required to renew waivers for additional 5-year, rather than 3-year periods.

- The law defined covered habilitation services, with respect to individuals receiving such services after discharge from a SNF or ICF, as services designed to assist individuals in acquiring, retaining, and improving the self-help, socialization, and adaptive skills necessary to reside successfully in home and community-based settings.

The OBRA 86 made a number of additional changes to the 2176 provisions including:

- Eligibility for home and community-based services was extended to all individuals who, but for the provision of such services, would require the level of care provided in a hospital, SNF or ICF, the cost of which would be reimbursed under Medicaid.

- In the case of a waiver that applied only to individuals with a particular illness or condition, the State could estimate the average per capita expenditure associated with this group of persons and not the expenditures associated with other individuals in hospitals, SNFs or ICFs.

- The following additional services were added under the waiver authority for the chronically mentally ill: day treatment or other partial hospitalization services; psychosocial rehabilitation services; and clinic services (whether or not furnished in a facility).

The OBRA 87 raised the limit on the number of persons who could be covered under a model home and community-based services waiver to 200. MCCA clarified that the Secretary could not limit the number of persons covered under a waiver to under 200 persons.

The OBRA 87 specified that in the case of a waiver that applied only to persons with developmental disabilities requiring ICF/MR services, the State could estimate the average per capita expenditure associated with just this group of persons. MCCA specified that this may be done without regard to the availability of beds for such inpatients.

The TAMRA removed the requirement for institutionalization prior to receiving waivered services for persons receiving such services under an illness or specific condition waiver.

The OBRA 90 included several amendments. It clarified that the Secretary did not have authority to limit the number of hours of respite care under a budget-neutral waiver. It also clarified requirements pertaining to documenting budget neutrality under a 2176 waiver for persons with mental retardation or related condition; States could, in the case of clients in an ICF/MR terminated from the Medicaid program, disregard the reduction in the number of beds at the facility.

C. Long-Term Care Services for the Elderly

The OBRA 87 established a new waiver authority, separate from the 2176 waiver authority. Enactment of this "1915(d) waiver" was in response to an issue which had arisen in connection with implementation of the 2176 authority. To meet the law's requirement that the average per capita expenditures under 2176 waiver programs not exceed average per capita expenditures that would be incurred in the absence of the waiver, HCFA required States to estimate the number of individuals who would otherwise be served in a Medicaid nursing home bed. HCFA used this estimate as a ceiling on the number of persons who could be served under the waiver. States that restricted the supply of nursing home beds were therefore limited in the number of persons they could enroll under the waiver.

The OBRA 87 therefore established a new waiver authority that allowed States, on a budget neutral basis, to provide a mix of home and community-based and institutional services to the elderly at risk of nursing home care. The budget neutrality formula limited States electing the waiver in 1988 and 1989 to a maximum 7 percent rate of growth in their institutional and noninstitutional long-term care outlays under Medicaid, compounded annually. The Secretary was required to promulgate, by October 1, 1989, indices for projecting increases in institutional and noninstitutional long-term care costs, as well as State-specific projections of increases in the number of residents over age 75. Upon promulgation, the test for budget neutrality would be the greater of: (1) the sum of the percentages yielded by these indices, and (2) 7 percent, compounded annually. MCCA modified the provision by specifying that the State specific projections were for persons over 65; it required the Secretary, by October 1, 1989, to develop a method of projecting the increases for persons over 75.

The TAMRA allowed a modification of a State's limit on expenditures under a waiver. The modification was to adjust for increased aggregate expenditures for nursing facility and home and community-based services for the aged which were attributable to enactment of legislation subsequent to OBRA 87. OBRA 90 required adjustment of expenditure estimates to take into account the costs of implementing nursing home reform.

D. Boarder Babies

The term boarder babies is used to apply to newborn babies, infected with AIDS or drug dependent, who are left at the hospital because their mothers are unable to care for them. MCCA authorized waivers from certain State plan requirements (comparability and statewideness) for States to provide part or all of the cost of specified services to certain children who would otherwise be likely to require hospital or nursing home care. Services which could be covered under a waiver were nursing care, respite care, physicians' services, prescribed drugs, medical devices and supplies, transportation services, and such other services requested by the State. Children who could be covered under such a waiver were those under age 5 who at the time of birth were infected with or tested positively for AIDS, had AIDS, or at the time of birth were dependent on heroin, cocaine, or phencyclidine. Adoption or foster care assistance had to be made available for these children. MCCA required States to provide certain assurances including an assurance that per capita expenditures would not exceed those which would have been spent in the absence of a waiver.

E. Provisions Relating to Health Maintenance Organizations and Other Prepaid Health Plans

The OBRA 81 permitted States to enter into prepaid or other risk arrangements with entities other than federally qualified HMOs, provided that such entities met certain requirements. The provision raised the existing ceiling on Medicare and Medicaid beneficiaries in HMOs from 50 percent to 75 percent of enrollment; the Secretary could waive this requirement in the case of public HMOs if he determined special circumstances warranted and the entity was taking reasonable efforts to enroll non-Medicare/Medicaid beneficiaries. The law required that enrolles under a risk arrangement be permitted to disenroll without cause on 1 month's notice. Further, the law added additional contract requirements relating to financial accountability, nondiscrimination on the basis of health status, termination provisions, and payment for emergency services furnished elsewhere. States were permitted to enter arrangements with federally qualified HMOs under which minimum enrollment periods of up to 6 months would be established, i.e., eligibility would be guaranteed even if the individual lost Medicaid eligibility during the period.

The DEFRA permitted the Secretary to waive or modify the 75 percent enrollment requirement in the case of a nonprofit federally qualified HMO in an underserved area which had at least 25,000 enrolles and which had previously received an enrollment waiver.

The DEFRA also permitted States to require Medicaid beneficiaries who enrolled in HMOs meeting certain requirements to remain in the HMO for up to 6 months unless the beneficiary had good cause to disenroll earlier. COBRA extended the 6-month guaranteed enrollment and restricted disenrollment provisions to certain federally-funded community, migrant, and Appalachian health centers.

The COBRA also provided that where a health insuring organization (HIO) arranged with other providers (through subcontract or otherwise) for the delivery of services to Medicaid beneficiaries, it was subject to the requirements applicable to HMOs or other prepaid entities. This provision applied even though the HIO itself did not itself deliver services.

The OBRA 86 required States to provide for an annual independent review of Medicaid services provided or arranged by each HMO, HIO, or other prepaid plan with which the State had entered a risk-based contract. The State could select a PRO or private accreditation body to perform this function. OBRA 87 provided that the 75 percent Federal matching rate for the cost of independent quality review of HMO care applied both to PROs and to other qualified review organizations.

The OBRA 86 required any HMO that was not a federally qualified HMO and was contracting with a State to provide services to Medicaid beneficiaries on a capitated or risk basis to report to the State a description of transactions between the organization and party in interest. Transactions required to be reported included: any sale, exchange or leasing of property; any furnishing for consideration of goods, services, or facilities (but not employees salaries); and any loans or extensions of credit. The information would be made available upon request to the Secretary, Inspector General, the Comptroller General, and the organization's enrolles. The Secretary was required to give prior approval of contracts in excess of $100,000 between States and entities contracting to provide services to Medicaid beneficiaries on a capitated or risk basis.

The OBRA 86 further provided for the imposition of civil monetary penalties for entities, contracting on a risk basis with States, under the following circumstances. Penalties would be imposed if the entity failed to provide required medically necessary items and services and such failure adversely affected the patients. OBRA 87 expanded the acts that would be subject to penalties to include imposition of excess premiums, acts to expel or refuse to reenroll individuals in violation of the law, practices which would reasonably be expected to have the effect of denying or discouraging enrollment of persons whose medical condition indicated the need for substantial future medical services, and misrepresenting or falsifying information. OBRA 87 authorized suspensions of enrollments and payments in addition to civil monetary penalties. MCCA incorporated technical modifications and increased the possible amount of civil monetary penalties under this section. Further, the law provided for a denial of Federal payments (in lieu of the suspension provisions) in cases where the Secretary determined a violation existed; the denial would remain in effect until the Secretary was satisfied that the basis for the determination was corrected.

The OBRA 90 included a number of HMO amendments. It specified that HMOs, HIOs and other prepaid plans participating on a risk basis would be subject to the same requirements relating to physician incentive plans as those made applicable to HMOs participating under Medicare. Medicare requirements precluded payments to induce physicians to reduce or limit medically unnecessary services, and included a requirement that physicians could not be placed at a substantial financial risk unless there was appropriate stop loss protection and the organization periodically surveyed beneficiaries to determine satisfaction with access and quality.

The OBRA 90 provided that the Secretary, when waiving the minimum 25-percent private enrollment rule for public entities, need not consider whether special circumstances warrant the waiver. Other OBRA 90 amendments extended to competitive medical plans the existing provisions relating to guaranteed enrollment and 6-month lock-in, and permitted automatic reenrollment in an HMO when an individual lost and then regained Medicaid eligibility within a 3 month period.

The OBRA 90 further provided that FQHCs that were not HMOs, but subcontracted with HMOs, had to be reimbursed for 100 percent of reasonable costs.

Public Law 102-276 authorized a waiver for the Dayton Area Health Plan of the requirements limiting the maximum number of Medicare and Medicaid beneficiaries in an HMO. Public Law 102-317 extended a similar waiver for the Tennessee Primary Care Network.

VI. ADMINISTRATION

Recent legislation included a number of provisions targeted toward improving the accuracy of eligibility determinations, improving collection of third party liabilities, and strengthening utilization review activities. In addition, Congress approved a provision requiring providers participating in Medicaid to notify patients of their rights (under State law) to make decisions about their health care, including the right to execute a living will or grant power of attorney to another individual.

A. Eligibility Determinations

1. *Quality Control/Target Error Rates*

The TEFRA deleted provisions, incorporated in the 1980 Appropriations Act, pertaining to target error rates for eligibility determinations and penalties for failure to fall below these levels. It established a 3 percent target error rate for erroneous excess payments beginning after March 30, 1983. It provided for the application of prospective fiscal sanctions for the 6-month period beginning April 1, 1983 and annually thereafter. The Secretary was provided discretion in applying the penalty, in whole or in part, for a State which made a good faith effort to meet the 3 percent target.

The COBRA required the Secretary to conduct a study of AFDC and Medicaid quality control programs. The Secretary was required to contract with the National Academy of Sciences to conduct a concurrent independent study for the same purpose. When the studies were completed, the Secretary was required to restructure these quality control programs and establish criteria for adjusting fiscal sanctions previously imposed.

The OBRA 87 prohibited the imposition of fiscal sanctions prior to July 1, 1988.

The OBRA 89 revised the AFDC quality control program, but left the Medicaid program intact.

The OBRA 90 required a report on error rates in determining eligibility for pregnant women and infants and excluded erroneous expenditures for these persons from the calculation of error rate penalties until 1 year after submission of the report.

2. Income and Eligibility Verification System

The DEFRA required States to have an income and eligibility verification system for use in administering Medicaid and other specified programs. The programs were required to request and make use of Internal Revenue Service unearned income and quarterly wage information. OBRA 86 clarified that the requirement that the use of such information be targeted toward the most productive uses, did not require States to use the information to verify the eligibility of all beneficiaries. The Immigration Reform and Control Act of 1986 required, effective October 1, 1988, all Medicaid applicants to declare in writing, under penalty of perjury, that they were a citizen or national of the U.S. or an alien in a satisfactory immigration status. In addition, States were required to verify with the Immigration and Naturalization Service, the immigration status of all aliens applying for Medicaid. MCCA exempted illegal aliens receiving treatment for emergency medical conditions from this requirement.

3. Presumptive Eligibility

The OBRA 86 permitted States to make ambulatory prenatal care available to pregnant women for a presumptive period of eligibility. The period would begin on the date on which a qualified provider determined (on the basis of preliminary information) that the family income fell below the applicable Medicaid standard. The period would end on the earlier of: (a) the day on which a determination was made on the application by the State agency; (b) 45 days after the provider made the determination; or (c) 14 days after the preliminary determination, if the woman did not file an application.

The OBRA 90 extended the time during which an application must be filed and extended the presumptive eligibility period to the date the State made the final eligibility determination.

4. Processing

The OBRA 90 required States to allow the processing of Medicaid applications for pregnant women and children at locations other than welfare offices.

5. Paternity Determinations

The OBRA 90 specified that pregnant women applying only for coverage for prenatal, delivery, and postpartum care were exempt from the general requirement that they cooperate with the State in establishing paternity and obtaining child support.

6. Disability Determinations

The OBRA 90 permitted States, for purposes of determining Medicaid eligibility, to make determinations of disability or blindness using Federal standards. State determinations would be effective until a final determination was made by the Social Security Administration (SSA).

B. Inapplicability of Certain State Plan Requirements

The OBRA 81 permitted a State, for a reasonable period of time, to (1) require individuals who overutilized services to use particular providers (sometimes referred to as "lock-in"); and (2) limit the participation of providers, which the State found (after notice and opportunity for a hearing) to have, in a significant number or proportion of cases, abused the program (sometimes referred to as "lock-out"). A restriction was permitted provided individuals eligible for a service had reasonable access (taking into account geographic location and travel time) to such services of adequate quality. The legislation also permitted States to enter into competitive bidding or other arrangements for the purchase of laboratory services or medical devices for Medicaid eligibles.

C. Required Coordination

The OBRA 89 required Medicaid plans to provide for coordination with the Special Supplemental Food Program for Women, Infants, and Children (WIC). The law required timely notification of the availability of WIC to all Medicaid eligibles who were pregnant, breastfeeding or postpartum women and children under age 5. Medicaid was further required to provide for the referral of such individuals to the agency administering WIC.

D. Advance Directives

The OBRA 90 required hospitals, nursing facilities, home health providers and HMOs participating in Medicaid to notify patients of their rights (under State law) to make decisions about their health care, including the right to execute a living will or to grant a power of attorney to another individual.

E. Third Party Liability Recoveries

Medicaid requires States to take reasonable measures to ascertain the legal liability of third parties (such as private insurers) to pay for services that Medicaid would otherwise have to pay for. If Medicaid has made payment for such care, the State is required to seek recovery from the third party. OBRA 81 modified the third-party recovery requirement by specifying that it only applied to cases where the amount of recovery could reasonably be expected to exceed the cost of taking action.

The DEFRA mandated States to require Medicaid applicants to assign to States their right to payment for medical support (as specified by a court or administrative order) and other medical care.

The COBRA made a number of additional modifications to the third party recovery requirements including: (a) specifying certain State actions for meeting the requirement that States take reasonable measures for ascertaining the legal liability of third parties; (b) requiring the Secretary to develop performance standards for assessing States' third party liability collection efforts which were to be integrated with and monitored as part of the Secretary's review of each State's Medicaid Management Information System (MMIS); (c) requiring individuals, as a condition of eligibility, to cooperate with the State in identifying, and providing information to assist the State in pursuing, any liable third parties unless such individual had good cause for refusing to cooperate; and (d) specifying that in the case of prenatal and preventive pediatric services (including EPSDT services), payment is to be made according to the usual payment schedule without regard to third party liability (with subsequent recovery efforts occurring where warranted).

F. Utilization Review/Peer Review

1. Recertification of SNF and ICF Patients

States are required to have an adequate utilization control program; as part of this program, physicians were required to recertify the continuing need for SNF and ICF stays. DEFRA modified existing recertification requirements. It required recertifications of SNF patients 30, 60, and 90 days after initial certification and every 60 days thereafter. ICF recertifications were required 60 days, 180 days, 12 months, 18 months, and 24 months after initial certification and every 12 months thereafter. OBRA 87 provided that these requirements would be eliminated when nursing home reform provisions were fully implemented on October 1, 1990. At this time, the SNF and ICF categories were combined and a new set of resident assessment and preadmission screening and annual resident review requirements was established.

2. Peer Review Organization Program

The TEFRA provided for the establishment of a Peer Review Organization (PRO) program. PROs were charged with the review of necessity, appropriateness, and quality of services provided under Medicare. TEFRA authorized the States to contract with PROs for Medicaid review and authorized 75 percent Federal matching for such purpose.

3. State Utilization Review Systems

The OBRA 86 temporarily prohibited the Secretary from issuing final regulations requiring States to implement second surgical opinion programs

(SSOPs) or inpatient hospital preadmission review programs. The prohibition would end 180 days after the submission of a report to Congress, based on a representative sample of States, on: (1) high cost or high volume procedures; (2) payment rates and aggregate payments for such procedures; (3) utilization rates of these procedures among Medicaid and non-Medicaid populations; (4) number of physicians performing these procedures and the number providing second opinions; and (5) steps States with mandatory SSOPs took to avoid access problems, particularly in rural areas. The report was to include a list of surgical procedures that the Secretary believed should be included in a mandatory SSOP. The report was due by October 1, 1988. By January 1, 1990, the Secretary was required to submit a report to Congress examining the utilization of selected medical treatments and surgical procedures by Medicaid beneficiaries to assess the appropriateness, necessity and effectiveness of such treatments and procedures. MCCA specified that the report due January 1, 1990 was to be an interim report, with a final report due by January 1, 1992.

The OBRA 90 prohibited the Secretary from issuing final regulations requiring the States to adopt ambulatory surgery, preadmission testing or same-day surgery programs until 180 days after submitting a report to Congress on the effects of such programs on access, quality, and costs of care. The Secretary was prohibited from issuing final regulations requiring States to adopt SSOPs.

VII. FINANCING

Financing amendments enacted since 1981 can be classified into one of four categories: temporary reductions in Federal matching payments, calculation of the Federal Medical Assistance Percentage (FMAP), increasing the payment limits for the territories, and treatment of voluntary contributions or provider-paid taxes.

A. Reduction in Medicaid Payments to States and Offset for Meeting Federal Medicaid Expenditure Targets

The OBRA 81 provided for reductions in Federal Medicaid payments to States. The amount of Federal matching payments to which a State was otherwise entitled was to be reduced by 3 percent in FY 1982, 4 percent in FY 1983, and 4.5 percent in FY 1984. A State could lower the amount of its reduction by 1 percentage point for each of the following: (1) operating a qualified hospital cost review program; (2) sustaining an unemployment rate exceeding 150 percent of the national average; or (3) demonstrating recoveries from fraud and abuse activities (and with respect to FY 1982, third party recoveries) equal to 1 percent of Federal payments. A State was entitled to a dollar for dollar offset in its reduction if total Federal Medicaid expenditures in a year fell below a specified target amount. The legislation also included several amendments designed to give States increased flexibility in implementing their Medicaid programs.

B. Federal Medical Assistance Percentage

The OBRA 81 required the Comptroller General, in consultation with the Advisory Committee for Intergovernmental Relations, to conduct a study of the FMAP.

The COBRA required an annual, rather than biennial calculation of the FMAP beginning with FY 1987. OBRA 87 provided that the change to the annual calculation would not apply to State Medicaid programs, in FY 1987 only, if the State would be adversely affected by the change.

C. Payments to Territories

The OBRA 81 increased, effective FY 1982, the annual ceilings on Federal payments to the territories. The ceiling for Puerto Rico was increased from $30 million to $45 million; the ceiling for the Virgin Islands was increased from $1 million to $1.5 million; and the ceiling for Guam was increased from $0.9 million to $1.4 million. The law also established a ceiling for the Northern Mariana Islands at $350,000.

The TEFRA authorized, effective FY 1983, Medicaid coverage in American Samoa, subject to the same 50 percent matching rate applicable for other territories, and established an annual expenditure limitation at $750,000. TEFRA gave the Secretary broad authority to waive or modify existing Medicaid requirements with respect to this jurisdiction.

The DEFRA increased the ceilings, effective FY 1984, as follows: Puerto Rico, $63.4 million; Virgin Islands, $2.1 million; Guam, $2.0 million; Northern Mariana Islands, $550,000; and American Samoa, $1.15 million.

The OBRA 87 increased the ceilings as follows: Puerto Rico, $73.4 million in FY 1988, $76.2 million in FY 1989, and $79.0 million in FY 1990 and subsequent years; Virgin Islands, $2.43 million in FY 1988, $2.515 million in FY 1989, and $2.6 million in FY 1990 and subsequent years; Guam, $2.320 million in FY 1988, $2.41 million in FY 1989 and $2.5 million in FY 1990 and subsequent years; Northern Mariana Islands, $636,700 in FY 1988, $693,350 in FY 1989, and $750,000 in FY 1990 and subsequent years; and American Samoa, $1.33 million in FY 1988, $1.39 million in FY 1989, and $1.45 million in FY 1990 and subsequent years.

The OBRA 87 also permitted the Secretary to waive most Medicaid requirements with respect to the Northern Mariana Islands.

D. Voluntary Contributions

Beginning in 1986, States developed programs to use funds donated by health care providers or taxes paid by these providers to draw greater Federal matching payments. The Administration first proposed to outlaw these financing mechanisms in 1988. The Congress delayed the Secretary's authority to regulate in this area several times. TAMRA prohibited the Secretary from issuing final regulations prior to May 1, 1989, which would change the treatment of voluntary contributions or provider-paid taxes utilized by the States to receive Federal matching funds. OBRA 89 extended the prohibition through December 31, 1990 while OBRA 90 extended the prohibition through December 31, 1991. OBRA 90 also permitted States to continue to receive matching payments for provider-paid taxes.

The Medicaid Voluntary Contribution and Provider-Specific Tax Amendments of 1991 prohibited the use of most provider donations or provider taxes that are not "broad-based" (such as taxes imposed solely on Medicaid revenues) although States using such revenues at the time were permitted to phase them out in 1992 and 1993. Total revenues from donations and taxes (whether or not broad-based) are limited to 25 percent of the State's share of Medicaid, again with exceptions for States that were relying more heavily on these revenues. The Act also prohibited the Secretary from restricting States' use of funds derived from State or local taxes (including funds appropriated to State-owned teaching hospitals) transferred from or certified by local government units (including units that are providers) unless the transfers exceed the 40 percent limit on local government sharing in Medicaid or stem from otherwise prohibited donations or taxes. As noted above, the Act also limited national aggregate spending for disproportionate share hospital payment adjustments.

VIII. QUALITY OF INSTITUTIONAL LONG-TERM CARE SERVICES

Congress enacted several amendments designed to improve the quality of services provided to residents in long term care facilities. Of particular importance were the nursing home reform provisions incorporated in OBRA 87 and subsequent amendments to that legislation.

A. Intermediate Care Facilities for the Mentally Retarded

The COBRA added a new section to the law dealing with Intermediate Care Facilities for the Mentally Retarded (ICFs/MR) correction and reduction plans. The section specified that if the Secretary found that an ICF/MR had substantial deficiencies which did not impose an immediate threat to the resident's health and safety, the State could elect to submit either a written correction plan or reduction plan. The correction plan had to identify deficiencies found during a validation survey and provide a timetable for correcting all staffing and/or physical plant deficiencies within 6 months. A reduction plan had to provide for permanently reducing the number of certified beds, within a maximum of 36 months, in order to permit any noncomplying buildings (or distinct part thereof) to be vacated and any staffing deficiencies to be corrected. COBRA further specified that the provision only applied to correction and reduction plans approved within 3 years of the effective date of final regulations. OBRA 87 specified that the implementing regulations were to be effective as if promulgated on the effective date of COBRA (April 7, 1986).

The TAMRA clarified that correction and reduction plans could be used to remedy deficiencies related to active treatment. Further, the application of the provision was extended to plans approved by the Secretary prior to January 1, 1990. No further extensions were enacted.

B. Review of SNF and ICF Services

The DEFRA made consistent state plan requirements for medical review for SNFs and independent professional review for ICFs.

C. Nursing Home Quality Improvements

The OBRA 87 contained major nursing home reform provisions for both Medicare and Medicaid. Effective October 1, 1990, all nursing facilities participating in Medicaid would have to meet a single set of requirements pertaining to the provision of services, residents' rights, administration and other matters.

The law established a new process, effective October 1, 1990, for State and Federal monitoring of nursing facility compliance with the Medicaid requirements. The Secretary was responsible for determining the compliance of State nursing facilities; States were responsible for determining the compliance of all other nursing facilities. The Secretary would conduct on-site validation surveys of at least 5 percent of the facilities surveyed by the State each year.

In general, certification would be based on a two-step survey process--an unannounced standard survey which would occur, on average, at least annually and an extended survey for facilities found during a standard survey to have provided substandard quality care.

The law expanded the remedies available to both the Secretary and the States for the purposes of deterring and sanctioning noncompliance with Medicaid requirements. The Secretary's new remedies were effective January 1, 1988, with respect to existing requirements for SNFs and ICFs; they were to apply with respect to compliance by nursing facilities with the new requirements when those took effect October 1, 1990. States were required to have the new remedies in place no later than October 1, 1989. The law detailed intermediate remedies that could be taken if a facility's deficiencies did not immediately jeopardize the health or safety of residents.

No changes were made in the existing law requirements for ICFs/MR or institutions for mental diseases. However, effective January 1, 1989, each State had to have in effect a preadmission screening program for all mentally ill or mentally retarded individuals to determine whether placement in a SNF or ICF was appropriate. The law also required that mentally retarded or mentally ill persons admitted before such date be reviewed on an annual basis to determine whether their care was appropriate. (The preadmission screening and annual resident review requirements are frequently referred to as PASARR requirements). Federal matching payments would not be available for persons not found to need placement. States were required to review all mentally ill or mentally retarded individuals in nursing facilities by April 1, 1990, to determine whether continued placement was appropriate. They were further required to arrange for the safe and orderly discharge and active treatment of residents for whom continued placement was inappropriate.

The OBRA 89 made a number of modifications to the nursing home reform provisions. Included were a number of provisions relating to nurse aide training. The law delayed from January 1, 1990 to October 1, 1990, the requirement that aides be trained and determined competent. It required the Secretary to issue proposed regulations on nurse aide training and competency evaluation programs not later than 90 days after enactment. It specified that training and evaluation programs must address the care of cognitively impaired residents. Further, the law required States to offer alternatives to written exams and prohibited the imposition of charges for training and competency evaluation programs. States were permitted to waive the competency evaluation (but not training requirements) in the case of an individual who, as of enactment, had served as nurse aide for at least 24 months for the same employer.

The OBRA 89 postponed until October 1, 1990, implementation of regulations relating to requirements for nursing facilities participating in Medicare or Medicaid. It also directed the Secretary to published proposed regulations for PASARR requirements within 90 days of enactment.

The OBRA 90 included a number of technical corrections to the nursing home reform provisions. It prohibited the Secretary from taking any compliance action against any State which made a good faith effort to comply with the nurse aid training requirements for any period prior to May 12, 1989. It also defined a nursing facility which would be prohibited from conducting a nurse aide training program to include a facility which, during the 2 previous years: (1) operated under a waiver of the nurse staffing requirements in excess of 48 hours per week; (2) was subject to an extended or partially extended survey; or (3) had been subject to certain sanctions.

The OBRA 90 contained several amendments to the PASARR requirements. It prohibited the Secretary from taking any compliance action against any State that had made a good faith effort to comply with the PASARR requirements with respect to any period prior to the effective date of Department of Health and Human Services (DHHS) guidelines (i.e., May 26, 1989). The law also modified the definition of mental illness for purposes of applying the PASARR requirements. The revised definition is "serious mental illness as defined by the Secretary in consultation with the National Institutes of Mental Health". The definition excluded individuals with a nonprimary diagnosis of dementia and primary diagnosis that was not a serious mental illness.

The OBRA 90 included several additional amendments. It clarified that a State could waive nurse staffing requirements only to the extent that a facility could not meet those requirements and required that notice of any nurse staffing waiver be given to residents, their families, and appropriate State agencies. The law also prohibited the Secretary from taking any compliance action against a State that made a good faith effort to comply with the enforcement requirements prior to the date the Secretary issued guidelines regarding establishment of remedies for facility noncompliance.

IX. FRAUD AND ABUSE

The OBRA 81 authorized the Secretary to assess a civil monetary penalty of up to $2,000 for fraudulent claims under Medicaid and Medicare and to impose an assessment of twice the amount of the fraudulent claim, in lieu of damages.

The OBRA 86 provided for a civil monetary penalty of $2,000 per patient if a hospital (or effective April 1, 1989, an entity delivering services on a risk basis) knowingly made a payment, directly or indirectly, to a physician as an inducement to reduce or limit services to Medicaid patients under the direct care of the physician. The Secretary was required to report to Congress by January 1, 1988 on incentive arrangements offered by HMOs and competitive medical plans. OBRA 87 delayed application of the provision to risk-based entities to April 1,1990. (See discussion under item V-E above relating to OBRA 90 requirements relating to physician incentive plans.)

The OBRA 86 contained several additional modifications to the existing civil monetary penalty and exclusion provisions applicable to both Medicare and Medicaid. It specified that when an individual had a prior conviction of a Federal crime charging fraud or false statements, and the current proceedings involved the same transactions, the individual was prevented from denying the elements affirmed in the previous trial. It authorized the official conducting a hearing to impose sanctions for misconduct that would interfere with the speedy, orderly, or fair conduct of a hearing. Further, the law clarified cases under which an individual would be considered convicted of a criminal offense for purposes of exclusion from the program.

The Medicare and Medicaid Patient and Program Protection Act of 1987 was designed to protect Medicare and Medicaid beneficiaries from unfit health practitioners and to recodify and strengthen the anti-fraud provisions in the Social Security Act. Under the law, the Secretary was required to exclude from Medicare and required to direct States to exclude from Medicaid any individual or entity convicted of a criminal offense related to delivery of services under these programs or convicted of a criminal offense related to neglect or abuse of patients in connection with the delivery of a health care item or service.

Under certain other specified circumstances, the Secretary was permitted to exclude individuals or entities from Medicare and could direct States to exclude them from Medicaid. These circumstances included: conviction of fraud in connection with a health care program; conviction relating to obstruction of an investigation of health care fraud, license revocation or suspension; exclusion or suspension unde Federal or State health care program; claims for excessive charges or unnecessary services; fraud, kickbacks or other prohibited activities; failure to make required disclosures; failure to supply requested information on subcontractors and suppliers; and failure to supply payment information. The

Secretary was required to specify the duration of the exclusion; mandatory exclusions were for a minimum of 5 years. A State was permitted to exclude any individual or entity from Medicaid for any reason for which the Secretary could have excluded an individual from participation in Medicare. A State had to exclude an HMO which could have been excluded from Medicare because of the conviction of the owners or managers for certain crimes or which had a substantial or contractual relationship with any individual or entity convicted of such crimes.

The 1987 law also required States to have a system of reporting information with respect to formal proceedings concluded against a health care practitioner or entity by a State licensing authority. The law further clarified and consolidated civil monetary and criminal penalty provisions.

The OBRA 89 included several technical clarifications. Exclusions could also apply to providers who lost the right to apply for or renew licenses on the same grounds as those whose licenses were revoked or suspended. The exception permitting payment for emergency services by excluded providers did not apply to services furnished in a hospital emergency room. Further, HMOs could not employ or contract with excluded providers for the provision of services.

X. ESTIMATED IMPACT OF LEGISLATION

The Congressional Budget Office (CBO) estimated the impact of each of the reconciliation bills at the time of their enactment. However, the numbers **cannot** be added together. The CBO baseline estimate in a year reflects economic assumptions at the time the estimate is made. Estimates of the impact of legislative changes are compared with that baseline. Any costs or savings attributable to passage of one reconciliation bill, as well as any changes in economic assumptions, are included in the current law CBO baseline for the next fiscal year. Tables IX-1 to IX-11 show the CBO estimates of changes in Federal Medicaid outlays which were made at the time of enactment of the 1981 to 1990 reconciliation bills and other legislation enacted during the period.[3]

The CBO estimated no change in the Medicaid baseline as a result of the enactment of the Medicaid Voluntary Contribution and Provider-Specific Tax Amendments of 1991 and the Veterans Health Care Act of 1992.

---

[3]CBO's estimate for TAMRA did not include an estimate of changes in Medicaid outlays; a TAMRA estimate is therefore not included in these tables.

TABLE IX-1. P.L. 97-35, Omnibus Budget Reconciliation Act of 1981 (OBRA 81), Congressional Budget Office Estimates of Changes in Medicaid Outlays Made at Time of Enactment, FY 1982 to FY 1984 (in millions of dollars)

	FY 1982	FY 1983	FY 1984
Medicaid provisions	- $890	- $870	- $1,000
Impact of Medicare provisions	- 44	- 50	- 52
Other	2	8	11
Total	- 932	- 912	- 1,041

Source: Congressional Budget Office. Unpublished table, Aug. 1981.

TABLE IX-2. P.L. 97-248, Tax Equity and Fiscal Responsibility Act of 1982 (TEFRA), Congressional Budget Office Estimates of Changes in Medicaid Outlays Made at Time of Enactment, FY 1983 to FY 1985 (in millions of dollars)

	FY 1983	FY 1984	FY 1985
Medicaid provisions:			
Copayments by Medicaid recipients	$ 45	$ 50	$ 56
Modification in lien provisions	165	180	200
Error rate sanctions	30	65	72
Coverage of disabled children at home	a	a	a
American Samoa	- 1	- 1	- 1
Subtotal, Medicaid provisions	239	294	327
Other items:			
Impact of Medicare provisions	1	46	122
Impact of AFDC provisions	16	20	25
Impact of penalty provisions of OBRA 81	0	- 30	- 30
Subtotal, other items	17	36	117
Total	256	330	444

aNegligible cost.

Source: U.S. Congress. House. *Tax Equity and Fiscal Responsibility Act of 1982.* Conference Report to Accompany H.R. 4961, Aug. 7, 1982. House Report No. 97-760, 97th Cong., 2d Sess., and conversation with CBO official, Sept. 1982. Washington, GPO, 1982.

TABLE IX-3. P.L. 98-369, Deficit Reduction Act of 1984 (DEFRA), Congressional Budget Office Estimates of Changes in Medicaid Outlays Made at Time of Enactment, FY 1984 to FY 1989
(in millions of dollars)

	FY 1984	FY 1985	FY 1986	FY 1987	FY 1988	FY 1989
Medicaid provisions:						
Clinical lab payments	-$10	-$49	-$57	-$67	-$60	-$69
Revaluation of assets	-2	-20	-40	-55	-80	-95
Pregnant women and children	0	40	90	140	195	260
Recertification of SNF and ICF care	-1	-6	0	1	1	1
Increased ceilings for territories	20	20	20	20	20	20
Payments for psychiatric hospital services	3	10	6	3	0	0
Assignment of rights to medical support	0	-7	-7	-8	-9	-10
Subtotal, Medicaid provisions	10	-12	12	34	67	107
Other items:						
Impact of Medicare provisions	0	-28	-6	27	42	45
Impact of AFDC provisions	--	145	195	205	235	245
Impact of SSI provisions	--	2	10	15	25	35
Other	--	0	-210	-240	-255	-275
Subtotal, other items	--	119	-11	7	47	50
Total	10	107	1	41	114	157

Source: Congressional Budget Office. Unpublished table, Aug. 1984.

TABLE IX-4. P.L. 99-272, Consolidated Omnibus Budget Reconciliation Act of 1985 (COBRA), Congressional Budget Office Estimates of Changes in Medicaid Outlays Made at Time of Enactment, FY 1987 to FY 1991

(in millions of dollars)

	FY 1987	FY 1988	FY 1989	FY 1990	FY 1991
Medicaid provisions:					
Services for pregnant women	$40	$40	$45	$45	$45
Third party liability	- 25	- 30	- 30	- 35	- 40
Revaluation of assets	25	30	35	40	45
Coverage start date for institutionalized persons	5	5	5	5	5
Coverage of children	5	5	5	5	5
Overpayment recovery	5	5	5	5	5
Subtotal, Medicaid provisions	55	55	65	65	65
Impact of other provisions	4	4	4	4	4
Total	59	59	69	69	69

Source: Congressional Budget Office. Unpublished table, Apr. 1986.

TABLE IX-5. P.L. 99-509, Omnibus Budget Reconciliation Act of 1986 (OBRA 86), Congressional Budget Office Estimates of Changes in Medicaid Outlays Made at Time of Enactment, FY 1987 to FY 1991
(in millions of dollars)

	FY 1987	FY 1988	FY 1989	FY 1990	FY 1991
Optional coverage of pregnant women and children	$25	$85	$110	$145	$185
Optional coverage of elderly and disabled	45	170	240	295	355
Respiratory care services	-2	0	0	0	0
Hold harmless for Medicaid matching percentages	50	0	0	0	0
Respite care pilot project	1	2	2	0	0
Presumptive eligibility	2	2	2	2	2
Total	121	259	354	442	542

Source: Congressional Budget Office. Unpublished table, Oct. 1986.

TABLE IX-6. P.L. 100-203, Omnibus Budget Reconciliation Act of 1987 (OBRA 87), Congressional Budget Office Estimates of Changes in Medicaid Outlays Made at Time of Enactment, FY 1988 to FY 1990

(in millions of dollars)

Provisions	FY 1988	FY 1989	FY 1990
Coverage for pregnant women & children	$15	$ 90	$105
Nursing home requirements:			
Increase in nurse staff requirements	0	0	0
Nurse aide training	0	35	55
Social worker requirements	0	0	1
Increase in administrative, recordkeeping and personnel costs	0	5	10
Other requirements on institution	0	0	10
New survey and certification requirement	0	3	25
Increased match for survey and certification	0	0	15
Subtotal, nursing home requirements	0	43	116
Payment adjustment for territories	8	14	17
Clinic services for homeless	15	30	35
Payments to disproportionate share hospitals	5	30	60
Community-based services for disabled children: technical amendment	1	2	2
Total	44	209	335

Source: Congressional Budget Office. Unpublished table, Dec. 1987.

TABLE IX-7. P.L. 100-360, Medicare Catastrophic Coverage Act of 1988, Congressional Budget Office Estimates of Changes in Medicaid Outlays Made at Time of Enactment, FY 1989 to FY 1993
(in millions of dollars)

	FY 1989	FY 1990	FY 1991	FY 1992	FY 1993
Offsets from Medicare provisions	$ 45	- $247	- $398	- $495	-$605
Medicaid buyin for Medicare	106	231	435	591	665
Spousal protection	- 6	358	339	210	229
Pregnant women/infants	5	50	125	160	195
OBRA 87 technical amendments/other	- 15	- 4	0	8	11
Net Medicaid effect	45	388	501	474	495

Source: Congressional Budget Office. Unpublished table, June 1988.

TABLE IX-8. P.L. 100-485, The Family Support Act of 1988, Congressional
Budget Office Estimates of Changes in Medicaid Outlays Made at Time of
Enactment, FY 1989 to FY 1993
(in millions of dollars)

	FY89	FY90	FY91	FY92	FY93	FY89-FY93
Mandate income withholding for child support	---	---	- $5	- $5	- $10	- $20
Mandate child support guidelines	---	a	- 5	- 10	- 15	- 30
JOBS program establishment	a	- 5	- 10	- 20	- 30	- 65
Add mandatory participation rate for JOBS	---	a	a	- 5	- 10	- 15
Extend Medicaid coverage for persons leaving AFDC	10	5	105	155	165	440
Mandate AFDC-UP	---	---	180	260	295	735
Related amendments	---	3	18	19	20	60
Demonstration projects	a	a	1	3	5	9
Miscellaneous	---	- 10	- 25	- 30	- 30	- 95
Total Medicaid	10	- 7	259	367	390	1,019

ªLess than $500,000.

Source: Congressional Budget Office. Unpublished table, 1988.

TABLE IX-9. P.L. 101-234, Medicare Catastrophic Coverage Repeal Act of
1989, Congressional Budget Office Estimates of Changes in Medicaid
Outlays Made at Time of Enactment, FY 1990 to FY 1994
(in millions of dollars)

	FY90	FY91	FY92	FY93	FY94	FY90-FY94
Medicaid offset	$242	$618	$832	$922	$1,029	$3,642

Source: Congressional Budget Office. Unpublished table, Jan. 1990.

TABLE IX-10. P.L. 101-239, Omnibus Budget Reconciliation Act of 1989, Congressional Budget Office Estimates of Changes in Medicaid Outlays Made at Time of Enactment, FY 1990 to FY 1994
(in millions of dollars)

	FY90	FY91	FY92	FY93	FY94	FY90-FY94
Coverage of pregnant women and children	$ 60	$150	$175	$190	$210	$785
Coverage of children up to 133 1/3% of poverty	50	120	145	170	185	670
Obstetrical and pediatric services	2	11	12	13	14	52
EPSDT	20	25	25	30	30	130
Federally qualified health centers	8	15	20	20	25	88
Nurse practitioners	---	---	1	1	2	4
WIC coordination	1	2	2	2	2	9
Pregnant women and children demo	10	10	10	0	0	30
Institutions for mental disease	---	0	0	0	0	---
Texas waiver	1	0	0	0	0	1
Hospice	1	2	2	5	5	15
Medicare premium buy-in for certain disabled	---	1	5	7	10	23
Other provisions	---	1	5	6	9	21
Miscellaneous technical provisions	---	---	---	---	---	---
Total Medicaid	153	337	402	444	492	1,828

Source: Congressional Budget Office. Unpublished table, Dec. 1990.

TABLE IX-11. P.L. 101-508, Omnibus Budget Reconciliation Act of 1990, Congressional Budget Office Estimates of Changes in Medicaid Outlays Made at Time of Enactment, FY 1991 to FY 1995
(in millions of dollars)

	FY91	FY92	FY93	FY94	FY95	FY91-FY95
Prescription drugs	-$70	-$330	-$415	-$505	-$610	-$1,930
Payment of group health plan premiums and cost-sharing	-85	-160	-205	-250	-305	-1,005
Medicare payments for low-income	35	15	55	85	195	385
Coverage of children	10	55	105	160	230	560
Outreach	9	50	55	55	60	229
Continuation of benefits through pregnancy or first year of life	15	30	35	35	40	155
Hospital payments	6	30	30	35	40	141
Presumptive eligibility	1	1	2	2	2	8
Paternity determinations	---	---	---	---	---	---
Error rate report and transition	---	---	0	0	0	---
Federally qualified health centers	3	4	4	4	4	19
Limitation on disallowance	0	12	0	0	0	12
Frail elderly	40	70	130	160	180	580
Community supported living arrangement services	5	10	20	30	35	100
Disregard of German reparation payments	---	1	1	1	1	4
Minn. personal care	1	1	1	1	0	4
Personal care services	0	0	0	0	25	25
Spenddown option	---	---	---	---	---	---
Frail elderly demonstration waivers	---	---	---	---	---	---
Low-income family coverage demonstrations	12	12	12	4	0	40
Respite care demonstration	2	2	0	0	0	4

TABLE IX-11. P.L. 101-508, Omnibus Budget Reconciliation Act of 1990,
Congressional Budget Office Estimates of Changes in Medicaid Outlays
Made at Time of Enactment, FY 1991 to FY 1995--Continued
(in millions of dollars)

	FY91	FY92	FY93	FY94	FY95	FY91-FY95
HIV positive demonstration	5	12	13	0	0	30
Advance directives	---	1	1	1	1	4
Quality of physicians' services	---	1	1	1	1	4
Nursing home reform technicals	11	1	1	1	1	15
Total Medicaid	0	-182	-154	-180	-100	-616

Source: Congressional Budget Office. Unpublished table, Dec. 1990.

APPENDIX: KEY DOCUMENTS RELATED TO PASSAGE OF MAJOR RECONCILIATION, ANTIFRAUD, AND CATASTROPHIC LEGISLATION, 1980-PRESENT

The following is a *selected* list of committee reports and conference reports related to major reconciliation, antifraud, and catastrophic legislation from 1980 to the present that have led to changes in the Medicaid program. In some cases, House and Senate reports were not issued; therefore, only the conference report is shown. The list is arranged in chronological order.

Omnibus Reconciliation Act of 1980, Public Law 96-499

U.S. Congress. House. Committee on Interstate and Foreign Commerce. *Medicare and Medicaid amendments of 1980*; report to accompany H.R. 4000. Washington, GPO, 1980. (96th Congress, 2d session. House. Report no. 96-589)

U.S. Congress. Senate. Committee on Finance. *Spending reductions: recommendations of the Committee on Finance required by the reconciliation process in section 3(a)(15) of H. Con. Res. 307, the first budget resolution for fiscal year 1981*. Washington, GPO, 1980. (96th Congress, 2d session. Senate. CP 96-36)

U.S. Congress. House. Committee on the Budget. *Omnibus reconciliation act of 1980*; report to accompany H.R. 7765. Washington, GPO, 1980. (96th Congress, 2d session. House. Report no. 96-1167)

U.S. Congress. House. Conference Committee. *Omnibus reconciliation act of 1980*; report to accompany H.R. 7765. Washington, GPO, 1980. (96th Congress, 2d session. House. Report no. 96-1479)

Omnibus Budget Reconciliation Act of 1981, Public Law 97-35

U.S. Congress. Senate. Committee on the Budget. *Omnibus reconciliation act of 1981*; report to accompany S. 1377. Washington, GPO, 1981. (97th Congress, 1st session. Senate. Report no. 97-139)

U.S. Congress. House. Committee on the Budget. *Omnibus reconciliation act of 1981*; report to accompany H.R. 3982. Washington, GPO, 1981. (97th Congress, 1st session. House. Report no. 97-158, v. II)

U.S. Congress. House. Conference Committee. *Omnibus budget reconciliation act of 1981*; report to accompany H.R. 3982. Washington, GPO, 1981. (97th Congress, 1st session. House. Report no. 97-208)

Tax Equity and Fiscal Responsibility Act of 1982, Public Law 97-248

U.S. Congress. Senate. Committee on Finance. *Tax equity and fiscal responsibility act of 1982*; report together with additional supplemental and minority views on H.R. 4961. Washington, GPO, 1982. (97th Congress, 2d session. Senate. Report no. 97-494)

U.S. Congress. House. Committee on Energy and Commerce. *Medicaid and Medicare part B budget reconciliation amendments of 1982*; report together with dissenting and supplemental views to accompany H.R. 6877. Washington, GPO, 1982. (97th Congress, 2d session. House. Report no. 97-757)

U.S. Congress. House. Conference Committee. *Tax equity and fiscal responsibility act of 1982*; report to accompany H.R. 4961. Washington, GPO, 1982. (97th Congress, 2d session. House. Report no. 97-760)

U.S. Congress. Senate. Conference Committee. *Tax equity and fiscal responsibility act of 1982*; report to accompany H.R. 4961. Washington, GPO, 1982. (97th Congress, 2d session. Senate. Report no. 97-530)

Deficit Reduction Act of 1984, Public Law 98-369

U.S. Congress. House. Committee on Energy and Commerce. *Medicare and Medicaid budget reconciliation amendments of 1983*; report together with supplemental and minority views to accompany H.R. 4136. Washington, GPO, 1983. (98th Congress, 1st session. House. Report no. 98-442)

U.S. Congress. Senate. Committee on Finance. *Deficit reduction act of 1984*; explanation of provisions approved by the Committee on March 21, 1984. Washington, GPO, 1984. (98th Congress, 2d session. Senate. S. Prt. 98-169)

U.S. Congress. House. Conference Committee. *Deficit reduction act of 1984*; report to accompany H.R. 4170. Washington, GPO, 1984. (98th Congress, 2d session. House. Report no. 98-861)

Consolidated Omnibus Budget Reconciliation Act of 1985, Public Law 99-272

U.S. Congress. House. Committee on Energy and Commerce. *Medicare and Medicaid budget reconciliation amendments of 1985*; report together with minority views to accompany H.R. 3101. Washington, GPO, 1985. (99th Congress, 1st session. House. Report no. 99-265)

U.S. Congress. Senate. Committee on the Budget. *Consolidated omnibus budget reconciliation act of 1985*; report to accompany S. 1730. Washington, GPO, 1985. (99th Congress, 1st session. Senate. Report no. 99-1

U.S. Congress. House. Conference Committee. *Consolidated omnibus budget reconciliation act of 1985*; report to accompany H.R. 3128. Washington, GPO, 1985. (99th Congress, 1st session. House. Report no. 99-453)

Omnibus Budget Reconciliation Act of 1986, Public Law 99-509

U.S. Congress. House. Committee on the Budget. *Omnibus budget reconciliation act of 1986*; report together with supplemental, additional, and minority views to accompany H.R. 5300. Washington, GPO, 1986. (99th Congress, 2d session. House. Report no. 99-727)

U.S. Congress. Senate. Committee on the Budget. *Sixth omnibus budget reconciliation act, 1986*; report together with additional and minority views to accompany S. 2706. Washington, GPO, 1986. (99th Congress, 2d session. Senate. Report no. 99-348)

U.S. Congress. House. Conference Committee. *Providing for reconciliation pursuant to section 2 of the concurrent resolution on the budget for fiscal year 1987*; report to accompany H.R. 5300. Washington, GPO, 1986. (99th Congress, 2d session. House. Report no. 99-1012)

Medicare and Medicaid Patient and Program Protection Act of 1987, Public Law 100-93

U.S. Congress. House. Committee on Energy and Commerce. *Medicare and Medicaid patient and program protection act of 1987*; report to accompany H.R. 1444. Washington, GPO, 1987. (100th Congress, 1st session. House. Report no. 100-85)

U.S. Congress. Senate. Committee on Finance. *Medicare and Medicaid patient and program protection act of 1987*; report to accompany S. 661. Washington, GPO, 1987. (100th Congress, 1st session. Senate. Report no. 100-109)

Omnibus Budget Reconciliation Act of 1987, Public Law 100-203

U.S. Congress. House. Committee on the Budget. *Omnibus budget reconciliation act of 1987*; report together with supplemental, additional, and minority views to accompany H.R. 3545. Washington, GPO, 1987. (100th Congress, 1st session. House. Report no. 100-391)

U.S. Congress. Senate. Committee on the Budget. *Reconciliation submissions of the instructed committees pursuant to the concurrent resolution on the budget for fiscal year 1988 (H. Con. Res. 93, Rept. No. 100-76).* Washington, GPO, 1987. (100th Congress, 1st session. Committee Print)

U.S. Congress. House. Conference Committee. *Omnibus budget reconciliation act of 1987*; report to accompany H.R. 3545. Washington, GPO, 1987. (100th Congress, 1st session. House. Report no. 100-495)

Medicare Catastrophic Coverage Act of 1988, Public Law 100-360

U.S. Congress. House. Committee on Energy and Commerce. *Medicare catastrophic protection act of 1987*; report together with dissenting views to accompany H.R. 2470. Washington, GPO, 1987. (100th Congress, 1st session. House. Report no. 100-105)

U.S. Congress. Senate. Committee on Finance. *Medicare catastrophic loss prevention act of 1987*; report to accompany S. 1127. Washington, GPO, 1987. (100th Congress, 1st session. Senate. Report no. 100-126)

U.S. Congress. House. Conference Committee. *Medicare catastrophic coverage act of 1988*; report to accompany H.R. 2470. Washington, GPO, 1988. (100th Congress, 2d session. House. Report no. 100-661)

Family Support Act of 1988, Public Law 100-485

U.S. Congress. House. Committee on Energy and Commerce. *Family support act of 1988*; report to accompany H.R. 1720. Washington, GPO, 1987. (100th Congress, 2d session. House. Report no. 100-159)

U.S. Congress. Senate. Committee on Finance. *Family support act of 1988*; report to accompany S. 1511. Washington, GPO, 1988. (100th Congress, 2d session. Senate. Report no. 100-377)

U.S. Congress. House. Conference Committee. *Family support act of 1988*; report to accompany H.R. 1720. Washington, GPO, 1988. (100th Congress, 2d session. House. Report no. 100-998)

Technical and Miscellaneous Revenue Act of 1988, Public Law 100-647

U.S. Congress. House. Committee on Ways and Means. *Technical and miscellaneous revenue act of 1988*; report to accompany H.R. 4333. Washington, GPO, 1988. (100th Congress, 2d session. House. Report no. 100-795)

U.S. Congress. Senate. Committee on Finance. *Technical and miscellaneous revenue act of 1988*; report to accompany S. 2238. Washington, GPO, 1988. (100th Congress, 2d session. Senate. Report no. 100-445)

U.S. Congress. House. Conference Committee. *Technical and miscellaneous revenue act of 1988*; report to accompany H.R. 4333. Washington, GPO, 1988. (100th Congress, 2d session. House. Report no. 100-1104)

Medicare Catastrophic Coverage Repeal Act of 1989, Public Law 101-234

U.S. Congress. House. Conference Committee. *Medicare catastrophic coverage repeal act of 1989*; report to accompany H.R. 3607. Washington, GPO, 1989. (101st Congress, 1st session. House. Report no. 101-378)

Omnibus Budget Reconciliation Act of 1989, Public Law 101-239

U.S. Congress. House. Committee on the Budget. *Omnibus budget reconciliation act of 1989*; report together with supplemental and additional views to accompany H.R. 3299. Washington, GPO, 1989. (101st Congress, 1st session. House. Report no. 101-247)

U.S. Congress. House. Conference Committee. *Omnibus budget reconciliation act of 1989*; report to accompany H.R. 3299. Washington, GPO, 1989. (101st Congress, 1st session. House. Report no. 101-386)

Omnibus Budget Reconciliation Act of 1990, Public Law 101-508

U.S. Congress. House. Committee on the Budget. *Omnibus budget reconciliation act of 1990*; report together with additional, minority, and dissenting views to accompany H.R. 5835. Washington, GPO, 1990. (101st Congress, 2d session. House. Report no. 101-881)

U.S. Congress. House. Conference Committee. *Omnibus budget reconciliation act of 1990*; report to accompany H.R. 5835. Washington, GPO, 1990. (101st Congress, 2d session. House. Report no. 101-964)

Medicaid Voluntary Contribution and Provider-Specific Tax Amendments of 1991, Public Law 102-234

U.S. Congress. House. Committee on Energy and Commerce. *The Medicaid moratorium amendment of 1991*; report to accompany H.R. 3595. Washington, GPO, 1991. (102d Congress, 1st session. House. Report no. 102-310)

U.S. Congress. House. Conference Committee. *Medicaid moratorium amendments of 1991*; report to accompany H.R. 3595. Washington, GPO, 1991. (102d Congress, 1st session. House. Report no. 102-409)

Veterans Health Care Act of 1992, Public Law 102-585

U.S. Congress. House. Committee on Veterans' Affairs. *Establishment of limits on prices of drugs procured by the Department of Veterans Affairs*; report to accompany H.R. 2890. Washington, GPO, 1991. (102d Congress, 1st session. House. Report no. 102-384, Part I)

U.S. Congress. House. Committee on Energy and Commerce. *The Medicaid drug rebate amendments of 1992*; report to accompany H.R. 2890. Washington, GPO, 1992. (102d Congress, 2d session. House. Report no. 102-384, Part 2)

U.S. Congress. Senate. Committee on Veterans' Affairs. *Veterans health programs improvement act of 1992*; report to accompany S. 2575. Washington, GPO, 1992. (102d Congress, 2d session. Senate. Report no. 102-401)

For final passage of H.R. 5193 with an explanation of the compromise agreement, see *Congressional Record*, October 8, 1992, S17872-S17904

CHAPTER X. MEDICAID PAYMENT AND BENEFICIARY INFORMATION, FISCAL YEAR 1991[1]

I. INTRODUCTION

The Medicaid program is a joint Federal-State government program that provides medical assistance to certain low-income and other specified groups of individuals. The program is separately administered by each State, the District of Columbia, and the outlying territories. Within broad Federal guidelines, each State determines who is covered, the type of services covered, and the method of reimbursement for these services. Consequently there is a substantial amount of variation among States in the number of people covered and the type of services used.

This chapter is a compendium of statistical tables that provides State-by-State beneficiary and service data for FY 1991, the most recent annual data available. The chapter provides supplementary data relevant to discussions in previous chapters of this report. Except where otherwise indicated, all the information reported in the tables found in this chapter is based on data reported to the Health Care Financing Administration (HCFA) by the States. Obvious errors in the data were corrected by HCFA. However, some inaccuracies still exist.

In FY 1991, 28.3 million people received medical assistance payments under the Medicaid program at a total cost (Federal, State and local spending) of $77 billion. About half of these beneficiaries were less than 21 years old. About 61 percent received some form of cash welfare in addition to Medicaid.

II. SOURCES OF STATISTICAL INFORMATION ABOUT MEDICAID

Information about the Medicaid program is collected on three distinct Federal forms: a State budget estimating form; the State's current financial management report; and the State statistical report (HCFA-2082).[2] The State

---

[1]This chapter was written by Richard Rimkunas.

[2]The State budget estimating form is HCFA Form 25; the current financial management report is HCFA Form 64. The formal title for the report that supplies the data detailed in this chapter is *Statistical Report on Medical Care: Eligibles, Recipients, Payments, and Services*, HCFA 2082. Additional information on Medicaid State plans, research and demonstration information, and ad hoc surveys of the States are also collected by HCFA. For additional (continued...)

budget estimating form and the State current financial management report are quarterly statistical documents used for budget purposes. The data contained in the following set of tables are from State statistical reports.

Since 1972, States have been required to submit HCFA Form 2082. Data for this report are generated from the State Medicaid Management Information System (MMIS). MMIS is a system maintained by States for claims processing. Information submitted on the HCFA Form 2082 includes the number of beneficiaries and amount of vendor payments by eligibility status, whether the beneficiary received cash assistance payments, the type of medical services used by beneficiaries, and some limited demographic characteristics. The HCFA Form 2082 represents the primary source of descriptive information about the Medicaid program.

Data from the HCFA Form 2082 covers the Federal fiscal year which begins October 1 and ends September 30. The annual reports are due to HCFA by January 15 each year and a limited set of data tables for the prior Federal fiscal year are usually available in the early summer. The 2082 form collects data aggregated by specified eligibility categories, service categories, and selected demographic characteristics. In FY 1991, all beneficiary and payment data for Rhode Island, Puerto Rico, and data for blind eligibles in Massachusetts were estimated by HCFA. FY 1991 marks the first year that information on Arizona's cost containment demonstration project (AHCCCS) is included in the annual data. (For a description of this program, see *Appendix G, Managed Care.*) Data provided by States using form 2082 do not include capitated payments. Since Arizona's project is primarily a capitation plan, its payment amounts on the statistical forms were much lower than the State's actual payments. As a result of this underreporting, all of Arizona's payments are excluded from the tables in this chapter. However, beneficiary information appears to be complete and is included in the tables.

The aggregate nature of the statistics reported on HCFA Form 2082 allows for some ambiguity in how information is reported between the States. States may not be entirely consistent in the classification of beneficiaries, service and other categories. These and other limitations with the form have been noted by the Office of Management and Budget (OMB). In July of 1991, a joint Department of Health and Human Services (HHS)-OMB task force recommended that:

> ... HCFA needs to improve its collection of data on actual Medicaid program expenditures; the current financial management report (HCFA 64) and statistical report (HCFA 2082) are not sufficiently

---

[2](...continued)
information on these sources see: U.S. Department of Health and Human Services. Health Care Financing Administration. Medicaid Bureau. *Medicaid State Profile Data (spDATA) System: Characteristics of Medicaid State Programs.* Appendix III: HCFA Data Systems. May 1992.

timely or detailed to provide satisfactory support for historical program analysis or the development of accurate budget estimates . . . .[3]

More recently a preliminary evaluation of form 2082 statistics looked at the data in terms of its consistency across time, its consistency with other Medicaid information, and its validity.[4] For some States the statistical information on the form was found to be inconsistent from one year to the next, and in variance with expenditure information from other sources. Furthermore, some States failed to follow HCFA reporting instructions. Despite these limitations, the HCFA Form 2082 is the best currently available source of detailed information for payments and beneficiaries that includes all States over the 1975 to 1991 period.

III. DEFINITIONS

A. Beneficiaries

As reported on the HCFA Form 2082, a beneficiary is defined as a Medicaid enrollee who had payments made on their behalf by Medicaid during the fiscal year. The actual services may have been provided in a prior fiscal year. In order to be counted as a beneficiary, payments may be made for: a covered medical service; a Medicare deductible or coinsurance amount for qualified Medicare beneficiaries, and capitation or premium payments for Medicaid beneficiaries enrolled in managed care plans.[5]

1. Receipt of Cash Welfare Payments

Tables 1 and 2 provide information on beneficiaries divided into five categories:

- individuals who receive Medicaid services and who also receive some form of cash assistance payments (i.e., Aid to Families with Dependent Children (AFDC), Supplemental Security Income (SSI) payments, mandatory or optional State supplements, and children receiving adoption assistance or foster care maintenance payments).

- individuals who receive Medicaid services and are categorically eligible for the program, but do not receive any cash assistance payments.

---

[3]See U.S. Executive Office of the President. Office of Management and Budget. *Mid-Session Review of the Budget.* July 15, 1991. p. 23.

[4]See Cherlow, Ann, Marilyn Rymer Ellwood, Embry Howell, Kay Miller, and Suzanne Dodds. *Data Quality in the Medicaid Statistical Information System (MSIS).* SysteMetrics/McGraw-Hill, Dec. 1991.

[5]While a beneficiary is anyone who is enrolled in a Medicaid managed care plan, the payment information reported in later tables excludes these capitation payment amounts.

Also included in this category are aliens receiving emergency assistance.

- individuals who receive Medicaid services and are medically needy (i.e., persons who are unable to cover the cost of their medical care and expenses and who meet the categorical requirements of the program). This is an optional category of eligibility.

- individuals who do not qualify as medically needy, but who are eligible for the program based on legislative changes effective prior to January 1, 1988. *Chapter IX, Recent Legislative History* highlights these eligibility categories. This group contains individuals who are eligible at a State's option. Individuals in this category include: persons receiving Medicaid through receipt of State supplementary payments, and aged, blind or disabled persons, pregnant women and infants eligible under the provisions of the Budget Reconciliation Acts of 1986 and 1987, the Deficit Reduction Act of 1984, the Tax Equity and Fiscal Responsibility Act of 1982 and other legislation.[6]

- individuals who receive Medicaid services and qualify for the program as a result of legislation effective on or after January 1, 1988. Qualified Medicare beneficiaries, and mandatory coverage of pregnant women and infants with low incomes would be included in this category.

In FY 1991, about 61 percent of all Medicaid beneficiaries also received some form of cash welfare payments. This can be compared with FY 1986, when 75 percent of all beneficiaries received these payments. This reduction in the share of beneficiaries receiving cash welfare is largely a result of the decoupling of Medicaid from the cash welfare system. For example, the 1991 beneficiary count includes 1.7 million beneficiaries who were eligible for Medicaid as a result of the eligibility expansions effective after January 1, 1988--expansions that base Medicaid eligibility on criteria that generally are distinct from those used by the cash welfare programs. Figure X-1 portrays the States by the share of Medicaid beneficiaries receiving cash welfare payments. Most States indicated that

---

[6]In order to attempt to isolate new eligibility groups, the HCFA Form 2082 added this and the subsequently discussed eligibility category to the statistical reporting form. Unfortunately, the use of the January 1, 1988 effective date does not allow for the analysis of the effect of particular eligibility expansions. As noted in *Chapter IX, Recent Legislative History*, some of the eligibility expansions (e.g., coverage of pregnant women and young children) were first introduced as optional coverage categories (i.e., States could choose to enroll individuals in these categories, but were not required). Subsequent legislation made the categories mandatory. These optional and mandatory expansions occurred prior to and subsequent to January 1, 1988. Instructions for the form require States to divide the group based on the effective date of legislation. In addition, some categories that in previous years were counted in the categorically needy no cash assistance group and the "other" group were moved to this category.

roughly 60 percent of beneficiaries also received cash payments. In 6 States and the District of Columbia over 70 percent of Medicaid beneficiaries also received cash assistance payments (see figure X-1). These States include: Rhode Island, New Jersey, Michigan, Georgia, Colorado, and New Mexico.

As can be seen in table X-2, payments per Medicaid beneficiary varied rather dramatically by eligibility category. Overall, the Medicaid program spent $2,752 per Medicaid beneficiary.[7] However, payments per medically needy beneficiary equalled $4,658, while payments per beneficiary receiving cash welfare were approximately 44 percent of this amount, $2,053. In addition to the variation among eligibility groups, the payment per beneficiary varies from a low of $1,607 in Mississippi to a high of $5,994 in Connecticut. It should be noted that overall payment per beneficiary estimates are influenced by many factors including: the different mix of beneficiaries, the types of services covered, and the reimbursement methods used by each State. Additional discussion of State variation in payments per beneficiary is provided in *Chapter II, Trends in Medicaid Payments and Beneficiaries.*

2. *Eligibility Groups*

Table X-3 divides beneficiaries into five groups based on the individual's eligibility category:

- *Children in low-income families.* This category includes both children who receive cash welfare payments and those who may qualify for Medicaid through the myriad other avenues of eligibility for low-income children, including the recent eligibility expansion categories. In this table a child is defined as an individual under the age of 18.[8]

- *Adults in low-income families.* This category represents individuals who are the "caretaker relatives" of individuals in low-income families. There is no lower or upper bound on an "adult's" age.

- *Low-income aged.* This group mainly consists of persons 65 years of age or older who either receive SSI or qualify for Medicaid because they meet the stricter eligibility guidelines in 209(b) States. Aged individuals who do not have enough resources to pay for their medical services and living expenses are also in this category.

- *Low-income disabled.* This category represents the blind and disabled who qualify for Medicaid, primarily as a result of SSI receipt. An

---

[7]All payment per beneficiary estimates contained in this report exclude Arizona.

[8]This age limit is a general rule. Under some circumstances in some States eligibility will extend beyond age 18. *Chapter III, Eligibility* highlights the States and circumstances where this happens. These children are also included in this category.

individual will be counted in this group regardless of age. Therefore, disabled children and adults will be counted in this category.

- *Others.* This group represents individuals who qualify for Medicaid through other eligibility criteria. It is a relatively small category representing less than 4 percent of the total.

Children and adults in low-income families make up 70 percent of the total number of Medicaid beneficiaries. Approximately 4.1 million beneficiaries are blind or disabled, roughly 14 percent of the total. Table X-3 provides the State-by-State distribution for these eligibility categories.

Figure X-4 highlights the dramatic difference in the payment per beneficiary using these eligibility categories. In FY 1991, the average payment per beneficiary for a low-income child on Medicaid was $902, the average payment per beneficiary for aged and disabled beneficiaries was about 8 times as large, $7,617 and $7,005 respectively. The variation among States for these payment categories is shown in table X-4.

3. Age of Beneficiary

Tables X-5 and X-6 provide information on beneficiaries by age; it ignores how these individuals become eligible for the program. The table divides the Medicaid beneficiary population into four categories:

- children under 6 years old;
- children who are 6 to 20 years old;
- adults who are 21 to 64 years old; and
- adults 65 years old or older

Children under the age of 21 represent about half (49 percent) of all Medicaid beneficiaries. This age group's overall share of the beneficiary population remains essentially unchanged from 1986. However, the share of children under age 6 has increased. In FY 1986, children under 6 represented 21.3 percent of all beneficiaries; in FY 1991 young children represented 23.5 percent of all beneficiaries. The total number of children in this table differs somewhat from table X-3 for two reasons. First, a child is defined in table X-5 as anyone under the age of 21, while in table X-3 a child is largely defined as anyone under age 18. Second, a share of those individuals who are counted as low-income disabled in table X-3 are counted in the child categories in table X-5.

Table X-6 highlights the difference in payments per beneficiary for each of these age groups. As in the previous table, benefit payments per child are substantially less than for adults and the aged. For example, payments per beneficiary for children age 6 and under equalled $1,157 as compared to payments per beneficiary for persons age 65 or older which equalled $7,087.

4. Race/Ethnicity of Beneficiary

Table X-7 provides information on the number of beneficiaries by racial/ethnic category. The table divides beneficiaries into:

- white, not of Hispanic origin;
- black, not of Hispanic origin;
- American Indian or Alaskan native;
- Asian or Pacific islander; and
- Hispanic

Whites comprised over 48 percent of the total Medicaid beneficiary population in States providing race/ethnicity information, blacks comprised 28 percent, Hispanics comprised 13 percent and 8 percent of the total was reported as unknown. In addition to this 8 percent, Arizona, Maine, Rhode Island, Puerto Rico, and the Virgin Islands did not provide information on the race/ethnicity of Medicaid beneficiaries.

Table X-8 provides race/ethnicity information on payments per beneficiary taking into account the beneficiary's age. Not only does this table exhibit the general pattern showing lower payments for children between the ages of 1 and 20 compared with other age groups, but the table shows a difference in payments per beneficiary between each racial/ethnic category. It should be noted that this summary comparison does not take into account the mix of services and method of reimbursement used for the payment of services for these beneficiary groups.

B. Payments

As portrayed in the following tables, Medicaid payments include expenditures on claims of providers for services provided to Medicaid beneficiaries; and any deductible or coinsurance amounts for Medicare qualified beneficiaries. The payment amounts exclude: administration and training costs; any State payments that do not meet Federal matching requirements; payments provided under the emergency assistance provisions of title IV; and capitation payments. Payments represent total spending for these services. That is, both the Federal and State/local share of payments.

C. Service Categories

Tables X-9 through X-13 provide State level information on Medicaid services. This classification is based on the billing category for the service. The following list provides broad descriptions of what services fall into individual categories.

Table X-9, Hospital Services:

Inpatient hospital services. Services that are provided in a hospital in the care and treatment of acute inpatient episodes. Nursing home type activities furnished by a hospital with "swing-bed" approval are excluded from this category.[9]

Outpatient hospital services. Preventive, diagnostic, therapeutic, rehabilitative or palliative services that are furnished to outpatients by a physician, dentist, or nurse midwife in a hospital.

Table X-10, Practitioner Services:

Physician services. Physician services include services provided and billed by a physician with the exception of lab and x-ray services. The services can be furnished in a physician's office, a beneficiary's home, nursing facility, hospital or elsewhere. The services in this category do not include services provided and billed by a hospital, clinic or laboratory.

Dental services. Diagnostic, preventive, or corrective procedures provided by a dentist including dental screening and dental clinic services. Services in this category exclude services provided as part of inpatient, outpatient hospital, non-dental clinic or laboratory services that are billed separately.

Other practitioner services. Services provided by practitioners other than physicians or dentists. Examples of such practitioners are: nurse practitioners, chiropractors, podiatrists, psychologists, optometrists, and private duty nurses. This category includes the cost of hearing aids and eyeglasses if they are directly billed by the professional. Prosthetic devices or other devices/services are counted in the other services categories. Services rendered by speech therapists, audiologists, opticians, physical therapists, and occupational therapists are excluded from this category and are included in the other care category.

Table X-11, Long-Term Care Services:

Nursing facility services. Services provided by a separate nursing facility, or a distinct part of a facility designated for nursing services, or a swing-bed hospital that has approval to provide nursing facility services. Services in this category combine those services that were reported in earlier years as separate categories: intermediate care facility services, and skilled nursing facility services.

Intermediate care facilities for the mentally retarded (ICFs/MR). Services provided for the mentally retarded or persons with related conditions in a designated ICF/MR.

Inpatient mental health services. Services to: individuals age 65 or older in an institution for mental diseases; and inpatient psychiatric facility services for persons under 22. An institution for mental diseases is a hospital

---

[9]Swing-beds are acute care hospital beds that can be used to provide long-term care services.

or other institution of 16 beds or more that is primarily engaged in treating individuals with mental disease.

Home health services. These are services provided at a beneficiary's place of residence. Services in this setting include: nursing services; home health aide services; physical therapy, occupational therapy, speech pathology and audiology services performed by a home health agency. Personal care services and home and community-based waiver services are also included in this category. Additionally, payment for medical supplies and equipment used in the home are included in this category.

Table X-12, Clinic and Related Services:

Clinic services. Preventive, diagnostic, therapeutic, rehabilitative or palliative items or services that are provided on an outpatient basis in a facility that is not part of a hospital. Services provided in physician and dental group practices are reported in the physician services and dental services categories. Services provided in Federally Qualified Health Centers (FQHC) are reported in this category.

Early and Periodic Screening. This category encompasses the two sets of screenings that comprise the Early and Periodic Screening provision of the EPSDT program within Medicaid: (1) periodic screenings to Medicaid eligibles under 21 that include a physical exam, immunizations, laboratory tests, and health education; and (2) interperiodic screenings that are medically necessary. Dental, hearing, or vision services that are part of these screening are excluded from this category and reported in the dental or other practitioner services categories.

Rural health clinics. Services provided in a rural health clinic, or services by a physician who has an agreement with the rural health clinic whether those services are provided in or away from the clinic, or services provided by a physician assistant, nurse practitioner, nurse midwife, or specialized nurse practitioner. In addition, part-time or intermittent visiting nurse care as well as supplies are included in this category.

Family planning services. Services defined under an individual State's plan for family planning services including: consultation, laboratory services, and other approved services and supplies.

Table X-13, Ancillary Services and Other Care:

Laboratory and x-ray services. Laboratory and radiological services that are provided by an independent laboratory, provided in an office or facility other than an inpatient or outpatient department or clinic. X-ray, laboratory or other radiological services provided by dentists or as part of family planning services are included in the dental or family planning service categories, respectively.

Prescribed drugs. Drugs for the cure, mitigation or prevention of disease prescribed by a physician or other licensed practitioner and dispensed by a licensed pharmacist or authorized practitioner.

Other care. Any medical services or remedial care that are within the scope of a State's Medicaid plan, but do not fall into the other designated service categories. Service and supplies that could be included in this category are: physical therapy, occupational therapy, services for persons with speech, hearing or language disorders, dentures, some prosthetic devices, some eyeglasses, diagnostic, screening, preventive and rehabilitative services not reported elsewhere, hospice services and transportation.

The figures provided with the service category tables highlight the wide variation in the size of the payments made for each service category, as well as the variation in the size of the payments made per beneficiary. In terms of total payments, the largest Medicaid service category is nursing home care ($20.7 billion), followed by inpatient hospital care ($19.8 billion), intermediate care for the mentally retarded ($7.7 billion), prescribed drugs ($5.4 billion) and physician services ($4.9 billion). These categories represent 76 percent of all Medicaid spending in FY 1991. On a per beneficiary basis the most expensive service categories are found in the long-term care service categories. Medicaid payment per beneficiary for beneficiaries in ICFs/MR equalled $52,791 per annum. Inpatient mental health services equalled $30,970, nursing home care $13,893 and home health services $5,070. On a per beneficiary basis, the least expensive service and supply categories include: early and periodic screenings ($83 per beneficiary), lab and x-ray services ($86 per beneficiary), and other practitioner services ($102 per beneficiary).

FIGURE X-1. Share of Medicaid Beneficiaries who also Receive Cash Welfare Payments, FY 1991

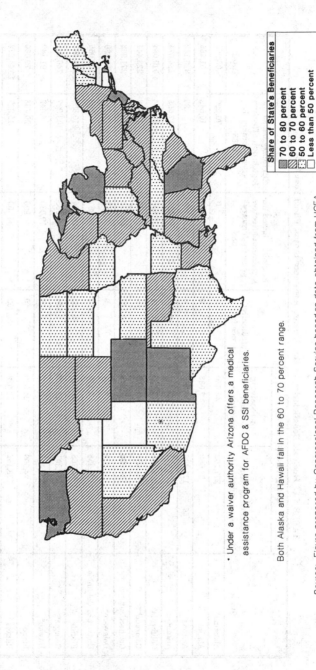

Share of State's Beneficiaries
- 70 to 80 percent
- 60 to 70 percent
- 50 to 60 percent
- Less than 50 percent

* Under a waiver authority Arizona offers a medical assistance program for AFDC & SSI beneficiaries.

Both Alaska and Hawaii fall in the 60 to 70 percent range.

Source: Figure prepared by Congressional Research Service based on data obtained from HCFA.

TABLE X-1. Medicaid Beneficiaries, by Maintenance Assistance Status, Fiscal Year 1991

State	Categorically needy		Medically needy	Eligibility based on legislation effective prior to January 1988	Eligibility based on legislation effective after January 1, 1988	Total
	Receiving cash assistance	Not receiving cash assistance				
Alabama[a]	277,109	48,530	0	0	76,520	403,255
Alaska	33,560	7,086	0	0	10,642	51,288
Arizona	177,406	16,236	0	119,464	36	313,142
Arkansas	169,475	23,391	13,625	60,625	17,558	284,674
California[a]	2,524,168	519,865	775,314	68,496	98,334	4,019,084
Colorado[a]	158,039	50,883	0	1,973	12,546	223,444
Connecticut	110,020	1,273	57,147	55,073	48,390	271,903
Delaware[a]	34,608	5,464	0	4,642	5,848	50,680
District of Columbia	79,258	9,115	6,916	4,251	525	100,065
Florida	782,768	87,038	48,233	120,494	210,350	1,248,883
Georgia[a]	537,301	42,973	2,514	46,833	103,937	746,241
Hawaii[a]	55,456	0	9,378	19,090	4,442	91,162
Idaho	24,006	24,560	0	996	20,498	70,060
Illinois	778,162	72,672	183,752	94,359	15,327	1,144,272
Indiana[a]	237,327	116,945	0	57,628	196	415,167
Iowa[a]	151,287	85,542	23,439	337	0	261,419

See notes at end of table.

TABLE X-1. Medicaid Beneficiaries, by Maintenance Assistance Status, Fiscal Year 1991–Continued

State	Categorically needy		Medically needy	Eligibility based on legislation effective prior to January 1988	Eligibility based on legislation effective after January 1, 1988	Total
	Receiving cash assistance	Not receiving cash assistance				
Kansas[a]	120,413	18,113	21,668	44,084	0	209,329
Kentucky[a][b]	365,762	27,395	51,433	38,090	33,931	525,497
Louisiana	429,252	61,705	13,026	79,373	57,206	640,562
Maine[a]	89,301	42,817	3,621	14,214	37	150,623
Maryland	251,553	15,546	64,469	29,364	1,588	362,520
Massachusetts	153,511	329,144	96,830	41,663	29,908	651,056
Michigan	821,769	65,399	157,940	37,107	30,318	1,112,533
Minnesota	259,053	22,475	131,434	8,434	342	421,738
Mississippi	320,585	34,487	0	19,591	95,021	469,684
Missouri[a]	241,867	187,679	0	4,337	62,222	503,310
Montana[a][b]	41,897	10,469	3,120	6,279	0	63,615
Nebraska	60,846	54,824	2,386	0	15,695	133,751
Nevada[a]	33,744	21,589	0	2,265	1,397	59,296
New Hampshire[a]	34,774	15,156	7,272	2,003	190	59,684
New Jersey[a][b]	460,723	88,893	4,958	28,333	20,677	614,073
New Mexico	114,342	31,010	0	7,114	9,529	161,995
New York	1,630,865	93,092	705,316	0	32,264	2,461,537

See notes at end of table.

TABLE X-1. Medicaid Beneficiaries, by Maintenance Assistance Status, Fiscal Year 1991--Continued

State	Categorically needy		Medically needy	Eligibility based on legislation effective prior to January 1988	Eligibility based on legislation effective after January 1, 1988	Total
	Receiving cash assistance	Not receiving cash assistance				
North Carolina	354,980	21,448	58,912	162,619	69,244	667,203
North Dakota[a]	27,737	5,741	17,696	0	768	52,539
Ohio	891,311	249,168	0	49,632	109,174	1,299,285
Oklahoma	195,077	52,186	13,578	479	43,339	304,659
Oregon	166,380	10,713	17,045	40,398	28,767	263,303
Pennsylvania	815,623	213,921	127,879	82,918	37,087	1,277,428
Rhode Island	127,789	15,711	19,299	905	0	163,704
South Carolina	237,023	4,523	4,972	31,496	97,219	375,233
South Dakota	32,761	4,715	0	6,815	12,854	57,145
Tennessee	415,203	78,014	73,337	115,655	15,202	697,411
Texas	1,034,052	203,478	63,383	94,236	333,480	1,728,629
Utah[a]	63,490	17,391	5,084	15,916	24,591	129,274
Vermont[a b]	40,971	25,108	4,472	0	0	70,699
Virginia	271,834	41,458	38,479	80,963	9,339	442,073
Washington[a]	354,241	93,477	24,843	31,624	680	506,279
West Virginia	197,795	43,460	9,046	0	33,407	283,708
Wisconsin[a]	254,575	138,892	16,284	597	2,753	415,942

See notes at end of table.

TABLE X-1. Medicaid Beneficiaries, by Maintenance Assistance Status, Fiscal Year 1991.-Continued

| State | Categorically needy | | | Eligibility based on legislation effective prior to January 1988 | Eligibility based on legislation effective after January 1, 1988 | Total |
	Receiving cash assistance	Not receiving cash assistance	Medically needy			
Wyoming[a]	23,781	12,899	0	0	0	36,804
Puerto Rico	296,190	324,486	580,523	0	0	1,201,199
Virgin Islands	4,398	217	6,930	0	177	11,722
50 States and the District of Columbia[a][b]	17,064,830	3,463,669	2,878,100	1,730,765	1,833,378	27,066,860
U.S. Total[a][b]	17,365,418	3,788,372	3,465,553	1,730,765	1,833,555	28,279,781

[a]Total beneficiary estimate includes some individuals with an unknown eligibility category.

[b]If an individual's eligibility status changes during the year, they may be counted in more than one category in this State.

NOTE: Medicaid beneficiaries are individuals who receive any Medicaid covered services during the year. Individuals eligible for Medicaid because of eligibility expansions associated with legislation effective prior to 1988 include individuals who receive Medicaid because of State supplemental payments, and those eligible as a result of provision in OBRA 86, OBRA 87, DEFRA, TEFRA, or earlier legislation (see Chapter IX, Recent Legislative History for details). Individuals eligible for Medicaid because of eligibility expansions associated with legislation in effect on or after January 1, 1988 include mandatory and optional coverage categories such as qualified Medicare beneficiaries (QMBs), and mandatory coverage of pregnant women and infants. All estimates represent figures reported by the States, except for Massachusetts, Rhode Island, and Puerto Rico-for these States HCFA provides estimates.

Source: Table prepared by the Congressional Research Service based on data contained on HCFA Form 2082.

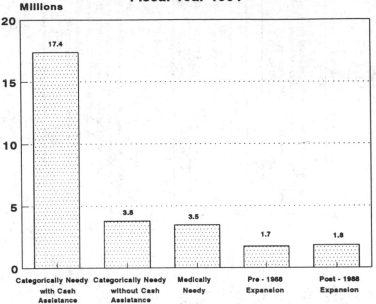

FIGURE X-2. Medicaid Beneficiaries
by Maintenance Assistance Status and Eligibility Group
Fiscal Year 1991

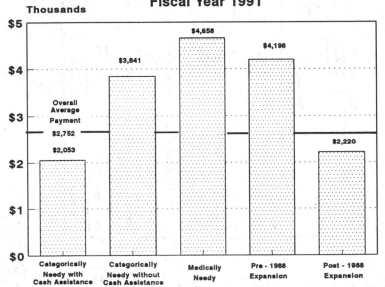

Medicaid Payments Per Beneficiary
by Maintenance Assistance Status and Eligibility Group
Fiscal Year 1991

Source: Figure prepared by Congressional Research Service based on data obtained from the Health Care Financing Adminstration.

TABLE X-2. Medicaid Payments Per Beneficiary, By Maintenance Assistance Status, Fiscal Year 1991

State[a]	Categorically needy		Medically needy	Eligibility based on legislation effective prior to January 1988	Eligibility based on legislation effective after January 1, 1988	Total
	Receiving cash assistance	Not receiving cash assistance				
Alabama[a]	$1,592	$ 5,649	$ 0	$ 0	$1,170	$1,997
Alaska	2,663	3,373	0	0	4,409	3,123
Arizona[b]	NA	NA	NA	NA	NA	NA
Arkansas	2,042	9,944	1,543	1,262	672	2,417
California[a]	1,595	1,404	2,628	1,591	6,168	1,886
Colorado[a]	2,347	5,034	0	11,928	1,770	3,011
Connecticut	1,642	13,264	5,542	16,592	4,171	5,997
Delaware[a]	2,782	1,130	0	15,780	1,657	3,671
District of Columbia	3,239	6,830	16,233	3,346	721	4,456
Florida	1,886	1,597	2,008	7,760	1,414	2,358
Georgia[a]	1,982	957	1,279	10,444	1,783	2,411
Hawaii[a]	1,180	0	3,909	6,580	1,793	2,606
Idaho	1,967	5,907	0	800	1,461	3,184
Illinois	1,814	833	6,002	1,503	931	2,387
Indiana[a]	2,608	7,919	0	1,922	491	4,003
Iowa[a]	2,349	4,322	1,725	448	0	2,930
Kansas[a]	1,954	1,526	4,265	4,287	0	2,642

See notes at end of table.

TABLE X-2. Medicaid Payments Per Beneficiary, By Maintenance Assistance Status, Fiscal Year 1991–Continued

| State | Categorically needy | | | Eligibility based on legislation effective prior to January 1988 | Eligibility based on legislation effective after January 1, 1988 | Total |
	Receiving cash assistance	Not receiving cash assistance	Medically needy			
Kentucky[a][c]	$1,966	$ 9,719	$ 2,359	$ 1,330	$ 1,137	$2,284
Louisiana	1,788	7,226	5,270	3,919	2,272	2,690
Maine[a]	2,162	7,075	3,645	1,875	573	3,561
Maryland	2,338	4,779	8,682	2,363	444	3,565
Massachusetts	6,140	1,691	9,132	3,152	10,485	4,344
Michigan	1,794	2,711	5,075	1,502	1,032	2,283
Minnesota	2,241	11,441	5,416	1,311	2,636	3,702
Mississippi	1,376	5,632	0	1,752	898	1,607
Missouri[a]	895	4,395	0	2,825	963	2,221
Montana[a][c]	2,088	7,670	4,974	889	0	3,037
Nebraska	2,473	3,858	4,487	0	1,092	2,915
Nevada[a]	1,280	5,916	0	2,248	575	3,005
New Hampshire[a]	2,512	9,279	8,385	710	7,705	4,898
New Jersey[a][c]	3,155	11,794	787	3,754	2,828	4,437
New Mexico	1,770	793	0	13,577	1,957	2,113
New York	3,902	1,566	10,135	0	2,209	5,577
North Carolina	1,739	4,722	8,018	1,996	3,929	2,679

See notes at end of table.

TABLE X-2. Medicaid Payments Per Beneficiary, By Maintenance Assistance Status, Fiscal Year 1991–Continued

| State | Categorically needy | | | Eligibility based on legislation effective prior to January 1988 | Eligibility based on legislation effective after January 1, 1988 | Total |
	Receiving cash assistance	Not receiving cash assistance	Medically needy			
North Dakota[a]	$3,219	$ 2,437	$6,813	$ 0	$2,929	$4,319
Ohio	1,437	7,104	0	1,228	4,961	2,812
Oklahoma	1,428	7,800	2,641	203	2,140	2,673
Oregon	1,500	719	1,305	7,559	1,478	2,531
Pennsylvania	2,001	5,780	2,520	1,551	3,161	2,690
Rhode Island	2,425	13,085	7,203	2,821	0	4,014
South Carolina	1,899	790	2,953	8,651	1,743	2,426
South Dakota	2,441	5,674	0	10,859	1,212	3,435
Tennessee	1,877	5,842	1,721	1,033	300	2,130
Texas	1,687	1,436	1,042	11,671	988	2,043
Utah[a]	1,958	1,306	3,880	6,312	1,706	2,408
Vermont[a c]	2,392	2,380	8,645	0	0	2,782
Virginia	2,176	5,091	7,849	1,305	871	2,756
Washington[a]	1,651	4,658	2,435	1,553	1,038	2,235
West Virginia	1,428	4,163	2,064	0	1,806	1,912
Wisconsin[a]	2,417	5,702	2,570	557	6,898	3,537
Wyoming[a]	1,907	3,456	0	0	0	2,450

See notes at end of table.

TABLE X-2. Medicaid Payments Per Beneficiary, By Maintenance Assistance Status, Fiscal Year 1991—Continued

| State | Categorically needy | | Medically needy | Eligibility based on legislation effective prior to January 1988 | Eligibility based on legislation effective after January 1, 1988 | Total |
	Receiving cash assistance	Not receiving cash assistance				
Puerto Rico	$ 120	$ 100	$ 135	$ 0	$ 0	$ 122
Virgin Islands	318	306	394	0	76	359
49 reporting States and the District of Columbia[a][c]	2,087	4,193	5,580	4,198	2,220	2,871
U.S. Total[a][c]	$2,053	$3,841	$4,658	$4,198	$2,220	$2,752

[a]Total beneficiary estimate includes some individuals with an unknown eligibility category.

[b]The Health Care Financing Administration does not report capitation payments for Arizona, therefore this estimate is unavailable.

[c]If an individual's eligibility status changes during the year, they may be counted in more than one category in this State.

NOTE: Medicaid beneficiaries are individuals who have any Medicaid covered services paid for during the year. Individuals eligible for Medicaid because of eligibility expansions associated with legislation effective prior to 1988 include individuals who receive Medicaid because of State supplemental payments, and those eligible as a result of provision in OBRA 86, OBRA 87, DEFRA, TEFRA, or earlier legislation (see Chapter IX, Recent Legislative History for details). Individuals eligible for Medicaid because of eligibility expansions associated with legislation in effect on or after January 1, 1988 include mandatory and optional coverage categories such as QMBs, and mandatory coverage of pregnant women and infants. All estimates represent figures reported by the States, except for Massachusetts, Rhode Island, and Puerto Rico–for these States HCFA provides estimates. Estimates are based on total (Federal and State) payments for services and supplies and exclude any administrative or other expenses. See the accompanying text for additional detail.

Source: Table prepared by the Congressional Research Service based on data contained on HCFA Form 2082.

FIGURE X-3. Medicaid Beneficiaries by Categorical Characteristics Fiscal Year 1991

Unduplicated Total = 28.3 Million

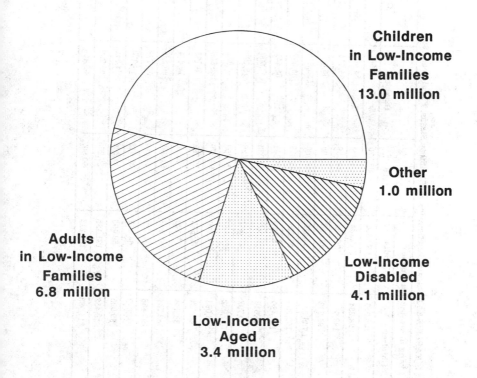

Children
in Low-Income
Families
13.0 million

Other
1.0 million

Adults
in Low-Income
Families
6.8 million

Low-Income
Disabled
4.1 million

Low-Income
Aged
3.4 million

Source: Figure prepared by Congressional Research Service based on data obtained from the Health Care Financing Administration.

TABLE X-3. Medicaid Beneficiaries, by Eligibility Status, Fiscal Year 1991

State	Living in low-income families[a]		Aged	Disabled	Other	Total
	Children	Adults				
Alabama	158,033	79,865	68,370	90,681	6,306	403,255
Alaska	28,284	15,234	3,368	4,402	0	51,288
Arizona	183,618	75,051	18,959	35,514	0	313,142
Arkansas	98,292	49,086	45,896	58,657	32,743	284,674
California	1,768,004	1,134,615	456,700	586,215	73,550	4,019,084
Colorado	100,854	56,225	31,813	30,502	4,050	223,444
Connecticut	122,430	4,481	43,085	68,441	33,466	271,903
Delaware	24,819	12,007	5,038	7,500	1,316	50,680
District of Columbia	50,702	22,662	11,426	15,199	76	100,065
Florida	581,922	284,836	174,852	184,832	22,441	1,248,883
Georgia	336,094	174,140	93,279	128,859	13,869	746,241
Hawaii	43,734	22,652	12,792	9,188	2,796	91,162
Idaho	34,344	17,123	7,586	10,484	523	70,060
Illinois	582,764	268,585	91,092	185,238	16,593	1,144,272
Indiana	195,456	104,383	48,484	63,773	3,071	415,167
Iowa	107,619	64,477	37,013	36,276	16,034	261,419
Kansas	99,095	56,495	24,646	24,042	5,051	209,329
Kentucky	219,452	121,135	57,260	102,298	25,352	525,497
Louisiana	314,083	139,213	90,807	96,459	0	640,562

See notes at end of table.

TABLE X-3. Medicaid Beneficiaries, by Eligibility Status, Fiscal Year 1991–Continued

State	Living in low-income families[a]		Aged	Disabled	Other	Total
	Children	Adults				
Maine	61,841	36,189	21,600	24,827	6,166	150,623
Maryland	177,523	79,177	43,903	54,914	7,003	362,520
Massachusetts	294,145	141,293	96,198	113,884	5,536	651,056
Michigan	563,754	310,348	85,930	152,501	0	1,112,533
Minnesota	210,293	104,574	54,512	41,560	10,799	421,738
Mississippi	225,502	87,907	67,966	87,162	1,147	469,684
Missouri	226,416	124,246	76,579	68,858	7,211	503,310
Montana	22,183	12,602	7,443	10,837	10,550	63,615
Nebraska	59,922	28,581	18,386	15,486	11,376	133,751
Nevada	26,461	14,100	8,303	8,662	1,770	59,296
New Hampshire	28,570	10,982	11,719	8,124	289	59,684
New Jersey	288,913	142,219	74,815	97,616	10,510	614,073
New Mexico	88,839	34,610	13,889	24,657	0	161,995
New York	1,095,225	497,347	335,948	351,080	181,937	2,461,537
North Carolina	302,847	173,410	109,796	81,149	1	667,203
North Dakota	21,554	11,287	10,343	6,576	2,779	52,539
Ohio	701,633	310,256	117,748	159,628	10,020	1,299,285
Oklahoma	143,424	68,050	53,629	38,511	1,045	304,659
Oregon	131,388	74,481	26,447	30,987	0	263,303

See notes at end of table.

TABLE X-3. Medicaid Beneficiaries, by Eligibility Status, Fiscal Year 1991--Continued

State	Living in low-income families[a]				Other	Total
	Children	Adults	Aged	Disabled		
Pennsylvania	593,179	299,853	135,382	193,910	55,104	1,277,428
Rhode Island	64,538	34,584	30,103	33,242	1,237	163,704
South Carolina	164,238	80,256	55,146	75,567	26	375,233
South Dakota	26,683	12,245	9,217	9,000	0	57,145
Tennessee	322,389	137,751	89,041	137,601	10,629	697,411
Texas	909,551	409,928	244,136	165,014	0	1,728,629
Utah	66,022	38,280	8,412	12,755	3,805	129,274
Vermont	31,233	19,114	10,499	9,281	572	70,699
Virginia	200,723	100,528	72,427	68,395	0	442,073
Washington	216,629	143,302	47,592	67,493	31,263	506,279
West Virginia	121,981	87,630	29,720	42,183	2,194	283,708
Wisconsin	165,073	77,611	66,001	80,577	26,680	415,942
Wyoming	20,144	9,749	3,044	3,201	666	36,804
Puerto Rico	409,832	360,709	0	53,976	376,682	1,201,199
Virgin Islands	6,277	2,946	1,125	800	574	11,722
50 States and the District of Columbia	12,622,415	6,414,755	3,358,340	4,013,798	657,552	27,066,860
U.S. Total	13,038,524	6,778,410	3,359,465	4,068,574	1,034,808	28,279,781

See notes below.

TABLE X-3. Medicaid Beneficiaries, by Eligibility Status, Fiscal Year 1991–Continued

ªIncludes individuals who are eligible because they meet poverty related income eligibility criteria, as well as cash assistance and medically needy criteria.

NOTE: All estimates represent figures reported by the States, except for Massachusetts, Rhode Island, and Puerto Rico–for these States HCFA provides estimates. Estimates for the number of disabled beneficiaries include beneficiaries eligible for the program who are blind. The "other" category can also include individuals with an unknown eligibility status. See text for additional detail.

Source: Table prepared by the Congressional Research Service based on data contained on HCFA Form 2082.

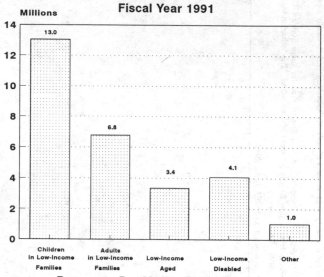

FIGURE X-4. Medicaid Beneficiaries by Categorical Characteristics Fiscal Year 1991

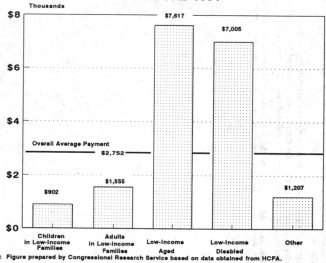

Payments Per Medicaid Beneficiary by Categorical Characteristics Fiscal Year 1991

Source: Figure prepared by Congressional Research Service based on data obtained from HCFA.

TABLE X-4. Medicaid Payments Per Beneficiary, by Eligibility Status, Fiscal Year 1991

State	Living in low-income families[a]		Aged	Disabled	Other	Total
	Children	Adults				
Alabama	$ 664	$1,499	$ 3,841	$ 3,410	$1,413	$1,997
Alaska	1,534	2,321	9,995	10,858	0	3,123
Arizona	NA	NA	NA	NA	NA	NA
Arkansas	811	1,050	4,788	4,744	1,793	2,417
California	648	1,418	4,251	4,652	2,120	1,886
Colorado	928	1,707	6,279	8,772	3,926	3,011
Connecticut	1,750	140	19,278	7,584	1,953	5,994
Delaware	996	1,893	11,355	10,491	2,058	3,671
District of Columbia	1,474	2,271	12,136	11,888	4,412	4,456
Florida	974	1,498	5,271	5,331	1,952	2,358
Georgia	794	2,242	5,190	4,973	1,222	2,411
Hawaii	838	1,816	7,974	6,083	660	2,606
Idaho	903	1,790	8,395	9,218	2,052	3,184
Illinois	719	1,123	6,644	7,340	2,754	2,387
Indiana	1,334	2,131	9,743	10,980	1,928	4,003
Iowa	970	1,885	5,919	8,076	1,747	2,930
Kansas	865	1,627	6,785	8,298	1,715	2,642
Kentucky	851	1,577	5,371	4,682	1,417	2,284

See notes at end of table.

TABLE X-4. Medicaid Payments Per Beneficiary, by Eligibility Status, Fiscal Year 1991—Continued

State	Living in low-income families[a]					Total
	Children	Adults	Aged	Disabled	Other	
Louisiana	$1,142	$2,130	$ 4,559	$ 6,780	$ 0	$2,690
Maine	945	1,736	9,834	7,667	1,996	3,561
Maryland	1,322	2,029	8,829	8,462	6,367	3,565
Massachusetts	1,371	2,084	11,584	8,887	727	4,344
Michigan	774	1,394	6,926	7,055	0	2,283
Minnesota	825	1,433	11,089	14,788	1,747	3,702
Mississippi	553	1,367	3,426	3,160	1,590	1,607
Missouri	827	1,098	5,570	5,275	613	2,221
Montana	788	1,506	8,434	6,977	1,743	3,037
Nebraska	835	1,480	7,751	8,559	1,974	2,915
Nevada	905	1,819	5,939	8,529	3,043	3,005
New Hampshire	951	1,414	12,829	12,160	1,820	4,898
New Jersey	974	2,640	11,835	11,561	5,122	4,437
New Mexico	799	1,506	6,062	5,471	0	2,113
New York	1,422	2,340	17,084	14,282	1,393	5,577
North Carolina	1,131	1,586	5,295	7,256	81	2,679
North Dakota	1,221	1,691	8,680	13,404	1,295	4,319
Ohio	1,033	1,495	10,102	7,929	943	2,812

See notes at end of table.

TABLE X-4. Medicaid Payments Per Beneficiary, by Eligibility Status, Fiscal Year 1991—Continued

State	Living in low-income families[a]		Aged	Disabled	Other	Total
	Children	Adults				
Oklahoma	$1,231	$1,776	$4,915	$6,541	$1,400	$2,673
Oregon	771	1,204	6,188	8,802	0	2,531
Pennsylvania	1,047	1,537	8,397	5,936	1,211	2,690
Rhode Island	952	1,585	8,363	8,587	2,918	4,014
South Carolina	888	1,784	4,242	5,124	4,842	2,426
South Dakota	1,071	1,345	7,744	8,875	0	3,435
Tennessee	922	1,592	4,290	4,031	3,011	2,130
Texas	723	1,537	5,036	6,152	0	2,043
Utah	840	2,021	6,273	9,619	808	2,408
Vermont	654	1,486	6,396	8,573	2,016	2,782
Virginia	905	1,694	6,025	6,288	0	2,756
Washington	733	1,688	7,876	4,970	654	2,235
West Virginia	540	1,257	5,585	4,498	4,892	1,912
Wisconsin	727	1,221	9,037	7,394	2,401	3,537
Wyoming	971	1,955	9,360	6,791	2,004	2,450
Puerto Rico	121	93	0	136	148	122
Virgin Islands	181	367	676	950	821	359

See notes at end of table.

TABLE X-4. Medicaid Payments Per Beneficiary, by Eligibility Status, Fiscal Year 1991--Continued

State	Living in low-income families[a]		Aged	Disabled	Other	Total
	Children	Adults				
49 reporting States and the District of Columbia[b]	$928	$1,638	$7,619	$7,099	$1,814	$2,871
U.S. Total[b]	$902	$1,555	$7,617	$7,005	$1,207	$2,752

[a]Includes individuals who are eligible because they meet poverty related income eligibility criteria, as well as cash assistance and medically needy criteria.

[b]The Health Care Financing Administration does not report capitation payments for Arizona, therefore this estimate is unavailable.

NOTE: All estimates represent figures reported by the States, except for Massachusetts, Rhode Island, and Puerto Rico--for these States HCFA provides estimates. Estimates for the disabled include beneficiaries eligible for the program who are blind. The "other" category can also include individuals with an unknown eligibility status. All payments per beneficiary reflect total (Federal, State and local) payments.

Source: Table prepared by the Congressional Research Service based on data contained on HCFA Form 2082.

FIGURE X-5. Medicaid Beneficiaries by Age, FY 1991

Total = 28.3 Million

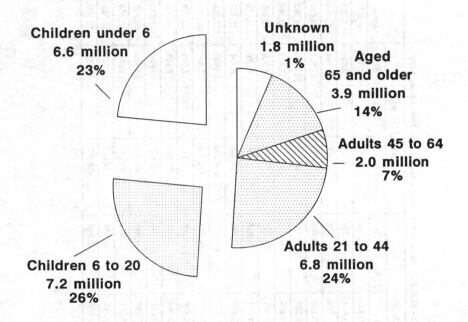

Children under 6
6.6 million
23%

Unknown
1.8 million
1%

Aged
65 and older
3.9 million
14%

Adults 45 to 64
2.0 million
7%

Children 6 to 20
7.2 million
26%

Adults 21 to 44
6.8 million
24%

NOTE: Arizona and Puerto Rico did not provide information on age
for Medicaid beneficiaries in FY 1991. Totals for these
States are included in the unknown category.

Source: Figure prepared by Congressional Research Service based
on data obtained from HCFA.

TABLE X-5. Medicaid Beneficiaries, by Age, Fiscal Year 1991

State	Children		Working age adults		Aged	Unknown	Total
	Under age 6	Age 6 to 20	Age 21 to 44	Age 45 to 64			
Alabama	100,825	91,838	87,292	35,107	87,169	1,024	403,255
Alaska	14,414	15,766	15,108	2,524	3,476	0	51,288
Arizona	NA	NA	NA	NA	NA	313,142	313,142
Arkansas	71,148	69,936	59,991	22,911	48,595	12,093	284,674
California	933,226	1,078,931	1,097,215	313,900	568,352	27,460	4,019,084
Colorado	60,215	60,003	57,637	13,281	32,308	0	223,444
Connecticut	70,061	74,167	67,672	16,918	43,085	0	271,903
Delaware	14,907	14,013	12,986	3,026	5,679	69	50,680
District of Columbia	27,463	27,329	24,768	8,404	12,101	0	100,065
Florida	257,377	246,727	364,124	107,629	273,026	0	1,248,883
Georgia	189,619	194,914	176,754	55,354	121,365	8,235	746,241
Hawaii	21,400	26,196	21,744	5,746	13,576	2,500	91,162
Idaho	22,703	17,376	17,829	3,937	8,215	0	70,060
Illinois	300,077	329,983	307,825	88,823	116,633	931	1,144,272
Indiana	107,294	109,659	107,319	30,049	58,883	1,963	415,167
Iowa	58,347	75,391	71,179	16,236	40,103	163	261,419
Kansas	50,115	60,740	57,687	14,819	25,515	453	209,329
Kentucky	113,975	145,520	136,005	49,582	73,698	6,767	525,497

TABLE X-5. Medicaid Beneficiaries, by Age, Fiscal Year 1991--Continued

State	Children		Working age adults		Aged	Unknown	Total
	Under age 6	Age 6 to 20	Age 21 to 44	Age 45 to 64			
Louisiana	183,057	178,250	143,871	44,470	90,914	0	640,562
Maine	28,819	43,269	40,513	12,735	24,724	563	150,623
Maryland	96,477	92,724	96,492	26,542	50,285	0	362,520
Massachusetts	136,185	177,225	164,881	50,094	112,879	9,792	651,056
Michigan	255,162	344,471	335,279	72,780	104,841	0	1,112,533
Minnesota	106,245	120,964	110,983	22,863	60,588	95	421,738
Mississippi	138,452	122,417	92,999	34,302	81,514	0	469,684
Missouri	128,042	125,970	124,826	37,217	81,628	5,627	503,310
Montana	12,056	18,391	18,017	4,886	8,639	1,626	63,615
Nebraska	37,096	39,084	31,090	7,796	18,685	0	133,751
Nevada	17,267	14,348	14,788	4,007	8,653	233	59,296
New Hampshire	14,474	15,137	15,933	3,869	10,059	212	59,684
New Jersey	138,437	179,536	156,629	42,022	92,844	4,605	614,073
New Mexico	49,824	41,100	38,340	10,302	18,565	3,864	161,995
New York	614,131	704,390	587,666	184,218	371,132	0	2,461,537
North Carolina	173,867	167,575	159,866	54,111	111,784	0	667,203
North Dakota	10,738	14,372	12,886	3,457	10,555	531	52,539
Ohio	326,034	404,068	353,069	83,011	133,103	0	1,299,285

TABLE X-5. Medicaid Beneficiaries, by Age, Fiscal Year 1991.–Continued

State	Children		Working age adults		Aged	Unknown	Total
	Under age 6	Age 6 to 20	Age 21 to 44	Age 45 to 64			
Oklahoma	68,617	87,933	71,458	21,459	55,445	0	304,659
Oregon	76,392	69,879	73,587	14,979	28,309	157	263,303
Pennsylvania	296,526	372,059	348,772	107,583	152,488	0	1,277,428
Rhode Island	NA	NA	NA	NA	NA	163,704	163,704
South Carolina	97,276	91,992	83,647	31,538	70,637	143	375,233
South Dakota	16,202	14,247	13,019	3,486	10,191	0	57,145
Tennessee	167,657	190,172	160,609	67,098	111,875	0	697,411
Texas	574,737	445,257	371,789	94,740	242,106	0	1,728,629
Utah	37,357	38,282	36,410	5,898	8,768	2,559	129,274
Vermont	14,427	20,059	19,898	5,514	10,706	95	70,699
Virginia	120,421	107,893	103,150	35,458	75,151	0	442,073
Washington	118,011	142,989	156,987	34,946	52,375	971	506,279
West Virginia	72,008	77,753	76,418	23,614	33,914	1	283,708
Wisconsin	85,200	105,834	113,150	30,948	78,551	2,259	415,942
Wyoming	10,885	11,248	10,015	1,538	3,070	48	36,804
Puerto Rico	NA	NA	NA	NA	NA	1,201,199	1,201,199
Virgin Islands	3,134	3,843	2,680	837	1,228	0	11,722

TABLE X-5. Medicaid Beneficiaries, by Age, Fiscal Year 1991–Continued

State	Children			Working age adults			Unknown	Total
	Under age 6	Age 6 to 20	Age 21 to 44	Age 45 to 64	Aged			
50 States and the District of Columbia	6,635,245	7,217,377	6,820,172	1,965,677	3,856,757		571,885	27,066,860
U.S. Total	6,638,379	7,221,220	6,822,852	1,966,514	3,857,985		1,773,084	28,279,781

NA = Not available.

NOTE: Tabulation based on age of beneficiary and therefore will differ from similar categories found in table X-1. For instance, a number of children and the aged in this table will be classified as disabled in table X-1. All estimates represent figures reported by the States. Estimates were not available for Arizona, Rhode Island and Puerto Rico.

Source: Table prepared by the Congressional Research Service based on data contained on HCFA Form 2082.

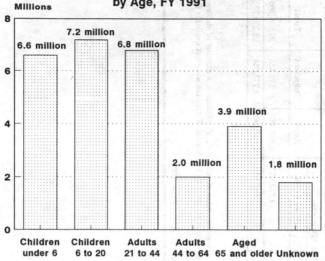

FIGURE X-6. Medicaid Beneficiaries by Age, FY 1991

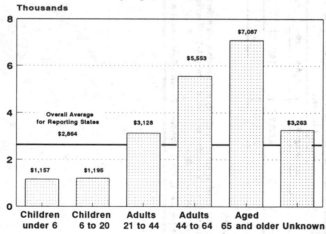

Payments Per Medicaid Beneficiary by Age, FY 1991

NOTE: Estimates exclude payments for Arizona, Rhode Island, Puerto Rico and the Virgin Islands. These States and entities did not provide information.
Source: Figure prepared by Congressional Research Service based on data obtained from HCFA.

TABLE X-6. Medicaid Payments Per Beneficiary, by Age, Fiscal Year 1991

State	Children		Working age adults		Aged	Unknown	Total
	Under age 6	Age 6 to 20	Age 21 to 44	Age 45 to 64			
Alabama	$ 947	$ 957	$2,217	$3,192	$ 3,619	$ 965	$1,997
Alaska	1,811	1,904	3,470	6,810	9,915	0	3,123
Arkansas	1,366	1,472	2,425	3,613	3,925	5,695	2,417
California	765	893	2,408	3,700	3,593	2,048	1,886
Colorado	1,127	1,669	3,776	6,295	6,301	0	3,011
Connecticut	1,328	1,682	7,469	7,486	18,105	0	5,994
Delaware	1,731	1,101	4,087	9,247	11,134	7,684	3,671
District of Columbia	2,066	1,258	5,283	9,427	11,954	0	4,456
Florida	1,200	1,324	2,242	3,591	4,051	0	2,358
Georgia	1,130	1,164	2,870	4,560	4,843	1,293	2,411
Hawaii	1,041	903	2,536	4,921	7,841	692	2,606
Idaho	1,302	1,723	3,695	7,352	8,367	0	3,184
Illinois	1,084	843	2,718	5,562	6,829	516	2,387
Indiana	1,553	1,900	4,277	8,550	9,614	2,419	4,003
Iowa	1,239	1,464	3,500	6,057	5,877	639	2,930
Kansas	826	1,449	3,071	5,098	6,675	1,270	2,642
Kentucky	1,100	1,202	2,414	4,134	4,934	490	2,284
Louisiana	1,376	1,583	3,527	5,997	4,567	0	2,690

TABLE X-6. Medicaid Payments Per Beneficiary, by Age, Fiscal Year 1991 –Continued

State	Children		Working age adults			Unknown	Total
	Under age 6	Age 6 to 20	Age 21 to 44	Age 45 to 64	Aged		
Maine	$1,214	%1,442	$3,487	$6,318	$8,769	$710	$3,561
Maryland	1,644	1,817	3,587	7,308	8,454	0	3,565
Massachusetts	1,561	1,650	4,173	6,837	10,761	7,990	4,344
Michigan	1,080	814	2,625	5,696	6,577	0	2,283
Minnesota	883	1,166	4,046	8,716	11,188	2,882	3,702
Mississippi	680	855	1,877	3,177	3,345	0	1,607
Missouri	1,067	861	2,247	3,960	5,406	649	2,221
Montana	1,095	1,399	2,880	5,730	8,120	2,618	3,037
Nebraska	1,121	1,232	3,311	6,695	7,759	0	2,915
Nevada	1,602	1,388	3,558	6,493	5,886	4,422	3,005
New Hampshire	1,104	993	4,521	9,944	14,938	2,678	4,898
New Jersey	1,422	1,397	5,208	9,474	11,330	2,448	4,437
New Mexico	874	1,186	2,567	4,685	5,397	786	2,113
New York	1,845	1,712	5,675	10,432	16,523	0	5,577
North Carolina	1,247	1,314	3,054	5,018	5,286	0	2,679
North Dakota	1,441	1,651	4,983	9,230	8,630	987	4,319
Ohio	1,415	1,036	2,671	6,260	9,846	0	2,812
Oklahoma	1,048	1,993	2,902	4,165	4,808	0	2,673

TABLE X-6. Medicaid Payments Per Beneficiary, by Age, Fiscal Year 1991–Continued

State	Children		Working age adults			Aged	Unknown	Total
	Under age 6	Age 6 to 20	Age 21 to 44	Age 45 to 64				
Oregon	$ 781	$1,097	$3,198	$5,579		$6,065	$252,498	$2,531
Pennsylvania	1,190	1,188	2,690	4,774		7,799	0	2,690
South Carolina	1,158	1,114	3,085	4,638		3,986	65,512	2,426
South Dakota	1,524	1,603	3,886	6,803		7,309	0	3,435
Tennessee	1,017	1,162	2,450	3,866		3,940	0	2,130
Texas	954	873	2,492	4,729		5,041	0	2,043
Utah	1,110	1,277	3,477	6,460		6,178	807	2,408
Vermont	887	1,011	3,170	5,875		6,346	2,343	2,782
Virginia	1,206	1,099	3,087	5,264		5,982	0	2,756
Washington	731	1,008	2,264	4,381		7,473	1,039	2,235
West Virginia	672	951	1,983	3,907		5,200	13,991	1,912
Wisconsin	981	1,290	3,151	6,267		8,887	1,044	3,537
Wyoming	1,425	983	2,572	5,967		9,306	2,195	2,450
Reporting States	1,157	1,195	3,128	5,533		7,087	3,263	2,864

NOTE: Tabulation based on age of beneficiary and therefore will differ from similar categories found in table X-1. For instance, a number of children and the aged in this table will be classified as disabled in table X-1. Information not available for Arizona, Rhode Island, Puerto Rico and Virgin Islands.

Source: Table prepared by the Congressional Research Service based on data contained on HCFA Form 2082.

FIGURE X-7. Medicaid Beneficiaries by Race/Ethnicity, Fiscal Year 1991

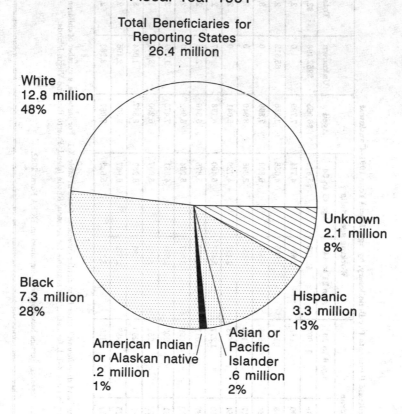

Total Beneficiaries for
Reporting States
26.4 million

White
12.8 million
48%

Unknown
2.1 million
8%

Black
7.3 million
28%

Hispanic
3.3 million
13%

American Indian
or Alaskan native
.2 million
1%

Asian or
Pacific
Islander
.6 million
2%

NOTE: Distribution excludes beneficiaries in Arizona, Maine, Rhode Island, Puerto Rico and the Virgin Islands.

Source: Figure prepared by Congressional Research Service based on data obtained from HCFA.

TABLE X-7. Medicaid Beneficiaries, by Race/Ethnicity, Fiscal Year 1991

State	White	Black	American Indian	Asian	Hispanic	Unknown	Total
Alabama	162,932	216,395	391	726	495	22,316	403,255
Alaska	26,541	3,671	17,691	1,544	1,227	614	51,288
Arizona	0	0	0	0	0	0	313,142
Arkansas	188,713	81,713	184	272	700	13,092	284,674
California	1,451,439	542,013	19,384	358,615	1,240,930	406,703	4,019,084
Colorado	122,012	23,566	2,111	3,782	69,002	2,971	223,444
Connecticut	124,622	65,413	271	2,376	73,963	5,258	271,903
Delaware	20,660	26,176	97	106	2,620	1,021	50,680
District of Columbia	2,038	95,397	0	0	0	2,630	100,065
Florida	569,917	454,877	720	4,522	146,026	72,821	1,248,883
Georgia	281,348	420,652	247	2,231	4,850	36,913	746,241
Hawaii	14,234	909	4,714	67,701	1,106	2,498	91,162
Idaho	61,644	309	1,738	214	6,155	0	70,060
Illinois	476,305	523,467	1,546	15,500	125,654	1,800	1,144,272
Indiana	300,900	101,346	279	1,048	8,677	2,917	415,167
Iowa	235,094	18,484	1,513	2,385	3,780	163	261,419
Kansas	149,160	42,261	2,637	4,791	10,063	417	209,329
Kentucky	431,443	67,715	525	108	425	25,281	525,497
Louisiana	197,588	408,810	0	0	0	34,164	640,562

TABLE X-7. Medicaid Beneficiaries, by Race/Ethnicity, Fiscal Year 1991–Continued

State	White	Black	American Indian	Asian	Hispanic	Unknown	Total
Maine	0	0	0	0	0	0	150,623
Maryland	148,741	200,638	633	6,022	4,510	1,976	362,520
Massachusetts	425,820	78,969	1,464	20,009	104,480	20,314	651,056
Michigan	675,449	358,566	4,927	9,556	34,931	29,104	1,112,533
Minnesota	316,384	41,139	22,453	24,571	16,039	1,152	421,738
Mississippi	136,583	330,143	901	1,637	372	48	469,684
Missouri	346,084	151,299	285	4	11	5,627	503,310
Montana	61,794	0	10	38	147	1,626	63,615
Nebraska	97,597	19,474	5,432	1,109	5,907	4,232	133,751
Nevada	38,160	13,805	1,249	696	4,754	632	59,296
New Hampshire	57,011	562	9	1,073	827	202	59,684
New Jersey	199,126	238,036	1,592	3,353	126,431	45,535	614,073
New Mexico	55,252	5,811	15,094	1,034	71,601	13,203	161,995
New York	646,802	444,692	4,404	15,338	336,440	1,013,861	2,461,537
North Carolina	303,686	340,106	15,036	1,750	5,190	1,435	667,203
North Dakota	39,783	343	11,005	428	441	539	52,539
Ohio	834,928	340,088	3,425	3,036	22,970	94,838	1,299,285
Oklahoma	208,514	59,190	27,822	1,378	7,755	0	304,659
Oregon	220,630	15,171	16,437	4,597	5,816	652	263,303

TABLE X-7. Medicaid Beneficiaries, by Race/Ethnicity, Fiscal Year 1991–Continued

State	White	Black	American Indian	Asian	Hispanic	Unknown	Total
Pennsylvania	768,729	393,458	828	17,022	87,173	10,218	1,277,428
Rhode Island	0	0	0	0	0	0	163,704
South Carolina	132,143	224,873	420	341	947	16,509	375,233
South Dakota	35,899	69	17,787	0	7	3,383	57,145
Tennessee	433,843	230,861	388	1,752	1,589	28,978	697,411
Texas	544,854	416,313	3,452	13,291	711,416	39,303	1,728,629
Utah	102,485	2,063	6,861	3,631	11,219	3,015	129,274
Vermont	69,780	287	138	215	81	198	70,699
Virginia	210,237	216,795	292	7,158	6,215	1,376	442,073
Washington	363,847	34,477	19,228	13,089	42,432	33,206	506,279
West Virginia	257,664	12,536	75	0	75	13,358	283,708
Wisconsin	225,347	36,205	11,336	12,992	11,549	118,513	415,942
Wyoming	28,662	764	2,092	1,134	3,515	637	36,804
Total for reporting States	12,802,424	7,299,907	249,123	632,175	3,320,513	2,135,249	27,066,860

NOTE: Racial/ethnic beneficiary information was not provided by Arizona, Maine, Rhode Island, Puerto Rico and Virgin Islands. Beneficiary counts are those reported by the States.

Source: Table prepared by the Congressional Research Service based on data contained on HCFA Form 2082.

618

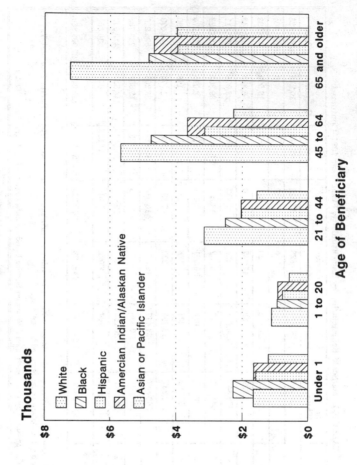

FIGURE X-8. Payments Per Medicaid Beneficiary, by Race/Ethnicity and Age, FY 1991

Thousands

- White
- Black
- Hispanic
- Amercian Indian/Alaskan Native
- Asian or Pacific Islander

$8
$6
$4
$2
$0

Under 1   1 to 20   21 to 44   45 to 64   65 and older

Age of Beneficiary

Source: Figure prepared by Congressional Research Service based on data obtained from HCFA.

TABLE X-8. Medicaid Payments Per Beneficiary by Race/Ethnicity and Age, Fiscal Year 1991

Age	White	Black	Hispanic	American Indian or Alaskan native	Asian or Pacific Islander	Total
Under 1	$1,661	$2,272	$1,589	$1,651	$1,208	$1,975
1 to 20	1,113	942	781	924	570	1,072
21 to 44	3,149	2,508	2,023	2,032	1,559	3,126
45 to 64	5,675	4,742	3,140	3,656	2,264	5,528
65 and older	7,228	4,810	3,952	4,651	3,967	7,076

NOTE: Medicaid payments per beneficiary are influenced by many additional factors not taken into consideration in these estimates. Among other factors payments per beneficiary will be influenced by a State's reimbursement methods, the mix of services used by each group of beneficiaries. Estimates contained in this table exclude beneficiary and payment information for Arizona, Maine, Rhode Island, Puerto Rico and the Virgin Islands. Racial/ethnic information was not provided by these States.

Source: Table prepared by the Congressional Research Service based on data contained on HCFA Form 2082.

FIGURE X-9. Total (Federal and State) Medicaid Payments
for Hospital Related Services, FY 1991

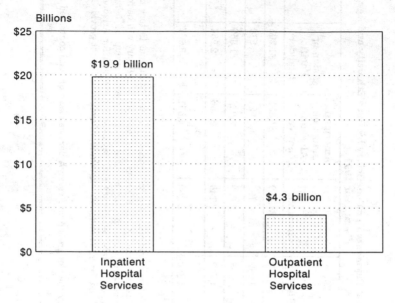

Medicaid Payments Per Beneficiary
for Hospital Related Services, FY 1991

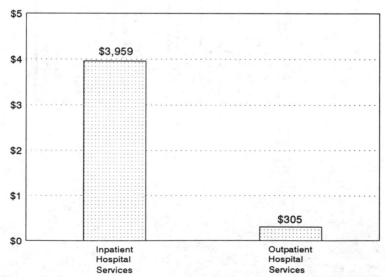

Source: Figure prepared by Congressional Research Service based on data obtained from HCFA.

TABLE X-9. Medicaid Payments for Hospital Services, Fiscal Year 1991

State	Inpatient hospital services	Outpatient hospital services	Hospital services total
Alabama	$ 176,378,877	$ 19,195,511	$ 195,574,388
Alaska	34,991,294	8,226,415	43,217,709
Arizona[a]	NA	NA	NA
Arkansas	142,608,682	25,504,571	168,113,253
California	2,812,177,684	383,623,050	3,195,800,734
Colorado	143,998,571	28,351,410	172,349,981
Connecticut	201,290,485	92,260,081	293,550,566
Delaware	53,374,557	13,138,990	66,513,547
District of Columbia	139,673,982	29,699,194	169,373,176
Florida	887,788,480	186,823,475	1,074,611,955
Georgia	493,214,478	146,560,314	639,774,792
Hawaii	47,140,803	12,081,152	59,221,955
Idaho	49,902,407	10,890,100	60,792,507
Illinois	807,088,696	98,142,608	905,231,304
Indiana	355,723,204	105,285,419	461,008,623
Iowa	175,618,021	49,123,282	224,741,303
Kansas	131,625,170	10,812,978	142,438,148
Kentucky	277,738,802	94,796,024	372,534,826
Louisiana	544,861,870	82,850,244	627,712,114
Maine	109,942,195	34,077,952	144,020,147
Maryland	403,999,337	98,095,490	502,094,827
Massachusetts	699,833,053	202,537,303	902,370,356
Michigan	678,723,467	156,743,288	835,466,755
Minnesota	205,969,274	41,333,867	247,303,141
Mississippi	218,484,964	59,850,751	278,335,715
Missouri	264,535,341	86,106,874	350,642,215
Montana	37,944,432	9,880,743	47,825,175
Nebraska	65,229,844	17,558,491	82,788,335
Nevada	56,818,875	9,444,062	66,262,937

See notes at end of table.

TABLE X-9. Medicaid Payments for Hospital Services, Fiscal Year 1991
--Continued--

State	Inpatient hospital services	Outpatient hospital services	Hospital services total
New Hampshire	$ 29,146,436	$ 14,035,777	$ 43,182,213
New Jersey	784,005,010	177,722,417	961,727,427
New Mexico	83,408,041	29,057,267	112,465,308
New York	3,287,926,056	660,129,868	3,948,055,924
North Carolina	464,837,156	85,139,478	549,976,634
North Dakota	33,202,458	10,286,671	43,489,129
Ohio	859,667,051	230,353,796	1,090,020,847
Oklahoma	213,172,602	28,352,161	241,524,763
Oregon	92,538,776	33,435,746	125,974,522
Pennsylvania	831,521,573	103,669,521	935,191,094
Rhode Island	285,169,699	24,324,440	309,494,139
South Carolina	249,644,375	34,343,816	283,988,191
South Dakota	43,477,944	8,908,636	52,386,580
Tennessee	331,609,182	134,774,043	466,383,225
Texas	923,620,373	220,300,473	1,143,920,846
Utah	94,160,439	14,283,007	108,443,446
Vermont	34,610,561	13,998,933	48,609,494
Virginia	284,040,831	94,940,332	378,981,163
Washington	240,088,098	75,899,360	315,987,458
West Virginia	160,162,780	19,748,785	179,911,565
Wisconsin	215,676,827	64,914,653	280,591,480
Wyoming	26,069,415	6,212,609	32,282,024
Puerto Rico	65,060,119	81,075,081	146,135,200
Virgin Islands	1,503,382	1,077,035	2,580,417
49 reporting States and the District of Columbia	19,784,432,528	4,197,825,428	23,982,257,956
U.S. Totals	$19,850,996,029	$4,279,977,544	$24,130,973,573

See notes at end of table.

TABLE X-9. Medicaid Payments for Hospital Services, Fiscal Year 1991
--Continued--

NA = Not available.

ᵃThe Health Care Financing Administration does not report capitation payments for Arizona, therefore this estimate is unavailable.

NOTE: All estimates represent figures reported by the States, except for Massachusetts, Rhode Island, and Puerto Rico--for these States HCFA provides estimates.

Source: Table prepared by the Congressional Research Service based on data contained on HCFA Form 2082.

FIGURE X-10. Total (Federal and State) Medicaid Payments for Practitioner Services, FY 1991

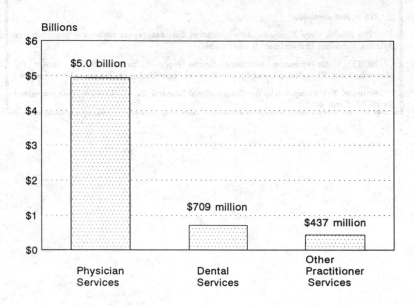

Medicaid Payments Per Beneficiary for Practitioner Services, FY 1991

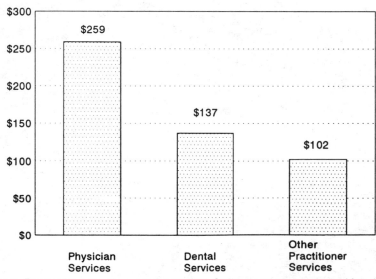

Source: Figure prepared by Congressional Research Service based on data obtained from HCFA.

TABLE X-10. Medicaid Payments for Practitioner Services, Fiscal Year 1991

State	Physician services	Dental services	Other practitioner services	Practitioner services total
Alabama	$ 77,706,184	$ 5,271,526	$ 2,235,634	$ 85,213,344
Alaska	28,854,742	4,853,206	1,115,619	34,823,567
Arizona[a]	NA	NA	NA	NA
Arkansas	65,802,641	4,198,150	3,373,853	73,374,644
California	689,672,092	19,083,900	73,877,233	782,633,225
Colorado	48,853,262	3,381,337	1,268,452	53,503,051
Connecticut	50,068,323	11,322,615	8,584,440	69,975,378
Delaware	10,415,835	466,589	735,617	11,618,041
District of Columbia	17,173,494	835,968	379,307	18,388,769
Florida	283,484,923	36,572,234	11,846,107	331,903,264
Georgia	231,363,592	25,701,365	11,609,216	268,674,173
Hawaii	35,680,248	8,046,913	2,224,263	45,951,424
Idaho	20,100,357	1,565,334	2,533,558	24,199,249
Illinois	181,459,244	41,901	18,377,608	199,878,753
Indiana	99,462,049	21,263,925	18,967,351	139,693,325
Iowa	66,118,891	18,708,063	5,632,818	90,459,772
Kansas	35,000,381	4,886,682	3,359,724	43,246,787

See notes at end of table.

TABLE X-10. Medicaid Payments for Practitioner Services, Fiscal Year 1991–Continued

State	Physician services	Dental services	Other practitioner services	Practitioner services total
Kentucky	$127,280,132	$ 22,920,304	$ 6,968,497	$157,168,933
Louisiana	164,451,476	22,512,182	8,097,232	195,060,890
Maine	21,847,100	5,367,680	3,455,696	30,670,476
Maryland	101,727,648	4,822,671	1,462,394	108,012,713
Massachusetts	140,855,172	31,268,607	7,998,231	180,122,010
Michigan	185,772,032	30,917,332	7,649,889	224,339,253
Minnesota	87,245,095	17,034,535	15,432,064	119,711,694
Mississippi	84,172,799	9,146,631	2,747,890	96,067,320
Missouri	55,519,193	13,134,135	3,821,182	72,474,510
Montana	15,597,300	3,386,929	2,639,279	21,623,508
Nebraska	38,227,760	5,174,421	4,580,742	47,982,923
Nevada	21,192,228	3,891,385	2,521,416	27,605,029
New Hampshire	7,933,379	1,249,539	1,516,714	10,699,632
New Jersey	68,954,353	26,034,676	6,635,983	101,625,012
New Mexico	46,430,831	3,864,614	1,967,655	52,263,100
New York	223,333,410	127,286,550	96,994,575	447,614,535
North Carolina	155,488,095	23,261,434	4,940,802	183,690,331
North Dakota	10,672,763	3,081,200	941,730	14,695,693

See notes at end of table.

TABLE X-10. Medicaid Payments for Practitioner Services, Fiscal Year 1991—Continued

State	Physician services	Dental services	Other practitioner services	Practitioner services total
Ohio	$186,028,807	$34,235,333	$21,471,911	$241,736,051
Oklahoma	57,973,066	6,920,212	5,068,162	69,961,440
Oregon	38,922,885	6,075,820	1,757,346	46,756,051
Pennsylvania	125,793,227	21,770,165	6,481,408	154,044,800
Rhode Island	7,743,069	2,633,095	1,131,942	11,508,106
South Carolina	91,360,754	7,981,829	4,758,301	104,100,884
South Dakota	13,165,337	867,317	492,870	14,525,524
Tennessee	171,520,630	17,067,388	7,579,642	196,167,660
Texas	387,351,452	30,005,299	19,860,117	437,216,868
Utah	33,557,388	4,739,668	2,221,324	40,518,380
Vermont	13,324,072	3,048,166	972,970	17,345,208
Virginia	109,665,920	6,912,623	3,946,425	120,524,968
Washington	117,038,182	31,627,393	7,985,859	156,651,434
West Virginia	45,177,249	3,954,625	1,675,996	50,807,870
Wisconsin	39,577,638	9,825,350	4,595,826	53,998,814
Wyoming	9,817,428	1,134,602	401,501	11,353,531
Puerto Rico	0	0	0	0
Virgin Islands	308,448	79,758	0	388,206

See notes at end of table.

TABLE X-10. Medicaid Payments for Practitioner Services, Fiscal Year 1991--Continued

State	Physician services	Dental services	Other practitioner services	Practitioner services total
49 reporting States and the District of Columbia	$4,945,934,128	$709,353,418	$436,894,371	$6,092,181,917
U.S. Total	$4,946,242,576	$709,433,176	$436,894,371	$6,092,570,123

aThe Health Care Financing Administration does not report capitation payments for Arizona, therefore this estimate is unavailable.

NOTE: All estimates represent figures reported by the States, except for Massachusetts, Rhode Island, and Puerto Rico--for these States HCFA provides estimates.

Source: Table prepared by the Congressional Research Service based on data contained on HCFA Form 2082.

FIGURE X-11. Total (Federal and State) Medicaid Payments for Long-Term Care Services, FY 1991

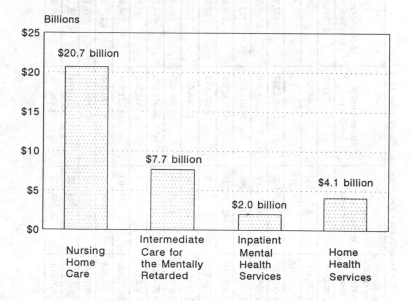

Medicaid Payments Per Beneficiary for Long-Term Care Services, FY 1991

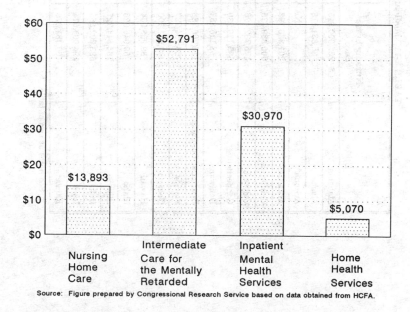

Source: Figure prepared by Congressional Research Service based on data obtained from HCFA.

TABLE X-11. Medicaid Payments for Long-Term Care Services, Fiscal Year 1991

State	Nursing home care	Intermediate care for the mentally retarded	Inpatient mental health services	Home health services	Long-term care services total
Alabama	$ 232,090,813	$ 72,228,858	$10,780,659	$ 47,479,938	$ 362,580,268
Alaska	35,831,316	11,047,835	6,511,032	2,505,523	55,895,706
Arizona[a]	NA	NA	NA	NA	NA
Arkansas	201,386,793	81,669,189	15,625,685	29,072,267	327,753,934
California	1,600,889,335	461,256,170	14,872,705	29,328,605	2,106,346,815
Colorado	176,732,498	51,124,572	17,651,262	67,614,522	313,122,854
Connecticut	690,119,230	224,952,148	42,090,381	147,786,165	1,104,947,924
Delaware	53,115,867	23,757,222	0	7,633,973	84,507,062
District of Columbia	113,766,788	37,796,084	21,991,034	13,208,639	186,762,545
Florida	766,934,727	169,060,202	11,688,181	42,358,433	990,041,543
Georgia	440,971,100	109,394,418	0	54,376,232	604,741,750
Hawaii	89,968,904	7,238,192	0	947,768	98,154,864
Idaho	59,046,926	33,997,053	854,869	10,621,919	104,520,767
Illinois	784,544,727	382,865,962	18,699,941	91,779,523	1,277,890,153
Indiana	533,002,369	192,204,444	51,252,612	20,704,070	797,163,495
Iowa	194,001,574	137,505,668	4,078,337	19,545,686	355,131,265
Kansas	160,481,370	97,379,816	20,153,372	12,324,019	290,338,577

See notes at end of table.

TABLE X-11. Medicaid Payments for Long-Term Care Services, Fiscal Year 1991--Continued

State	Nursing home care	Intermediate care for the mentally retarded	Inpatient mental health services	Home health services	Long-term care services total
Kentucky	$ 270,197,665	$ 57,325,273	$ 27,313,101	$ 71,655,303	$ 426,491,342
Louisiana	319,545,675	235,707,301	49,112,507	11,354,396	615,719,879
Maine	181,928,161	48,405,144	9,465,044	28,239,383	268,037,732
Maryland	344,784,526	60,483,827	47,412,354	31,465,097	484,145,804
Massachusetts	936,492,071	112,067,617	41,526,286	231,580,797	1,321,666,771
Michigan	555,201,308	192,890,989	72,491,254	112,200,484	932,784,035
Minnesota	614,351,993	268,744,306	21,253,395	103,090,632	1,007,440,326
Mississippi	182,973,304	57,663,620	2,174,898	5,665,429	248,477,251
Missouri	347,597,473	103,774,496	7,272,354	25,118,850	483,763,173
Montana	59,252,567	14,695,211	8,812,942	1,204,654	83,965,374
Nebraska	137,993,597	30,259,112	6,310,851	9,746,837	184,310,397
Nevada	44,096,928	14,658,596	392,151	7,291,954	66,439,629
New Hampshire	141,769,171	1,768,474	7,040,261	50,132,063	200,709,969
New Jersey	823,083,257	279,966,657	50,630,495	193,374,785	1,347,055,194
New Mexico	86,222,951	34,285,756	4,811,965	3,119,719	128,440,391
New York	3,326,788,325	1,508,345,231	1,035,560,305	1,866,109,265	7,736,803,126

See notes at end of table.

TABLE X-11. Medicaid Payments for Long-Term Care Services, Fiscal Year 1991.–Continued

State	Nursing home care	Intermediate care for the mentally retarded	Inpatient mental health services	Home health services	Long-term care services total
North Carolina	$ 423,119,753	$243,038,039	$ 37,122,562	$111,806,851	$ 815,087,205
North Dakota	76,685,763	40,467,140	3,362,325	23,749,367	144,264,595
Ohio	1,222,957,622	389,113,788	223,233	32,946,644	1,645,241,287
Oklahoma	213,454,302	108,645,291	45,190,276	36,460,938	403,750,807
Oregon	129,441,615	98,026,752	12,646,716	94,110,061	334,225,144
Pennsylvania	1,021,109,722	452,493,141	122,390,901	13,213,362	1,609,207,126
Rhode Island	166,233,941	66,307,665	7,687,468	49,923,123	290,152,197
South Carolina	167,442,334	144,240,561	24,584,763	33,949,838	370,217,496
South Dakota	60,143,145	26,875,807	4,222,700	15,909,086	107,150,738
Tennessee	361,863,678	101,674,282	24,602,806	11,870,588	500,011,354
Texas	899,821,195	472,481,944	0	148,781,478	1,521,084,617
Utah	13,147,278	37,029,158	41,717,235	23,960,477	115,854,148
Vermont	52,707,451	20,441,958	684,738	17,810,496	91,644,643
Virginia	315,254,911	133,039,417	15,260,768	45,223,942	508,779,038
Washington	354,464,067	17,385,429	2,642,968	6,192,198	380,684,662
West Virginia	130,356,934	41,606,519	6,442,678	3,508,141	181,914,272

See notes at end of table.

TABLE X-11. Medicaid Payments for Long-Term Care Services, Fiscal Year 1991--Continued

State	Nursing home care	Intermediate care for the mentally retarded	Inpatient mental health services	Home health services	Long-term care services total
Wisconsin	$ 558,028,707	$ 169,940,510	$ 32,670,072	$ 82,595,367	$ 843,234,656
Wyoming	27,791,872	2,195,424	364,684	713,969	31,065,949
Puerto Rico	0	0	0	0	0
Virgin Islands	0	0	0	5,031	5,031
49 States and the District of Columbia	20,699,187,599	7,679,522,268	2,009,647,126	4,101,362,856	34,489,719,849
Totals	$20,699,187,599	$7,679,522,268	$2,009,647,126	$4,101,367,887	$34,489,724,880

ªThe Health Care Financing Administration does not report capitation payments for Arizona, therefore this estimate is unavailable.

NOTE: All estimates represent figures reported by the States, except for Massachusetts, Rhode Island, and Puerto Rico--for these States HCFA provides estimates.

Source: Table prepared by the Congressional Research Service based on data contained on HCFA Form 2082.

FIGURE X-12. Total (Federal and State) Medicaid Payments
for Clinic and Related Services, FY 1991

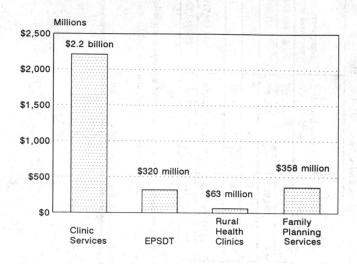

Medicaid Payments Per Beneficiary
for Clinic and Related Services, FY 1991

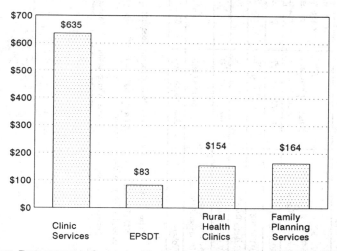

Source: Figure prepared by Congressional Research Service based on data obtained from HCFA.

TABLE X-12. Medicaid Payments for Clinic and Related Services, Fiscal Year 1991

State	Clinic services	Early and periodic screening	Rural health clinics	Family planning services	Clinic and related services total
Alabama	$ 16,171,949	$ 5,233,939	$ 3,234,346	$ 5,557,990	$ 30,198,224
Alaska	6,012,034	195,825	54,650	361,647	6,624,156
Arizona[a]	NA	NA	NA	NA	NA
Arkansas	23,644,373	6,792,661	0	1,037,386	31,474,420
California	270,420,859	69,556,414	20,959,052	27,234,084	388,170,409
Colorado	33,641,224	4,052,871	2,717,011	7,917,777	48,328,883
Connecticut	22,496,911	449,491	5,390	2,413,045	25,364,837
Delaware	537,661	169,128	0	297,972	1,004,761
District of Columbia	24,529,530	306,932	0	617,772	25,454,234
Florida	45,053,636	8,785,359	7,930,245	7,441,065	69,210,305
Georgia	35,369,726	14,029,439	41,079	24,678,212	74,118,456
Hawaii	1,832,381	1,648,504	0	199,244	3,680,129
Idaho	2,882,954	589,265	140,367	1,269,606	4,882,192
Illinois	18,334,103	19,906,361	620,825	12,087,358	50,948,647
Indiana	34,126,707	879,890	0	6,457,864	41,464,461
Iowa	3,631,197	408,056	228,197	3,762,122	8,029,572
Kansas	16,040,968	167,081	131,082	2,959,576	19,298,707
Kentucky	58,303,840	2,177,652	1,111,768	10,181,818	71,775,078

See notes at end of table.

TABLE X-12. Medicaid Payments for Clinic and Related Services, Fiscal Year 1991–Continued

State	Clinic services	Early and periodic screening	Rural health clinics	Family planning services	Clinic and related services total
Louisiana	$ 16,085,153	$18,805,818	$ 0	$ 6,725,471	$ 41,616,442
Maine	11,440	1,454,026	1,592,027	2,460,338	5,517,831
Maryland	35,623,971	5,435,614	95,482	8,259,687	49,414,754
Massachusetts	103,276,414	2,512,054	0	8,232,525	114,020,993
Michigan	225,457,066	7,790,253	0	16,521,369	249,768,688
Minnesota	27,406,729	3,180,882	0	2,186,766	32,774,377
Mississippi	4,906,161	6,703,726	142,767	4,356,999	16,109,653
Missouri	37,728,650	2,543,051	142,225	4,014,276	44,428,202
Montana	4,410,381	895,932	0	815,528	6,121,841
Nebraska	2,366,639	2,343,240	0	1,830,133	6,540,012
Nevada	357,542	624,598	14,816	0	996,956
New Hampshire	13,217,857	311,764	327,004	1,144,824	15,001,449
New Jersey	56,543,429	1,039,602	0	7,514,158	65,097,189
New Mexico	2,791,690	996,828	1,228,357	1,123,398	6,140,273
New York	478,151,863	20,929,255	0	42,963,769	542,044,887
North Carolina	25,086,320	5,965,270	3,456,907	12,361,316	46,869,813
North Dakota	3,225,980	181,915	143,494	706,332	4,257,721

See notes at end of table.

TABLE X-12. Medicaid Payments for Clinic and Related Services, Fiscal Year 1991–Continued

State	Clinic services	Early and periodic screening	Rural health clinics	Family planning services	Clinic and related services total
Ohio	$104,924,244	$ 8,801,983	$1,887,818	$26,547,339	$142,161,384
Oklahoma	12,394,970	3,208,695	66,349	3,448,118	19,118,132
Oregon	24,540,985	25,102,098	361,759	2,757,660	52,762,502
Pennsylvania	74,443,841	6,080,319	5,195,491	17,347,528	103,067,179
Rhode Island	0	665,539	145,477	771,517	1,582,533
South Carolina	37,390,045	4,589,721	261,540	7,890,796	50,132,102
South Dakota	3,870,727	2,020,841	657,433	699,428	7,248,429
Tennessee	48,261,532	7,036,500	316,682	10,154,584	65,769,298
Texas	4,200,764	9,112,572	1,590,108	31,439,114	46,342,558
Utah	17,384,862	455,318	120,484	818,100	18,778,764
Vermont	6,483,995	228,234	441,206	662,462	7,815,897
Virginia	36,390,367	26,208,241	17,669	4,806,898	67,423,175
Washington	89,229,787	5,448,509	309,693	4,030,543	99,018,532
West Virginia	50,247,984	1,939,565	6,591,784	1,160,405	59,939,738
Wisconsin	46,669,195	1,989,444	246,027	7,508,056	56,412,722
Wyoming	1,533,482	346,106	2,847	2,167,229	4,049,664
Puerto Rico	0	0	0	0	0

See notes at end of table.

TABLE X-12. Medicaid Payments for Clinic and Related Services, Fiscal Year 1991--Continued

State	Clinic services	Early and periodic screening	Rural health clinics	Family planning services	Clinic and related services total
Virgin Islands	$ 0	$ 24,275	$ 0	$ 47,090	$ 71,365
49 reporting States and the District of Columbia	2,207,644,118	320,296,381	62,529,458	357,901,204	2,948,371,161
U.S. Totals	$2,207,644,118	$320,320,656	$62,529,458	$357,948,294	$2,948,442,526

ªThe Health Care Financing Administration does not report capitation payments for Arizona, therefore this estimate is unavailable.

NOTE: All estimates represent figures reported by the States, except for Massachusetts, Rhode Island, and Puerto Rico--for these States HCFA provides estimates.

Source: Table prepared by the Congressional Research Service based on data contained on HCFA Form 2082.

FIGURE X-13. Total (Federal and State) Medicaid Payments
for Ancillary and Other Services, FY 1991

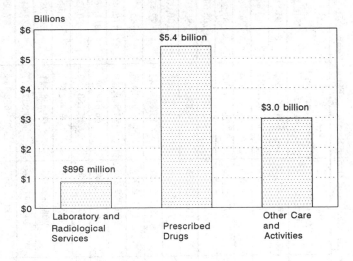

Medicaid Payments Per Beneficiary
for Ancillary and Other Services, FY 1991

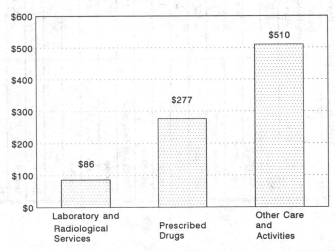

Source: Figure prepared by Congressional Research Service based on data obtained from HCFA.

TABLE X-13. Medicaid Payments for Ancillary and Other Services, Fiscal Year 1991

State	Laboratory and radiological services	Prescribed drugs	Other care and activities	Total
Alabama	$ 4,886,159	$ 76,064,912	$ 50,937,802	$ 131,888,873
Alaska	501,965	7,580,080	11,551,311	19,633,356
Arizona[a]	NA	NA	NA	NA
Arkansas	6,270,703	67,082,664	13,897,262	87,250,629
California	156,983,869	667,392,734	281,218,987	1,105,595,590
Colorado	5,221,888	43,638,855	36,630,663	85,491,406
Connecticut	3,228,802	75,118,718	57,712,331	136,059,851
Delaware	1,311,430	9,773,997	11,328,144	22,413,571
District of Columbia	3,776,982	17,110,049	24,990,436	45,877,467
Florida	77,581,527	276,909,226	124,099,310	478,590,063
Georgia	4,925,880	160,447,195	46,614,081	211,987,156
Hawaii	3,279,359	20,057,668	7,183,882	30,520,909
Idaho	2,774,229	15,976,430	9,902,977	28,653,636
Illinois	33,023,481	203,362,055	60,833,411	297,218,947
Indiana	30,023,374	142,141,008	50,282,277	222,446,659
Iowa	1,242,720	64,645,567	21,692,444	87,580,731

See notes at end of table.

TABLE X-13. Medicaid Payments for Ancillary and Other Services, Fiscal Year 1991--Continued

State	Laboratory and radiological services	Prescribed drugs	Other care and activities	Total
Kansas	$10,973,969	$ 36,721,420	$ 9,969,561	$ 57,664,950
Kentucky	27,896,737	111,386,790	33,040,480	172,324,007
Louisiana	33,958,494	160,185,889	49,024,497	243,168,880
Maine	4,183,204	38,370,703	45,547,670	88,101,577
Maryland	5,204,672	77,754,038	65,618,256	148,576,966
Massachusetts	11,698,350	154,531,201	143,905,612	310,135,163
Michigan	37,000,628	208,388,883	52,338,455	297,727,966
Minnesota	8,492,249	85,655,723	59,926,101	154,074,073
Mississippi	3,978,433	86,631,141	25,317,703	115,927,277
Missouri	5,872,032	99,369,991	61,332,199	166,574,222
Montana	1,136,158	14,372,264	18,184,780	33,693,202
Nebraska	4,563,067	33,188,482	30,473,214	68,224,763
Nevada	1,309,667	10,863,477	4,692,155	16,865,299
New Hampshire	1,498,351	14,701,265	6,558,808	22,758,424
New Jersey	15,065,704	186,349,352	47,800,706	249,215,762
New Mexico	2,078,187	26,338,569	14,520,018	42,936,774

See notes at end of table.

TABLE X-13. Medicaid Payments for Ancillary and Other Services, Fiscal Year 1991--Continued

State	Laboratory and radiological services	Prescribed drugs	Other care and activities	Total
New York	$46,958,889	$524,698,035	$482,276,706	$1,053,933,630
North Carolina	39,584,720	125,411,106	26,949,701	191,945,527
North Dakota	2,174,165	11,307,248	6,748,943	20,230,356
Ohio	43,124,323	260,488,410	230,659,404	534,272,137
Oklahoma	7,067,360	58,134,128	14,815,620	80,017,108
Oregon	9,664,179	48,180,487	48,963,498	106,808,164
Pennsylvania	28,557,888	293,441,746	312,654,993	634,654,627
Rhode Island	623,763	26,531,006	17,166,002	44,320,771
South Carolina	6,221,514	63,439,773	32,187,235	101,848,522
South Dakota	1,144,148	10,684,661	3,165,573	14,994,382
Tennessee	44,846,423	144,580,884	67,488,932	256,916,239
Texas	97,036,313	247,615,290	38,887,423	383,539,026
Utah	690,580	21,613,773	5,440,455	27,744,808
Vermont	201,104	17,254,421	13,844,703	31,300,228
Virginia	10,458,983	104,199,762	28,063,333	142,722,078
Washington	21,192,633	102,608,558	55,264,866	179,066,057

See notes at end of table.

TABLE X-13. Medicaid Payments for Ancillary and Other Services, Fiscal Year 1991--Continued

State	Laboratory and radiological services	Prescribed drugs	Other care and activities	Total
West Virginia	$ 3,754,602	$ 43,125,816	$ 23,036,174	$ 69,916,592
Wisconsin	20,761,782	120,975,029	95,036,619	236,773,430
Wyoming	1,594,026	6,751,444	3,080,739	11,426,209
Puerto Rico	0	0	0	0
Virgin Islands	84,913	849,078	228,804	1,162,795
49 reporting States and the District of Columbia	895,599,665	5,423,151,923	2,982,856,452	9,301,608,040
Totals	$895,684,578	$5,424,001,001	$2,983,085,256	$9,302,770,835

[a]The Health Care Financing Administration does not report capitation payments for Arizona, therefore this estimate is unavailable.

NOTE: All estimates represent figures reported by the States, except for Massachusetts, Rhode Island, and Puerto Rico--for these States HCFA provides estimates.

Source: Table prepared by the Congressional Research Service based on data contained on HCFA Form 2082.

CHAPTER XI. REPORTS TO CONGRESS
AND SELECTED BIBLIOGRAPHY[1]

I. REPORTS AND STUDIES REQUIRED BY LEGISLATION

Reports and studies required by legislation from the Secretary of Health and Human Services (HHS), the Prospective Payment Assessment Commission, and the Physician Payment Review Commission:

Topic	Due Date

ICF/MR REDUCTION PLANS

Secretary of HHS shall submit to Congress a study   Issued
on the implementation and results of permitting
intermediate care facilities for the mentally
retarded to submit correction and reduction plans.
(Section 9516 of Public Law 99-272, COBRA 1985)

HOME HEALTH PROSPECTIVE PAYMENT DEMONSTRATION

Secretary of HHS shall submit to Congress an   Issued
interim report on the result of demonstration
projects assessing alternative methods of paying
home health agencies on a prospective basis for
services furnished under the Medicare and Medicaid
programs. (Section 4027(a) of Public Law 100-203,
OBRA 1987)

QUALITY OF CARE

Secretary of HHS shall submit an interim report to   Issued
Congress on the results of a study of the utilization
of selected medical treatments and surgical
procedures by Medicaid beneficiaries to assess the
appropriateness, necessity, and effectiveness of such
treatments and procedures. (Section 9432(c) of
Public Law 99-509, OBRA 1986)

---

[1]This chapter was written by Dawn Nuschler.

Topic	Due Date

UTILIZATION AND QUALITY CONTROL PEER REVIEW ORGANIZATION PROGRAM

Secretary of HHS shall submit to Congress a report on the administration, impact, and cost of the utilization and quality control peer review organization (PRO) program. (Section 1161 of the Social Security Act as amended by section 143 of Public Law 97-248)

Issued

MEDICAID ELIGIBILITY QUALITY CONTROL (MEQC) NEGATIVE CASE ACTION STUDY

Secretary of HHS shall report to Congress the results of a study of the quality control system for the Medicaid program under title XIX of the Social Security Act. The study shall examine how best to operate such system in order to obtain information which will allow program managers to improve the quality of administration, and provide reasonable data on the basis of which Federal funding may be withheld for States with excessive levels of erroneous payments. (Section 12301 of Public Law 99-272, COBRA 1985)

Issued

INSTITUTIONS FOR MENTAL DISEASES

Secretary of HHS shall report to Congress the results of a study of the implementation, under current provisions, regulations, guidelines, and regulatory practices under title XIX of the Social Security Act, of the exclusion of coverage of services to certain individuals residing in institutions for mental diseases, and the costs and benefits of providing services in public subacute psychiatric facilities. (Section 6408(a)(2) of Public Law 101-239, OBRA 1989)

Pending as of September 1992

Topic	Due Date

*FY 1990 UTILIZATION AND
QUALITY CONTROL PEER REVIEW
ORGANIZATION PROGRAM*

Secretary of HHS shall submit to Congress a report on the administration, impact, and cost of the utilization and quality control peer review organization (PRO) program. (Section 1161 of the Social Security Act as amended by section 143 of Public Law 97-248)

Pending as of September 1992

ERRORS IN ELIGIBILITY DETERMINATIONS

Secretary of HHS shall report to Congress on error rates by States in determining eligibility of individuals described in subparagraph (A) or (B) of section 1902(l)(1) of the Social Security Act for medical assistance under plans approved under title XIX of such Act. Such report may include data for medical assistance provided before July 1, 1989. (Section 4607(a) of Public Law 101-508, OBRA 1990)

Pending as of September 1992

PAYMENTS FOR VACCINES

Secretary of HHS shall report to Congress the results of a study of the relationship between State medical assistance plans and Federal and State acquisition and reimbursement policies for vaccines and the accessibility of vaccinations and immunization to children. (Section 4401(d)(5) of Public Law 101-508, OBRA 1990)

Pending as of September 1992

*HOME HEALTH PROSPECTIVE
PAYMENT DEMONSTRATION*

Secretary of HHS shall submit to Congress a final report on the result of demonstration projects assessing alternative methods of paying home health agencies on a prospective basis for services furnished under the Medicare and Medicaid programs. (Section 4027(a) of Public Law 100-203, OBRA 1987)

Issued

Topic	Due Date

PRIOR APPROVAL PROCEDURES

Secretary of HHS and the Comptroller General shall report to Congress the results of a study of prior approval procedures utilized by State medical assistance programs conducted under title XIX of the Social Security Act, including the appeals provisions under such programs and the effects of such procedures on beneficiary and provider access to medications covered under such programs. (Section 4401(d)(3) of Public Law 101-508, OBRA 1990)

Pending as of September 1992

ADEQUACY OF PAYMENT RATES TO PHARMACISTS

Secretary of HHS shall report to Congress on the results of a study on the adequacy of current reimbursement rates to pharmacists under each State medical assistance program conducted under title XIX of the Social Security Act and the extent to which reimbursement rates under such programs have an effect on beneficiary access to medications covered and pharmacy services under such programs. (Section 4401(d)(4) of Public Law 101-508, OBRA 1990)

December 31, 1991 *(Note: Due date subject to change)*

EXTENSION OF BENEFITS TO PREGNANT WOMEN AND CHILDREN DEMONSTRATION

Secretary of HHS shall submit to Congress an interim report on demonstration projects to study the effect of allowing States to extend Medicaid to pregnant women and children not otherwise qualified to receive Medicaid benefits. The report shall evaluate the effect of each project with respect to access to health care, private health care insurance coverage, costs with respect to health care, and developing feasible premium and cost-sharing policies. (Section 6407(g)(2) of Public Law 101-239, OBRA 1989)

Pending as of September 1992

Topic	Due Date

QUALITY OF CARE

Secretary of HHS shall submit a final report to Congress on the results of a study of the utilization of selected medical treatments and surgical procedures by Medicaid beneficiaries in order to assess the appropriateness, necessity, and effectiveness of such treatments and procedures. (Section 9432(c) of Public Law 99-509, OBRA 1986 as amended by section 411 of Public Law 100-360, MCCA)

Pending as of September 1992

STUDY ON STAFFING REQUIREMENTS IN NURSING FACILITIES

Secretary of HHS shall report to Congress on the appropriateness of establishing minimum caregiver to resident ratios and minimum supervisor to caregiver ratios for skilled nursing facilities serving as providers of services under title XVIII of the Social Security Act and nursing facilities receiving payments under a State plan under title XIX of the Social Security Act, and shall include in such study recommendations regarding appropriate minimum ratios. (Section 4801(b) of Public Law 101-508, OBRA 1990)

Pending as of September 1992

FY 1991 UTILIZATION AND QUALITY CONTROL PEER REVIEW ORGANIZATION PROGRAM

Secretary of HHS shall submit to Congress a report on the administration, impact, and cost of the utilization and quality control peer review organization (PRO) program. (Section 1161 of the Social Security Act as amended by section 143 of Public Law 97-248)

Pending as of September 1992

Topic	Due Date

MEDICAID DRUG REBATE PROGRAM

Secretary of HHS shall report to Congress on ingredient costs paid under this title for single source drugs, multiple source drugs, and nonprescription covered outpatient drugs; the total value of rebates received and number of manufacturers providing such rebates; how the size of such rebates compare with the size or rebates offered to other purchasers of covered outpatient drugs; the effect of inflation on the value of rebates required under this section; trends in prices paid under this title for covered outpatient drugs; and Federal and State administrative costs associated with compliance with the provisions of this title. (Section 4401(a) of Public Law 101-508, OBRA 1990)

Issued

STAFFING REQUIREMENTS

Secretary of HHS shall report to Congress on the progress made in implementing nursing facility staffing requirements, including the number and types of waivers approved and the number of facilities which have received waivers. (Section 4211(k) of Public Law 100-203, OBRA 1987)

January 1, 1993

STATE UTILIZATION REVIEW SYSTEMS

Secretary of HHS shall report to Congress an analysis of the procedures for which programs for ambulatory surgery, preadmission testing, and same-day surgery are appropriate for patients who are covered under the State Medicaid plan, and the effects of such programs on access of such patients to necessary care, quality of care, and costs of care. (Section 4755(b) of Public Law 101-508, OBRA 1990)

January 1, 1993

Topic	Due Date

EXTENSION OF BENEFITS TO LOW-INCOME FAMILIES DEMONSTRATION

Secretary of HHS shall submit to Congress an interim report on the status of demonstration projects to study the effect of allowing States to extend Medicaid coverage to low-income families not otherwise qualified to receive Medicaid benefits. The report shall evaluate the effect of the projects with respect to access to, and costs of, health care; private health care insurance coverage; and premiums and cost-sharing. (Section 4745(a)(b)(c) of Public Law 101-508, OBRA 1990)

January 1, 1993

EXTENSION OF MUNICIPAL HEALTH SERVICE DEMONSTRATION

Secretary of HHS shall submit a report to Congress on the waiver program with respect to the quality of health care, beneficiary costs, and such other factors as may be appropriate. (Section 402(a) of the Social Security Amendments of 1967; amended by section 9215 of Public Law 99-272, COBRA; as amended by section 6135 of Public Law 101-239, OBRA 1989)

December 31, 1993

PROSPECTIVE DRUG UTILIZATION REVIEW

Secretary of HHS shall submit to Congress a report on demonstration projects to evaluate the efficiency and cost-effectiveness of prospective drug utilization review (as a component of on-line, real-time electronic point-of-sales claims management) in fulfilling patient counseling and in reducing costs for prescription drugs. (Section 4401(c)(1) of Public Law 101-508, OBRA 1990)

January 1, 1994

Topic	Due Date

EXTENSION OF BENEFITS TO PREGNANT WOMEN AND CHILDREN DEMONSTRATION

Secretary of HHS shall submit to Congress a final report on demonstration projects to study the effect of allowing States to extend Medicaid to pregnant women and children not otherwise qualified to receive Medicaid benefits. The report shall evaluate the effect of each project with respect to access to health care, private health care insurance coverage, costs with respect to health care, and developing feasible premium and cost-sharing policies. (Section 6407(g)(2) of Public Law 101-239, OBRA 1989)

January 1, 1994

COST-EFFECTIVENESS OF REIMBURSEMENT FOR PHARMACISTS' COGNITIVE SERVICES DEMONSTRATION

Secretary of HHS shall submit a report to Congress on the results of a demonstration project to evaluate the impact on quality of care and cost-effectiveness of paying pharmacists under title XIX of the Social Security Act, whether or not a drug is dispensed, for drug use review services. (Section 4401(c)(2) of Public Law 101-508, OBRA 1990)

January 1, 1995

EXTENSION OF BENEFITS TO LOW-INCOME FAMILIES DEMONSTRATION

Secretary of HHS shall submit to Congress a final report on the status of demonstration projects to study the effect of allowing States to extend Medicaid coverage to low-income families not otherwise qualified to receive Medicaid benefits. The report shall evaluate the effect of the projects with respect to access to, and costs of, health care; private health care insurance coverage; and premiums and cost-sharing. (Section 4745(a)(b)(c) of Public Law 101-508, OBRA 1990)

January 1, 1995

Topic	Due Date

DEMONSTRATION PROJECT TO PROVIDE MEDICAID COVERAGE FOR HIV-POSITIVE INDIVIDUALS

Secretary of HHS shall report to Congress on the results of an evaluation of the comparative costs of providing services to individuals who have tested positive for the presence of HIV virus at an early stage after detection of such virus and those that are treated at a later stage after such detection. (Section 4747 of Public Law 101-508, OBRA 1990)	Report due 6 months after termination of demonstration

PROSPECTIVE PAYMENT ASSESSMENT COMMISSION (ProPAC) STUDY OF MEDICAID PAYMENTS TO HOSPITALS

The Commission shall submit a report to Congress on a study of hospital payment rates under State plans for medical assistance under title XIX of the Social Security Act, and shall specifically examine in such study the relationship between payments under such plans and payments made to hospitals under title XVIII of such Act, and the financial condition of hospitals receiving payments under such plans, with particular attention to hospitals in urban areas which treat large numbers of individuals eligible for medical assistance under title XIX of such Act and other low-income individuals. (Section 4002(g)(4) of Public Law 101-508, OBRA 1990)	Issued

PHYSICIAN PAYMENT REVIEW COMMISSION (PPRC) STUDY OF PHYSICIAN FEES UNDER MEDICAID

The Commission shall conduct a study on physician fees under State Medicaid programs established under title XIX of the Social Security Act. The Commission shall specifically examine in such study the adequacy of physician reimbursement under such programs, physician participation in such programs, and access to care by Medicaid beneficiaries. (Section 6102(d)(8) of Public Law 101-239, OBRA 1989)	Issued

II. SELECTED BIBLIOGRAPHY

The bibliography lists in reverse chronology *selected* reports from 1989 to the present by the following government agencies: General Accounting Office, Health Care Financing Administration, Congressional Budget Office, Office of Technology Assessment, Congressional Research Service, and Office of Inspector General (Department of Health and Human Services). Congressional hearings are also included, as well as journal articles cited in this source book. Other selected reports of topical importance to the Medicaid program are also listed.

A. General Accounting Office Reports

U.S. General Accounting Office. Welfare to work: implementation and evaluation of transitional benefits need HHS action; report to congressional requesters. Sept. 29, 1992. Washington, GAO, 1992. GAO/HRD-92-118, B-248840

"In addition to describing how States are delivering transitional benefits, an objective of our review was to determine the extent to which the eligible population is receiving either transitional child care or transitional Medicaid benefits. For our analysis, benefit utilization rates are defined as the ratio of recipients who received the transitional benefit for at least 1 month to recipients who left Aid to Families With Dependent Children due to increased earnings. Because of limitations in the data that are discussed below, we recommend caution in the use of the estimates."

----- D.C. government: District Medicaid payments to hospitals; fact sheet for the Committee on the District of Columbia, House of Representatives. Aug. 24, 1992. Washington, GAO, 1992. GAO/GGD-92-138FS, B-249162

This fact sheet determines "(1) the causes of the legal action taken by District of Columbia hospitals against the District Medicaid program and (2) whether the District could be using Federal Medicaid money to fund other District programs."

----- Medicaid: Oregon's managed care program and implications for expansions; report to the Chairman, Subcommittee on Health and the Environment, Committee on Energy and Commerce, House of Representatives. June 19, 1992. Washington, GAO, 1992. GAO/HRD-92-89, B-246496

"This report reviews the Oregon Medicaid managed care program and the State's proposal to expand the program as part of a larger demonstration. The report reviews issues of access, quality of care, and financial oversight."

----- Medicaid: ensuring that noncustodial parents provide health insurance can save costs; report to the Chairman, Committee on Government Operations, House of Representatives. June 17, 1992. Washington, GAO, 1992. GAO/HRD-92-80, B-246421

Recommends that "Congress require, as a condition of Federal participation in their child support programs, that States enact laws enabling the programs to enforce health insurance requirements on employers, such as is done with income withholding for cash support."

----- Access to health care: States respond to growing crisis; report to congressional requesters. June 16, 1992. Washington, GAO, 1992. GAO/HRD-92-70, B-245950

This report "describes comprehensive plans to provide universal access to coverage, programs to extend access to specific groups, and efforts to control costs by reforming payment mechanisms."

----- Veterans' benefits: savings from reducing VA pensions to Medicaid-supported nursing home residents; report to the Chairman, Committee on Veterans' Affairs, U.S. Senate. Dec. 1991. Washington, GAO, 1991. GAO/HRD-92-32, B-246372

"As a result of OBRA 1990, VA should be able to reduce pensions by about $174 million annually for veterans receiving Medicaid-supported nursing home care . . . VA has not fully implemented the OBRA 1990 legislation. By not adequately controlling the case review process, VA did not reduce all affected veterans' pensions. VA is planning changes that eventually should identify all veterans' cases where pensions should be reduced. If the proposed legislation reducing survivor benefits passes, significant potential savings can occur."

----- Medicaid: changes in drug prices paid by VA and DOD since enactment of rebate provisions; report to congressional committees. Sept. 1991. Washington, GAO, 1991. GAO/HRD-91-139, B-245667

In this report, GAO focuses on "how VA and DOD prescription drug prices had changed and what effect the changes had on agency costs."

----- Medicaid expansions: coverage improves but State fiscal problems jeopardize continued progress; report to the Chairman, Committee on Finance, U.S. Senate. June 1991. Washington, GAO, 1991. GAO/HRD-91-78, B-243156

This report "examine[s] the effects of the recent Federal legislation, focusing particularly on changes affecting low-income women and children. The analysis also addresse[s] States' concerns, by examining the extent to which Medicaid contributes to their fiscal stress."

----- Substance abuse treatment: Medicaid allows some services but generally limits coverage; report to congressional requesters. June 1991. Washington, GAO, 1991. GAO/HRD-91-92, B-243725

This report "review[s] Federal guidance to the States on Medicaid coverage of substance abuse treatment services, the types of Medicaid services available in States, the level of Federal and State spending, and barriers that may exist to obtaining treatment reimbursed by Medicaid."

----- Medicaid: alternatives for improving the distribution of funds; fact sheet for the Honorable Dale Bumpers, U.S. Senate. May 20, 1991. Washington, GAO, 1991. GAO/HRD-91-66FS, B-205047

Recommends a revised formula to improve how Medicaid funds are distributed among the States, based on total taxable resources and number of people in poverty. Describes this formula and several other options.

----- Trauma care: lifesaving system threatened by unreimbursed costs and other factors; report to the Chairman, Subcommittee on Health for Families and the Uninsured, Committee on Finance, U.S. Senate. May 17, 1991. Washington, GAO, 1991. GAO/HRD-91-57, B-242551

"Provides information on the reasons hospitals in major urban areas withdraw from trauma care systems that serve people with life-threatening injuries."

----- Medicaid: HCFA needs authority to enforce third-party requirements on States. Apr. 11, 1991. Washington, GAO, 1991. GAO/HRD-91-60

Explains "the need for better compliance with and enforcement of Medicaid third-party liability requirements and for Congress to authorize HCFA to withhold Federal matching funds when States do not comply."

----- Rural hospitals: Federal efforts should target areas where closures threaten access to care. Feb. 15, 1991. Washington, GAO, 1991. GAO/HRD-91-31FS

Finds that "most rural hospital closures did not significantly reduce access to care, but in some areas closures did appear to worsen access, especially for Medicaid [beneficiaries] and the uninsured."

----- Early success in enrolling women made eligible by Medicaid expansions. Feb. 1991. Washington, GAO, 1991. GAO/PEMD-91-10

Reports on the "success of State Medicaid programs in implementing coverage of low-income pregnant and postpartum women who were made eligible by expansions of the Federal Medicaid law in 1986 and 1987."

----- Medicaid: millions of dollars not recovered from Michigan Blue Cross/Blue Shield; report to the Chairman, Committee on Government Operations, House of Representatives. Nov. 30, 1990. Washington, GAO, 1990. GAO/HRD-91-12, B-239899

Finds that "since August 1988, Michigan has made recovery on none of the medical claims it paid for Medicaid [beneficiaries] with BC/BS benefits," despite Federal laws requiring State agencies to seek recovery from responsible third-party private insurers.

----- Medicaid: legislation needed to improve collection from private insurers. Nov. 30, 1990. Washington, GAO, 1990. GAO/HRD-91-25, B-238267

"While State officials found it hard to pinpoint losses resulting from their payment systems, . . . the problem may be substantial--perhaps millions of dollars in losses each year--and growing."

----- Long-term care insurance: proposals to link private insurance and Medicaid need close scrutiny; report to the Chairman, Subcommittee on Health and Long-Term Care, Select Committee on Aging, House of Representatives. Sept. 10, 1990. Washington, GAO, 1990. GAO/HRD-90-154, B-240641

Evaluates proposed State demonstration projects involving planning grants to California, Connecticut, Indiana, Massachusetts, New Jersey, New York, Oregon, and Wisconsin.

----- Nursing homes: admission problems for Medicaid recipients and attempts to solve them; report to the Honorable Howard M. Metzenbaum, U.S. Senate. Sept. 5, 1990. Washington, GAO, 1990. GAO/HRD-90-135, B-232993

"Includes information on the types of reforms that have been implemented in various States and factors that influence States' willingness to improve access for Medicaid [beneficiaries]."

----- Medicaid: oversight of health maintenance organizations in the Chicago area: report to the Honorable Cardiss Collins. Aug. 27, 1990. Washington, GAO, 1990. GAO/HRD-90-81, B-237798

Assesses "the adequacy of Health Care Financing Administration and Illinois oversight of the quality of care provided to Medicaid [beneficiaries] by Chicago-area health maintenance organizations."

----- Home visiting: a promising early intervention strategy for at-risk families; report to the Chairman, Subcommittee on Labor, Health and Human Services, Education and Related Agencies, Committee on Appropriations, U.S. Senate. July 11, 1990. Washington, GAO, 1990. GAO/HRD-90-83, B-238294

"On the basis of an extensive examination of selected home visiting programs nationwide and in Europe, GAO concluded that home visiting can be an effective strategy for delivering or improving access to early intervention services that can help at-risk families become healthier and more self-sufficient." GAO recommended that Congress "establish as an optional Medicaid service, prenatal and postnatal home-visiting services for high-risk women, and home-visiting services for high-risk infants."

----- Medicare: comparative analyses of payments for selected hospital services: report to the Subcommittee on Health, Committee on Ways and Means, House of Representatives. July 6, 1990. Washington, GAO, 1990. GAO/HRD-90-108, B-239657

"Compared Medicare payment rates for selected inpatient hospital services with Medicaid payments for these same services in California, New York, and Ohio."

----- Medicaid: sources of information on mental health services; report to the Honorable Daniel K. Inouye. May 7, 1990. Washington, GAO, 1990. GAO/HRD-90-100, B-239070

"This report identifies sources of information on the types of mental health services offered under each State's Medicaid program. GAO found that several federal agencies publish data about Medicaid and mental health expenditures, and numbers of recipients of services for each State. However, these agencies publish little information about the specific mental health services available to Medicaid [beneficiaries] in each State."

----- Medicare and Medicaid: more information exchange could improve detection of substandard care; report to the Administrator, Health Care Financing Administration, Department of Health and Human Services. Mar. 7, 1990. Washington, GAO, 1990. GAO/HRD-90-29, B-237781

"Peer review organizations, Medicare carriers, and State Medicaid agencies do not routinely exchange information about physicians they have identified as providing unnecessary or poor quality care. GAO recommends that the Health Care Financing Administration require these groups to routinely exchange such information."

----- Medicaid: Federal oversight of Kansas facility for the retarded inadequate; report to the Subcommittee on the Handicapped, Committee on Labor and Human Resources, U.S. Senate. Sept. 29, 1989. Washington, GAO, 1989. GAO/HRD-89-85, B-230468

GAO finds that HCFA improperly reinstated the Winfield State Hospital and Training Center in the Medicaid program in March 1987.

----- Medicaid: States expand coverage for pregnant women, infants, and children; report to the Honorable Ronnie G. Flippo. Aug. 16, 1989. Washington, GAO, 1989. GAO/HRD-89-90, B-236032

As a result of options provided in the Omnibus Budget Reconciliation Acts of 1986 and 1987, most States have expanded Medicaid programs for this population. The Medicare Catastrophic Coverage Act made mandatory the OBRA 86 option that States cover pregnant women and infants with family incomes at or below the Federal poverty level.

----- ADP systems: better control over States' Medicaid systems needed: report to the Secretary of Health and Human Services. Aug. 2, 1989. Washington, GAO, 1989. GAO/IMTEC-89-19

"The Health Care Financing Administration (HCFA) and the States depend heavily on automated systems to manage and control the annual $48 billion in Medicaid program costs . . . GAO reviewed HCFA's procedures for ensuring Federal funding for States' automated systems will lead to the benefits expected by the Congress in making such funding available."

----- Health care: nine States' experiences with home care waivers: report to the Chairman, Committee on Finance, U.S. Senate. July 14, 1989. Washington, GAO, 1989. GAO/HRD-89-95, B-231228

Gives information "on States' experiences in applying for, renewing, and administering Medicaid waivers to permit payment for home care provided to chronically ill children." Study involved nine States (California, Texas, Florida, Georgia, Maine, Maryland, Minnesota, Mississippi, and Ohio).

----- Medicaid: recoveries from nursing home residents' estates could offset program costs. Mar. 7, 1989. Washington, GAO, 1989. GAO/HRD-89-56, B-226448

"GAO studied Medicaid nursing home programs in eight states, focusing particular attention on the estate recovery program operated by Oregon. The objective was to discover the potential financial impact of such programs on Medicaid and whether they provide a mechanism that is acceptable to the elderly for sharing the costs of nursing home care."

----- Medicaid: some recipients neglect to report U.S. savings bond holdings; report to congressional committees. Jan. 18, 1989. Washington, GAO, 1989. GAO/HRD-89-43, B-232864

Examines "how U.S. savings bond holdings of Medicaid applicants are determined during the eligibility process . . . the effectiveness of States' policies and procedures for verifying savings bond holdings. Also, determine[s] the extent of savings bond holdings by Medicaid [beneficiaries] residing in Massachusetts nursing homes."

B. Health Care Financing Administration Documents

U.S. Department of Health and Human Services. Health Care Financing Administration. Medicaid Bureau. Medicaid State Profile Data (spDATA) System: Characteristics of Medicaid State Programs--Volume I, National Comparisons. Washington, GPO, May 1992. HCFA Pub. No. 02178

"The Medicaid program is a major funding source of health care for America's poor and disabled. A rapid increase in Medicaid expenditures in recent years has focused attention on the need for a database with current, comprehensive information on all State Medicaid programs. *Medicaid State Profile Data (spDATA) System: Characteristics of Medicaid State Programs* provides details on State Medicaid programs. This report includes data generated from the Health Care Financing Administration's (HCFA's) new data system, spDATA, and data collected through the research efforts of the National Governors' Association (NGA). This report . . . primarily contains information from Medicaid State plans. Volume I introduces the spDATA System, presents national tables of selected State plan characteristics, and summarizes Medicaid program policy changes tracked by NGA."

----- Office of Research and Demonstrations. Status report: research and demonstrations in health care financing, fiscal year 1991 edition. Washington, GPO, Mar. 1992. HCFA Pub. No. 03323

"This report provides basic information on active intramural and extramural projects in a brief format. These projects are used to assess new methods and approaches for providing quality health care while containing costs, and they often provide the basis for making critical policy decisions on health care financing issues . . . This is the twelfth edition of the *Status Report*. Updated editions are produced on an annual basis. The information presented should be of use to policy officials, health planners, and researchers in examining the range of research and demonstration activities that are undertaken by ORD and the implications of results and findings."

----- Office of Research and Demonstrations. Program statistics: Medicare and Medicaid data book, 1990. Washington, GPO, Mar. 1991. HCFA Pub. No. 03314

This report "presents a broad overview of the Medicare and Medicaid programs . . . Data and analyses are presented for enrollees and recipients by demographic characteristics and basis of eligibility on use and expenditures for selected services. Administration and financing of the programs are discussed . . . Information on Medicare carriers and intermediaries and Medicaid agencies and fiscal agents is included." (Note: Medicare data for calendar year 1986 and Medicaid data for fiscal year 1986 are presented in the report.)

----- Office of Research and Demonstrations. The health care financing system and the uninsured. Washington, GPO, Apr. 1990.

"This study assesses the problems of the uninsured, underinsured, and persons at risk of incurring catastrophic expenses, and provides an analysis of the impact of alternative policy approaches on these problems and other aspects of the health care system . . . A wide variety of options to extend insurance coverage to the uninsured were analyzed . . . Some options result in large shifts of sources of insurance among insured populations as well, with many people dropping nongroup coverage in favor of Medicaid or employment-based insurance."

----- Bureau of Data Management and Strategy. 1989 data users conference proceedings. Washington, GPO, Sept. 1989. HCFA Pub. No. 03293

"This document contains the proceedings of the first Health Care Financing Administration's Data Users Conference. The goals of the Conference were to provide an overview of the type of Medicare and Medicaid data that is available in HCFA; and to share experiences in using HCFA data to study the effectiveness of the health care delivery system."

C. Health Care Financing Review Articles

Merzel, Cheryl, Stephen Crystal, Usha Sambamoorthi, et al. New Jersey's Medicaid waiver for acquired immunodeficiency syndrome. Health care financing review, v. 13, spring 1992: 27-44.

"This article contains data from a study of New Jersey's home and community-based Medicaid waiver program for persons with symptomatic human immunodeficiency virus illness. Major findings include lower hospital costs and utilization for waiver participants compared with general Medicaid acquired immunodeficiency syndrome admissions in New Jersey. Average program expenditures were $2,400 per person per month. Based on study findings, it is evident that the waiver program is an important means of providing financial benefits and access to services and that comprehensive case management is a critical factor in assuring program quality."

Cost-containment issues, methods, and experiences. Health care financing review 1991 annual supplement, Mar. 1992, HCFA Pub. No. 03322

"This Annual Supplement of the *Health Care Financing Review* focuses on cost containment. Underlying cost trends are analyzed and the range of demand and supply-side solutions to constraining health care costs, along with the attendant consequences, are discussed. The entire range of solutions, from all-payer ratesetting systems to voucher approaches to coordinated care arrangements, is presented . . . Health care currently consumes 1 of every 8 dollars of our total production and, by the year 2000, will consume 1 of every 6 dollars. The information presented here is intended to contribute to the current debate on improving access and increasing efficiency in our $700 billion health care sector."

Andrews, Roxanne, Margaret Keyes, and Penelope Pine. Longitudinal patterns of California Medicaid recipients with acquired immunodeficiency syndrome. Health care financing review, v. 13, winter 1991: 1-12.

"In this study, the authors examine the longitudinal experience, annual trends, and subpopulation differences in Medicaid use and expenditures for persons with acquired immunodeficiency syndrome (AIDS) in California from 1983 through 1986. About two-thirds of adult males were enrolled in Medicaid within 1 month of their AIDS diagnosis. These recipients averaged approximately 20-percent higher lifetime expenditures than those enrolled at a later time. Monthly expenditures were higher in the beginning of enrollment and prior to death than in the months in between. From 1983 through 1986, there was a shift of care from inpatient to outpatient settings. In 1986, children and adult females had higher median expenditures than did adult males."

Schlenker, Robert E. Comparison of Medicaid nursing home payment systems. Health care financing review, v. 13, fall 1991: 93-109.

"This article summarizes the main findings of a study comparing three generic Medicaid nursing home payment systems: case-mix, facility-specific, and class-rate. The major comparative analyses examined patient-level case mix and quality, facility-level costs, Medicaid payment rates, and profitability. The study also analyzed case-mix payment systems in greater detail, emphasizing the earlier systems. The results suggest advantages and disadvantages for all system types and highlight important considerations for policyplanners, particularly in States considering case-mix systems. The article concludes with a discussion of issues important to further research on nursing home payment."

Buchanan, Robert J., R. Peter Madel, and Dan Persons. Medicaid payment policies for nursing home care: a national survey. Health care financing review, v. 13, fall 1991: 55-72.

"This research gives a comprehensive overview of the nursing home payment methodologies used by each State Medicaid program. To present this comprehensive overview, 1988 data were collected by survey from 49 States and the District of Columbia. The literature was reviewed and integrated into the study to provide a theoretical framework to analyze the collected data. The data are organized and presented as follows: payment levels, payment methods, payment of capital-related costs, and incentives in nursing home payment. [The article] conclude[s] with a discussion of the impact these different methodologies have on program cost containment, quality, and recipient access."

Sonnefeld, Sally T., Daniel R. Waldo, Jeffrey A. Lemieux, et al. Projections of national health expenditures through the year 2000. Health care financing review, v. 13, fall 1991: 1-27.

"In this article, the authors present a scenario for health expenditures during the 1990s. Assuming that current laws and practices remain unchanged, the Nation will spend $1.6 trillion for health care in the year 2000, an amount equal to 16.4 percent of that year's gross national product. Medicare and Medicaid will foot an increasing share of the nation's health bill, rising to more than one-third of the total. The factors accounting for growth in national health spending are described as well as the effects of those factors on spending by type of service and by source of funds."

Andrews, Roxanne, Elicia Herz, Suzanne Dodds, et al. Access to hospital care for California and Michigan Medicaid recipients. Health care financing review, v. 12, summer 1991: 99-104.

"This article is a comparison of the characteristics of hospitals serving the general population and Medicaid [beneficiaries] in California and Michigan, using data from Medicaid uniform claims files and the American Hospital Association Annual Survey for 1984. A greater concentration of discharges in a small number of "high Medicaid volume" urban and rural hospitals in each State was observed for Medicaid [beneficiaries] compared with the general population. In addition, discharge data suggest that Supplemental Security Income crossovers (individuals covered by both Medicaid and Medicare) and other [beneficiaries] (mostly children not enrolled in the Aid to Families with Dependent Children program) receive inpatient care in different hospitals from the general population as well as from other Medicaid eligibility groups. Medicaid cost-containment policies and differential access to hospital care are discussed."

Brown, E. Richard and Michael R. Cousineau. Loss of Medicaid and access to health services. Health care financing review, v. 12, summer 1991: 17-26.

"In this article, the authors assessed the effects of the loss of Medicaid eligibility on access to health services by the medically indigent population in two California counties. An historically derived baseline of health services received by each county's medically indigent adults under Medicaid was compared with the volume of services provided by the county to the same population after they lost Medicaid eligibility. The baseline figures were used as an "expected" volume of services which can be compared with the actual, or "observed," volume of services. The analysis found fewer hospital discharges than expected in Los Angeles and much fewer outpatient visits than expected in Orange County, suggesting that these groups experienced substantial reduction in access related to loss of Medicaid eligibility."

Howell, Embry M., Elicia J. Herz, Ruey-Hua Wang, et al. A comparison of Medicaid and non-Medicaid obstetrical care in California. Health care financing review, v. 12, summer 1991: 1-15.

"The use of prenatal care and rates of low birth weight were examined among four groups of women who delivered in California in October 1983. Medicaid paid for the deliveries of two groups, and two groups were not so covered. The analyses suggest that longer Medicaid enrollment improved the use of prenatal care. The association between prenatal care and birth weight was less clear. For women under Medicaid, measures of infant and maternal morbidity, hospital characteristics, and Medicaid eligibility were all statistically related to charges, payments, and length of stay for the delivery hospitalization."

Medicaid: innovations and opportunities. Health care financing review 1990 annual supplement, Dec. 1990, HCFA Pub. No. 03311

Includes articles on "trends and data issues, quality of care, program management issues, maternal and child health, AIDS, special populations, and program expansions. The topics were chosen to offer insight, ideas, and information to help shape responsible and creative Medicaid initiatives."

Dubay, Lisa C. Changes in Medicare skilled nursing facility benefit admissions. Health care financing review, v. 12, winter 1990: 27-35.

"In this article, the changes in Medicare skilled nursing facility (SNF) benefit admissions from 1983 through 1985 are examined and factors that influence changes in access since the implementation of Medicare's prospective payment system are analyzed. During this period, use of the SNF benefit increased nationally by 21 percent. Multivariate analysis is used to determine factors associated with changes in admissions. Changes in SNF benefit admissions were found to be negatively associated with changes in area hospitals' lengths of stay and changes in hospitals' discharges. Medicaid reimbursement policies were also shown to affect changes in utilization."

Gohmann, Stephan F., and Robert L. Ohsfeldt. Medicaid payment rates for nursing homes, 1979-86. Health care financing review, v. 12, winter 1990: 55-66.

"The issue of the cost containment effects of payment systems on per diem payments by Medicaid to nursing homes is addressed. Estimates of real payment rates as a function of broadly defined payment system classifications and economic and demographic variables using State-level data are presented. Little support for the notion that prospective payment systems substantially restrain payment rates for intermediate care facilities is found, but some model specifications indicate possible cost savings associated with prospective payment systems for skilled nursing facilities. Significant methodological concerns that need to be addressed in future research on the cost containment effects of payment systems are also discussed."

Holahan, John. Hospital back-up days: impact on joint Medicare and Medicaid beneficiaries. Health care financing review, v. 12, winter 1990: 67-73.

"In this article the question of whether nursing home market characteristics affect the ability of hospitals to discharge patients to nursing homes is examined. Also examined is the question of whether joint Medicare and Medicaid beneficiaries have a more difficult time being placed than do other patients. The principal conclusions are first, that the nursing home bed supply and the type of Medicaid payment system affect the ability of hospitals to discharge patients to nursing homes. Joint Medicare and Medicaid beneficiaries have a more difficult time being placed in nursing homes in States with fewer beds and more restrictive Medicaid payment policies, and joint beneficiaries do not appear to have longer stays in hospitals. Rather, they have a greater likelihood of being discharged to home."

Welch, W. Pete. Giving physicians incentives to contain costs under Medicaid. Health care financing review, v. 12, winter 1990: 103-112.

"In this article, the risk arrangements in Medicaid programs that put physicians at risk are summarized. These programs--partial capitation and health insuring organizations--pay physicians a capitation amount to cover some or all physician services. Physicians also receive part of the savings from reduced hospitalization. Most of these programs have successfully lowered Medicaid costs. They could serve as models for other Medicaid programs, State-level programs to cover people ineligible for Medicaid, and programs abroad, such as in the United Kingdom."

Heinen, LuAnn, Peter D. Fox, and Maren D. Anderson. Findings from the Medicaid competition demonstrations: a guide for States. Health care financing review, v. 11, summer 1990: 55-67.

"The Medicaid Competition Demonstrations were initiated in 1983-84 in six States (California, Florida, Minnesota, Missouri, New Jersey, and New York). State experiences in implementing the demonstrations are presented in this article. Although problems of enrolling Medicaid [beneficiaries] in prepaid plans or with primary care case managers under these demonstrations proved challenging to States, lessons were learned in three key areas: program design and administration, health plan and provider relations, and beneficiary acceptance. Therefore, States considering similar programs in the future could benefit from these findings."

Leibowitz, Arleen, and Joan L. Buchanan. Setting capitations for Medicaid: a case study. Health care financing review, v. 11, summer 1990: 79-85.

"This article examines the methodology New York State used to set capitation rates for a Medicaid health maintenance organization. By examining the methods used and the assumptions made in a particular case, some general lessons are drawn about the ratesetting process. Greater reliance on statewide data to assure fair and statistically stable estimates is needed. Although the article focuses on one State and its ratesetting for one particular plan (Health Care Plus), the issues raised have general interest for other plans and for other States concerned with the setting of capitation rates for Medicaid enrollees in prepaid plans."

Coburn, Andrew F., Elizabeth H. Kilbreth, Richard H. Fortinsky, et al. Impact of the Maine Medicaid waiver for the mentally retarded. Health care financing review, v. 11, spring 1990: 43-50.

"To evaluate the impact of Maine's Medicaid waiver for the mentally retarded, baseline and 1-year followup data were obtained for 191 waiver clients and a comparison population of 115 persons excluded from the program because of enrollment limits. Program effectiveness was evaluated through measures of changes in clients' personal and community living skills. Medicaid and other data were used to establish individual and aggregate costs. It was found that the waiver program is a cost-effective alternative to intermediate care placements but that client screening is necessary to limit the enrollment of clients not at risk of institutional placement."

Klingman, David, Penelope L. Pine, and James Simon. Outcomes of surgery under Medicaid. Health care financing review, v. 11, spring 1990: 1-16.

"In this study, health outcomes during the 6-month period following surgery are examined for all Medicaid [beneficiaries] in Michigan and Georgia who underwent selected surgical procedures between July 1, 1981, and June 30, 1982. Readmissions were somewhat more prevalent in both States for hysterectomy, cholecystectomy, appendectomy, and myringotomy. On almost all measures in both States, levels of post-surgical utilization, expenditure, and complications were higher among females, older patients, Supplemental Security Income enrollees, and those with higher levels of presurgical utilization and longer and more costly surgical stays. The results further demonstrate the utility of claims data in monitoring outcomes of surgery."

Freund, Deborah A., Louis F. Rossiter, Peter D. Fox, et al. Evaluation of the Medicaid competition demonstrations. Health care financing review, v. 11, winter 1989: 81-97.

"In 1983, the Health Care Financing Administration funded a multiyear evaluation of Medicaid demonstrations in six States. The alternative delivery systems represented by the demonstrations contained a number of innovative features, most notably capitation, case management, limitations on provider choice, and provider competition. Implementation and operation issues as well as demonstration effects on utilization and cost of care, administrative costs, rate setting, biased selection, quality of care, and access and satisfaction were evaluated. Both primary and secondary data sources were used in the evaluation. This article contains an overview and summary of evaluation findings on the effects of the demonstrations."

McDevitt, Roland D., and Benson Dutton. Expenditures for ambulatory episodes of care: the Michigan Medicaid experience. Health care financing review, v. 11, winter 1989: 43-55.

"It is widely accepted that ambulatory care furnished in hospital outpatient department (OPD) settings is more costly than similar care furnished in office settings, but few researchers have explored whether practice patterns differ between the two settings. Differences in practice patterns may account for differences in the overall cost of care associated with these settings. Diagnosis-specific episodes of care were used to compare the costs of treating disease episodes in OPDs and offices. The findings suggest that OPD care is more costly not only because of price, but also because continuity of care is less common and the likelihood of hospital admission is substantially greater."

Adams, E. Kathleen, Marilyn Rymer Ellwood, and Penelope L. Pine. Utilization and expenditures under Medicaid for Supplemental Security Income disabled. Health care financing review, v. 11, fall 1989: 1-24.

"Recently available data on major disabling conditions of the Supplemental Security Income disabled are used to examine 1984 patterns of Medicaid expenditures in California, Georgia, Michigan, and Tennessee. Results indicate that 37-58 percent of these expenditures are for enrollees whose major disabling condition involves mental retardation or other mental disorders. This pattern occurs because a high proportion of disabled enrollees have these conditions, rather than high expenses per enrollee. Annual Medicaid expenditures per enrollee were highest for the disabled with neoplasms, blood disorders, and genitourinary conditions. Expenditures per enrollee were higher for younger enrollees and lower for those dually enrolled in Medicare."

Buczko, William. Hospital utilization and expenditures in a Medicaid population. Health care financing review, v. 11, fall 1989: 35-47.

"In this article, regression analysis is used to examine the determinants of the probability of a hospital visit, the number of hospitalizations, and the total inpatient hospital expenditures for Medicaid enrollees in the States of California, Michigan, New York, and Texas who were continuously enrolled throughout 1980."

McCall, Nelda, E. Deborah Jay, and Richard West. Access and satisfaction in the Arizona Health Care Cost Containment System. Health care financing review, v. 11, fall 1989: 63-77.

"The Arizona Health Care Cost Containment System is an alternative to Medicaid's acute medical care coverage. The results of the study indicate few differences in access and satisfaction between the two groups of beneficiaries on access to care, reported use of services, or satisfaction with the care received."

Pascal, Anthony, Marilyn Cvitanic, Charles Bennett, et al. State policies and the financing of acquired immunodeficiency syndrome care. Health care financing review, v. 11, fall 1989: 91-104.

"State policies, with respect to the operation of Medicaid programs and the regulation of private health insurance, affect who gets what care, how much is spent, and who ultimately pays. A RAND Corporation study was used to assess States and the District of Columbia in terms of the effects of their Medicaid and health insurance regulations on people with acquired immunodeficiency syndrome and other human immunodeficiency virus-related illnesses. State characteristics are used to explain the individual State policy rankings."

Howell, Embry M., and Gretchen A. Brown. Prenatal, delivery, and infant care under Medicaid in three States. Health care financing review, v. 10, summer 1989: 1-15.

"Medicaid services and expenditures were analyzed for care during the prenatal, delivery, and post-delivery periods in three States--California, Georgia, and Michigan. Uniform data were used from the Health Care

Financing Administration's Medicaid Tape-to-Tape project, 1983-84. Results indicate that from 16 to 24 percent of all births in the States of the study, during the study period, were financed by Medicaid. Overall, the study showed that more than one-half of expenditures for the study population were for the delivery hospitalization, and less than 12 percent were for prenatal care. As expected, a substantial portion of expenditures were for high-cost deliveries, up to 41 percent of total delivery payments. From 33 to 41 percent of total Medicaid expenditures for Aid to Families with Dependent Children were for pregnancy, delivery, and newborn care in 1983."

Lindsey, Phoebe A. Medicaid utilization control programs: results of a 1987 study. Health care financing review, v. 10, summer 1989: 79-92.

"Medicaid agencies use both second surgical opinion programs (SSOP's) and inpatient hospital preadmission review programs to control utilization of services and thus program expenditures. This article reports on the 13 mandatory and 7 voluntary SSOP's and the 21 inpatient preadmission review programs, based on responses from 44 State Medicaid agencies."

Ray, Wayne A., Charles F. Federspiel, David K. Baugh, et al. Experience of a Medicaid nursing home entry cohort. Health care financing review, v. 10, summer 1989: 51-63.

"Long-term care cost-containment policies have focused on reducing the numbers of persons entering nursing homes. To provide insight and background for such efforts, the authors studied the experience of Medicaid nursing home entry cohorts in three individual States. They found substantial interstate variation in rates of nursing home entry and subsequent patterns of discharge, suggesting the operation of fundamentally different policies for provision of Medicaid nursing home services. Analysis of the cost effectiveness and quality of care implications of these policies may provide guidance for future cost-containment efforts."

Vertrees, James C., Kenneth G. Manton, and Gerald S. Adler. Cost effectiveness of home and community-based care. Health care financing review, v. 10, summer 1989: 65-78.

"Medicaid section 2176 waivers allow States to provide home and community-based care to Medicaid eligibles who, but for these services, would enter Medicaid-funded nursing homes. One of the conditions required by Congress for granting these waivers is that this substitution results in no additional Medicaid spending (budget neutrality). The results of case studies of two of these waiver programs, one in California and one in Georgia, are presented in this article."

D. Congressional Budget Office Reports

U.S. Congress. Congressional Budget Office. The economic and budget outlook: an update. Washington, GPO, Aug. 1992.

"The Congressional Budget Office projects that the Federal budget deficit will reach $314 billion in fiscal year 1992--up from last year's record of $269 billion but well below previous estimates. The improvement in the budget outlook is only superficial, however, and stems largely from delays in approving additional funds to clean up the savings and loan mess. The deficit will shrink modestly over the next two or three years as the temporary effects of the recession and spending for deposit insurance fade away. But, by 1997, if no action is taken to reduce spending or raise taxes, the deficit will return to current levels."

----- Factors contributing to the growth of the Medicaid program. Washington, GPO, May 1992.

"This Congressional Budget Office staff memorandum analyzes recent trends in the Medicaid program and its projected growth through 1996. It discusses some of the policies, legal decisions, and other factors that may be contributing to rising Medicaid expenditures."

----- Selected options for expanding health insurance coverage. Washington, GPO, July 1991.

"At a time of rapidly rising health expenditures, concern over international competitiveness, and large budget deficits, it is difficult to fashion acceptable methods of providing health insurance for the medically uninsured. This study analyzes two major approaches for substantially reducing the number of uninsured people. One would expand employment-based coverage, and the other would cover more people under Medicaid."

----- Policy choices for long-term care. Washington, GPO, June 1991.

"This study analyzes policy choices for long-term care. In particular, it addresses the projected growth in total and Federal spending on long-term care under current law. It also examines alternative ways to increase financial protection for people who require extensive care and to broaden the range of services available to them."

E. Office of Technology Assessment Reports

U.S. Congress. Office of Technology Assessment. Evaluation of the Oregon Medicaid proposal: summary. Washington, GPO, 1992.

"The goals of the OTA study were to describe and analyze the specifics of the proposed program and to discuss its most likely implications for the Federal Government, the State of Oregon, and Medicaid beneficiaries. The role of the report is not to critique the existing Medicaid program in detail Rather, it is to examine the proposed program and especially its relevance to issues of particular interest to the Federal Government: the impact of the program on Medicaid beneficiaries, in whom the Federal Government (as a copayer) has a fiduciary interest; and the potential usefulness of Oregon's program if applied in other States and other contexts."

----- Adolescent health--volume I: summary and policy options. Washington, GPO, Apr. 1991. OTA-H-468

"This report . . . reviews the physical, emotional, and behavioral health status of contemporary American adolescents, including adolescents in groups considered to be in special need: adolescents living in poverty, adolescents from racial and ethnic minority groups and Native American adolescents; and adolescents in rural areas."

----- Adolescent health--volume II: background and the effectiveness of selected prevention and treatment services. Washington, GPO, 1991. OTA-H-466

Topics include prevention and services related to selected adolescent health concerns, AIDS and other sexually transmitted diseases, mental health problems, and alcohol, tobacco, and drug abuse.

----- Children's dental services under the Medicaid program. Washington, GPO, Sept. 1990. OTA-BP-H-78

"This study compares the dental manuals of seven State Medicaid programs with a set of 'basic' dental services (which comprise shared components of various well-accepted dental guidelines) to see if States allow these particular services. In addition, OTA surveyed practicing dentists in each of these seven States to see if dentists provide these 'basic' services to children under the Medicaid program in their State and, if not, what problems they encountered in trying to provide them."

----- Health care in rural America. Washington, GPO, Sept. 1990. OTA-H-434

"This report focuses on trends in the availability of primary and acute health care in rural areas and factors affecting those trends . . . The report itself examines in detail the issues faced by rural facilities providing health services and by physicians and other rural health personnel. To provide examples of how these issues may play out, it also discusses in more depth two specific groups of services: maternal and infant health services and mental health services."

----- The effectiveness of drug abuse treatment: implications for controlling AIDS/HIV infection. Washington, GPO, 1990.

"This OTA Background Paper has a dual role: it examines evidence for the effectiveness of treatment for drug abuse and evaluates the role of drug abuse treatment and a strategy to prevent HIV spread. Because most IV drug users are not in treatment, the study also examines other approaches to HIV prevention among this high-risk group."

----- Indian adolescent mental health. Washington, GPO, Jan. 1990. OTA-H-446

"This Special Report focuses on current knowledge about the mental health problems of American Indian and Alaska Native adolescents and the service systems that have evolved to treat such problems."

----- Rural emergency medical services. Washington, GPO, Nov. 1989. OTA-H-445

"This report finds that many State EMS (Emergency Medical Services) systems are fragmented and lacking resources to remedy EMS problems in rural areas. Many rural EMS programs lack specialized EMS providers, have inadequate EMS transportation and communications equipment, and are not part of a planned regional EMS system."

----- Adolescent health insurance status: analyses of trends in coverage and preliminary estimates of the effects of an employer mandate and Medicaid expansion on the uninsured: background paper for the Office of Technology Assessment's project on adolescent health prepared under contract by Richard Kronick. Washington, GPO, July 1989. OTA-BP-H-56

Examines the health insurance status of adolescents, age 10 to 18 years, using data from the Current Population Survey, including March 1988 data from new questions from the health insurance supplement.

F. Congressional Research Service Materials

U.S. Library of Congress. Congressional Research Service. Health insurance; issue brief by Mark Merlis. [Washington] Updated regularly. CRS Issue Brief IB91093

This paper provides an overview of a variety of health insurance issues of concern to Congress. Among these concerns are gaps in public and private health benefits coverage which result in large numbers of uninsured and underinsured individuals and families. There is strong congressional interest in controlling health care costs because of the effect on the Federal budget (chiefly through Medicare and Medicaid), on access to care for the uninsured, and on the competitiveness of employers who offer health benefits or the willingness of those employers to continue to offer benefits. In addition, there has been interest in expanding coverage through State and Federal insurance mandates and expansions of Medicaid program coverage.

----- Health insurance: summaries of legislation in the 102nd Congress; issue brief by Mark Merlis. [Washington] Updated regularly. CRS Issue Brief IB92102

The 102nd Congress is considering a wide variety of legislative alternatives for expanding access to health insurance and controlling health spending. Pending legislation incorporates widely different approaches. Comprehensive proposals would establish Federal or State public health insurance programs, mandate that all employers extend health insurance benefits or pay a tax, or assist the uninsured in buying private coverage through tax credits or other means. More incremental proposals would ease some of the perceived barriers to coverage for particular populations, such as small employer groups.

----- Long-term care for the elderly; issue brief by Richard J. Price and Carol O'Shaughnessy. [Washington] Updated regularly. CRS Issue Brief IB88098

Financing and providing for long-term care for the elderly is an important issue for the Congress for a number of reasons. Paying for long-term care services, especially nursing home care, can represent a catastrophic expenditure that impoverishes many elderly persons and their families. In addition, significant Federal resources are devoted to nursing home care through the Medicaid program, while only limited funding supports home and community-based services that the elderly and their families prefer over institutional care. This paper explores the major considerations related to this timely topic.

----- Prescription drug prices: should the Federal Government regulate them?; issue brief by Gary Guenther. [Washington] Updated regularly. CRS Issue Brief IB92097

A sharp escalation in the rate of increase in prescription drug prices since the early 1980s, coupled with the high initial prices charged by manufacturers for new breakthrough drugs in recent years, has sparked a lively debate in the Congress over whether the Federal Government should regulate prescription drug prices.

----- Medicaid: recent trends in beneficiaries and spending, by Kathleen King, Richard Rimkunas, and Dawn Nuschler. [Washington] Mar. 27, 1992. CRS Report 92-365 EPW

This report discusses Medicaid spending and beneficiary trends from FY 1987 through FY 1991 and projections from FY 1992 through FY 1997. It also discusses factors contributing to very rapid rates of growth in Medicaid spending, including: rapid increases in the number of Medicaid beneficiaries; inflation; increased reimbursement for selected Medicaid services; and changes in States' sources for Medicaid revenues.

----- The President's health care reform proposal, by the Health Section/Education and Public Welfare Division. [Washington] Mar. 5, 1992. CRS Report 92-285 EPW

On February 6, 1992, President Bush issued his Comprehensive Health Care Reform program, a plan designed to make health care more accessible by making health insurance more affordable and the health care system more efficient. The program uses market forces to implement reforms that build on our current health care system. This report describes and analyzes the President's plan. Financing provisions are not included, although suggested Medicare and Medicaid changes could produce savings in these programs.

----- Medicaid: financing, trends, and the President's FY 1993 budget proposals, by Melvina Ford. [Washington] Feb. 12, 1992. CRS Report 92-168 EPW

Mirroring the rapid increases in health care spending generally, Medicaid is one of the fastest growing items in both Federal and State budgets. Federal spending for Medicaid is expected to increase by 38 percent between fiscal years 1991 and 1992 and by another 16.5 percent in FY 1993. President Bush's FY 1993 budget proposes to limit growth in "mandatory" programs but would make only modest changes to Medicaid totalling $104 million in savings. Enactment of the President's legislative proposals would reduce Federal Medicaid spending from the $84.5 billion projected under current law to $84.396 billion in FY 1993.

----- Community supported living arrangements services for persons with developmental disabilities, by Mary F. Smith. [Washington] Revised Dec. 12, 1991. CRS Report 91-870 EPW (Revision of CRS Report 90-540 EPW)

The Omnibus Budget Reconciliation Act of 1990, P.L. 101-508, authorized a new limited option under the Medicaid program to permit from two to eight States to provide "community supported living arrangements services" for individuals with developmental disabilities. The purpose of the program is to assist these persons in the activities of daily living necessary to permit them to live in a family home or integrated community-based environment. Federal Medicaid expenditures for this program were limited to $10 million for FY 1992, and funding is to increase annually to $35 million for FY 1995. Eight States have been selected to implement this program.

----- Medicaid: provider donations and provider-specific taxes, by Mark Merlis. [Washington] Oct. 2, 1991. CRS Report 91-722 EPW

Medicaid is a program of medical assistance for certain low-income persons, with joint Federal and State financing. Recently, States have used funds donated by health care providers or taxes paid by those providers to draw greater Federal matching payments. The Administration has issued new regulations, effective January 1992, that would restrict these practices. This report provides a history of the State donation and tax programs, including past Administration and congressional efforts to regulate them, along with a summary of the new Federal rules and their potential impact on States.

----- Homeless mentally ill persons: problems and programs, by Edward R. Klebe. [Washington] Apr. 12, 1991. CRS Report 91-344 EPW

Mentally ill persons and persons with substance abuse problems make up a substantial percentage of the homeless population of the United States, with estimates ranging from 20 to 40 percent of the total. This report focuses on background information concerning mental illness and substance abuse among the homeless population and on the Federal programs including Medicaid that provide health and related services for this population.

----- Medicaid: reimbursement for outpatient prescription drugs, by Melvina Ford. [Washington] Mar. 7, 1991. CRS Report 91-235 EPW

Medicaid purchases over 12 percent of all prescription drugs sold in the U.S. at an annual cost of nearly $3.7 billion. Medicaid pays retail prices; other large purchasers receive discounts from drug manufacturers. The Omnibus Budget Reconciliation Act of 1990 (OBRA 90) substantially reforms Medicaid reimbursement for outpatient prescription drugs in all States. This report provides background on the new law which requires drug manufacturers to give rebates to Medicaid programs and expands access to drug products for Medicaid beneficiaries.

----- Characteristics of nursing home residents and proposals for reforming coverage of nursing home care, by Richard Price, Richard Rimkunas, and Carol O'Shaughnessy. [Washington] Sept. 24, 1990. CRS Report 90-471 EPW

This report analyzes data from the 1985 National Nursing Home Survey on resident length of stay patterns and levels of impairment. It also presents data on sources of payment for nursing home care. The two most often used sources of payment for nursing home care are residents' own income and Medicaid. Average length of stay varies among payment sources. For example, residents who used Medicaid as a source of payment tended to have longer length of stays than other residents.

----- Rationing health care, by Kathleen King. [Washington] July 12, 1990. CRS Report 90-346 EPW

This report discusses the concept of rationing health care and the extent of rationing in the current health care delivery system. Health care rationing has two meanings: (1) denying services to those who are unable to pay for them (price rationing); and (2) denying services, even those that might be beneficial, to those who are willing to pay (non-price rationing). Government policies do not explicitly ration health care by ability to pay. However, Government means-tested eligibility standards for Medicaid implicitly ration health care by ability to pay. Evidence also indicates that ability to pay is an implicit, but important, consideration in determining whether individuals have access to health care services in the private sector. Similarly, non-price measures also affect access and availability of health care services.

----- Medicare and Medicaid nursing home reform provisions in the Omnibus Budget Reconciliation Act of 1987, P.L. 100-203, by Richard Price. [Washington] Revised Jan. 16, 1990. CRS Report 90-80 EPW (Revision of CRS Report 89-463 EPW)

The Omnibus Budget Reconciliation Act of 1987 (OBRA 87) contained provisions that comprehensively reform the requirements nursing homes must meet in order to participate in Medicare and/or Medicaid. These provisions are divided into three major parts: (1) requirements that nursing homes must meet in order to participate; (2) provisions revising the survey and certification process for determining whether nursing homes comply with these requirements; and (3) provisions expanding the range of sanctions and penalties that HCFA and the States may impose against noncompliant nursing homes. Implementation of these provisions is to be phased in from 1988 through 1991, with major sections of the new law becoming effective October 1, 1990. This report summarizes the provisions as they are contained in the Medicare and Medicaid statutes and discusses a variety of issues that have arisen in the implementation of the new law.

G. Office of Inspector General Reports

U.S. Department of Health and Human Services. Office of Inspector General. Apparent inconsistency in Medicaid law--patients in private psychiatric facilities. Washington, May 17, 1991. A-09-90-00126

"Recommends that HCFA describe an apparent inconsistency in Federal law when it reports to Congress on the implementation of the Medicaid exclusion for patients in institutions for mental diseases (IMDs). Some of these patients are receiving Supplemental Security Income payments (SSI) and, as recipients of Federal cash assistance, are eligible for medical assistance under the Medicaid law. The Medicaid law, however, specifically prohibits payments for services to patients in IMDs who are over the age of 22 and under the age of 65."

----- States increase their use of revenues generated by provider tax and donation programs as the States' share of Medicaid expenditures. Washington, May 10, 1991. A-14-91-01010

This report "explain[s] States' use of donations and tax payments from health care providers as a means of enlarging the amount of State Medicaid payments and thereby increasing the amount of Federal Medicaid matching funds, and recommend[s] action by HCFA and Congress to restrict such practice."

----- Medicaid expansions for prenatal care: State and local implementation. [All findings are based on information as of January 1991) OEI-06-90-00160

"This inspection describes State and local efforts to implement eligibility expansions for Medicaid-covered prenatal care and to overcome barriers to accessibility and availability of prenatal care."

----- Use of donations and provider tax revenue as the State share of Medicaid expenditures. Washington, Oct. 1990. A-14-90-01009

This report presents survey results on "four basic categories of Medicaid provider tax/donation programs that are currently being used to supplement the States' shares of financial participation in their Medicaid programs. These categories are: hospital donation programs--Alabama, California, Georgia and Tennessee; taxes on provider operating costs or revenues--Florida, Kentucky, Ohio, South Carolina, and Texas; provider licenses and fees--Connecticut, Maine, New Hampshire, South Carolina, Tennessee and Vermont; and eligibility case worker administrative costs--California, Missouri, South Carolina and Texas."

H. Congressional Hearings

U.S. Congress. Senate. Committee on Finance. HCFA regulation restricting use of Medicaid provider donations and taxes. Hearing, 102nd Congress, 1st Session. S. Hrg. 102-580. Washington, GPO, 1992.

----- House of Representatives. Committee on Energy and Commerce. Subcommittee on Oversight and Investigations. Medicaid program investigation (part 1). Hearings, 102nd Congress, 1st Session. Comm. Pub. No. 102-91. Washington, GPO, 1992.

----- House of Representatives. Committee on Energy and Commerce. Subcommittee on Health and the Environment. State financing of Medicaid. Hearings, 102nd Congress, 1st Session. Comm. Pub. No. 102-79. Washington, GPO, 1992.

----- Senate. Committee on Finance. Subcommittee on Health for Families and the Uninsured. Medicaid/Medicare financing and implementation of certain programs. Hearing, 102nd Congress, 1st Session. S. Hrg. 102-392. Washington, GPO, 1992.

----- House of Representatives. Committee on Energy and Commerce. Subcommittee on Health and the Environment. Oregon Medicaid rationing experiment. Hearing, 102nd Congress, 1st Session. Comm. Pub. No. 102-49. Washington, GPO, 1991.

----- House of Representatives. Select Committee on Aging. Subcommittee on Health and Long-Term Care. Helping elders avoid nursing homes: a promising new approach. Hearing, 102nd Congress, 1st Session. Comm. Pub. No. 102-822. Washington, GPO, 1991.

----- House of Representatives. Committee on Government Operations. Subcommittee on Human Resources and Intergovernmental Relations. Medicaid funding crisis. Hearing, 101st Congress, 2nd Session. Washington, GPO, 1991.

----- Senate. Committee on Finance. Subcommittee on Health for Families and the Uninsured. Medicaid prescription drug pricing. Hearings, 101st Congress, 2nd Session. S. Hrg. 101-1261. Washington, GPO, 1991.

----- House of Representatives. Committee on Energy and Commerce. Subcommittee on Health and the Environment. Medicaid budget initiatives. Hearings, 101st Congress, 2nd Session. Comm. Pub. No. 101-206. Washington, GPO, 1991.

----- House of Representatives. Committee on the Budget. Task Force on Health Resources. Health care crisis: problems of cost and access for children of color. Hearings, 101st Congress, 2nd Session. Comm. Pub. No. 5-15. Washington, GPO, 1991.

----- House of Representatives. Committee on the Budget. Task Force on Health Resources. Health care crisis: problems of cost and access. Hearings, 101st Congress, 2nd Session. Comm. Pub. No. 5-13. Washington, GPO, 1991.

----- House of Representatives. Committee on Ways and Means. Subcommittee on Health. Health insurance options: proposals from the provider community. Hearings, 101st Congress, 2nd session. Comm. Pub. No. 101-106. Washington, GPO, 1990.

----- House of Representatives. Committee on Energy and Commerce. Subcommittee on Health and the Environment. Wage rates for nursing facilities personnel. Hearings, 101st Congress, 2nd session (on H.R. 1649). Comm. Pub. No. 101-180. Washington, GPO, 1990.

----- House of Representatives. Committee on Government Operations. Human Resources and Intergovernmental Relations Subcommittee. Quality of care provided by Medicaid physicians in New York. Hearings, 101st Congress, 2nd Session. Washington, GPO, 1990.

----- House of Representatives. Select Committee on Aging. Medicare and Medicaid's 25th anniversary--much promised, accomplished, and left unfinished. Hearings, 101st Congress, 2nd Session. Comm. Pub. No. 101-778. Washington, GPO, 1990.

----- House of Representatives. Committee on Energy and Commerce. Subcommittee on Health and the Environment. AIDS issues (part 3). Hearings, 101st Congress, 2nd Session. Comm. Pub. No. 101-162. Washington, GPO, 1990.

----- Senate. Committee on Finance. Health care coverage for children. Hearings, 101st Congress, 1st Session. Comm. Pub. No. 101-568. Washington, GPO, 1990.

----- House of Representatives. Committee on Energy and Commerce. Subcommittee on Health and the Environment. Medicare and Medicaid initiatives. Hearings, 101st Congress, 1st Session. Comm. Pub. No. 101-46. Washington, GPO, 1989.

----- House of Representatives. Select Committee on Aging. Medicare and Medicaid budget priorities in the 1990s. Hearings, 101st Congress, 1st Session. Comm. Pub. No. 101-724. Washington, GPO, 1989.

----- House of Representatives. Committee on Energy and Commerce. Subcommittee on Health and the Environment. Health insurance coverage and reform. Hearings, 101st Congress, 1st Session. Comm. Pub. No. 101-18. Washington, GPO, 1989.

I. Other Reports and Journal Articles

Medicaid financing crisis: balancing responsibilities, priorities, and dollars. Background papers prepared for a roundtable discussion sponsored by the Kaiser Commission on the Future of Medicaid, held in Washington, D.C., July 21, 1992.
   "As fiscal constraints at the Federal and State level are compounded by pressure to expand access to health care services for the low-income population, the current Medicaid financing crisis has become an area of critical concern to Federal and State policymakers alike. Although there is consensus that Medicaid has become a 'budget buster,' there is not a clear understanding of the factors contributing to the increased growth and the implications of these factors on future program structure and potential reform . . . The purpose of this roundtable is to discuss findings from Commission sponsored research on the contribution of various factors to Medicaid cost increases and financing problems and to explore the implications of these findings on current and future policy."

Medicaid provider tax and donation issues: the Federal debate. Health Policy Alternatives, Inc. Washington, D.C., July 1992.

"The report first sets the stage for the 1991 debate by reviewing the history of Medicaid provider donation and tax programs, as well as the history of a number of other matters that had a bearing on the debate. These include the general economic decline and fiscal problems confronting the States, and a series of Medicaid program issues and Federal budget rules that affected the debate. Second, the report reviews the 1991 debate including the administration's proposed budget, the explosive growth in the provider-based financing programs, the administration's initial regulatory proposal and its rejection by the States and the Congress, the negotiations between the Nation's governors and administration over the issue, and the final agreement. The report concludes with an assessment of the issues and reasons for the outcome that occurred, as well as the potential for further action."

St. Peter, Robert F., Paul W. Newacheck, and Neal Halfon. Access to care for poor children. Journal of the American medical association, v. 267, May 27, 1992: 2760-2764.

"While Medicaid does improve access to care for poor children, it does not ensure them access to the same locations and continuity of care as that available to other children. Recent changes in the Medicaid program may address some of these inequities, but others are likely to remain."

U.S. Department of Commerce. Bureau of the Census. Current Population Reports, Series P-70, No. 29. Health insurance coverage: 1987-1990 (selected data from the Survey of Income and Program Participation). Washington, GPO, May 1992.

"This report uses data from the Survey of Income and Program Participation (SIPP) to examine issues related to health insurance coverage. The report has two major points of focus. First, it presents quarterly estimates of the extent and type of health insurance coverage (and the characteristics of those who lacked insurance) from the first quarter of 1989 to the fourth quarter of 1990 . . . Secondly, the report examines the extent to which people are covered by health insurance over a 28-month period beginning in October 1986."

Mayes, Linda C., Richard H. Granger, Marc H. Bornstein, et al. The problem of prenatal cocaine exposure: a rush to judgment. Journal of the American medical association, v. 267, Jan. 15, 1992: 406-408.

"At present no reliable national estimates of the extent or patterns of cocaine use during pregnancy exists . . . For policymakers, social agencies, and health and educational institutions, we recommend a suspension of judgment about the developmental outcome of cocaine-exposed babies until solid scientific data are available. Whatever the damage from prenatal exposure to cocaine may prove to be, outcome will not be improved by an attitude that assumes that exposed children cannot be helped or that they are different from other children."

The effects of the AIDS epidemic on traditional Medicaid populations. Santa Monica, California, Rand Corporation, 1992.

"This study identifies the changes in State Medicaid systems that result from the spread of HIV-related diseases. Research suggests that a substantial share of the costs for AIDS patient care falls on Medicaid. This share is expected to rise as the intravenous drug user share of the AIDS caseload grows, as therapies continue to lengthen survival time, and as private health insurers become more successful in screening out people likely to develop AIDS symptomatology."

Medicaid: intergovernmental trends and options. U.S. Advisory Commission on Intergovernmental Relations. Washington, The Commission, 1992.

This report tries to "identify the major trends in Medicaid in terms of the program's size, structure, clientele, and services, and its ability to respond to emerging needs. The Commission's recommendations . . . are necessarily in the form of 'band-aid' fixes for Medicaid's problems."

Braveman, Paula A., Susan Egerter, Trude Bennett, et al. Differences in hospital resource allocation among sick newborns according to insurance coverage. Journal of the American medical association, v. 266, Dec. 18, 1991: 3300-3308.

"Sick newborns without insurance received fewer inpatient services than comparable privately insured newborns with either indemnity or prepaid coverage. This pattern was observed across all hospital ownership types. Mean stay was 15.7 days for all privately insured newborns (15.6 days for those with indemnity and 15.7 days for those with prepaid coverage), 14.8 days for Medicaid-covered newborns, and 13.2 days for uninsured newborns. Length of stay, total charges, and charges per day were 16 percent, 28 percent, and 10 percent less, respectively, for the uninsured than for all privately insured newborns. Resources for newborns covered by Medicaid were generally greater than for the uninsured and less than for the privately insured. Both uninsured and Medicaid-covered newborns were found to have more severe medical problems than the privately insured."

Lefkowitz, D., and A. Monheit. Health insurance, use of health services, and health care expenditures. Agency for Health Care Policy and Research (AHCPR), Public Health Service. AHCPR Pub. No. 92-0017. National Medical Expenditure Survey Research Findings 12. Rockville, Maryland, Dec. 1991.

"The focus of the report is on the relationship between insurance coverage and the use of health services, total expenditures, total out-of-pocket payments, and the proportion of medical care expenditures paid out of pocket. This relationship is examined separately for persons of different ages, for persons at different family income levels relative to poverty, and for persons reporting their health status as either fair/poor or excellent/good."

Stern, Robert S., Joel S. Weissman, and Arnold M. Epstein. The emergency department as a pathway to admission for poor and high-cost patients. Journal of the American medical association, v. 266, Oct. 23/30, 1991: 2238-2243.

"Our data indicate that patients with lower socioeconomic status are more likely than other patients to use the emergency department as their means of access to the hospital and that patients admitted via the emergency department use far more resources than patients in the same diagnosis related group admitted by other means. Hospitals that make emergency department services more available may be more likely to hospitalize socioeconomically disadvantaged patients and may be at a substantial financial disadvantage under per-case reimbursement systems such as Medicare."

Fossett, James W., Chang H. Choi, and John A Peterson. Hospital outpatient services and Medicaid patients' access to care. Medical care, v. 29, Oct. 1991: 964-976.

"This article examines the relationship between the use of hospital outpatient services by Medicaid patients, Medicaid physician fees, and the use of office-based physician services. Past research has indicated that the use of outpatient facilities by Medicaid patients substitutes for care by private physicians and might be reduced by raising physician fees, but these studies may be estimated at too high a level of geographic aggregation and include many outpatient services that are not substitutes for office-based physician care. The results in this study, which are estimated using LISREL on county level Medicaid claims data from the State of Illinois, provide little evidence that outpatient care substitutes for care by physicians or that raising physician fees would reduce inappropriate outpatient usage by Medicaid patients."

Brown, Lawrence D. The national politics of Oregon's rationing plan. Health affairs, v. 10, summer 1991: 28-51.

"In 1989, the State of Oregon passed legislation intended to achieve near-universal coverage by defining a new basic benefit package for a subset of Medicaid [beneficiaries], requiring employers to offer at least that basic package to their workers, and creating a pool to extend coverage to uninsurables. Because the basic benefit package would explicitly exclude services deemed to be insufficiently cost-effective, the plan has sparked a lively debate about health care "rationing." And because the proposed modifications to Medicaid cannot proceed unless the Federal Government waives certain requirements, the rationing debate is now crystallizing in Washington, D.C. This article tries to explain what the debate is about and indicates its larger policy significance."

Quadagno, Jill, Madonna Harrington Meyer, and J. Blake Turner. Falling into the Medicaid gap: the hidden long-term care dilemma. Gerontologist, v. 31, Aug. 1991: 521-526.

"This study describes the income, health, and functional capacity of older Florida residents who fall into the Medicaid gap--those whose incomes are too high to obtain eligibility for Medicaid yet too low to cover the cost of nursing home care as private pay patients--and examines the strategies adopted by their primary caregivers. Our findings suggest that few strategies succeed in alleviating this all but unresolvable problem, that those caught in the gap receive inadequate medical care, and that their primary caregivers face tremendous financial and emotional burdens with little hope for relief."

Improving Medicaid estimates: report of HHS-OMB task force. Washington, July 10, 1991.

The HHS-OMB Management Review Task Force was formed to "address continuing and largely unanticipated increases in Medicaid spending . . . A set of four fact-finding teams analyzed why Medicaid estimates have been so inaccurate; examined the deficiencies in the current Federal/State estimating process that allow such discrepancies to occur without prior notice, as well as possible corrective measures; looked at ways to work more closely with the States to understand the unique policy dynamics of the program in each State; and used the results of the review to improve Federal Medicaid tracking efforts and to evaluate better the fiscal impact of future Medicaid policy changes."

Physician payment under Medicaid. Washington, Physician Payment Review Commission, July 1991.

This report "examine[s] the adequacy of physician fees, physician participation, and beneficiary access to care . . . [It] presents new information and introduces the Commission's goal for Medicaid payment policy. In the Commission's view, Medicaid beneficiaries, whose care is largely financed by the Federal Government, should enjoy access to care comparable to that of beneficiaries of other federally financed programs, most notably Medicare. Yet although access to mainstream medical care for Medicaid beneficiaries should be an objective of the program, such access will remain elusive as long as fee levels for physicians' services are substantially below those paid by Medicare and other payers."

Brennan, Troyen A., Liesi E. Hebert, Nan M. Laird, et al. Hospital characteristics associated with adverse events and substandard care. Journal of the American medical association, v. 265, June 26, 1991: 3265-3269.

"This study based on data in more than 30,000 medical records from 51 randomly chosen hospitals in New York, constitutes a comprehensive analysis of medical injury and malpractice litigation. We now present information regarding hospital characteristics that are associated with adverse events (AEs), i.e., injuries caused by medical intervention as distinct from the disease process, and with the fraction of AEs caused by negligence or substandard care."

Mussman, Mary G., Lu Zawistowich, Carol S. Weisman, et al. Medical malpractice claims filed by Medicaid and non-Medicaid recipients in Maryland. Journal of the American medical association, v. 265, June 12, 1991: 2992-2994.

"Several databases available in Maryland are used to investigate whether Medicaid [beneficiaries] are more likely than other persons to engage in medical malpractice litigation. All malpractice claims filed during 1985 and 1986 were updated for outcomes through 1989 and described with regard to the payer status of claimants. The proportion of claims filed by persons enrolled in Medicaid before and/or during the alleged malpractice incident was lower than the proportion of State residents enrolled in Medicaid. In addition, the proportion of obstetric claims filed by Medicaid [beneficiaries] was identical to their proportion of hospital discharges for obstetric services during the period in which the incidents occurred."

Carey, Timothy S., Kathi Weis, and Charles Homer. Prepaid versus traditional Medicaid plans: lack of effect on pregnancy outcomes and prenatal care. Health services research, v. 26, June 1991: 165-181.

"Enrollment of Medicaid [beneficiaries] into capitated, case-managed systems has been advocated as a method of controlling cost. We studied prenatal care and birth outcomes for women and children enrolled in Aid to Families with Dependent Children (AFDC) in two capitated programs in Santa Barbara, California and Jackson County, Missouri (Prepaid), compared with similar but fee-for-service comparison medical communities in Ventura County, California and St. Louis, Missouri (FFS)."

Lewin-Epstein, Noah. Determinants of regular source of health care in black, Mexican, Puerto Rican, and non-Hispanic white populations. Medical care, v. 29, June 1991: 543-557.

"Multinomial logit analysis is used to estimate the likelihood of having a particular kind of regular source of care. The findings demonstrated considerable ethnic group differences. In particular, blacks tend to utilize hospital facilities as a result of past constraints and their current dependence on public insurance programs. Mexicans are the least likely to have a regular source of care due to social and cultural barriers such as language, migration status, and low community participation. The implications of social isolation associated with poverty are also examined and discussed."

Medicaid patients' access to office-based obstetricians. Journal of health care for the poor and underserved, v. 1, spring 1991.

Discusses the availability of office-based obstetric care to Illinois Medicaid patients.

Schwartz, Anne, David C. Colby, and Anne Lenhard Reisinger. Variation in Medicaid physician fees. Health affairs, v. 10, spring 1991: 131-139.

"The extent of variation in physician fee levels across States suggests that Medicaid beneficiaries in different States may face different degrees of access to medical care simply because of where they reside. While we have not attempted here to account for the causes of this variation beyond differences in practice costs, which appear to have little effect on the variation, the amount of variation in Medicaid physician fees is striking. This variation may reflect different policy choices made by each State. The data indicate significant opportunity to reduce the variation in fee levels among States and bring Medicaid fee levels closer to those of other insurers, as an avenue for reducing differential access to care."

Zedlweski, Sheila, and John Holahan. Expanding Medicaid to cover uninsured Americans. Health affairs, v. 10, spring 1991: 45-61.
"This article examines the effects of alternative Medicaid expansion strategies . . . Microsimulation methods [are used] to estimate the cost and coverage implications of Medicaid expansion proposals that would cover nonelderly, noninstitutionalized individuals up to selected percentages of the poverty line. The analysis provides estimates of the number and characteristics of people affected, as well as implications for federal and state budgets . . . The full expansion costs and net costs of different types of buy-in arrangements [as well as] . . . the implications of combining employer mandates with expansions [are shown]."

Rovner, Julie. Cost of Medicaid puts States in tightening budget vise. Congressional quarterly weekly report, v. 49, May 18, 1991: 1277-1284.
". . . the more lawmakers and administration officials look to Medicaid as a potential savior for the uninsured, the more problems they find with how it is carrying out its original mission. What began a generation ago as a program to help the nation's poorest people is being overwhelmed by forces that its planners never expected."

Hannan, Edward L., Harold Kilburn, Joseph F. O'Donnell, et al. Interracial access to selected cardiac procedures for patients hospitalized with coronary artery disease in New York State. Medical care, v. 29, May 1991: 430-441.
"This study examines black/white differences in the utilization of three cardiac procedures (coronary angiography, coronary artery bypass graft, and coronary angioplasty) for patients hospitalized with coronary artery disease in New York State in the first 6 months of 1987. In contrast with previous studies, disease stages are used to control for severity of illness in addition to various severity proxies. Another methodological difference is that patient episodes (a fixed period of time after an initial hospital admission) are used as the unit of analysis rather than discharges to accurately account for patients whose initial visit is to a hospital not certified to perform the procedure. After controlling for severity using logistic regression analysis, whites were found to undergo significantly more of each of the procedures than blacks (odds ratios of 1.25, 2.06, and 1.69 for angiography, bypass graft, and angioplasty, respectively). These significant differences existed for most levels of the various control variables."

Orr, Suezanne T., Evan Charney, John Straus, et al. Emergency room use by low income children with a regular source of health care. Medical care, v. 29, Mar. 1991: 283-286.
"The data reported in this article suggest that the enrollment of indigent children in sources of primary health care does not totally eliminate use of the emergency room. At the same time, these data also demonstrate that use of the emergency room comprises a relatively small percentage of all health care visits."

Little, Jane Sneddon. Medicaid. Federal Reserve Bank of Boston New England economic review, Jan.-Feb. 1991: 27-50.

"This article will begin by reviewing why governments have a role in providing health care for their citizens. Because the forces driving Medicaid spending nationally affect individual States, the next sections will explain why the Medicaid program has become a substantial burden for Massachusetts and other State governments and why that burden is likely to increase. The article will then examine why Massachusetts' Medicaid expenditures are well above average and will outline some choices that policymakers may be forced to consider in the immediate future."

Annual report to Congress, 1991. Washington, Physician Payment Review Commission, 1991.

With the transition to payment under the Medicare fee schedule set to begin in 1992, this report "considers numerous policy ad technical issues concerning implementation. These include refinements in the scale of relative work, modifications in the methods of calculating the practice expense and malpractice expense components of the relative value scale, and calculation of the budget-neutral conversion factor." Also "considers methods for adjusting and allocating practice and malpractice expenses, geographic payment areas, payment to nonphysician practitioners, and payment to assistants-at-surgery."

Beyond rhetoric: a new American agenda for children and families; final report of the National Commission on Children. Washington, 1991.

The National Commission on Children was created by Congress and the President "to assess the status of children and families in the United States and propose new directions for policy and program development." Its mission was "to design an action agenda for the 1990s and to build the necessary public commitment and sense of common purpose to see it implemented." The Commission presents its findings, conclusions, and recommendations in this final report.

Hill, Ian T., and Janine M. Breyel. Caring for kids. Washington, National Governors' Association, 1991.

"To determine the scope and nature of State efforts to improve child health, the National Governors' Association surveyed State Medicaid and Maternal and Child Health program officials during the spring and summer of 1990. This report presents detailed information on States' responses to OBRA-89 and OBRA-90 and offers insights on how States can achieve further progress in improving the accessibility and effectiveness of their health care programs for children."

Solloway, Michele R., and Connie Wessner. Major changes in State Medicaid programs 1990. Washington, Intergovernmental Health Policy Project, George Washington University, 1991.

"Individual State profiles show changes in benefits and service coverage, eligibility, reimbursement, management, or in Medicaid-related strategies. An introductory overview summarizes 1990 State Medicaid legislative action across the U.S."

Summer, Laura. Limited access: health care for the rural poor. Washington, Center on Budget and Policy Priorities, 1991.

Covers topics including the health status of rural and urban residents, the use of health care services, the availability of health care providers in rural areas, health insurance, Federal health programs for low income residents in rural areas, and the Medicaid program.

Schlesinger, Mark, and Karl Kronebusch. The failure of prenatal care policy for the poor. Health affairs, v. 9, winter 1990: 91-111.

"This study develops a set of empirical models that assess the relative merits of the Medicaid strategy in the current policy environment and estimates the magnitude of the various possible side effects. A study of this sort requires data and a strategy of analysis that differs from most prior studies of prenatal care. Despite extensive research on the effectiveness of prenatal care for reducing low birthweight and subsequent developmental disorders, there is relatively little published research on the factors that influence access to prenatal care."

Hudson, Terese. Lawsuits can pave rocky road to adequate Medicaid payment. Hospitals, Dec. 5, 1990: 34-37.

"*Wilder et al v. The Virginia Hospital Association* is about to go to trial. *Wilder* is the case that resulted in the Supreme Court's June ruling affirming hospitals' right to sue State governments for inadequate Medicaid reimbursement. A Federal court in Richmond must now decide whether Virginia's payment plan adequately reimburses the State's hospitals. And with momentum of their own, individual hospitals and State hospital associations are pressing hard for fair Medicaid reimbursements."

Azevedo, David. Which third parties pay you the most? Medical economics, Nov. 26, 1990: 144-157.

"Income from Medicare, Medicaid, Blue Shield, and commercial insurers fell 4 percentage points between 1986 and 1989. The share of revenue coming from patients' pockets also declined; our survey shows that in 1989, patients paid only 19 percent of doctors' bills themselves, down from 21 percent in 1986. With more and more corporations supposedly shifting health costs on to employees, this decline is surprising. One partial explanation may be that employers are forcing workers to pay part of their health insurance premiums, not more of their doctor bills."

Green, Jesse, and Peter S. Arno. The 'Medicaidization' of AIDS. Journal of the American medical association, v. 264, Sept. 12, 1990: 1261-1266.

"Among patients with the acquired immunodeficiency syndrome (AIDS) who were hospitalized in New York City, San Francisco, Calif, and Los Angeles, Calif, from 1983 through 1988, we observed a marked shift in the payer distribution toward Medicaid and away from private insurance. This trend, which we refer to as the "Medicaidization" of AIDS, occurred among whites as well as blacks and Hispanics and increased the burden on public hospitals and emergency rooms. "Medicaidization" jeopardizes access to office-based primary care because of very low reimbursement rates that are paid to physicians by Medicaid relative to private insurance. Policies designed to prevent the loss of employment-based private insurance would slow or reverse the trend to public financing. Increasing Medicaid reimbursement will improve access to care."

Wenneker, Mark B., Joel S. Weissman, and Arnold M. Epstein. The association of payer with utilization of cardiac procedures in Massachusetts. Journal of the American medical association, v. 264, Sept. 12, 1990: 1255-1260.

"To investigate the importance of the payer in the utilization of in-hospital cardiac procedures, we examined the care of 37,994 patients with Medicaid, private insurance, or no insurance who were admitted to Massachusetts hospitals in 1985 with circulatory disorders or chest pain. Using logistic regression to control for demographic, clinical, and hospital factors, we found that the odds that privately insured patients received angiography were 80 percent higher than uninsured patients; the odds were 40 percent higher for bypass grafting and 28 percent higher for angioplasty. Medicaid patients experienced odds similar to those of uninsured patients for receiving angiography and bypass, but had 48 percent lower odds of receiving angioplasty. In addition, the odds for Medicaid patients were lower than for privately insured patients for all three cardiac procedures. These findings suggest that insurance status is associated with the utilization of cardiac procedures. Future studies should determine the implications these findings have for appropriateness and outcome and whether interventions might improve care."

A call for action; final report and supplement of the U.S. Bipartisan Commission on Comprehensive Health Care (The Pepper Commission). Washington, GPO, Sept. 1990. S. Prt. 101-114 and 101-115.

"Based on a shared view that current conditions are unconscionable and that public action is urgent, the Commission unanimously agreed that all Americans should have access to affordable health and long-term care coverage in an efficient and effective system . . . This report lays out the problems the Commission believes the nation must solve and the Commission's blueprint to guarantee all Americans affordable, high-quality health care and long-term care when they need it."

Ball, Judy K., Joyce V. Kelly, and Barbara J. Turner. Third-party financing for AIDS hospitalizations in New York. AIDS and public policy journal, v. 5, spring 1990: 51-58.

Analyzes nearly 6,000 AIDS discharges from Greater New York hospitals in 1985. "Nearly 40 percent reported private insurance, primarily Blue Cross, as the primary source of payment. About 45 percent reported public insurance, primarily Medicaid. Approximately 11 percent of AIDS discharges were reported as self-pay; presumably, these patients had no insurance coverage." Warns that proposals to accord AIDS special treatment under Medicare could be costly.

Epstein, Arnold M., Robert S. Stern, and Joel S. Weissman. Do the poor cost more? A multihospital study of patients' socioeconomic status and use of hospital resources. New England journal of medicine, v. 322, Apr. 19, 1990: 1122-1128.

"... we found that the patients of the lowest socioeconomic status had hospital stays 3 to 30 percent longer than those of patients of higher status, the differences varying with the hospital and the indicator of socioeconomic status ... Hospital charges were 1 to 18 percent higher for the patients of lowest socioeconomic status than for those of higher status ... When we adjusted for age, illness, and DRG, the patients of lowest socioeconomic status had longer stays than those of higher status in 14 of 15 comparisons ... and higher charges in 13 of 15 comparisons ... The differences between patients of high and low status ranged up to 21 percent for length of stay and 13 percent for charges. Our findings suggest that hospitalized patients of lower socioeconomic status have longer stays and probably require more resources. Supplementary payments to hospitals for the treatment of poor patients merit further consideration."

Chavkin, Wendy. Drug addiction and pregnancy: policy crossroads. American journal of public health, v. 80, Apr. 1990: 483-487.

Society has responded to the problem of pregnant women taking drugs "in three different ways: criminal prosecution of the mother; allegations of child neglect against the mother with interruption of maternal custody; and drug treatment. The purpose of this article is to explore each of these policy approaches in an effort to ascertain whether each furthers the goal of reducing drug use during pregnancy and improving maternal and infant health and well-being."

Stafford, Randall S. Cesarean section use and source of payment: an analysis of California hospital discharge abstracts. American journal of public health, v. 80, Mar. 1990: 313-315.

"This study assessed the relation between payment source and cesarean section use by analyzing California data on hospital deliveries. Of 461,066 deliveries in 1986, cesarean sections were performed in 24.4 percent. Women with private insurance had the highest cesarean section rates (29.1 percent). Successively lower rates were observed for women covered by non-Kaiser health maintenance organizations (26.8 percent), Medi-Cal (22.9 percent), Kaiser (19.7 percent), self-pay (19.3 percent), and Indigent Services (15.6 percent). Vaginal birth after cesarean (VBAC) occurred more than twice as frequently in women covered by Kaiser (19.9 percent) and Indigent Services (24.8 percent), compared to those with private insurance (8.1 percent). Sizable, although less pronounced, associations between payment source and cesarean section use were noted for the indications of breech presentation, dystocia, and fetal distress. Accounting for maternal age and race/ethnicity did not alter these findings. Variations in the use of cesarean section have a substantial financial impact on health care payors."

Liu, Korbin, Pamela Doty, and Kenneth Manton. Medicaid spenddown in nursing homes. Gerontologist, v. 30, Feb. 1990.

"This paper employs information from nationally representative surveys to examine the incidence and causes of Medicaid spenddown among disabled elderly persons. About 10 percent of nursing home discharges experience 'asset spenddown,' the process of converting from private pay to Medicaid. In contrast, over 50 percent of nursing home patients remain private pay throughout their stays. In addition, becoming a Medicaid patient is more common among community residents than among nursing home residents. Implications of findings for health care policies are discussed."

Hellinger, Fred J. Updated forecasts of the costs of medical care for persons with AIDS, 1989-93. Public health reports, v. 105, Jan.-Feb. 1990: 1-12.

"The lifetime medical care cost of treating a person with AIDS is estimated to be about $75,000 (all estimates are in 1988 dollars) assuming that the average length of survival is 15 months and that the intensity of care (that is, the cost of medical care per month) does not fall as longevity rises. This total, $75,000, reflects recent increases in the length of survival and the diffusion of costly drug therapies (for example, AZT and aerosol pentamidine). This study forecasts that the cumulative lifetime medical care costs of treating all people diagnosed with AIDS during a given year to be about $3.3 billion in 1989, $4.3 billion in 1990, $5.3 billion in 1991, $6.5 billion in 1992, and $7.8 billion in 1993."

Annual report to the President and the Congress. National Commission on AIDS, Washington, 1990.

"The National Commission on AIDS was established to promote the development of a national consensus on policy concerning AIDS and to study and make recommendations for a consistent national policy on AIDS and the human immunodeficiency virus. The Commission holds public meetings, visits many regions of the country to hold public forums and solicits expert testimony in an attempt to better understand the challenges posed by the HIV/AIDS epidemic."

Demkovich, Linda. The States and the uninsured: slowly but surely, filling the gaps. Prepared for the National Health Policy Forum. Washington, National Health Policy Forum, and Intergovernmental Health Policy Project, George Washington University, 1990.

"While there has been talk of 'a Federal solution' to the problem of ensuring access to health care, huge deficits and a lack of consensus about the best approach to adopt seem to rule that out any time soon. Thus, it has fallen to the States--in the face of severe budget problems of their own-- to craft solutions, and they are indeed meeting the challenge. This background brief focuses on some of the innovative initiatives that the States have undertaken over the last several years to try and bridge the gaps in insurance coverage."

Healthy mothers, healthy babies: supplement to a compendium of program ideas for serving low-income women. Healthy Mothers, Healthy Babies Coalition. Subcommittee on Low-Income Women. Washington, U.S. Health Resources and Services Administration, Maternal and Child Health Bureau, 1990. DHHS Publication No. HRS-M-CH 90-6

This report includes information on improvements in the Medicaid program--expanding access for pregnant women and children--and recent policy recommendations.

Hill, Ian T. Improving State Medicaid programs for pregnant women and children. Health care financing review 1990 annual supplement: 75-87.

"States have moved to further improve programs by streamlining eligibility systems, enhancing outreach initiatives, attempting to recruit obstetrical providers into participating in Medicaid, and adding enriched nonmedical prenatal benefits to their State plans."

Jencks, Stephen F. and M. Beth Benedict. Accessibility and effectiveness of care under Medicaid. Health care financing review 1990 annual supplement: 47-56.

This article "suggest[s] a framework for assessing the accessibility, appropriateness, and outcomes of care to Medicaid [beneficiaries] and review[s] studies in these areas. Evidence is limited, and variation among States and the paucity of national data pose further problems. There is evidence that Medicaid [beneficiaries] receive less medically necessary care (e.g., prenatal care) than the insured, but evidence on the quality of their care is limited. Differences in payment rates between Medicaid and private insurance appear to explain only part of the variance. Studies have demonstrated major direct effects of diminished access on health status. Evaluation of program changes should focus on health outcomes rather than counts of services rendered."

Moffitt, Robert, and Barbara Wolfe. The effect of the Medicaid program on welfare participation and labor supply. National Bureau of Economic Research, Cambridge, Mass., 1990. (Working paper no. 3286)

"Medicaid has strong and significant effects on labor supply and welfare participation that are negative and positive in sign, respectively, but which are concentrated in the tail of the distribution with the highest expected medical expenditures. We also find that the availability and level of private health insurance have very large effects opposite in sign to those of Medicaid."

Report number one: failure of U.S. health care system to deal with HIV epidemic. National Commission on AIDS, Washington, 1990.

"While AIDS is not the cause of the health care system's disarray, it may well be the crisis that could pressure responsible national action to correct its serious shortfalls." Warns that increasing numbers of AIDS cases will be low-income people, including many women and children, with no insurance either public or private.

Solloway, Michele R. Major changes in State Medicaid and indigent care programs, 1989. Washington, Intergovernmental Health Policy Project, George Washington University, 1990.

This report "offers a guide to States' approaches and initiatives in the financing and delivery of care to the poor adopted during the 1989 legislative period."

Solomon, David J., Andrew J. Hogan, Reynard R. Bouknight, et al. Analysis of Michigan Medicaid costs to treat HIV infection. Public health reports, v. 104, Sept.-Oct. 1989: 416-424.

"Men were found to have twice as many claims as women, and men's claims cost about three times as much. A higher percentage of women than men (91 percent versus 37 percent) received pre-HIV paid services, indicating a higher percentage of women were at least initially receiving Medicaid for reasons other than an HIV-related disability. Diagnostic categories that accounted for the bulk of the HIV-related health care utilization included infectious and parasitic diseases, acquired immunodeficiency syndrome, diseases of the respiratory system, and non-HIV-specific immunity disorders. Inpatient hospitalization accounted for more than 75 percent of the payments, followed by physician costs (11 percent), pharmacy costs (5 percent), and outpatient costs (3 percent). A total of 45, or about 22 percent of the [beneficiaries], received zidovudine (AZT) prescriptions at an average monthly cost of $404."

Arno, Peter S., Douglas Shenson, Naomi F. Siegel, et al. Economic and policy implications of early intervention in HIV disease. Journal of the American medical association, v. 262, Sept. 15, 1989: 1493-1498.

"Effective early intervention in HIV disease may alter the course of one of the most devastating epidemics in modern history. Unless policymakers and public health and medical leaders begin to plan now for its impact, however, early intervention will only invite further chaos and disarray in the U.S. health care system."

Andrulis, Dennis P., Virginia Beer Weslowski, and Larry S. Gage. The 1987 U.S. hospital AIDS survey. Journal of the American medical association, v. 262, Aug. 11, 1989: 784-794.

". . . Estimated cost for AIDS inpatient care during 1987 was $486 million; Medicaid represented the primary payer. Regional and ownership comparisons for this year and between 1985 and 1987 indicated significant differences in utilization, payer source, and financing. Results suggest major differences in reimbursement and losses related to payer source or lack of insurance, with many hospitals that serve large numbers of low-income persons with AIDS encountering moderate to severe financial shortfalls. We conclude that increasing concentrations of persons with AIDS in relatively few hospitals in large cities may make it more difficult to secure the broader political base necessary to obtain adequate support for treatment."

Gould, Jeffrey B., Becky Davey, and Randall S. Stafford. Socioeconomic differences in rates of cesarean section. New England journal of medicine, v. 321, July 27, 1989: 233-239.

"The rates of primary cesarean section were highest among non-Hispanic whites (20.6 percent), intermediate among Asian Americans (19.2 percent) and blacks (18.9 percent), and lowest among Mexican Americans (13.9 percent). Significant socioeconomic differences in these rates were observed in all four groups. We conclude that the rates of primary cesarean section vary directly with socioeconomic status and that this association cannot be accounted for by differences in maternal age, parity, birth weight, race, ethnic group, or complications of pregnancy or childbirth."

Weissman, Joel, and Arnold M. Epstein. Case mix and resource utilization by uninsured hospital patients in the Boston metropolitan area. Journal of the American medical association, v. 261, June 23/30, 1989: 3572-3576.

"We found that the overall case mix severity index (based on expected length of stay per diagnosis related group) for uninsured patients was 30 percent higher in public hospitals and 8 percent higher in major teaching hospitals compared with other institutions. Across all hospitals, the severity index of uninsured patients was similar to that of insured patients. However, after adjusting for diagnosis related group case mix, uninsured patients had, on average, 7 percent shorter stays (5.36 vs 5.79 days) and underwent 7 percent fewer procedures (1.16 vs 1.25) than Blue Cross patients, the differences varying with hospital type. Uninsured patients also had shorter stays on average than Medicaid patients (5.36 vs 5.87 days), but they underwent a similar number of procedures. These results suggest that patients who lack insurance may receive unequal treatment even after being hospitalized."

Newacheck, Paul W. Chronically ill children and their health care needs. Caring, v. 8, May 1989.

Discusses the prevalence of chronic illness in children, health needs of disabled children, and paying for health care services.

Cohen, Joel W. Medicaid policy and the substitution of hospital outpatient care for physician care. Health services research, v. 24, Apr. 1989: 33-66.

"This article explores the effects of reimbursement and utilization control policies on utilization patterns and spending for physician and hospital outpatient services under State Medicaid programs. The empirical work shows a negative relationship between the level of Medicaid physician fees relative to Medicare and private fees, and the numbers of outpatient care recipients, suggesting that outpatient care substitutes for physician care in States with low fee levels. In addition, it shows a positive relationship between Medicaid physician fees and outpatient spending per [beneficiary], suggesting that in low-fee States outpatient departments are providing some types of care that could be provided in a physicians office. Finally, the analysis demonstrates that reimbursement and utilization control policies have significant effects in the expected directions on aggregate Medicaid spending for physician and outpatient services."

Chasnoff, Ira J., Dan R. Griffith, Scott MacGregor, et al. Temporal patterns of cocaine use in pregnancy. Journal of the American medical association, v. 261, Mar. 24/31, 1989: 1741-1744.

"Seventy-five cocaine-using women enrolled in a comprehensive perinatal care program were divided into two groups: those who used cocaine in only the first trimester of pregnancy (group 1) and those who used cocaine throughout pregnancy (group 2). Perinatal outcomes of these pregnancies were compared with perinatal outcomes of a matched group of obstetric patients with no history or evidence of substance abuse. Group 2 women had an increased rate of preterm delivery and low-birth-weight infants as well as an increased rate of intrauterine growth retardation. Group 1 women had rates of these complications similar to the drug-free group. Mean birth weight, length, and head circumference for term infants were reduced in only the group 2 infants. However, both groups of cocaine-exposed infants demonstrated significant impairment of orientation, motor, and State regulation behaviors on the Neonatal Behavioral Assessment Scale."

Zuckerman, Barry, Deborah A. Frank, Ralph Hingson, et al. Effects of maternal marijuana and cocaine use on fetal growth. New England journal of medicine, v. 320, Mar. 23, 1989: 762-768.

Concludes "that the use of marijuana or cocaine during pregnancy is associated with impaired fetal growth and that measuring a biologic marker of such use is important to demonstrate the association."

Aging in America: the Federal Government's role. Washington, Congressional quarterly, 1989.

Separate chapters examine the composition of today's elderly population, Social Security, Medicare and Medicaid, catastrophic costs, and long-term care.

Institute of Medicine. Committee on Utilization Management by Third Parties. Controlling costs and changing patient care?: the role of utilization management. Washington, National Academy Press, 1989.

The focus of this report is "on the private sector, and the effectiveness of this new system of bringing patient-level and system-level concerns together on cutting costs."

Institute of Medicine. Council on Health Care Technology. Care of the elderly patient: policy issues and research opportunities. Washington, National Academy Press, 1989.

This report addresses research and policy issues surrounding home and community care of the elderly as well as system resources and constraints.

Short, Pamela Farley, Joel C. Cantor, and Alan C. Monheit. The dynamics of Medicaid enrollment. Inquiry, v. 25, winter 1988: 504-516.

"This longitudinal study examines transitions on and off Medicaid in the 1984 Panel of the Survey of Income and Program Participation. A majority of those enrolled at the outset, but just 43 percent of those enrolled at any time during the 32-month survey, remained on Medicaid throughout. While slightly less than half of those departing the program subsequently enjoyed improved employment, private insurance, and higher incomes, nearly half were still poor and 55 percent became uninsured, indicating that persons who lost their Medicaid cards were in real danger of being without insurance and financial access to health care--a serious disincentive to get off welfare."

APPENDIX A. MEDICAID, THE POOR, AND HEALTH INSURANCE[1]

I. INTRODUCTION

In 1991, the number of persons in families with income below the poverty threshold reached 35.7 million, the largest number since the mid-1960s. Based on information from the Current Population Survey (CPS), a survey that asks questions on a respondent's income as well as Medicaid coverage, more than 47 percent of the poor (individuals with incomes below the Federal poverty threshold) were covered by Medicaid in 1991. This represents a 16 percent increase over the 1986 coverage rate of 41 percent. Medicaid is the largest single source of health insurance for the poor. However, as earlier chapters of this report have pointed out, not all of the poor are beneficiaries of Medicaid and not all Medicaid beneficiaries are poor. Because of changes in who is eligible for Medicaid, Medicaid's coverage rate of poor children is substantially higher than in the past. This has a large impact on Medicaid's overall coverage rate of the poor.

This appendix provides estimates of Medicaid coverage of the poor and near-poor (individuals with incomes less than 185 percent of Federal poverty thresholds). It focuses on whom among the poor and near-poor are covered by Medicaid or other forms of health insurance. Some of the more important findings are:

- While roughly 47 percent of the poor have Medicaid coverage, another 24 percent are covered by other forms of health insurance. Roughly 29 percent of the poor have no health insurance.

- Most people still qualify for Medicaid as a result of Aid to Families with Dependent Children (AFDC) or Supplemental Security Income (SSI) receipt. Eligibility criteria used in these programs vary by the State an individual lives in, whether anyone in the family is employed and how long they have been employed.

- Medicaid's mandated eligibility expansions have resulted in mandatory eligibility thresholds for children and pregnant women that link eligibility to the Federal poverty guideline

---

[1]This appendix was written by Richard Rimkunas.

in all States. These guidelines are higher than the AFDC income limits.[2]

- Linking Medicaid eligibility to Federal poverty guidelines for pregnant women and children not only allows for coverage of the increasing share of the nation's poor children in female-headed families, but also allows for health insurance protection for children and pregnant women in two-parent families that may be adversely affected by economic downturns.

- Between 1988 and 1991 the number of poor children covered by Medicaid increased by over 33 percent from 7 million to 9.4 million. This increase is largely the result of increased Medicaid coverage of children under age 7.

- The myriad avenues to Medicaid coverage result in the health program's coverage rate varying for different groups of the poor. In 1991, it is estimated that 66 percent of poor children were covered by Medicaid. The coverage rate for poor women of child bearing age (18-44) is estimated to be 48 percent. The coverage rate for poor men between the age of 18 and 44 is 16 percent;

- Young adults have a greater chance of being without health insurance. For young women, Medicaid appears to fill a gap in private coverage, for males this is not the case. The share of young men and women with private health insurance is about equal. However, greater Medicaid coverage rates for females results in a lower share of females between the ages of 18 and 44 without health insurance, when compared to men;

- Despite the important role Medicaid plays in providing health insurance coverage for the poor and near-poor, for most Americans health insurance coverage is a product of labor force attachment. One result of this phenomenon is that a disproportionate share of the poor and near-poor, individuals with weak ties to the labor force are uninsured.

Whether a poor or near-poor person is covered by Medicaid depends on whether the individual meets the criteria associated with the program's needs test. As noted in *Chapter III, Eligibility*, there are two sets of factors associated with this eligibility test: a categorical test and an income test. The first determines who among the poor are potentially eligible; the second, includes an explicit test of income (and assets) to determine if the level of poverty faced by

---

[2]While mandatory income levels are uniform across States, many States expand coverage beyond these mandatory levels for pregnant women and infants. This results in additional interstate variation.

the individual is below a predetermined cutoff. While this appendix focuses on an individual's family income and whether the individual is covered by Medicaid, a large number of people will not be covered by Medicaid because they don't meet the other eligibility factors. For example, most nonaged nondisabled childless couples and single individuals will be ineligible for Medicaid since they fail to fall into any of the potential categories of Medicaid coverage. In 1991, roughly 32 percent of the poor lived in families with no related children. These are individuals that generally do not meet the program's categorical eligibility criteria.

For those individuals who are categorically eligible there are many avenues to Medicaid eligibility, each with its own set of income criteria. For instance, individuals who qualify for Medicaid because they are cash welfare recipients face one set of income criteria; the "medically needy" (individuals with large medical or other expenses) face a different set of criteria; pregnant women, infants, and children face still another set.

This appendix clarifies who the poor are, why some are eligible for Medicaid, and why others are not. The first part of the appendix describes how poverty is defined, how likely individuals in certain demographic groups are to be poor, and the makeup of the poor population. The second part of the appendix describes the relationship between Medicaid coverage, the poor, and near-poor. It briefly describes the eligibility rules associated with AFDC and SSI, recent eligibility expansions, and how the income limits for these avenues to eligibility are related to the poverty level. It provides estimates of Medicaid coverage rates for the poor and nonpoor based on an analysis of the CPS. The final section of the appendix focuses on the uninsured.

The estimates presented in this appendix are based upon information contained in the CPS. The CPS allows us to make estimates for the noninstitutionalized poor. These estimates exclude one segment of the Medicaid population that is part of the program's statistical reporting forms--those in institutions such as nursing homes and intermediate care facilities for the mentally retarded. Since the focus of the CPS is different from the focus of Medicaid's statistical reporting forms, the estimates of the number of persons covered by Medicaid in this appendix will differ from the beneficiary information contained in earlier chapters of this report. Additional information on the CPS estimates is contained in an addendum to this appendix.

II. WHO ARE THE POOR

A. Defining Poverty

Using information from the CPS, the Census Bureau estimates the number of poor based upon a family's annual pretax cash income. Cash income includes income from earnings, interest, public and private pensions, child support and alimony; income from social insurance programs like social security and unemployment compensation; and income from cash assistance programs like AFDC, and SSI.

Individuals are considered to be poor when their family's annual cash pretax income is below a predefined poverty threshold. The poverty threshold is a statistical measure that attempts to indicate the level of cash income needed by a family to purchase a "minimally adequate" market basket of goods and services on an annual basis.[3] The threshold is adjusted for family size and updated each year for inflation. While the cost of living may vary from location to location, the poverty thresholds do not; the threshold is a nationwide standard of poverty. Using the poverty thresholds, a family of 3 would have to have an income level below $10,860 to be considered poor in 1991. All estimates of the number of poor contained in this appendix are based on these Census Bureau poverty thresholds.

While this comparison of family income to the poverty threshold will be used in our estimates of the poverty population, families with incomes below the poverty threshold do not automatically become eligible for needs-tested benefit programs. Of direct importance to this discussion, these poverty thresholds are not used to determine eligibility for Medicaid or the cash assistance programs (e.g., AFDC, SSI).

A simplified version of these Census Bureau statistical thresholds is prepared by the Secretary of Health and Human Services (HHS) to be used in the administration of a number of means-tested programs.[4] These DHHS income levels are usually referred to as the "Federal poverty income guidelines."[5] As noted in *Chapter III, Eligibility*, Medicaid eligibility for children, pregnant women, and some of the aged are tied to these guidelines.

---

[3]Originally developed in 1961, the threshold represented three times the annual cost of the U.S. Dept. of Agriculture's (USDA) 1961 Economy Food Plan. The USDA economy food plan specified quantities of food groups that together met nutritional goals (Recommended Daily Allowances (RDAs)). The multiplier used in building the threshold is based on a 1955 USDA food consumption survey that found, on average, food costs represented one-third of a family's after tax cash income.

[4]Some federally funded health programs that use this guideline include the Maternal and Child Health Services block grants, Community Health Centers, and Migrant Health Centers. For a detailed description of the programs that used these guidelines see: U.S. Library of Congress. Congressional Research Service. *Cash and Noncash Benefits for Persons with Limited Incomes: Eligibility Rules, Recipient and Expenditure Data, FY 1988-90.* CRS Report for Congress No. 91-741 EPW, by Vee Burke. Washington, Sept. 30, 1991.

[5]The Federal poverty guidelines are a variant of the Census Bureau thresholds. The Census Bureau thresholds are revised by: 1) rounding the dollar amounts off; 2) standardizing the dollar difference between different family sizes; 3) creating individual poverty guidelines for families greater than nine; and 4) creating separate guidelines for Alaska and Hawaii. This procedure was developed by the Community Services Administration (CSA) and approved by the Office of Management and Budget (OMB). Since OBRA 81 (Public Law 97-35) which abolished CSA, the guidelines have been updated by DHHS.

However, it should be noted that an individual's eligibility is based on monthly income and a prorated threshold, not on annual income. Estimates of the poor are based on a family's annual income.

This difference between income used in determining eligibility and the income accounting on the CPS causes some complication in interpreting the estimates in this appendix. Some people can have low incomes for part of the year and qualify for Medicaid. In other parts of the year their income can exceed the poverty threshold. This may result in their reported annual income exceeding the poverty threshold, but for part of the year they were covered by Medicaid. The result is that some of these people will be classified as nonpoor, yet also report Medicaid coverage.

Table A-1 displays the Census Bureau poverty thresholds for 1991 and the Federal poverty guidelines for 1992.

TABLE A-1. Selected Poverty Measures for Families, 1991 and 1992

Family size	1991 Census Bureau poverty threshold	HHS 1992 poverty guidelines		
		States[a]	Alaska	Hawaii
One person[b]	$ 6,932	$ 6,810	$ 8,500	$ 7,830
Two persons[c]	8,865	9,190	11,480	10,570
Three persons	10,860	11,570	14,460	13,310
Four persons	13,924	13,950	17,440	16,050
Five persons	16,456	16,330	20,420	18,790
Six persons	18,587	18,710	23,400	21,530
Seven persons	21,058	21,090	26,380	24,270
Eight persons	23,605	23,470	29,360	27,010
Nine persons	27,942[f]	25,850[d]	32,340[e]	29,750[f]

[a]Federal poverty guidelines for the 48 continental States and the District of Columbia.

[b]Different poverty thresholds apply to individuals below 65 years of age and over 65 years of age. For an individual below 65, the threshold equals $7,086; for an individual 65 or older the threshold equals 6,532.

[c]Different poverty thresholds apply to householders below 65 years of age and over 65 years of age. For an individual below 65, the threshold equals $9,165; for an individual 65 or older the threshold equals 8,241.

[d]For family units with more than 8 members add $2,380 for each additional member.

[e]For family units with more than 8 members add $2,980 for each additional member.

[f]For family units with more than 8 members add $2,740 for each additional member.

NOTE: All Census Bureau poverty thresholds represent the weighted average threshold for a family. In estimating poverty the thresholds will vary depending on the presence and number of related children under 18 years old in the household.

Source: Table prepared by the Congressional Research Service based on information obtained from the Census Bureau, and Dept. of Health and Human Services. Annual Update of the HHS Poverty Income Guidelines. *Federal Register*, Feb. 14, 1992. p. 5455.

B. The Incidence of Poverty--1991[6]

In 1991, an estimated 14.2 percent of the population (35.7 million) had incomes below the poverty threshold. However, the incidence of poverty varied among different demographic groups. For example, children are more likely to be poor than other age groups. The poverty rate for children under 18 in 1991 was 21.8 percent, the rate for working age adults (individuals between 18 and 64 years of age) was 11.4 percent, and the rate for the aged (individuals 65 years or older) was 12.4 percent. The poverty rate also varied by race and ethnicity. The rate of poverty for blacks was 32.7 percent, that for Hispanics was 28.7 percent, and that for whites was 11.3 percent. Whether an individual is in a single parent or two parent family also affects their likelihood of being poor. The poverty rate for individuals in single parent female-headed families was 39.7 percent, the rate in two parent families was 7.2 percent. Figure A-1 provides a comparison of these poverty rates for selected demographic groups.

1. Poverty and the Aged

The 1991 aged poverty rate (12.4 percent) increased from its historical low of 11.4 percent in 1989. This increase largely comes as a result of the recent recession affecting individuals who still have some attachment to the labor market (for instance, the poverty rate for those between ages 65 and 74 increased from 8.8 percent in 1989 to 10.6 percent in 1991). While the poverty rate for those 75 and over actually declined slightly (from 15.4 percent in 1989 to 15.0 percent in 1991).

Over the long term the aged poverty rate has declined. In 1959, the aged poverty rate of 35.2 percent was the highest of any age group. Between 1959 and 1973, the aged poverty rate consistently fell. Between 1973 and 1989 the rate continued to decline, but with some fits and starts. The rate declined from 15.3 percent in 1973 to its historical low of 11.4 in 1989. There are a number of factors associated with the long-term decline in the rate. First, there has been a substantial expansion of social security benefits. The program's expansion has occurred in two ways: 1) with an increase in the number of individuals receiving the benefits, and 2) with larger benefits awarded. The number of retired workers, dependents of retired workers, and their survivors has grown tremendously since the early 1960s. Wage growth in the overall economy has resulted in increased initial benefits for social security recipients. In addition, numerous ad hoc benefit increases occurred during the 1960s and 1970s; and since 1975, cost of living adjustments (COLAs) have protected these benefits against price inflation. Additional income support for the aged has occurred with the expansion of private pension programs.

---

[6]For a discussion of the limitation of these estimates see the addendum to this appendix.

FIGURE A-1.
Selected Poverty Rates, 1991

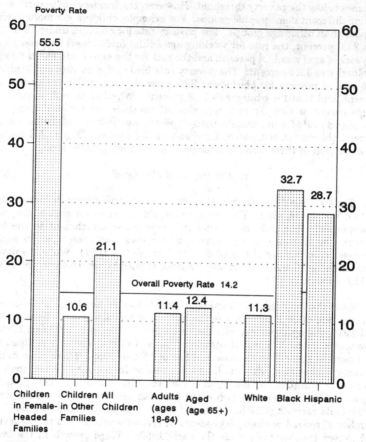

NOTE: Child rates are for children living with relatives. Working age adults are ages 18-64. Aged are individuals 65 years and older.

Source: Figure prepared by Congressional Research Service based on an analysis of the March 1992 CPS.

It should be kept in mind, that despite the reduction in the overall poverty rate for this group, the aged poverty rate is still higher than the rate of other adults, and that some segments of the aged are likely to experience poverty more than others. For instance, the poverty rate for aged women (15.5 percent) is almost twice the rate of aged men (7.9 percent); and the poverty rate for those 75 years old and older (15.0 percent) is 42 percent higher than that of those between 65 and 74 years old (10.6 percent).

Furthermore, while the rate of poverty among the aged has declined, a sizable share of the aged have incomes near the poverty level. For instance, 19.7 percent of all the aged have incomes below 125 percent of poverty threshold, and 33.9 percent have incomes below 175 percent of the poverty threshold. Comparable statistics for working age adults (persons age 18 to 64 years of age) are: 15.1 percent and 23.5 percent, respectively.

2. Poverty and Children[7]

In 1991, more than 1 out of every 5 children (21.1 percent) lived in a family with annual income below the poverty threshold. This high overall poverty rate for children continues a long term trend. Since 1974, the poverty rate for children has been the highest of any age group. At least two factors affect child poverty.

First, the overall child poverty rate has been influenced by an almost continuous increase in the number of children living in single parent, female-headed families. From 1959 to 1991, the share of children living in female-headed families has increased from about 10 percent to more than 22 percent. The poverty rate for children in these single parent families has been very high. For example, in 1959 the poverty rate for children in female-headed families was 72.2 percent. Since 1959, the poverty rate for this group of children has dropped, but it still equalled 55.5 percent in 1991, an incidence rate more than 5 times as high as the rate for children in other families.

The impact of these high incidence rates is seen in the changing composition of who poor children are. In 1959, roughly 24 percent of all poor children lived in families headed by a single mother. By 1965, children in these families comprised 32 percent of poor children, by 1970--46 percent. Since 1972, children in single parent families headed by a female represented a majority of all poor children.[8] In 1991, 59 percent of all poor children lived in families

---

[7]In this discussion poverty rates are provided for related children under 18. These estimates will differ from estimates based solely on an individual's age. The estimates reported here exclude some children under 18 who may be living in homes without any relatives.

[8]The high poverty rate for all other families reduced the share of poor children who lived in female families between 1979 and 1983. In 1983, poor children in female-headed families equalled 50.3 percent of all poor children, but their share increased again until the late 1980s.

headed by a single mother. Figure A-2 portrays this trend in the incidence and composition of child poverty.

A second factor influencing the child poverty rate is more cyclical in nature. That is the poverty rate for two parent families. While, the poverty rate for children in two parent families is substantially lower than the rate for children in single parent female-headed families, the rate for these families is much more sensitive to fluctuations in the economy. Since most families with children are headed by working-age adults, it is not surprising that this poverty rate sways with economic upturns and downturns. This is largely a result of the stronger labor force attachment of these families. For instance, a large share of the increase in child poverty from 1979 to 1983 was a result of an increase in the poverty rates for children in two parent families. As can be seen in figure A-2, in 1978 the poverty rate for children in male present families was low, 7.9 percent. By 1983 the poverty rate for children in these families increased to 13.5 percent. Between 1983 and 1988, with an improved economy the poverty rate for these children declined from 13.5 to 10.0 percent. However, since 1988 the rate for children in these families has increased, reaching 10.7 percent in 1990 and 10.6 percent in 1991.[9]

The relative effect of changing poverty rates in two-parent families versus single parent families can be seen by comparing the effect of a 1 percent increase in the poverty rate for children in female-headed families with the effect of a 1 percent increase in the poverty rate for children in other families. In 1991, a 1 percent increase in the incidence of poverty among children in female-headed families adds about 145,000 children to the poverty count. Likewise, a 1 percent increase in the poverty rate for all other families adds 503,000 children to the ranks of the poor. While poverty rates for two-parent families are lower, fluctuations can add or remove a substantial number of children from poverty's ranks.

3. Poverty, Race and Ethnicity

The incidence of poverty among blacks and Hispanics is considerably higher than that of whites. In 1991, the poverty rates for blacks (32.7) was almost 3 times as high as the rate for whites (11.3), the poverty rate for Hispanics was more than 2.5 times as high (28.7 percent). This higher incidence of poverty among minorities leads to a disproportionate share of minorities living in poverty. While 12.5 percent of the total population are black, 28.7 percent of the poor are black; while 8.8 percent of the population is Hispanic, 17.8 percent of the poor population is Hispanic.

---

[9]In an analysis of the factors contributing to the changes in the poverty status of families between 1979 and 1989, the largest single factor affecting married couple families with children was change in "market income." See U.S. Congress. House. Committee on Ways and Means. *Overview of Entitlement Programs: 1991 Green Book.* WMCP No. 102-9. Washington, GPO, May 7, 1991.

FIGURE A-2.
Poverty Rates for Children by Type of Family, 1959-1991

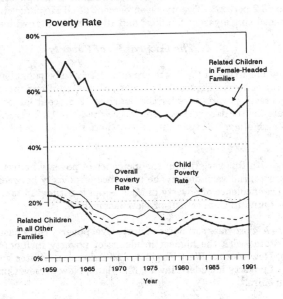

Source: Figure prepared by Congressional Research Service based on data from Bureau of Census.

Number of Poor Children, by Family Type, 1959-1991

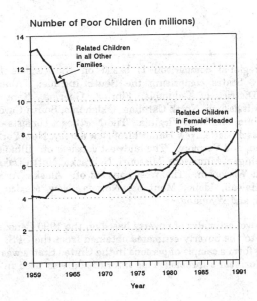

Source: Figure prepared by Congressional Research Service based on data from Bureau of Census.

704

For blacks, an important factor in this high poverty rate is the large number of children living in single parent families. In 1991, 55 percent of black children lived in female-headed single parent families; the poverty rate for this group was 68.2 percent. Twenty-seven percent of all Hispanic children lived in female-headed single parent families; and 16 percent of all white children.

4. The Geography of Poverty

Individuals living in the South are more likely to be poor than in any other region of the country. Figure A-3 provides estimates of regional poverty rates. The 16.0 percent poverty rate for the South is 12 percent larger than the 14.3 percent rate for the West, 21 percent larger than the 13.2 percent rate for the Midwest, and almost 31 percent larger than the 12.2 percent rate in the Northeast.[10]

Along with this variation in the incidence of poverty between the regions, there is substantial variation in the incidence of poverty between States. For instance, the incidence of poverty in Mississippi is estimated to be more than 3 times that found in Connecticut or New Hampshire.

Figure A-4 provides estimates of State level poverty rates based on the 1990 Census. States with the highest incidence of poverty include: Mississippi, Louisiana, New Mexico, West Virginia, and Arkansas. States with the lowest incidence of poverty include: Hawaii, Maryland, New Jersey, Connecticut, and New Hampshire.[11]

---

[10]This regional comparison is based on the Census Bureau regional definitions. States comprising the South include: Alabama, Arkansas, Delaware, District of Columbia, Florida, Georgia, Kentucky, Louisiana, Maryland, Mississippi, North Carolina, Oklahoma, South Carolina, Tennessee, Texas, Virginia, and West Virginia. The Northeast consists of: Connecticut, Maine, Massachusetts, New Hampshire, New Jersey, New York, Pennsylvania, Rhode Island, and Vermont. The Midwest consists of: Illinois, Indiana, Iowa, Kansas, Michigan, Minnesota, Missouri, Nebraska, North Dakota, Ohio, South Dakota, and Wisconsin. The West consists of: Alaska, Arizona, California, Colorado, Hawaii, Idaho, Montana, Nevada, New Mexico, Oregon, Utah, Washington, and Wyoming.

[11]State level estimates of poverty based on the 1990 Census are not strictly comparable to the poverty estimates obtained from the CPS. Using the 1990 Census long form a sample of persons in the United States was asked questions on their prior year's income. This information was used in preparing these estimates.

FIGURE A-3. Regional Poverty Rates, 1991

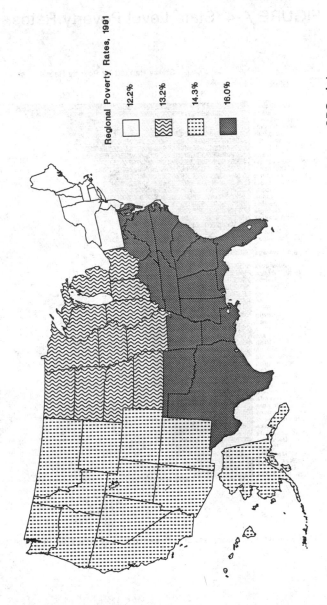

Regional Poverty Rates, 1991

☐ 12.2%

▨ 13.2%

▧ 14.3%

■ 16.0%

Source: Chart prepared by Congressional Research Service, based on CPS data.

FIGURE A-4. State Level Poverty Rates, 1989

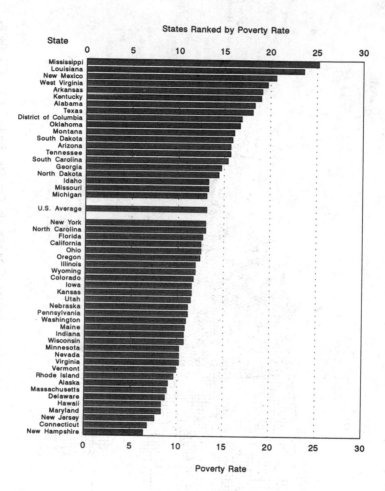

Source: Figure prepared by Congressional Research Service based on 1990 Census data.

These State poverty figures reflect variation in poverty rates in urban, suburban and rural settings. Poverty is much more likely to occur in rural (non metropolitan) areas (16.1 percent in 1991), than in metropolitan areas (13.7 percent). Furthermore within metropolitan areas, there is a significant difference between the incidence of poverty in central cities (20.2 percent) and suburban areas (9.6 percent).

C. The Composition of the Poor Population--1991

Another perspective on poverty is gained by examining the composition of the poverty population. Figure A-5 portrays selected demographic characteristics of the poor in 1991. A number of important characteristics of the poor can be seen in these figures. First, roughly 40 percent of the poor are children under 18; another major share of the poor (49 percent) are working age adults, and 11 percent of the poor are aged. Looking at the race and ethnicity of the poor, about 50 percent of the poor are non-Hispanic white, 28 percent are black, and 18 percent are of Hispanic origin. Finally, looking at the geographic distribution of the poor, about 4 out of every 10 poor persons reside in the South. Each remaining region--the Midwest, the West, and the Northeast-- contains about 2 out of every 10 poor persons.

708

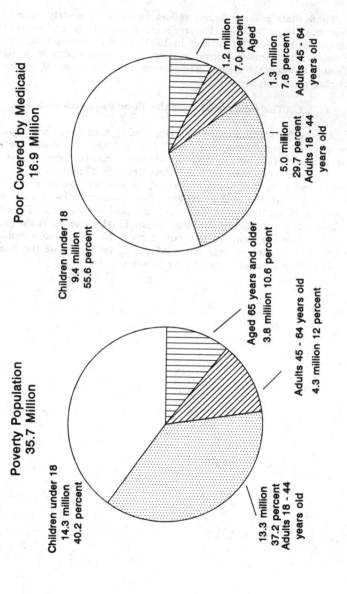

FIGURE A-5.
Composition of the Poor and the Poor Covered
by Medicaid, 1991

Poverty Population
35.7 Million

Poor Covered by Medicaid
16.9 Million

Children under 18
14.3 million
40.2 percent

Children under 18
9.4 million
55.6 percent

13.3 million
37.2 percent
Adults 18 - 44
years old

5.0 million
29.7 percent
Adults 18 - 44
years old

Adults 45 - 64 years old
4.3 million 12 percent

1.3 million
7.8 percent
Adults 45 - 64
years old

Aged 65 years and older
3.8 million 10.6 percent

1.2 million
7.0 percent
Aged

FIGURE A-5. Composition of the Poor and the Poor Covered by Medicaid, 1991--Continued

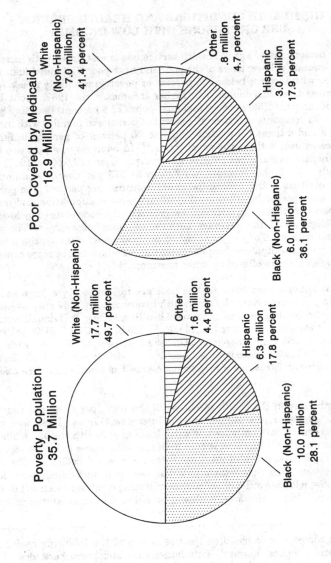

Poverty Population
35.7 Million

White (Non-Hispanic)
17.7 million
49.7 percent

Other
1.6 million
4.4 percent

Hispanic
6.3 million
17.8 percent

Black (Non-Hispanic)
10.0 million
28.1 percent

Poor Covered by Medicaid
16.9 Million

White (Non-Hispanic)
7.0 million
41.4 percent

Other
.8 million
4.7 percent

Hispanic
3.0 million
17.9 percent

Black (Non-Hispanic)
6.0 million
36.1 percent

Source: Figure prepared by Congressional Research Service based on analysis of the March 1992 Current Population Survey.

III. HEALTH CONDITIONS AND HEALTH SERVICE
USE OF PERSONS WITH LOW INCOME

For persons under age 65, health service use is associated with increasing levels of income. A lower share of the poor and near-poor (i.e., individuals living in families with incomes below 125 percent of poverty) are likely to use health care services than individuals with higher incomes.[12] In 1987, about three-fourths of the poor (75.6 percent) and near-poor (77.8 percent) used any health services, this compares with over 87 percent of persons in families with incomes between 2 and 4 times the poverty line, and 90 percent of persons in families with incomes over 4 times the poverty line.[13] In addition, the poor are likely to have higher average health expenditures per user ($2,024 in 1987) than individuals with higher incomes, ($1,225 to $1,373 per user). A number of factors contribute to this differential in expenditures per person. The poor are likely to have poorer health than that of the general population and may be more expensive to treat. In addition, a segment of the poor covered by Medicaid became eligible for the program because of some disability. These are individuals who are likely to have higher medical costs. Finally, the poor are more likely to use outpatient hospital departments which can be more expensive than comparable care offered by other providers.[14]

These summary statistics for the poor are influenced by a large share of this group not being covered by any health insurance. In 1987 only 63 percent of the poor without health insurance used health services. Individuals with any form of public health insurance (i.e., Medicaid, Medicare, CHAMPUS, or VA) are more likely to use health services. Almost 82 percent of the poor with some form of public health insurance used health services. *Appendix H, Medicaid as Health Insurance: Measures of Performance*, provides additional information on this topic.

Information on the health condition of the poor, per se, is not routinely analyzed. However, the annual Health Interview Survey (HIS) does allow analysts to control for family income when looking at health status. While this does not control for family size, it does highlight differences in health status by income. Figure A-6 provides incidence rates for selected health conditions by family income. The figure highlights the fact that individuals with lower incomes have a higher incidence of such debilitating conditions as heart disease, arthritis and ulcers. However, it should be noted that these statistics do not

---

[12]This comparison is based on the use of any of the following health care services and supplies: hospital, ambulatory care and home care, dental and vision services, prescribed medicine and medical equipment purchases.

[13]Estimates are taken from Lefkowitz, D., and A. Monheit. *Health Insurance, Use of Health Services, and Health Care Expenditures.* Agency for Health Care Policy and Research (AHCPR). AHCPR Publication No. 92-0017. National Medical Expenditure Survey Research Findings 12. Rockville, Maryland., Dec. 1991.

[14]Ibid., p. 5.

highlight a causal link between poverty and health condition. That is, the figure does not answer the question as to whether the higher incidence among low-income persons occurs because of their lower income, or their condition precludes these individuals from working thereby lowering their income.

FIGURE A-6.
Number of Reported Arthritic Conditions Per 1,000 Persons by Age and Family Income level, 1989

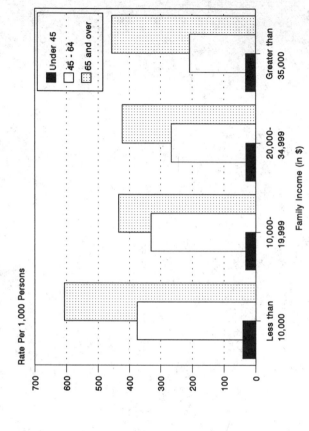

Source: Figure prepared by Congressional Research Service based on information from the 1989 Health Interview Survey.

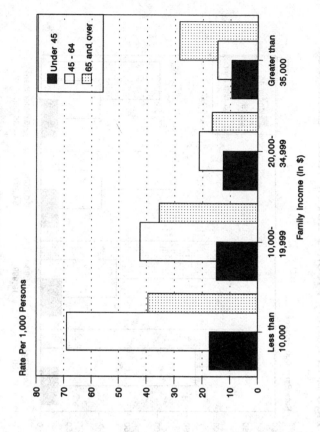

FIGURE A-6.
Number of Reported Ulcers Per 1,000 Persons
by Age and Family Income Level, 1989--Continued

Rate Per 1,000 Persons

Family Income (in $)

Under 45
45 - 64
65 and over

Source: Figure prepared by Congressional Research Service based on information from the
1989 Health Interview Survey.

FIGURE A-6.

Number of Reported Heart Disease Cases Per 1,000 Persons by Age and Family Income Level, 1989--Continued

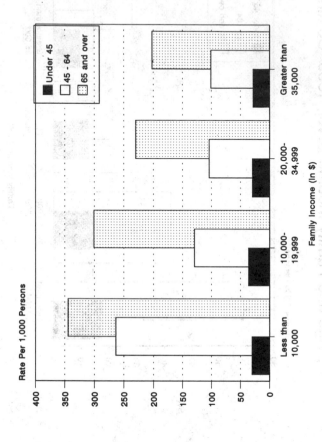

Rate Per 1,000 Persons

Family Income (In $)

Legend:
- Under 45
- 45 - 64
- 65 and over

Source: Figure prepared by Congressional Research Service based on information from the 1989 Health Interview Survey.

IV. THE POOR AND MEDICAID COVERAGE, 1991

Medicaid's coverage rate of the poor is influenced by who the poor are, whether a large share meet the categorical requirements of the program and how the means-tested component of program eligibility varies depending on an individual's eligibility status.

A. Medicaid Coverage Rate of the Poor, 1991

Based on information contained in the CPS, more than 47 percent of the poor (16.9 million) were covered by Medicaid during 1991.[15] Another 24 percent of the poor (8.6 million) were covered by other forms of public or private health insurance, while roughly 29 percent of the poor (10.2 million) reported having no health insurance at all. Tables A-2 and A-3 provide the distribution of health insurance coverage for the poor by selected demographic characteristics. Figure A-7 provides a graphic description of health insurance coverage of the poor.

1. Demographic Characteristics

Table A-2 highlights Medicaid's role as the sole payor of medical services for the nonaged poor. In 1991, 43 percent of the nonaged poor relied on Medicaid as their **only** source of health insurance. An additional 4 percent report that they were covered by Medicaid and some other form of health insurance sometime during the year. Since no questions were asked about dual insurance coverage, we can not determine if this coverage occurred at the same time.[16] Medicare's almost universal coverage of the aged means that Medicaid is not likely to be the sole payor of most medical services for the aged poor. In the CPS sample, almost all the aged poor who were covered by Medicaid sometime during 1991 were also covered by Medicare.

Roughly 66 percent of poor children under 18 are covered by Medicaid, this is the highest coverage rate of any age group. About 36 percent of working age poor adults (18-64) are covered by Medicaid, while 31 percent of the aged poor are covered.[17]

---

[15]It should be noted that these estimates are for the noninstitutionalized poor covered by Medicaid. Not all Medicaid beneficiaries are poor and some persons who are covered by Medicaid will have annual incomes in excess of the poverty threshold.

[16]See *Chapter V, Reimbursement* on reimbursement of dual covered beneficiaries and *Appendix C, Medicaid, Long-Term Care, and the Elderly* on the role of dual coverage for aged Medicaid beneficiaries.

[17]It should be noted that the CPS does not sample individuals in institutions. Since a sizable portion of the aged Medicaid population resides in long-term care institutions (see *Appendix C, Medicaid, Long-Term Care, and the Elderly*) the overall coverage rate for Medicaid coverage of the aged poor should be viewed with some caution.

Children and pregnant women are more likely to be covered by Medicaid as a result of: 1) Medicaid's link to the cash assistance programs; and 2) expanded eligibility that targets Medicaid coverage toward poor young children (i.e., currently children under age 9) and pregnant women. The avenue to Medicaid coverage for poor working age adults and older children (children 9 through 18) is likely to come through AFDC eligibility or some of the optional eligibility categories that rely on AFDC income standards. The disabled and the elderly poor are likely to receive Medicaid as a result of SSI eligibility.[18]

Sixty-nine percent of the poor in single-parent families with children are covered by Medicaid. These single parent families are much more likely to qualify for AFDC. This is a coverage rate that is 1.7 times the coverage rate of the poor in two parent families with children (40.3 percent). While there is a substantial difference in the coverage rate between persons in these two family types, an important aspect of this comparison should be pointed out. The Medicaid coverage rate for persons in two parent families is much higher than it has been in the past (e.g., in 1986 only about 31 percent of persons in these poor families had Medicaid coverage). This is probably the result of both the expansion of Medicaid coverage to children based on poverty-related eligibility guidelines and to a lesser extent the expansion of the AFDC-UP (Unemployed Parent) program to all States (see *Chapter III, Eligibility*).

Not all of the poor in families with children qualify for Medicaid. For example, the recent eligibility expansions do not provide coverage to the husband in a two parent family, nor to the mother except when pregnant. Likewise, AFDC eligibility criteria limit recipients of the welfare payments to the parent(s) and all related children under 18. Generally, other individuals in these families, like older siblings, aunts, uncles, and grandparents would not be eligible.[19] The result of the myriad sets of eligibility rules is that 43 percent of all persons in poor families with children were not covered by Medicaid in 1991. Most of these persons are either older children (between the ages of 7 and 17) or adults.

---

[18]In addition, the medically needy eligibility criteria are likely to play a major role for the institutionalized disabled and elderly.

[19]Despite this definition of the AFDC unit, some States extend Medicaid eligibility to related children between the ages of 18 and 21. See *Chapter III, Eligibility* for more information.

TABLE A-2. Number of the Poor with Medicaid, or Other Health Insurance Coverage, by Selected Characteristics, 1991

Selected characteristics	Medicaid			Other health insurance	No health insurance	Total
	Only	And other health insurance	Total			
	(number of persons in thousands)					
Age:						
Under 18	8,421	967	9,388	2,017	2,935	14,341
18 - 44	4,436	574	5,010	2,707	5,562	13,280
45 - 64	973	329	1,320	1,387	1,618	4,306
65 and over	*	1,178	1,187	2,490	104	3,781
Family type:						
Families with related children under 18						
Single parent	9,118	961	10,079	1,680	2,814	14,573
Two parent	3,345	623	3,968	2,301	3,576	9,846
Families without related children under 18						
Husband/wives	234	232	466	1,097	795	2,358
Single individuals	1,142	1,231	2,373	3,522	3,036	8,931
Race/ethnicity:						
White (non-Hispanic)	5,456	1,532	6,988	5,839	4,912	17,741

See notes at end of table.

TABLE A-2. Number of the Poor with Medicaid, or Other Health Insurance Coverage, by Selected Characteristics, 1991–Continued

	Medicaid			Other health insurance	No health insurance	Total
	Only	And other health insurance	Total			
Selected characteristics	(number of persons in thousands)					
Black (non-Hispanic)	5,142	949	6,091	1,666	2,282	10,040
Hispanic	2,595	427	3,022	751	2,566	6,339
Other (non-Hispanic)	646	140	786	343	459	1,588
Total	13,840	3,048	16,888	8,600	10,220	35,708

*Number too small to report.

NOTE: All figures are estimates of the noninstitutionalized poverty populations. All estimates are subject to the limitations of the data and methods employed in their calculations. Details may not add to total due to rounding.

Source: Table prepared by the Congressional Research Service based on data contained in the Mar. 1992 Current Population Survey.

TABLE A-3. Percentage Share of the Poor with Medicaid, or Other Health Insurance Coverage, by Selected Characteristics, 1991

Selected characteristics	Medicaid			Other health insurance	No health insurance	Total
	Only	And other health insurance	Total			
	Coverage rates:					
Age:						
Under 18	58.7%	6.7%	65.5%	14.15%	20.5%	100.0%
18-44	33.4	4.3	37.7	20.4	41.9	100.0
45-64	22.6	7.6	30.2	32.2	37.6	100.0
65 and over	*	31.2	31.4	65.9	2.8	100.0
Family type:						
Families with related children under 18:						
Single parent	62.6	6.6	69.2	11.5	19.3	100.0
Two parent	34.0	6.3	40.3	23.4	36.3	100.0
Families without related children under 18:						
Husband/wife	9.9	9.8	19.8	46.5	33.7	100.0
Single individuals	12.8	13.8	26.6	39.4	34.0	100.0
Race/ethnicity:						
White (non-Hispanic)	30.8	8.6	39.4	32.9	27.7	100,0

See notes at end of table.

TABLE A-3. Percentage Share of the Poor with Medicaid, or Other Health Insurance Coverage, by Selected Characteristics, 1991.--Continued

Selected characteristics	Medicaid			Other health insurance	No health insurance	Total
	Only	And other health insurance	Total			
				Coverage rates:		
Black (non-Hispanic)	51.2	9.5	60.7	16.6	22.7	100.0
Hispanic	40.9	6.7	47.7	11.9	40.5	100.0
Other (non-Hispanic)	40.7	8.8	49.5	21.6	28.9	100.0
Total	38.8	8.5	47.3	24.1	28.6	100.0

*Number too small to report.

NOTE: All figures are estimates of the noninstitutionalized poverty population. All estimates are subject to the limitations of the data and methods employed in their calculations. Details may not add to total due to rounding.

Source: Table prepared by the Congressional Research Service based on data contained in the Mar. 1992 Current Population Survey.

FIGURE A-7. Health Insurance Status of the Poor, 1991

Total Poor = 35.7 Million

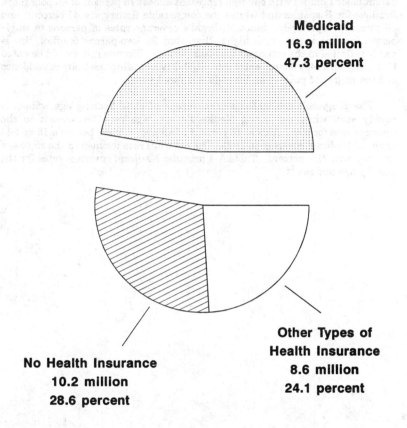

Medicaid
16.9 million
47.3 percent

Other Types of
Health Insurance
8.6 million
24.1 percent

No Health Insurance
10.2 million
28.6 percent

Source: Figure prepared by Congressional Research Service
based on data contained in the March 1992 Current Population Survey.

Racial/ethnic coverage rates are partly influenced by the share of two-parent families and single parent families with incomes below poverty that make up these demographic groups. Sixty-one percent of poor blacks are covered by Medicaid; 48 percent of poor Hispanics; and 39 percent of poor whites. Single parent black families with children represent almost 75 percent of all poor black families; for Hispanics and whites the comparable figures are 47 percent; and 43 percent, respectively. Since Medicaid's coverage rates of persons in single parent families are so much higher than that for two-parent families, this is partly reflected in the estimates for black persons. However, it should be noted that many different factors enter into eligibility including the State of residence and the degree of poverty an individual is faced with.

The program's recent focus on coverage of child bearing age women is readily seen when comparing Medicaid's coverage rate for women to the coverage rate for men. Almost 48 percent of all poor women between 18 and 44 reported Medicaid coverage in 1991. The coverage rate for men in the same age category was 21.7 percent. Table A-4 provides Medicaid coverage rates for the poor by age and sex.[20]

---

[20]Recent eligibility expansions directed at young children should result in coverage rates close to 100 percent of the poor. The estimates provided in this and subsequent tables rely on self-reported health insurance and income status. A rate less than 100 percent may be the result of under-reporting of income and or health insurance status, or differences in accounting practices for income between the CPS and Medicaid eligibility. Furthermore, individuals may have never applied for Medicaid coverage and therefore not know they are eligible for the coverage.

TABLE A-4. Medicaid Coverage Rate of the Poor, by Sex and Age, 1991
(persons in thousands)

Age	Males			Females			Total		
	People covered by Medicaid	Poor persons	Percent of poor	People covered by Medicaid	Poor Persons	Percent of poor	People covered by Medicaid	Poor persons	Percent of poor
<7	2,505	3,386	74.0%	2,335	3,181	73.4%	4,840	6,568	74.0%
7-17	2,185	3,819	57.2	2,363	3,955	59.7	4,548	7,773	58.5
18-44	1,125	5,175	21.7	3,886	8,105	47.9	5,011	13,280	37.7
45-64	409	1,687	14.2	893	2,619	34.1	1,302	4,306	30.2
65+	286	1,015	28.2	901	2,766	32.6	1,187	3,781	31.4
Total	6,510	15,082	43.2	10,398	20,626	50.4	16,908	35,708	47.4

NOTE: All figures are estimates of the noninstitutionalized poverty populations. All estimates are subject to the limitations of the data and methods employed in their calculations. Details may not sum to totals due to rounding. Estimates of persons covered by Medicaid include those individuals reporting either Medicaid as the only source of health insurance or Medicaid and some other form of health insurance.

Source: Table prepared by the Congressional Research Service based on data contained in the Mar. 1992 Current Population Survey.

724

2. *Geographic Characteristics*

Given the tremendous degree of variability in State Medicaid plans it is not surprising that Medicaid coverage rates of the poor vary by region and geographic place. More than 56 percent of the poor in the Northeast rely on Medicaid as a form of health insurance, this compares with 52 percent in the Midwest, 44 percent in the West, and 42 percent in the South (table A-5).

TABLE A-5. Medicaid Coverage Rate of the Poor by Region, 1991
(persons covered in thousands)

Region	Medicaid Only	And other health insurance	Total	Other health insurance	No health insurance	Total
Midwest	3,480	678	4,157	2,024	1,808	7,989
Northeast	2,772	708	3,480	1557	1,141	6,177
South	4,693	1,123	5,816	3,406	4,561	13,783
West	895	540	3,435	1,614	2,710	7,759
Total	13,840	3,048	16,888	8,600	10,220	35,708
Coverage rates:						
Midwest	43.6%	8.5%	52.0%	25.3%	22.6%	100%
Northeast	44.9	11.5	56.3	25.2	18.5	100
South	34.1	8.2	42.2	24.7	33.1	100
West	37.3	7.0	44.3	20.8	34.9	100
Total	38.8	8.5	47.3	24.1	28.6	100

NOTE: All figures are estimates, subject to the limitations of the data and methods employed in their calculations. All estimates of the number of persons are in thousands. Details may not sum to total due to rounding.

Source: Table prepared by the Congressional Research Service based on information contained on the Mar. 1992 Current Population Survey.

3. The Degree of Poverty and Medicaid Coverage

The likelihood of a poor person being covered by Medicaid is closely related to the degree of poverty a family is facing. Individuals in families with income equal to less than 75 percent of the poverty threshold are much more likely to be covered by Medicaid than those individuals with income closer to the poverty line. For instance, 54.1 percent of the poor with income less than one-half of the poverty line are covered, while 35.6 percent of those with incomes that are less than poverty but greater than three-quarters of the poverty threshold are covered.

In 1991, almost 39 percent of the poor had incomes less than half of the poverty threshold. This group's large share of the poverty population and its relatively high Medicaid coverage rates result in this income group representing 45 percent of the total poor covered by Medicaid. Table A-6 presents information on the number of poor, the share of the poor covered by Medicaid and other health insurance, and the composition of those covered by Medicaid taking into account an individual's degree of poverty.

TABLE A-6. Medicaid and Other Insurance Coverage of the Poor Population
(number of persons in thousands)

Family income in relation to poverty threshold	Medicaid			Other health insurance	No health insurance	Total
	Only	And other health insurance	Total			
Less than 50 percent	6,924	690	7,614	2,387	4,059	14,059
50 to 74 percent	4,400	875	5,275	2,242	2,884	10,400
75 to less than 100 percent	2,516	1,484	4,000	3,971	3,277	11,248
Total	13,840	3,049	16,888	8,600	10,220	35,708
Insurance coverage rates (in percents)						
Less than 50 percent	49.3%	4.9%	54.2%	17.0%	28.9%	100%
50 to 74 percent	42.3	8.4	50.7	21.6	27.7	100
75 to less than 100 percent	22.4	13.2	35.6	35.3	29.1	100
Total	38.8	8.5	47.3	24.1	28.6	100

NOTE: All figures are estimates, subject to the limitations of the data and methods employed in their calculations. All estimates of the number of persons are in thousands. Details may not sum to total due to rounding.

Source: Table prepared by the Congressional Research Service based on information contained on the Mar. 1992 Current Population Survey.

B. A Comparison of Medicaid Coverage Rates of the Poor, 1979-1991

The statutorily mandated eligibility expansion of the late 1980s and recent AFDC caseload increases have affected the share of the poor who are covered by Medicaid. In 1987, 41.6 percent of the poor were covered by Medicaid, by 1991 the share of the poor covered increased to 47.3 percent. Most of this increase is the result of a larger share of poor children being covered by Medicaid. As table A-7 and figure A-8 depicts, the 1991 Medicaid coverage rate for the poor is the highest rate over the last 11 years.[21] This coverage rate occurs despite a recent increase in the number of poor.

The coverage trend between 1988 and 1991 shows a rather marked change from the coverage rates of earlier years. Between 1979 and 1983, the share of the poor covered by Medicaid dropped from 39 percent to 37 percent. This occurred while there was a sudden and rather dramatic increase in the number of poor between 1979 and 1983. (The number of poor increased from 26 to 35 million over this period.) Between 1984 and 1986 there were only minor fluctuations in the share of the poor covered by Medicaid. Throughout the mid-1980s the share of the noninstitutionalized poor hovered around 40 percent. However, since 1988 the share of the poor covered by Medicaid has grown to more than 47 percent.

---

[21]Estimates of the share of the poor with Medicaid coverage prior to 1987 are not comparable to those in the subsequent period. This is because of a change in the CPS questions about health insurance coverage. The basic difference in the two set of questionnaires deals with health insurance coverage of children and employment based coverage of adults. This questionnaire change had the effect of increasing the estimate of the number of children covered by Medicaid. Comparisons between the 1986 and 1987 estimates are confounded by these changes in the survey.

FIGURE A-8.
Number of Non Institutionalized Poor Covered by Medicaid, 1979-1991

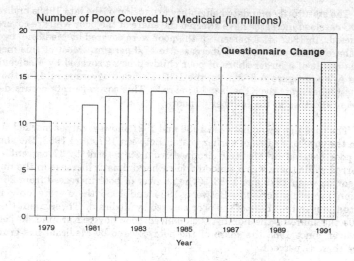

Number of Poor Covered by Medicaid (in millions)

Medicaid Coverage Rate of the Non Institutionalized Poor
1979-1991

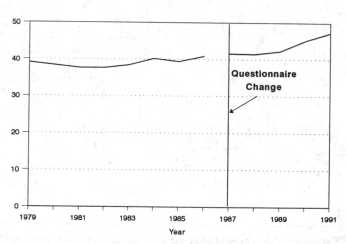

Source: Figure prepared by Congressional Research Service based on data from selected years of the March Current Population Survey.

TABLE A-7. Medicaid Coverage Rate for the Poor and
Total Population, 1979-1991

Year	All persons covered	Total population	Percent of total	Poor persons covered	Poor persons	Percent of poor
1979	18,357	222,903	8.3%	10,185	26,072	39.1%
1980[b]						
1981	19,459	227,157	8.6	11,968	31,822	37.6
1982	18,924	229,412	8.2	12,926	34,398	37.6
1983[a]	19,307	231,612	8.3	13,534	35,267	38.4
1984	19,421	233,816	8.3	13,531	33,700	40.2
1985	19,281	236,594	8.1	12,984	33,064	39.3
1986	19,769	238,554	8.3	13,232	32,370	40.9
Questionnaire change[c]						
1987	20,111	240,982	8.3	13,418	32,221	41.6
1988	20,674	243,530	8.5	13,185	31,745	41.5
1989	21,073	245,992	8.6	13,326	31,534	42.3
1990	24,160	248,644	9.7	15,175	33,585	45.2
1991	26,739	251,179	10.6	16,888	35,708	47.3

[a]Estimate based upon analysis of original Current Population Survey (CPS) information. The Census Bureau has subsequently revised these tapes. These estimates do not reflect the Census Bureau re-estimates.

[b]Comparable estimates for 1980 are not available.

[c]Beginning with the March 1988 CPS questionnaire additional and different questions on health insurance were asked of respondents. Estimates from earlier years are not strictly comparable.

NOTE: Estimates are of the noninstitutionalized population.

Source: Table prepared by the Congressional Research Service based on an analysis of March CPS data for selected years.

The recent dramatic increases in Medicaid's coverage rate of the poor are greatly influenced by changes in the coverage rate of poor children. Table A-8 provides estimates of the share of noninstitutionalized poor children covered by Medicaid. Between 1988 and 1991 the number of poor children covered by Medicaid increased by 33 percent, from 7 million to 9.4 million. In 1991, almost two out of every three poor children were covered by Medicaid. This increase is largely a result of large coverage increases for young children. In 1988, Medicaid covered 61 percent of poor children under the age of 7. In 1991, the share of children covered in this age group increased to 74 percent.[22] Because of the incremental nature of eligibility expansion, coverage rates for older children do not show the same dramatic increase. For most of these older children, Medicaid eligibility is still linked to receipt of cash assistance or income near cash assistance levels for the medically needy. In 1988, Medicaid covered 52 percent of children between the ages of 7 and 17. By 1991 the share of these older children covered by the program increased, but only to 59 percent. Some of the increase in older children is probably associated with AFDC caseload increases. In addition, some of the poor children in this age group, those born after September 30, 1983, fall within mandated Medicaid coverage expansions.

[22]Recent eligibility expansions directed at this age group should result in 100 percent coverage rates. The estimates provided in the table rely on self reported health insurance status. Individuals may have never applied for Medicaid coverage and therefore not know they are eligible for coverage. See *Appendix B, Medicaid and Maternal and Child Health* for a discussion of what some States are doing to reach this population. The lower than expected coverage rate may also occur because of underreporting of income and/or health insurance status on the survey.

TABLE A-8. Medicaid Coverage Rate for Noninstitutionalized Poor Children, 1979-1991 (children in thousands)

Year	Poor children under 7			Poor children 7-17			All poor children		
	Covered by Medicaid	All poor children	Percent of poor children	Covered by Medicaid	All poor children	Percent of poor children	Covered by Medicaid	All poor children	Percent of poor children
1979	2,030	4,078	49.8%	2,973	6,300	47.2%	5,004	10,377	48.2%
1980[a]									
1981	2,635	5,222	50.5	3,176	7,283	43.6	5,811	12,505	46.5
1982	2,997	5,764	52.0	3,432	7,883	43.5	6,429	13,647	47.1
1983[b]	3,160	6,046	52.3	3,532	7,761	45.5	6,692	13,807	48.5
1984	3,004	5,886	51.0	3,618	7,534	48.0	6,622	13,419	49.3
1985	3,060	5,733	53.4	3,509	7,728	48.2	6,569	13,011	50.5
1986	3,124	5,611	55.7	3,553	7,265	48.9	6,676	12,876	51.8
Questionnaire change[c]									
1987	3,531	5,763	61.3	3,622	7,080	51.2	7,153	12,843	55.7
1988	3,580	5,753	62.2	3,490	6,702	52.1	7,070	12,465	56.8
1989	3,678	5,852	62.9	3,450	6,738	51.2	7,128	12,590	56.6
1990	4,353	6,298	69.1	3,960	7,133	55.5	8,313	13,431	61.9
1991	4,840	6,568	73.7	4,548	7,773	58.5	9,388	14,341	65.5

See notes at end of table.

TABLE A-8. Medicaid Coverage Rate for Noninstitutionalized Poor Children, 1979-1991–Continued

[a]Comparable estimates for 1980 are not available.

[b]Estimate based upon analysis of original Current Population Survey information. The Census Bureau has subsequently revised these tapes. These estimates do not reflect the Census Bureau re-estimates.

[c]Beginning with the March 1988 CPS questionnaire additional and different questions on health insurance were asked of respondents. Estimates from earlier years are not strictly comparable.

NOTE: Estimates are of the noninstitutionalized population. Detail may not sum to total due to rounding.

Source: Table prepared by the Congressional Research Service based on an analysis of March CPS data for selected years.

C. Medicaid, Welfare Dynamics and Transitional Coverage

Analysis of the CPS allows for a snapshot picture of who receives Medicaid, but does not allow us to explore how people get Medicaid or leave the program. Once someone is on Medicaid, how long are they likely to stay covered, what events lead to Medicaid enrollment and what events are likely to result in the person leaving the program?

A number of studies suggest that a sizable share of Medicaid beneficiaries are enrolled for short periods. One Census Bureau study looking at health insurance coverage in calendar year 1987 found that about 57 percent of those with Medicaid at any time during the year had continuous coverage over the 12 month period. About 18 percent were covered from 1 to 4 months.[23] Lengthening the period of investigation, from 12 months to 28 months (covering the time from 1987 to 1989) alters the length of coverage distribution. About 41 percent of those with Medicaid coverage at any point in the study period had continuous coverage for the 28 months, while 20 percent were covered by Medicaid from 1 to 6 months. Figure A-9 provides the distribution of persons by length of time on Medicaid coverage for the 28 month investigation period.

Persons in continuous poverty are more likely to have long stays on Medicaid rolls than persons in families that fall into and then climb out of poverty. For example, the Census Bureau study classifies individuals by the number of months in which family income fell below the poverty threshold. Fifty-two percent of persons in families with income below poverty for all 28 months of the study period had continuous Medicaid coverage. In contrast, about 2 percent of persons in families with 1 to 6 months of poverty income had continuous Medicaid coverage. Since not all of the poor are categorically eligible for Medicaid some individuals in families with income below the poverty threshold for the 28 month period were never covered by Medicaid (25 percent).[24]

---

[23]U.S. Dept. of Commerce. Bureau of the Census. *Health Insurance Coverage 1987-90.* [By] Short, Kathleen. Current Population Reports. Household Economic Studies, Series P-70, no. 29. May 1992.

[24]However, it should be noted that this does not preclude coverage by private health insurance or other public health insurance programs.

FIGURE A-9.
Length of Medicaid Coverage Over a
28 Month Period, 1987-1989

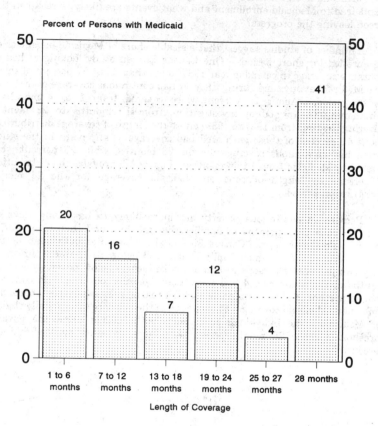

Percent of Persons with Medicaid

Length of Coverage

Source: Figure prepared by Congressional Research Service based on data contained
in K. Short, "Health Insurance Coverage 1987-90" Census Bureau
Current Population Reports. Series P-70, No. 29.

Another study exploring coverage patterns over a 32-month period (covering a period from the fall of 1983 through the summer of 1986) found that about 43 percent of those ever enrolled in Medicaid over the study period were enrolled for all of the period.[25] Results from this second study highlighted the importance of the receipt of cash assistance payments for many Medicaid beneficiaries. A strong indicator of whether an individual was likely to have continuous coverage over the study period appeared to be the receipt of cash assistance, either AFDC or SSI payments, at the start of the period. About two-thirds of those receiving AFDC at the start of the period had continuous Medicaid coverage, while three-fourths of those persons with SSI payments at the start of the period had continuous Medicaid coverage. In contrast, only about 23 percent of those individuals receiving unemployment compensation at the start of period had continuous Medicaid coverage.[26]

Results from this longitudinal study suggests that the program affects two rather distinct populations. A sizable share of Medicaid enrollees appears to be from the ranks of workers who, because of job loss, reduced work hours, or reduced hourly wages, find themselves eligible for Medicaid. About 22 percent of those persons becoming eligible for Medicaid were in middle or high income families prior to their Medicaid coverage. A second group of Medicaid enrollees face more long-term economic hardships. About half of new Medicaid entrants were living in families with income below the poverty threshold prior to Medicaid enrollment.[27]

Further analysis suggests that economic change appears to be an important factor leading to Medicaid enrollment. More than 48 percent of those enrolling in Medicaid faced reduced employment (job loss, reduced hours, or reduced hourly wages) prior to enrollment. Another 12 percent experience some other decrease in family income. Changes in family status, for example, the loss of a spouse, childbirth, or other changes in family size were experienced by 22 percent of Medicaid enrollees. About 17 percent of new enrollment was unexplained. This last group of individuals may have incurred some disability, or experienced high medical bills prior to their entrance. Unfortunately, the survey that this analysis is based on did not provide information on these type of conditions.

Increased income plays an important role for many people leaving Medicaid. About 45 percent of those people losing Medicaid coverage experienced an improvement in their employment status. This might result from new

---

[25]Short, Pamela, J. Cantor, and A. Monheit. The Dynamics of Medicaid Enrollment. *Inquiry*, 25(1), winter, 1988: 504-516.

[26]The authors of these estimates note that the estimates can be influenced by a number of factors including: the way the sample was constructed, the survey design not distinguishing between Medicaid and State indigent care programs, and the correction of missed reported coverage status over time.

[27]This analysis is based on the income status of the individual in the 8-month period prior to Medicaid enrollment.

employment (14.6 percent), increased hours worked (13.9 percent), or increased hourly wages (16.5 percent). Another 14 percent of people leaving Medicaid's rolls experienced some other increase in family income. But leaving Medicaid's rolls should not be viewed as an improvement in a persons health insurance status. A majority of those leaving Medicaid became uninsured.[28]

This last finding suggests that with the increased income from employment some individuals may face both the loss of AFDC benefits, and the loss of Medicaid coverage. This loss of insurance coverage has been viewed as a major barrier to leaving welfare rolls and seeking employment. For persons who find work that excludes health insurance benefits, the loss of Medicaid coverage could act as a greater work disincentive than the loss of AFDC payments.

Concern about Medicaid's work disincentive effect has prompted the establishment of "transitional coverage" eligibility requirements. States will either provide Medicaid coverage or pay health insurance premiums, deductibles and coinsurance amounts for an individual for up to 1 year after a family leaves AFDC rolls because of increased earned income. Eligibility for transitional coverage during this period will continue if a family continues to have a dependent child, does not have gross monthly earnings in excess of 185 percent of poverty and continues to report those earnings on a quarterly basis. For additional details on transitional coverage, see *Chapter III, Eligibility*.

The number of studies investigating the work disincentive role of Medicaid is quite small. Perhaps the most useful relies on program data from two States, Georgia and California, but covers a period when Medicaid's transitional coverage policies were different from current law.[29] First, the authors found that few mothers who were eligible for Medicaid because of receipt of AFDC or AFDC-UP actually received transitional coverage upon leaving Medicaid. The authors suggest that this lack of transitional coverage occurs because individuals did not report higher earnings to the welfare office. These former beneficiaries no longer received benefits because their exit from Medicaid was classified by State administrators as a result of "recipient initiative." This is a catchall term for persons who left for unknown reasons. These findings suggest that for many exits, increased earnings were never reported to Medicaid administrators. The former beneficiary never bothered to apply for the transition coverage. Program administrators had no way of knowing whether individuals were actually eligible for the transition coverage or not.

The authors of this study went on to develop a model of welfare exits. Results from the statistical model suggest that expected high medical costs are associated with a lower probability of welfare exits. However, this finding does not unequivocally show that Medicaid has a work disincentive effect. A number

---

[28]It should be noted that this analysis covers a period prior to many of the eligibility expansions aimed at pregnant women and young children discussed earlier. It is not clear to what extent these changes would affect these findings.

[29]Ellwood, David T., and E. Kathleen Adams et al. *Medicaid Mysteries: Medicaid and Welfare Dynamics*. SysteMetrics/McGraw-Hill, Apr. 1990.

of other factors can affect these results. For example, if a person is sick or disabled they may be unable to work, unable to leave Medicaid's rolls, but still have high medical costs.

D. Comparing Medicaid's Income Eligibility Criteria to the Federal Poverty Guidelines[30]

There are many avenues to Medicaid coverage. But all have "toll booths" that individuals must pass. Perhaps the most important factor to consider is that Medicaid limits program coverage to certain types of individuals. This partly stems from the program's historical connection to the cash assistance programs, AFDC and SSI. These means-tested programs have always focused on the poor who are unable to work. Besides income criteria, additional program criteria are employed in considering who is eligible for these cash assistance payments. For example, in the AFDC program three criteria in addition to the explicit income test must be passed. These include: 1) being a child or caretaker; 2) the dependency criteria and 3) the resource criteria. In order to receive AFDC payments a needy child and their mother or caretaker must be deprived of support because the child's father is absent from home, is unable to work or is deceased, or in the case of two parent families, the father may be unemployed (AFDC-UP families). The resource criteria sets a level for the amount of assets a family can have and still be eligible for AFDC.[31]

Under SSI, an individual must meet the definition of "need" by being aged, blind or disabled as well as having income below the maximum allowable levels. In addition, the SSI program has asset limits.

Medicaid's recent eligibility expansions (see *Chapter III, Eligibility* or *Chapter IX, Recent Legislative History*) while broadening income and resource eligibility, continue to maintain the program's focus on children, their caretakers who do not work, the aged and disabled.

Another aspect in Medicaid's coverage of the poor is associated with the different means-tests employed in the program. The income eligibility threshold that is applicable to one set of individuals may be different from the income threshold applicable to others. For example, all children under 6 who live in families with incomes at or below 133 percent of the Federal poverty guidelines

---

[30]The discussion provided in this section concentrates on income eligibility guidelines for noninstitutionalized persons. Detailed discussion on eligibility for guidelines for those in nursing homes, intermediate care facilities for the mentally retarded (ICFs/MR), other institutions and home and community-based waiver settings are provided in *Chapter III, Eligibility*. The primary purpose of the following discussion is to relate income eligibility guidelines to the Federal poverty guidelines. Additional detail can be found in *Chapter III, Eligibility*.

[31]See *Chapter III, Eligibility* for details on these criteria.

are eligible for Medicaid.[32] Eligible children between ages 6 and 9 (in 1992) must live in families with incomes at or below 100 percent of poverty. Generally, children over age 9 qualify for Medicaid when family income is within the AFDC limits or medically needy limit, if the State employs this eligibility option. The AFDC program income eligibility standards vary from State to State and by family size (table A-10 shows these standards for a family of three). In almost all States the AFDC income criteria is less than the poverty guidelines. The picture is complicated further by the program's optional coverage standards. The poverty-related income criteria for infants must be at least 133 percent of poverty, but at a State's option, it can be as high as 185 percent of the poverty guideline. Many States have income cutoffs for infants exceeding the 133 percent minimum (see *Appendix B, Medicaid and Maternal and Child Health*).

Still another feature of Medicaid eligibility revolves around what income and assets are used in determining eligibility. The income used varies somewhat from category to category. The best example of this is seen when comparing the definition of income used of those Medicaid enrollees who become eligible through the receipt of cash assistance payments and the definition of income used for those enrollees who qualify because they are medically needy. A family's gross monthly cash income minus some disregards is the income used in determining AFDC (and Medicaid eligibility). For the medically needy, an individual's gross cash income may not be directly related to their Medicaid eligibility. Rather, these individuals qualify for Medicaid because their medical expenses are so high that their net income (i.e., income after medical expenses) is below the State's maximum allowable income level.[33] While the effective maximum allowable net income for these individuals is below the poverty guidelines in most States, a medically needy family's gross income may exceed the categorical eligibility income limits associated with the cash assistance programs and the poverty threshold.

1. AFDC Income Limits and the Poverty Guidelines[34]

Definitions of needs, payment levels, resource and income limits for State AFDC programs vary from State to State. The maximum allowable income associated with AFDC eligibility and recipiency is based on a State's "need

---

[32]At a State's option this eligibility limit can be set as high as 185 percent of the poverty guidelines.

[33]Those medical expenses that are considered in the calculation include: Medicare premiums and cost sharing charges, and services covered under a State's Medicaid plan or recognized under State law but not included in the plan. See *Chapter III, Eligibility* for additional details.

[34]A detailed discussion of AFDC eligibility and payment levels can be found in U.S. Library of Congress. Congressional Research Service. *Aid to Families with Dependent Children (AFDC): Need Standards, Payment Standards, and Maximum Benefits for Families*. CRS Report for Congress No. 91-849, by Carmen Solomon, Nov. 26, 1991 (updated regularly). Washington, 1991.

standard" and "payment standard." States define a monthly needs standard; this is the income amount that the individual State decides as necessary for purchasing such items as food, clothing, shelter, household supplies and personal care items. Actual AFDC payment amounts are based on the State's payment standard and a family's countable income. The State's payment standard can be equal to or less than the needs standard.

In order to be eligible for AFDC payments and automatically eligible for Medicaid, a family must pass two income tests: 1) a gross income test, and 2) a countable income test:

- **Gross income test.** The gross income test compares a family's gross income to the State's *needs* standard. An AFDC applicant's or recipient's gross monthly income can not exceed 185 percent of the State's *needs* standard.

- **Countable income test.** An *applicant's* countable income must be less than the State's *needs* standard. An AFDC *recipient's* countable income must be less than the State's *payment* standard.

The AFDC program provides incentives for labor force participation of its recipients using two means: 1) States must offer a job opportunities and basic skills program; and, 2) a different definition of countable income is used for recipients than the definition of income used in determining program eligibility. An applicant's countable income is defined as gross income minus child care costs up to $175 per child, and a standard earned income allowance of $90 a month. For a recipient the income disregards used in the countable income definition include an additional element, the work incentive bonus. Like the AFDC applicant, an AFDC recipient is allowed to deduct child care costs, and the $90 standard allowance. But in addition, during the first year on a job, a work incentive bonus is allowed. This bonus varies based on the length of employment. During the first 4 months of a job the bonus is equivalent to the first $30 of earned income and one-third of the earnings after the child care and standard deductions are taken. For the remaining 8 months the bonus is equivalent to $30. After 12 months there is no longer a work incentive bonus. Since these work disregards vary by the length of employment, an AFDC recipient's maximum allowable income will also vary depending on how long they have worked and received AFDC.

A State's payment standard is linked to the State's need standard. In some States the need standard equals the payment standard. However, in many States the payment standard is an amount below the need standard. The relationship between the need standard and payment is based on a formula. These formula vary from State to State.[35] States that set payment standards below the need standard can be grouped into two categories: States where the payment standard is a percentage of the need standard; and States that set the

---

[35]Ibid., for a discussion of the alternative payment standard methodologies used by the States.

payment standard equal to a percentage of the need standard minus countable income.[36] In the former States the payment standard determines Medicaid eligibility. In the later States the maximum AFDC payment is determined by the payment standard, but the more liberal need standard determines Medicaid eligibility.

As a result of these complex set of rules, the maximum allowable income levels used to determine Medicaid eligibility for AFDC families vary by State, by family size, and by the length of time in employment. Table III-2 in *Chapter III, Eligibility* illustrates this point; it shows the State by State variation in the maximum AFDC payment amounts for a family of three in January 1992.

Families relying solely on AFDC payments as their only source of income will have income levels below the poverty guidelines in all 50 States. Families with a member in their first 4 months of employment, depending on the State they reside in, can have income ranging from 36 percent of poverty to 125 percent of poverty. Seven States allow combined AFDC payments and earned income to exceed the poverty guidelines for these first 4 months of employment. The maximum allowable income after 12 months of employment falls between these two extremes, ranging between 25 percent and 84 percent of poverty.

This brief discussion of maximum allowable income levels associated with AFDC receipt indicates that categorical eligibility income standards alone can not guarantee universal Medicaid coverage for the poor. Even when the most liberal work disregards are in effect, during the first 4 months of employment, families with incomes below the Federal poverty guidelines may not qualify for AFDC payments and be categorically eligible for Medicaid in some States.

2. Medically Needy Income Thresholds and the Poverty Guidelines

The maximum AFDC payment amount is important for non-AFDC families. Individuals with incomes greater than the income thresholds used in the AFDC program may still be eligible for Medicaid if they live in a State that provides for the optional coverage category referred to as "medically needy" and meet the State's medically needy criteria for the program. First, like their cash assistance counterparts, these individuals must be in families that meet the categorical eligibility criteria (i.e., single parent families, aged, or disabled). In addition, these individuals must either have incomes below the medically needy thresholds or incur medical expenses that reduce their income to levels that are close to the thresholds used in the AFDC program for a family of comparable

---

[36]The difference in the payment formula is:

$$PS = NS \times RR; \text{ } versus \text{ } PS = (NS\text{-}CI) \times RR.$$
Where:
PS = Payment standard;
CI = Countable income;
NS = Need standard; and
RR = Rate reduction.

size. The medically needy income level can not exceed 133-1/3 percent of the maximum AFDC payment amount for a family of the same size in the State. As of January 1992, the medically needy income eligibility threshold ranged from 26 percent to 97 percent of the Federal poverty guidelines. However, it should be remembered that the medically needy income thresholds are for income after medical expenses are deducted, and not gross income.

In those States that define their AFDC payment standard as a percentage of the need standard minus countable income, the medically needy income threshold can be less than the applicable AFDC eligibility level for a family of the same size. This occurs because the medically needy level is based on the State's maximum **payment** amount and the AFDC/Medicaid eligibility level is based on the relatively more liberal **need** standard. In January of 1992 this occurred in Georgia, Kentucky, Maine, Michigan, Oklahoma, South Carolina, Tennessee and Utah.[37]

3. SSI Income Thresholds and the Federal Poverty Guidelines

The SSI program provides monthly cash payments to the blind, disabled and aged. These cash assistance payments consist of a basic Federal payment plus in some States, a State supplemental payment. Most States provide Medicaid coverage automatically to recipients of Federal SSI payments. However, States do have the option of using more restrictive eligibility rules.[38]

In order to qualify for Federal SSI benefits an individual must meet program eligibility criteria about blindness, age, or disability and have countable income less than the maximum allowable income limits provided in table A-9. The regular Federal SSI benefit guarantees a minimum income to all SSI recipients; at its option a State can supplement this Federal benefit. The result of the regular Federal benefit is that the maximum allowable income levels associated with Medicaid eligibility for SSI beneficiaries effectively stays around 74 percent of the Federal poverty guidelines for an individual (83 percent for a couple residing in the community) because both the SSI level and the poverty guidelines use the same cost of living adjustment.[39] For many States these income levels measured as a share of the poverty threshold are higher than those in the AFDC program. State supplements can increase this level. For example, Connecticut's State supplement raises an individual's income to 132 percent of the poverty guideline.

---

[37]Maine and Michigan's medically needy income standard is less than the 133-1/3 maximum. If the medically needy income standard equalled this maximum, the State's medically needy standard would exceed the effective AFDC eligibility level.

[38]See *Chapter III, Eligibility* for a discussion of how these eligibility rules are administered.

[39]Because Hawaii's poverty guideline is different from the 48 States, its SSI maximum benefit is less than the 74 percent.

Like the AFDC program, the SSI program disregards some earned income. This earned income disregard results in maximum allowable income amounts for working SSI recipients exceeding the poverty guideline in all States. In September 1991 about 4.6 percent of SSI recipients receiving federally administered payments had some form of earned income. Most of these (88.2 percent) were eligible for SSI because of a disability or blindness.

TABLE A-9. Maximum SSI Benefit Levels, for Individuals and Couples, January 1992

State	Individual (living in the community)		Couple (living in the community)	
	SSI income (maximum benefit)	Percent of poverty guideline	SSI income (maximum benefit)	Percent of poverty guideline
Alabama	422	74	633	83
Alaska	784	111	1161	121
Arizona[a]	422	74	633	83
Arkansas	422	74	633	83
California	645	114	1190	155
Colorado	478	84	956	125
Connecticut	747	132	1094	143
Delaware	422	74	633	83
District of Columbia	437	77	663	87
Florida	422	74	633	83
Georgia	422	74	633	83
Hawaii	427	65	642	73
Idaho	492	87	678	89
Illinois[b]				
Indiana	422	74	633	83
Iowa	422	74	633	83
Kansas	422	74	633	83
Kentucky	422	74	633	83
Louisiana	422	74	633	83
Maine	432	76	648	85
Maryland	422	74	633	83
Massachusetts	551	97	835	109
Michigan	436	77	654	85
Minnesota[c]	503	89	762	99
Mississippi	422	74	633	83
Missouri	422	74	633	83
Montana	422	74	633	83
Nebraska	452	80	681	89
Nevada	458	81	707	92
New Hampshire	449	79	654	85
New Jersey	453	80	658	86
New Mexico	422	74	633	83
New York	508	90	736	96
North Carolina	422	74	633	83
North Dakota	422	74	633	83
Ohio	422	74	633	83
Oklahoma	486	86	761	99
Oregon	424	75	633	83
Pennsylvania	454	80	682	89
Rhode Island	489	86	760	99
South Carolina	422	74	633	83
South Dakota	437	77	648	85
Tennessee	422	74	633	83
Texas	422	74	633	83
Utah	427	75	644	84
Vermont[d]	487	86	751	98
Virginia	422	74	633	83

See notes at end of table.

744

TABLE A-9. Maximum SSI Benefit Levels, for Individuals and Couples,
January 1992--Continued

State	Individual (living in the community)		Couple (living in the community)	
	SSI income (maximum benefit)	Percent of poverty guideline	SSI income (maximum benefit)	Percent of poverty guideline
Washington[e]	450	79	655	86
West Virginia	422	74	633	83
Wisconsin	515	91	779	102
Wyoming	442	78	673	88
Minimum State	422	65	633	73
Maximum State	784	132	1190	155

[a]Arizona's Medicaid program provides benefits under a waiver agreement.

[b]Illinois determines SSI benefit on a case-by-case basis.

[c]Payment level for Hennepin County. State has two geographic payment levels.

[d]State has two geographic payment levels--highest is shown in table.

[e]Sum paid in King, Pierce, Snohomish, and Thurston Counties.

NOTE: Allowable monthly income amount can exceed maximum SSI payment. For beneficiaries receiving Social Security an additional $20 of income is allowed because of income exclusions. For the working disabled, blind, and aged, additional work-related income and expenses can be deducted from gross monthly income. These maximum benefit amounts are for aged persons. In most States these maximums apply also to blind or disabled SSI recipients who are living in their own households; but some States provide different benefit schedules for each category.

Source: Table prepared by the Congressional Research Service.

4. Poverty-Related Coverage for Pregnant Women, Infants, and Children

Changes in the mid to late 1980s in income eligibility have eliminated many of the complicated income thresholds for infants, young children and pregnant women. In all States, the changes in income eligibility have resulted in substantially higher income eligibility thresholds for those meeting the categorical criteria. As noted in *Chapter III, Eligibility*, income eligibility that is linked to the Federal poverty guideline sets income standards equal to:

- 133 percent of poverty for pregnant women;

- 133 percent of poverty for children up to age 6;

- up to 185 percent of poverty, at State option, for infants; and

- 100 percent of poverty for children aged 6 to 19, born after September 30, 1983.

Appendix B, Medicaid and Maternal and Child Health provides a listing of those States using the higher income eligibility criteria for infants.

These different sets of income guidelines mean that the income criteria relative to the poverty guidelines will vary depending on the eligibility status of the individual. Table A-10 shows the AFDC, medically needy and poverty related income guidelines by State as a percentage of the Federal poverty guideline. In eight States, the medically needy income guidelines fall below the eligibility levels for AFDC. For these States, individuals who must "spend down" their income through the payment of high medical expenses are left with less income after these expenses than an AFDC family.

TABLE A-10. A Comparison of Selected Medicaid Income Eligibility Thresholds, January 1992
(in percentages)

State	AFDC income thresholds			Medically needy threshold[b]	Poverty guideline related thresholds		
	Effective eligibility level[a]	First 4 months of employment	After 12 months of employment		Pregnant women and infants	Children up to age 6	Children ages 7 to 9[c]
Alabama	15.5	35.7	24.8		133.0	133.0	100.0
Alaska	76.6	125.0	84.1		133.0	133.0	100.0
Arizona[d]	34.6	64.4	44.0		140.0	133.0	100.0
Arkansas	21.2	44.2	30.5	28.5	185.0	133.0	100.0
California	68.8	120.4	81.3	96.9	185.0	133.0	100.0
Colorado	43.7	78.0	53.0		133.0	133.0	100.0
Connecticut	60.3	118.2	79.9	80.2	185.0	133.0	100.0
Delaware	35.1	65.0	44.4		160.0	133.0	100.0
District of Columbia	42.4	76.1	51.8	56.5	185.0	133.0	100.0
Florida	31.4	59.6	40.8	31.4	150.0	133.0	100.0
Georgia	44.0	78.4	53.3	38.9	133.0	133.0	100.0
Hawaii	60.0	100.9	68.2	60.0	185.0	133.0	100.0
Idaho	32.7	61.5	42.0		133.0	133.0	100.0
Illinois	38.1	69.6	47.4	51.0	133.0	133.0	100.0
Indiana	29.9	57.3	39.2		150.0	133.0	100.0
Iowa	44.2	78.7	53.5	58.7	185.0	133.0	100.0
Kansas	41.1	78.1	53.1	48.7	133.0	133.0	100.0
Kentucky	54.6	94.3	63.9	31.9	185.0	133.0	100.0
Louisiana	19.7	42.0	29.0	26.8	133.0	133.0	100.0
Maine	59.4	101.6	68.8	47.5	185.0	133.0	100.0
Maryland	39.1	71.1	48.4	45.8	185.0	133.0	100.0
Massachusetts	60.1	96.4	65.2	80.4	185.0	133.0	100.0
Michigan	60.9	83.9	56.9	58.8	185.0	133.0	100.0
Minnesota	55.2	95.2	64.5	73.5	185.0	133.0	100.0

See notes at end of table.

TABLE A-10. A Comparison of Selected Medicaid Income Eligibility Thresholds, January 1992--Continued

(in percentages)

	AFDC income thresholds			Medically needy threshold[b]	Poverty guideline related thresholds		
State	Effective eligibility level[a]	First 4 months of employment	After 12 months of employment		Pregnant women and infants	Children up to age 6	Children ages 7 to 9[c]
Mississippi	38.2	69.7	47.5		185.0	133.0	100.0
Missouri	30.3	57.9	39.6		133.0	133.0	100.0
Montana	40.4	73.1	49.8	45.9	133.0	133.0	100.0
Nebraska	37.8	69.1	47.1	51.0	133.0	133.0	100.0
Nevada	36.1	70.3	47.9		133.0	133.0	100.0
New Hampshire	53.5	92.7	62.9	63.9	133.0	133.0	100.0
New Jersey	44.0	78.4	53.3	58.7	185.0	133.0	100.0
New Mexico	33.6	62.9	42.9		185.0	133.0	100.0
New York	59.8	102.3	69.2	77.8	185.0	133.0	100.0
North Carolina	28.2	54.8	37.5	38.1	185.0	133.0	100.0
North Dakota	41.6	74.9	50.9	45.1	133.0	133.0	100.0
Ohio	34.6	64.4	44.0		133.0	133.0	100.0
Oklahoma	48.9	65.5	44.7	47.6	133.0	133.0	100.0
Oregon	47.7	84.0	57.0	63.6	133.0	133.0	100.0
Pennsylvania	43.7	78.0	53.0	48.4	133.0	133.0	100.0
Rhode Island	57.5	98.6	66.8	76.9	185.0	133.0	100.0
South Carolina	45.6	80.9	55.0	29.4	185.0	133.0	100.0
South Dakota	41.9	75.3	51.2		133.0	133.0	100.0
Tennessee	44.2	78.7	53.5	25.9	185.0	133.0	100.0
Texas	19.1	41.1	28.4	27.7	185.0	133.0	100.0
Utah	55.7	96.0	65.0	55.6	133.0	133.0	100.0
Vermont	69.8	117.2	79.1	93.3	185.0	133.0	100.0
Virginia	30.2	67.5	46.1	37.1	133.0	133.0	100.0

See notes at end of table.

TABLE A-10. A Comparison of Selected Medicaid Income Eligibility Thresholds, January 1992–Continued
(In percentages)

State	AFDC income thresholds			Medically needy threshold[b]	Poverty guideline related thresholds		
	Effective eligibility level[a]	First 4 months of employment	After 12 months of employment		Pregnant women and infants	Children up to age 6	Children ages 7 to 9[c]
Washington	55.1	95.1	64.4	67.4	185.0	133.0	100.0
West Virginia	25.8	51.2	35.2	30.1	150.0	133.0	100.0
Wisconsin	53.7	92.9	63.0	71.5	155.0	133.0	100.0
Wyoming	37.3	68.5	46.7		133.0	133.0	100.0
Minimum State	15.5	35.7	24.8	25.9	133.0	133.0	100.0
Maximum State	76.6	125.0	84.1	96.9	185.0	133.0	100.0

[a] In most States this eligibility level corresponds to the maximum payment amount. In a few States this eligibility threshold is higher than the maximum payment amount.

[b] States with no entry for the medically needy income threshold have not incorporated this optional eligibility category as part of their State's Medicaid plan.

[c] Poverty-related guidelines for children born after Sept. 30, 1983 and between the ages of 7 and 19.

[d] Arizona provides Medicaid coverage under a waiver option.

NOTE: All figures are based on Federal poverty guidelines for a family of three ($11,570); in Alaska this guideline equals $14,460; and in Hawaii this guideline equals $13,310. AFDC maximum benefit amounts assume a standard deduction of $90 and no child care expenses.

Source: Table prepared by the Congressional Research Service (CRS) based on information collected by CRS and the National Governors' Association.

For the noninstitutionalized aged the likely avenue onto Medicaid's rolls is either through receipt of SSI or spending down because of medical need. Table A-11 provides a comparison of the SSI income guidelines for aged couples with the medically needy income guidelines for a family of two. In every State with a medically needy option, except New York and Vermont, the net income levels for Medicaid coverage because of medical need is lower than the income levels under SSI for a couple living in the community. In those States where medically needy levels are below the SSI levels, couples who qualify for Medicaid because they are medically needy will have less income after the payment of their medical expenses than their counterparts who are eligible as a result of SSI eligibility.

The difference in available income occurs because the medically needy threshold is based upon AFDC maximum payment amounts. Most States do not make adjustments for the cost of living in AFDC payment amounts. The federally administered SSI program does. Over time, if a State does not adjust its AFDC levels for inflation, the medically needy level can fall further below the SSI levels.

TABLE A-11. A Comparison of the Medically Needy Monthly Protected Income Levels with SSI Maximum Benefits for Couples, January 1992

State	SSI income (maximum benefit)	Percent of poverty guideline	Protected income threshold	Percent of poverty guideline
Alabama	633	83%		
Alaska	1,161	121		
Arizona[a]	633	83		
Arkansas	633	121	217	28%
California	1,190	83	750	98
Colorado	956	83		
Connecticut	1,094	155	629	82
Delaware	633	243		
District of Columbia	633	87	428	56
Florida	633	83	241	31
Georgia	633	83	317	41
Hawaii	642	73	531	60
Idaho	678	89		
Illinois			358	47

See notes at end of table.

TABLE A-11. A Comparison of the Medically Needy Monthly Protected Income Levels with SSI Maximum Benefits for Couples, January 1992--Continued

State	SSI maximum benefit (living in the community)		Medically needy (living in the community)	
	SSI income (maximum benefit)	Percent of poverty guideline	Protected income threshold	Percent of poverty guideline
Indiana	633	83		
Iowa	633	83	483	63
Kansas	633	83	466	61
Kentucky	633	83	267	35
Louisiana	633	83	192	25
Maine	648	85	341	45
Maryland	633	83	400	52
Massachusetts	835	109	650	85
Michigan	654	85	541	71
Minnesota	762	99	583	76
Mississippi	633	83		
Missouri	633	83		
Montana	633	83	417	54
Nebraska	681	89	392	51
Nevada	707	92		
New Hampshire	654	85	608	79
New Jersey	658	86	433	57
New Mexico	633	83		
New York	736	96	742	97
North Carolina	633	83	317	41
North Dakota	633	83	400	52
Ohio	633	83		
Oklahoma	761	99	359	47
Oregon	633	83	526	69
Pennsylvania	682	89	442	58
Rhode Island	760	99	600	78
South Carolina	633	83	225	29

See notes at end of table.

TABLE A-11. A Comparison of the Medically Needy Monthly Protected Income Levels with SSI Maximum Benefits for Couples, January 1992--Continued

State	SSI maximum benefit (living in the community)		Medically needy (living in the community)	
	SSI income (maximum benefit)	Percent of poverty guideline	Protected income threshold	Percent of poverty guideline
South Dakota	648	85		
Tennessee	633	83	192	25
Texas	633	83	211	28
Utah	644	84	430	56
Vermont	751	98	758	99
Virginia	633	83	308	40
Washington	655	86	575	75
West Virginia	633	83	275	36
Wisconsin	779	102	592	77
Wyoming	673	88		
Minimum State	633	73	192	25
Maximum State	1,190	155	758	99

ªArizona provides Medicaid services under a State waiver.

NOTE: Allowable monthly income amount can exceed maximum SSI payment. For beneficiaries receiving Social Security an additional $20 of income is allowed because of income exclusions. For the working disabled, blind, and aged, additional work-related income and expenses can be deducted from gross monthly income.

Source: Table prepared by the Congressional Research Service.

V. MEDICAID'S ROLE AS A SOURCE OF HEALTH INSURANCE

In terms of the number of people covered, Medicaid is a sizable health insurance program. In 1991, 10.7 percent of the noninstitutionalized U.S. population was covered by Medicaid. More than 12 percent of all women are covered by Medicaid and more than 20 percent of all children under 18 are covered.

In comparison, Medicare, the federally supported and administered health insurance program for the aged and the disabled, provided coverage to 13.1 percent of the U.S. population.

While these federally financed programs cover a sizable portion of the U.S. population, most Americans receive health insurance coverage through employer based health insurance. Based on an analysis of the March 1992 CPS, nearly 181 million persons had some form of private health insurance. Another 9.8

million were covered by CHAMPUS, VA, or a military health plan, leaving 35.4 million Americans (14.1 percent) without any form of health insurance.

A. The Uninsured and Family Income

Of the 35.4 million without health insurance, 10.2 million or 29 percent live in families with income below the poverty threshold. Another 25 percent live in families with income between 100 and 185 percent of poverty. Both of these groups represent a disproportionately large share of those without health insurance. However, 43 percent of those without health insurance report family income equal to or greater than 185 percent of poverty. In contrast, most Medicaid beneficiaries have low incomes. Eighty-five percent of all beneficiaries indicated that their income was below 185 percent of poverty. Table A-12 compares the distribution of individuals with Medicaid, and individuals without health insurance coverage by income to poverty ratios in 1991.

TABLE A-12. Distribution of Persons with No Health Insurance and with Medicaid by the Ratio of Family Income to Poverty Threshold

Family income relative to poverty ratio	Covered by Medicaid	Percent of Medicaid population[a]	Without any health insurance	Percent of total population	Total
Poor	16,888	63.2%	10,220	28.9%	35,708
100 percent to less than 133 percent	3,306	12.4	4,217	11.9	15,554
133 percent to less than 185 percent	2,706	10.1	5,851	16.6	25,744
185 percent and greater	3,840	14.4	15,071	42.6	174,174
Total	26,739	100.0	35,358	100.0	251,179

[a]Medicaid population includes only noninstitutionalized persons.

NOTE: Estimates are of the noninstitutionalized population. All estimates of the number of persons covered are in thousands. Detail may not add to total due to rounding.

Source: Table prepared by the Congressional Research Service based on an analysis of the Mar. 1992 Current Population Survey.

For the nonpoor, private insurance is the primary source of health insurance coverage, for the poor Medicaid performs that role. Figure A-10 compares insurance coverage rates for the poor and nonpoor by insurance type. This figure highlights some different aspects of health insurance coverage. First, the dominant role Medicaid plays in providing coverage for the poor is readily apparent in the chart. Second, it shows the large share of the poor without any form of health insurance. This later estimate suggests that Medicaid's categorical eligibility criteria play an important role in determining whether Medicaid will be an insurance source for an individual. Looking at additional demographic factors of the uninsured will help clarify this point.

FIGURE A-10.
Health Insurance Coverage Rates by Poverty Status, 1991

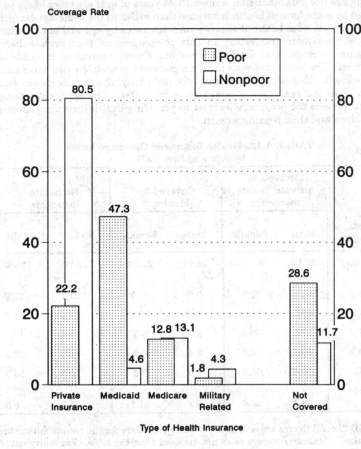

Source: Figure prepared by Congressional Research Service based on
March 1992 Current Population Survey.

B. Health Insurance Coverage by Sex

The share of males without health insurance (15.8 percent) is somewhat higher than that of females (12.4 percent). But this overall rate hides an important dichotomy in coverage rates between the two sexes. Women of child bearing age (for this discussion women 18-44 years of age) are more likely to be covered by some form of health insurance than males in the same age category. Table A-13 provides health insurance coverage rates by age and sex. Perhaps what is even more interesting in this comparison is that private health insurance coverage rates for both sexes are almost equivalent in these age categories. The large difference in coverage rates between the two sexes exists for Medicaid. Medicaid coverage rates for child bearing age females are much higher than the analogous coverage rates for males. The Medicaid coverage pattern reflects the program's interest in providing health insurance coverage to children and child bearing women.

TABLE A-13. Health Insurance Coverage Rates by Age and Sex, 1991

Age category	Covered by private health insurance		Covered by Medicaid		No health insurance	
	Male	Female	Male	Female	Male	Female
Less than 18	70.1%	69.7%	19.9%	20.7%	12.7%	12.4%
18-24	61.8	62.3	5.5	14.7	31.1	22.9
25-34	69.2	71.1	4.2	12.4	24.6	15.8
35-44	77.6	79.6	3.7	6.5	16.3	12.4
45-59	80.8	80.3	3.4	6.0	12.5	12.1
60-64	79.6	75.0	4.6	7.2	10.9	14.2
65 and older	69.2	66.6	7.2	11.1	1.0	0.9

NOTE: All figures are estimates. Coverage rates are for the noninstitutionalized population. Medicare coverage rates are excluded from the table. For individuals 55 years old and older Medicare plays an important role as a source of health insurance coverage.

Source: Table prepared by the Congressional Research Service based on an analysis of the Mar. 1992 Current Population Survey.

As this table suggests, individuals between the ages of 18 and 24 are much more likely to be uninsured than younger or older age categories. This lack of coverage comes largely as the result of no longer being dependents on their parents' private health insurance policies, no longer being considered as part of a Medicaid/AFDC filing unit, and perhaps having an entry level job that does not have health insurance benefits, or only having part time employment.

C. Labor Force Attachment and Health Insurance Coverage

The importance of labor force attachment in determining health insurance coverage can be seen in table A-14. This table highlights health insurance coverage rates by labor force attachment for individuals 16 to 64 years old. Two points are apparent from the table. First, full time, year round attachment to the labor force reduces the chances that a person will have no health insurance coverage. Eleven percent of full year, year round workers report no health insurance coverage. This compares with a rate of 24 percent for persons with part year or part time labor force attachment, and 22 percent for individuals who did not work during the year. While labor force attachment is an important indicator of health insurance coverage, not all workers have health insurance. Seventy-five percent of working age adults without health insurance had some ties to the labor market. Thirty-two percent of these adults had full time, year round labor force attachments but also had no health insurance.

TABLE A-14. Labor Force Attachment and Health Insurance Coverage for Individuals Aged 16 to 64, 1991

Work status	Covered by Medicaid	Coverage rate	No health insurance	Coverage rate	Total
Full time, year round	777	1.0%	8,842	11.2%	78,908
Full time, not year round	3,341	6.7	11,980	24.1	49,752
Did not work	7,251	22.3	7,012	21.5	32,612
Total	11,375	7.1	27,834	17.3	161,272

NOTE: All estimates are in thousands. Number of persons includes only individuals between the ages of 16 and 64. Estimates are of the noninstitutionalized population.

Source: Table prepared by the Congressional Research Service based on an analysis of the Mar. 1992 Current Population Survey.

D. The Uninsured and Other Demographic Characteristics

Table A-15 provides some additional details on the number of individuals without health insurance. More persons in the South are without health insurance than in any other region of the country. More than 17 percent of those in the South are without health insurance. More than 16 percent of those in the West are without health insurance. About 1 in 10 persons in the Northeast and Midwest are without any form of health insurance. These coverage rate differences result in 41 percent of the uninsured living in the South, 25 percent in the West, 18 percent in the Midwest, and 16 percent in the Northeast.

TABLE A-15. The Number of Uninsured, by Selected Demographic Characteristics, 1991
(numbers in thousands)

Selected characteristic	Individuals without insurance coverage	Percent of total	Total
Region:			
Midwest	6,261	10.4%	60,371
Northeast	5,283	10.4	50,788
South	14,900	17.4	85,891
West	8,915	16.5	54,129
Family type:			
Families with related children under 18:			
Single parent	6,137	19.3	31,733
Two parent	13,336	12.6	106,058
Families without related children under 18:			
Husband/wife	5,781	9.1	63,735
Single individuals	10,104	20.4	49,653
Race/ethnicity:			
White (non-Hispanic)	20,373	10.8	189,106
Black (non-Hispanic)	6,341	20.6	30,799
Hispanic	6,962	31.6	22,068
Other (non-Hispanic)	1,682	18.3	9,206
Total	35,358	14.1	251,279

NOTE: All figures are estimates. Coverage rates are for the noninstitutionalized population.

Source: Table prepared by the Congressional Research Service based on an analysis of the Mar. 1992 Current Population Survey.

ADDENDUM--LIMITATION OF CURRENT POPULATION SURVEY ESTIMATES

The estimates of Medicaid coverage contained in this appendix are based on information contained on March Current Population Surveys from 1980 through 1992. Among other items, this survey asks questions on family income and health insurance coverage. Retrospective reporting of the family's income and health insurance coverage during the prior year is provided by each respondent. For example, responses from the March 1992 survey provide information on income and health status for calendar year 1991. There are some important limitations to these data.

First, since the CPS relies on retrospective reporting of an individual's health insurance coverage for any time during the last year it does not allow us to provide any details on dual insurance coverage. By looking at responses on the survey we can determine whether an individual reports more than one form of health insurance coverage, but there is no way to determine if coverage from both sources occurred at the same time. For many of the poor, Medicaid was their only source of coverage, but almost all of the aged respondents with Medicaid coverage also reported that they had Medicare coverage. There may be an important dichotomy between the nonaged respondents with more than one form of health insurance and aged respondents. For many of the aged, dual coverage seems likely. For the nonaged, coverage of Medicaid and another form of health insurance coverage may be a result of: 1) the person moving onto or off of Medicaid's roll sometime during the calendar year and acquiring some other form of health insurance; or 2) the person having dual coverage.

The retrospective reporting used on the CPS survey has also raised some controversy. Some analysts have argued that CPS respondents provide information on their health insurance coverage at the time of the interview, rather than the retrospective reporting period asked in the question. This perspective is based on a comparison of estimates from the CPS and other surveys. Since many factors can account for these inter-survey differences, this comparison is inconclusive. The estimates presented in this appendix assume that respondents answered the health insurance coverage questions as they were asked, and do not substitute their current health insurance status for their status of last year.

The CPS estimates of income and program coverage are generally less than comparable to estimates from administrative records and other sources such as the National Income Product Account. This underreporting of program receipt and income is the result of a number of factors. For the Medicaid population, one important factor is that the CPS provides estimates of the noninstitutionalized population. This means that Medicaid beneficiaries in nursing homes and intermediate care facilities for the mentally retarded (ICFs/MR) will not be found in the CPS sample. Differences in Medicaid coverage between the CPS and other sources may also come as a result of respondents failing to report health insurance coverage or incorrectly reporting the information. In some instances, the Census Bureau imputes insurance status to individuals to reconcile some of these problems. No additional adjustments have been made in the estimates reported in this appendix.

Third, the health insurance coverage questions have undergone a change. Beginning with the March 1988 CPS, two additional questions were added to the survey on health insurance coverage. These questions specifically dealt with the health insurance status of children in the household. Survey respondents were effectively asked twice about the health insurance coverage of children in the household. Combining responses from these new questions on children's health insurance coverage with the other survey questions results in: 1) a reduction in the estimates of the number of individuals without health insurance; and 2) increases in the number of children with health insurance. It should be noted that this change in the questionnaire means that estimates of health insurance coverage prior to 1987 are not comparable to those in subsequent years. Additionally, responses to the added questions have resulted in inconsistent response patterns for some individuals. That is, for one series of health insurance questions a respondent may report no Medicaid coverage, but for the other questions the same respondent may say they have coverage. The estimates contained in this appendix were prepared under the assumption that a positive response to any health insurance question means the individual has that health insurance coverage (even if in a subsequent response they say they do not have the coverage).

Finally, the CPS estimates contained in this appendix are based on a national sample. As a result they will differ from the figures that would have been obtained if a census had been taken. Since the figures are based on a sample they should be considered estimates and some degree of sampling error is associated with them. Generally, the degree of error associated with the estimates increases as the number of respondents in a category decreases.

APPENDIX B. MEDICAID AND MATERNAL AND CHILD HEALTH[1]

SUMMARY

Since the mid-1980s, Medicaid eligibility has been expanded gradually to enhance access to services to pregnant women and children. The link between Medicaid and welfare has been severed for this population; recently established eligibility standards now apply in all States and the District of Columbia. All pregnant women and children to age 6 with incomes up to 133 percent of the Federal poverty level are now eligible for Medicaid. An infant born to a woman eligible for Medicaid is eligible for services throughout the first year of life so long as the child is in the mother's household and the mother would be eligible if she were pregnant. Other Medicaid reforms expand eligibility for older children on a nationwide basis. Children to age 19 in families with incomes up to 100 percent of the Federal poverty level are eligible for Medicaid if they were born after September 30, 1983. Thus, all poor children will be eligible for Medicaid in the year 2002.

Although congressional interest has centered on reducing financial barriers to medical care, there have been concerns that mere extension of Medicaid coverage may not ensure that all mothers and children will receive appropriate services. Other actions have been taken to simplify the Medicaid application process and remove non-financial barriers to access to services. Some of these actions address problems of a shortage of providers available to serve this population.

Although data are not presently available to evaluate the effects of recent Medicaid changes, they are believed to have resulted in significant progress toward eliminating barriers to health care for mothers and children.

Changes made to the early and periodic screening, diagnostic, and treatment program (EPSDT) for Medicaid-eligible individuals under age 21 were designed to allow children to receive treatment for conditions detected in screening.

Beyond the prenatal and routine preventive and primary care, Medicaid offers special services to children who are chronically ill or disabled.

Efforts have been made to coordinate Medicaid eligibility and benefits with those of the other major sources of Federal support for perinatal and child

---

[1]This appendix was written by Melvina Ford.

61-899 O—93——26

health care. The maternal and child health block grant program, the special supplemental food program for women, infants, and children, and community and migrant health centers all play a role in providing services to poor women and children.

I. HEALTH STATUS OF PREGNANT WOMEN AND CHILDREN

Health care for pregnant women, infants, and children has been a subject of congressional interest for decades. Major factors contributing to this interest in the 1980s have been: (1) failure to meet 1990 national health objectives for maternal and child health, (2) concern over the Nation's infant mortality rate and the relatively high costs of poor pregnancy outcomes vis a vis prenatal care, (3) the number of individuals who lack health insurance and financial access to health care, and (4) the immunization status of young children--brought to national attention by outbreaks of preventable diseases.

In 1980, the U.S. Public Health Service (PHS) issued 226 objectives for improving health and reducing health risks in the United States by the year 1990. The goals for maternal and child health reflected general indicators of the health of the country and the care of children. Infant mortality rate is often used as an indicator of the general health of a Nation's population; immunization status of children is often used as an indicator of the overall adequacy of child health care. PHS objectives for maternal and child health included reducing the infant mortality rate to 9 deaths per 1,000 live births, and reducing the incidence of low birthweight (referring to infants born weighing less than 5.5 pounds) to 5 percent of all live births. Objectives for child health included reducing reported cases of measles to under 500 per year, and completion by 90 percent of American children, of the basic childhood immunization series by age 2. The basic series includes vaccinations against such diseases as measles and whooping cough. By 1985, it was clear that these objectives for improving the health of mothers, infants, and children could not be reached by 1990.

In 1990, the infant mortality rate in the United States was 9.1 deaths in the first year of life per 1,000 live births. This rate was the lowest ever, but higher than the rates of many other industrialized countries. For minorities, and residents of inner cities and some rural areas, rates are considerably higher. The 1990 rates in some cities exceeded 20 deaths per 1,000 live births. A leading contributor to infant death is low birthweight. In 1990, the low birthweight rate for the country was 6.9 percent, the same rate observed in 1980 and slightly higher than the rate of 6.8 percent in 1989. Low birthweight infants are 40 times more likely to die in the first month of life than larger babies. Among those who survive, there are concerns for lasting illness and permanent disability. There is evidence that prenatal care is an important factor in pregnancy outcomes. Women who receive continuing prenatal care that is begun early in pregnancy are about half as likely to bear low birthweight babies than other women. Several studies have found the cost of providing comprehensive prenatal care to be considerably less than the cost of providing medical care associated with poor birth outcome. The Institute of Medicine

(IOM) estimated in 1985 that, for every $1 spent on prenatal care, $3.38 could be saved in costs of care for a low birthweight infant.[2] The U.S. Office of Technology Assessment (OTA) estimated that $14,000 to $30,000 could be saved for every low birthweight birth averted.[3]

Although 95 percent of American children entering school or enrolled in licensed child care centers are fully immunized against preventable childhood diseases, immunization rates among children of preschool age are considerably lower. The Centers for Disease Control (CDC) estimates that only 70 percent to 80 percent of children under age 2 have received the full series of childhood immunizations. Rates in some inner city and rural areas are estimated to be only 40 percent to 50 percent. These immunization rates of American children under age 2 compare unfavorably with rates of young children in other developed countries. For example, 100 percent of 1 year old children in Denmark, and 98 percent of 1 year olds in Sweden and Switzerland have been fully immunized against polio. The percentages of 1 year old children who are fully immunized against polio drop to 96 percent in Hong Kong, Mexico, and North Korea.[4]

The major health care needs of pregnant women and young children are primary and preventive care, including prenatal care, to prevent the occurrence of mortality and morbidity, detect problems in early presymptomatic stages, and to provide treatment that can prevent complications of illness. The American College of Obstetricians and Gynecologists recommends that prenatal care begin as early in pregnancy as possible and consist of 13 visits for a normal 40-week pregnancy.[5] From birth through adolescence, most children need regular, routine preventive health care that includes screening, immunizations, anticipatory guidance, and health education. Some children need care and treatment for acute episodes while other children need services for chronic illnesses. Over the last few years, Medicaid eligibility and service coverage rules have been altered to help States address these needs.

National health promotion and disease prevention objectives have been set for the year 2000. 2000 objectives for maternal and child health include:

- reduce the infant mortality rate to 7 per 1,000 live births;
- reduce low birthweight to 5 percent of live births;

---

[2]Institute of Medicine. *Preventing Low Birthweight*. National Academy Press. Washington, 1985.

[3]U.S. Congress. Office of Technology Assessment. *Healthy Children: Investing in the Future*. Washington, GPO, Feb. 1988. p. 85.

[4]These data attributed to UNICEF were reported in *The Health of America's Children*, Children's Defense Fund, Washington, 1991.

[5]American College of Obstetricians and Gynecologists. *Standards for Obstetric-Gynecologic Services*. Washington, 1989. 7th edition.

- increase to 90 percent the proportion of women who receive prenatal care in the first trimester of pregnancy;
- increase to 90 percent the proportion of infants who receive routine care; and
- increase to 90 percent the proportion of 2 year olds who have received appropriate immunization services.[6]

Medicaid will be a major factor in achieving the Nation's objectives for 2000.

II. THE ROLE OF MEDICAID

Surveys conducted by the Alan Guttmacher Institute indicate that in 1985 630,000 deliveries, 17 percent of all births in the United States, were covered by Medicaid.[7] [8] There are no data that show how many of these women were covered by Medicaid prior to delivery. There is evidence that pregnant women who are covered by Medicaid get insufficient prenatal care, but better prenatal care than women who are uninsured.

In a 1987 study, the U.S. General Accounting Office (GAO) found that privately insured women generally began prenatal care earlier and made more visits for care than Medicaid beneficiaries or uninsured women. However, Medicaid beneficiaries began care earlier and made more visits than the uninsured. The American Academy of Pediatrics (AAP) and the American College of Obstetricians and Gynecologists (ACOG) recommend that prenatal care begin as early in pregnancy as possible; with an uncomplicated pregnancy, they recommend that a woman be examined approximately every 4 weeks for the first 28 weeks of pregnancy, and more frequently thereafter.[9]

Table B-1 shows the trimester in which prenatal care began for Medicaid beneficiaries and uninsured women in the GAO study. As shown on table B-2, more of the Medicaid beneficiaries than uninsured women in the GAO study made the recommended number of prenatal visits; fewer of the Medicaid beneficiaries had the lowest number of visits. Overall, GAO found that 81 percent of privately insured, 36 percent of Medicaid beneficiaries, and 32 percent of uninsured women obtained adequate prenatal care. Of the babies born to the

---

[6]U.S. Dept. of Health and Human Services. Public Health Service. *Healthy People 2000: National Healthy Promotion and Disease Prevention Objectives.* DHHS Publication No. (PHS) 91-50212. Washington, 1991.

[7]Gold, Rachel Benson, Asta-Marie Kenney, and Susheela Singh. *Blessed Events and the Bottom Line,* The Alan Guttmacher Institute, 1987.

[8]At present, more recent data are not available on the numbers of pregnancies or deliveries supported by Medicaid. However, States have been required to collect such information and report annually beginning with fiscal year 1991.

[9]American Academy of Pediatrics and American College of Obstetricians and Gynecologists. *Guidelines for Perinatal Care, Third Edition.* Washington, 1992.

women interviewed by GAO, 12.4 percent were of low birthweight.[10] In this study, the most commonly cited barrier to early and frequent prenatal care was lack of money to pay for the care.

About 11 million children under age 21 are covered by Medicaid. Children who are covered by health insurance are more likely than others to have routine doctor visits and a regular source of health care. Since the enactment of the Medicaid program, utilization of health care services by poor children has approximated that of nonpoor children.[11] As shown in figure B-1, poor children are more likely to obtain timely routine care if they have Medicaid coverage.

---

[10]U.S. Congress. General Accounting Office. *Prenatal Care: Medicaid Recipients and Uninsured Women Obtain Insufficient Care*. GAO/HRD-87-137, Sept. 1987. Washington, 1987.

[11]Budetti, Peter P., John Butler, and Peggy McManus. Federal Health Program Reforms: Implications for Child Health Care, *Milbank Memorial Fund Quarterly*, v. 60, no. 1, winter 1982.

TABLE B-1. Time of First Prenatal Visit by Medicaid Beneficiaries and Uninsured Women, 1986 to 1987

(Number and percent of women by trimester in which care began)

Insurance status	Trimester of pregnancy:								Total
	First		Second		Third		No care		
	Number of women	Percent	Number of women	Percent	Number of women	Percent	Number of women	Percent	
Medicaid	301	49.8	244	40.3	54	8.9	6	1.0	605
Uninsured	221	40.0	235	42.6	72	13.0	24	4.3	522
Total	522	45.1	479	41.4	126	10.9	30	2.6	1,157

NOTE: Estimates include pregnancies with self-reported medical complications. Specifically, the first trimester includes 190 such cases, second trimester includes 147 such cases, third trimester includes 34 such cases, and no care includes 2 such cases.

TABLE B-2. Number of Prenatal Visits by Medicaid Beneficiaries and Uninsured Women, 1986 to 1987

(Number and percent of women by range of visits)

Insurance status	Number of visits:								Total
	Less than 4 visits		5 to 8 visits		9 to 12 visits		13 or more		
	Number of women	Percent	Number of women	Percent	Number of women	Percent	Number of women	Percent	
Medicaid	68	11.2	153	25.3	197	32.6	187	30.9	605
Uninsured	106	19.2	124	22.4	179	32.4	143	25.9	522
Total	174	15.0	277	23.9	376	32.5	330	28.5	1,157

NOTE: Estimates include pregnancies with self-reported medical complications. Specifically, less than 4 visits includes 30 such cases, 5-8 visits includes 63 such cases, 9-12 includes 123 such cases and 13+ includes 157 such cases. It should also be noted that in 30 cases no prenatal visits took place. These 30 cases: 6 by Medicaid women and 24 by the uninsured are contained in the less than 4 visit category.

Source: U.S. General Accounting Office. *Prenatal Care: Medicaid Recipients and Uninsured Women Obtain Insufficient Care*, Sept. 1987, appendix VII, table VII.1, p. 110; and appendix VI, table VI.1, p. 108.

FIGURE B-1. Share of Children Receiving Timely Routine Care,
by Health Insurance and Poverty Status, 1988

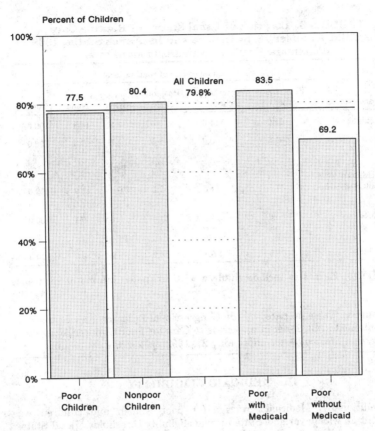

Source: Figure prepared by Congressional Research Service based on St. Peter, et al.,
Access to Care for Poor Children, *Journal of the American Medical Association,*
May 27, 1992, p. 2762.

Table B-3 shows the location of usual sources of routine care. Poor children with Medicaid are far less likely to lack a source of routine care than poor children without Medicaid. However, poor children are far less likely to receive routine care in a physician's office. This may reflect the shortage of private physicians in inner city areas and some rural areas.

TABLE B-3. Location of Usual Source of Routine Care for Children under 18, by Income and Insurance Status, 1988
(Percentage of children with usual routine care)

Insurance status	Usual source of routine care					
	Physician office	Community clinic	Hospital clinic	Other	None	Total
Poor children	52.0	14.6	9.6	8.9	14.8	100.0
Nonpoor children	81.5	3.2	3.0	4.5	7.9	100.0
Poor children without Medicaid	47.3	14.5	7.3	9.0	21.9	100.0
Poor children with Medicaid	55.9	14.7	11.5	8.8	9.1	100.0
All children	75.5	5.5	4.2	5.2	9.6	100.0

NOTE: Estimates include children with unknown income or insurance status.

Source: Table prepared by the Congressional Research Service based on data contained in St. Peter et al. Access to Care for Poor Children, *Journal of the American Medical Association*, May 27, 1992. p. 2763.

III. MEDICAID ELIGIBILITY

Traditionally, Medicaid coverage for poor women and children was dependent on widely variable State income eligibility thresholds. In all States, women and children who received cash welfare benefits under the Aid to Families with Dependent Children (AFDC) program were automatically eligible for Medicaid. In many States however, women were not eligible for AFDC unless they already had children. Some poor children were ineligible for AFDC because they did not meet the categorical definition of "dependency". Such children may have lived in two-parent families, or they may have been in foster homes or institutions. For individuals who were eligible, services varied according to the limitations that States imposed on amount, scope, and duration of services as well as differences in services States chose to cover beyond the federally required minimum.

Between 1975 and 1988, the average AFDC income eligibility threshold fell from 71.4 percent of poverty to 48 percent of poverty for a family of three.[12] In January 1992, the average AFDC income threshold for a family of three was 43.6 percent of the Federal poverty level.[13] During the 1980s Congress acted to sever the link between cash welfare and Medicaid eligibility for poor pregnant women, infants, and children. Over several years of targeted expansion, Medicaid has become a major source of federally supported maternal and child health care.

- OBRA 86 permitted States to extend Medicaid eligibility to poor pregnant women and infants with family incomes above AFDC levels but below a State established level up to 100 percent of the Federal poverty level.

- OBRA 87 permitted States to extend Medicaid coverage to pregnant women and infants with household incomes up to 185 percent of the Federal poverty level. The 1987 Act also permitted immediate coverage for children up to age 5 with household incomes up to 100 percent of poverty.

- The Medicare Catastrophic Coverage Act of 1988 (MCCA) required States to cover pregnant women and infants with incomes below 100 percent of poverty.

- OBRA 89 superseded the expansions mandated by MCCA. It required States to provide Medicaid coverage to pregnant women and children to age 6 from households with incomes up to 133 percent of poverty ($15,388 for a family of 3 in 1992).[14]

- OBRA 90 required States to phase in Medicaid coverage of children to age 19, born after September 30, 1983, in families with incomes under 100 percent of the Federal poverty level.

As of January 1992, 22 States and the District of Columbia covered pregnant women and infants up to the optional maximum 185 percent level; 6 other States covered pregnant women and infants at levels above the minimum 133 percent but below the maximum income level allowed. The income levels applicable to pregnant women and infants in each State are shown on table B-4.

---

[12]National Commission to Prevent Infant Mortality. *Death Before Life: The Tragedy of Infant Mortality*. Appendix. Washington, 1988. (Hereafter cited as National Commission to Prevent Infant Mortality, *Death Before Life*)

[13]National Governors' Association. MCH Update: State Coverage of Pregnant Women and Children, Jan. 1992.

[14]In the 1992 HHS poverty guidelines for all States (except Alaska and Hawaii) and the District of Columbia, the poverty guideline for a family of three is $11,570.

Recently, States have begun to take advantage of a provision now termed the 1902(r)(2) option. Enacted in 1988, the provision specifies that the income and resource methodology used in determining eligibility of pregnant women and children may be less restrictive, and shall be no more restrictive than the methodology under the most closely related eligibility category.

For pregnant women and children, the most closely related cash assistance program is AFDC. In determining financial eligibility for AFDC, States are required to disregard certain income and resources. Determinations are made on the basis of "countable" income--income that remains after disregards have been applied. Because of the disregards, individuals may qualify for Medicaid even though gross household income is higher than the eligibility threshold.

States can extend Medicaid benefits to people who would not otherwise be eligible by allowing various disregards that are not used in AFDC determinations. For example, States may disregard parental income of pregnant teens who live with their parents, or disregard a State-established amount for child care expenses. Since January 1992, the State of Washington has disregarded all income over the AFDC payment standard but under the Federal poverty line to offer Medicaid eligibility to an additional 9,000 children in the State. In July 1993, Minnesota plans to begin disregarding percentages of the Federal poverty level so that pregnant women and children to age 19 will be eligible for Medicaid if their family incomes are under 275 percent of poverty.[15]

---

[15]Fox, Harriette B. The Section 1902(r)(2) Option to Provide Medicaid Eligibility to Additional Children and Pregnant Women, memorandum to State Maternal and Child Health Program Directors, State Directors of Programs for Children with Special Health Needs, State Medicaid Directors, and Other Interested Parties, July 27, 1992.

**TABLE B-4. Optional Income Eligibility Thresholds for
Pregnant Women and Infants, January 1992**

State	Optional income eligibility level as a share of Federal poverty guideline
Alabama	NA
Alaska	NA
Arizona[a]	140
Arkansas	185
California	185
Colorado	NA
Connecticut	185
Delaware	160
District of Columbia	185
Florida	150
Georgia	NA
Hawaii	185
Idaho	NA
Illinois	NA
Indiana	150
Iowa	185
Kansas	150
Kentucky	185
Louisiana	NA
Maine	185
Maryland	185
Massachusetts	185
Michigan	185
Minnesota	185
Mississippi	185
Missouri	NA
Montana	NA
Nebraska	NA
Nevada	NA
New Hampshire	NA
New Jersey	185
New Mexico	185
New York	185
North Carolina	185

See notes at end of table.

TABLE B-4. Optional Income Eligibility Thresholds for Pregnant Women and Infants, January 1992--Continued

State	Optional income eligibility level as a share of Federal poverty guideline
North Dakota	NA
Ohio	NA
Oklahoma	NA
Oregon	NA
Pennsylvania	NA
Rhode Island	185
South Carolina	185
South Dakota	NA
Tennessee	185
Texas	185
Utah	NA
Vermont	185
Virginia	NA
Washington	185
West Virginia	150
Wisconsin	155
Wyoming	NA

*Arizona provides Medicaid services through a waiver program.

NOTE: NA = Not applicable. These States did not use eligibility option in Jan. 1992.

Source: National Governors' Association, 1992.

Amendments to Medicaid law severed the link between welfare and Medicaid eligibility, gradually expanded the number of pregnant women and children State Medicaid programs are permitted and required to cover, and established a uniform income floor among States in coverage of this population. However, eligibility expansion did not guarantee access to appropriate health care.

The process for determining eligibility may have been a barrier to receipt of Medicaid benefits. Lengthy application forms used for the cash welfare programs require extensive documentation and substantiation of income, assets, family composition, and other details. The complexity and the processing time could have discouraged many from filing an application unless there were serious health problems. Denials of eligibility due to failure to comply with procedural requirements (e.g., keeping appointments or completing forms) have been more common than denials for excess income or resources.[16] A deterrent to applying for Medicaid that has been mentioned by some observers is the welfare stigma associated with applying only for health care benefits in welfare offices.[17]

Initiatives were instituted to overcome these liabilities.

Optional assets tests. Under an option provided by OBRA 86, 48 States have dropped asset or resource tests from determinations of poverty-related eligibility for pregnant women and children. Without asset tests, the application and documentation requirements are simplified and there is less chance that applications will be rejected for failure to comply with AFDC procedures and documentation requirements. Dropping asset tests ensures that low-income pregnant women and children in families with modest resources are not denied coverage.

Presumptive eligibility. To enable early entry and continuity in prenatal care, OBRA 86 established the presumptive eligibility option under which certain providers, such as federally qualified health centers or local health departments, may make a preliminary determination that a low-income pregnant woman is potentially eligible for Medicaid. The woman may then receive immediate ambulatory services related to the pregnancy with a guarantee that providers will be reimbursed. Presumptive eligibility status ends on the last day of the month following the month in which the presumptive determination is made if the woman does not file a formal Medicaid application in that time. Otherwise, a presumptive eligibility period ends on the date on which a final eligibility determination is made. If a woman is ultimately determined ineligible for Medicaid coverage, reimbursement is made for prenatal services furnished by a qualified provider during the presumptive eligibility period.

---

[16]National Commission to Prevent Infant Mortality, *Death Before Life.*

[17]National Forum on the Future of Children and Families. *Including Children and Pregnant Women in Health Care Reform.* Washington, National Academy Press, 1992.

In the first year of its availability, the presumptive eligibility option was used by only seven States. By January 1992, 26 States were using the option with a simple form developed for completion by a provider. Originally, Medicaid law required that a woman make a formal application for Medicaid eligibility within 14 days after a presumptive eligibility determination was made. States noted that because women were not following through with regular applications for Medicaid, there was a poor ratio of conversions to full eligibility. OBRA 90 amended Medicaid law to allow the longer filing time stated above. It is difficult to determine the level of conversions from presumptive eligibility to full eligibility because some women determined presumptively eligible for Medicaid were found later to be eligible for AFDC cash benefits. These women were not counted among conversions.

Some States may be reluctant to establish presumptive eligibility programs because of other changes that need to be made in their Medicaid operations. Qualified providers must be designated and trained to determine presumptive eligibility. Computer systems have to be modified to pay the qualified providers for ambulatory prenatal care services furnished to individuals who are presumptively eligible. Some States may have found it easier to expedite formal Medicaid applications and/or shorten the forms used for them.

Outstationed eligibility workers. Some low-income women may not be aware that Medicaid coverage is available to them, or may find it difficult to arrange work or household schedules to visit a welfare office to apply. Potential beneficiaries are reported to be alienated, and deterred from participating, by the stigma associated with welfare offices. OBRA 90 requires States to accept and begin processing applications from pregnant women and children under 18 at locations other than those used for receipt and processing of cash assistance applications, including federally qualified health centers and disproportionate share hospitals. This allows women to apply for Medicaid coverage at the places they receive care, such as local health departments, hospital prenatal programs, or community health centers.

A determination made by an outstationed eligibility worker at a health service site differs from the presumptive eligibility determination which results in temporary Medicaid coverage for ambulatory services. The former permits a final eligibility determination to be made on the basis of information given at the provider's location, and does not require that an applicant make subsequent contact with a welfare office.

Mail-in applications. Some States have eliminated the need for a personal interview with an eligibility worker when applying for Medicaid coverage. These States allow the completion of eligibility applications for pregnant women and children by mail and telephone.

Shortened application form. With the elimination of assets tests from eligibility considerations, States were able to reduce applications to collect only the information needed for poverty-related eligibility for pregnant women and children. Instead of using the lengthy complex application form that may be used for cash assistance programs, 33 States use a shortened application form for pregnant women and children who are eligible for Medicaid solely due to family income. The shorter form can be more easily completed by applicants and processed by agencies, thereby potentially reducing the time for eligibility determination.

Expedited eligibility systems. To avoid the long processing time in eligibility determinations, some States assign priority to processing applications made on behalf of poverty-related pregnant women. Priorities take effect after all required documentation has been submitted.

Continuation of benefits. This provision guarantees Medicaid coverage throughout a pregnancy. Ordinarily, a Medicaid beneficiary can lose eligibility in any month in which family income exceeds a State's income standards. States were permitted to continue coverage for a pregnant woman through the end of the second full month beginning after the end of her pregnancy, even if the woman would otherwise become ineligible during that period. OBRA 90 converted this option to a mandate except in the case of a woman who was provided ambulatory care during a presumptive eligibility period and was subsequently found to be ineligible. After regular Medicaid eligibility has been established, a pregnant woman is deemed to continue to be eligible as a poverty-related beneficiary throughout her pregnancy and postpartum period regardless of a change in income.

An infant born to a woman eligible for and receiving Medicaid remains eligible throughout the first year of life so long as the child remains in the mother's household and the mother remains eligible for Medicaid, or would be eligible if she were pregnant. So that coverage will not be denied until the mother informs her local welfare office of the birth of a child, Medicaid statute requires that the mother's Medicaid eligibility identification number serve as the child's identification number unless a separate number is issued.

Newborn referral form. To facilitate the issuance of a separate identification number for an infant, some States provide hospitals with referral forms. After a Medicaid beneficiary delivers, the hospital in which she delivers completes a referral form and sends it to the appropriate local agency. This practice is intended to assure that the infant's eligibility is in place for a full year instead of terminating with the mother's eligibility after the allowed post partum period.

Hospital services for infants. State Medicaid programs may limit the number of covered inpatient hospital days. (See *Chapter V, Reimbursement.*) For infants up to age 1 in any hospital, and children up to age 6 in hospitals that serve a disproportionate number of low-income persons, States are prohibited from imposing durational limits for medically necessary services. States with prospective payment systems (under which payment rates are established in advance and may not reflect the hospital's actual costs for covered services) are required to provide for an adjustment in payment amounts for medically necessary services involving exceptionally high costs or exceptionally long lengths of stay. These requirements protect services to premature infants and older children with catastrophic conditions. States may not impose dollar limits on inpatient hospital services to infants up to age 1. If an infant is in the hospital when the first birthday is reached, the prohibition applies until the child is discharged.

Table B-5 shows the strategies each State is using to streamline the eligibility process for pregnant women, infants, and children.

TABLE B-5. Strategies to Streamline State Eligibility, by State, in Effect as of January 1992

State	Dropped assets test	Presumptive eligibility	Shortened application[a]	Expedited eligibility	Mail-in eligibility	Newborn referral form
			Type of strategy:			
Alabama	Yes		Yes	Yes	Yes	
Alaska	Yes			Yes	Yes	
Arizona[b]	Yes			Yes		
Arkansas	Yes	Yes	Yes			Yes
California						
Colorado	Yes	Yes	Yes		Yes	Yes
Connecticut	Yes	Yes			Yes	
Delaware	Yes		Yes			
District of Columbia	Yes	Yes				Yes
Florida	Yes	Yes	Yes			
Georgia	Yes		Yes	Yes	Yes	Yes
Hawaii	Yes	Yes	Yes		Yes	Yes
Idaho	Yes	Yes	Yes			
Illinois	Yes[c]	Yes	Yes			

See notes at end of table.

TABLE B-5. Strategies to Streamline State Eligibility, by State, in Effect as of January 1992–Continued

State	Dropped assets test	Presumptive eligibility	Shortened application[a]	Type of strategy: Expedited eligibility	Mail-in eligibility	Newborn referral form
Indiana	Yes		Yes		Yes	
Iowa		Yes	Yes[c]			
Kansas	Yes			Yes		
Kentucky	Yes		Yes		Yes	Yes
Louisiana	Yes	Yes	Yes			Yes
Maine	Yes	Yes			Yes	
Maryland	Yes	Yes	Yes			Yes
Massachusetts	Yes	Yes	Yes		Yes	Yes
Michigan	Yes		Yes		Yes	
Minnesota	Yes		Yes	Yes	Yes	
Mississippi	Yes		Yes			
Missouri	Yes	Yes	Yes			
Montana	Yes	Yes				

See notes at end of table.

TABLE B-5. Strategies to Streamline State Eligibility, by State, in Effect as of January 1992--Continued

State	Type of strategy:					
	Dropped assets test	Presumptive eligibility	Shortened application[a]	Expedited eligibility	Mail-in eligibility	Newborn referral form
Nebraska	Yes	Yes			Yes	
Nevada	Yes					
New Hampshire	Yes					
New Jersey	Yes	Yes	Yes			
New Mexico	Yes	Yes	Yes		Yes	
New York	Yes	Yes				
North Carolina	Yes	Yes	Yes	Yes		
North Dakota					Yes	
Ohio	Yes		Yes	Yes	Yes	
Oklahoma	Yes	Yes				
Oregon	Yes		Yes	Yes		
Pennsylvania	Yes	Yes				Yes
Rhode Island	Yes					Yes

See notes at end of table.

TABLE B-5. Strategies to Streamline State Eligibility, by State, in Effect as of January 1992—Continued

State	Dropped assets test	Presumptive eligibility	Shortened application[a]	Expedited eligibility	Mail-in eligibility	Newborn referral form
South Carolina	Yes		Yes		Yes	Yes
South Dakota	Yes		Yes			
Tennessee	Yes	Yes	Yes		Yes	Yes
Texas	Yes[c]	Yes	Yes			
Utah	Yes	Yes			Yes	
Vermont	Yes		Yes	Yes	Yes	Yes
Virginia	Yes		Yes	Yes	Yes	
Washington	Yes		Yes	Yes	Yes	
West Virginia	Yes		Yes	Yes	Yes	
Wisconsin	Yes	Yes	Yes	Yes		
Wyoming	Yes					
Total States using strategy	48	26	33	14	23	14

[a] In some States (e.g., New York) applicants are instructed to eliminate parts of the standard form in lieu of a shortened form. This information may not be reflected in the table.

[b] Arizona's Medicaid program operates under a demonstration program.

[c] State plans to implement strategy in the future.

Source: National Governors' Association. Jan. 1992.

IV. REDUCING NON-FINANCIAL BARRIERS TO CARE

Providing insurance coverage through Medicaid is necessary, but not sufficient to assure that pregnant women and children receive comprehensive and preventive health care. For many, limited Medicaid program participation of obstetricians and pediatricians is a barrier to appropriate and timely care. Some potential beneficiaries are not aware that subsidized care and benefits are available to them. Medicaid law has been amended to address the shortage of private providers available to serve pregnant women and children who are eligible for Medicaid. Some States have instituted outreach campaigns to identify potential eligibles and assist them in applying for benefits.

A. Providers

Practitioners. Obstetrician/gynecologists have historically had low rates of Medicaid participation. With recent changes in the profession, some of these specialists have ceased obstetrical practice altogether, some have reduced the high-risk obstetrical care they will perform, and some have reduced their overall number of deliveries.[18] These changes have had a profound effect on the availability of care to low-income pregnant women during the same period that Medicaid has expanded eligibility for them. Pediatricians have historically had relatively high rates of Medicaid participation. However, between 1978 and 1989, the percentage of pediatricians who did not care for children enrolled in Medicaid increased from 15 percent to 23 percent.[19] Observers generally agree that low Medicaid payment is a barrier to physicians' participation. However, many believe that fee increases would not substantially influence participation because other factors may be more important. For obstetricians, the cost of malpractice insurance is seen as a major reason for nonparticipation. For physicians in general, there are administrative issues such as billing complexities and payment delays. Finally, there is a perception of Medicaid patients as high risk individuals who do not keep appointments well, and are more likely than other patients to sue their providers. This perception persists despite the lack of supportive data. The Office of Technology Assessment (OTA) examined the available evidence and concluded that Medicaid patients do not sue more, and may sue less than would be expected.[20] Concern about an inadequate supply of providers has led to mandatory coverage of services furnished by a variety of qualified providers, as well as special attention to payment levels for the specialists whose services are most needed by pregnant women and children.

---

[18]James W. Fossett et al. Medicaid Patients' Access to Office-Based Obstetricians. *Journal of Health Care for the Poor and Underserved,* v. 1, no. 4, spring 1991.

[19]B.K. Yudkowsky, Cartland, J.D.C., and Flint, S.S. Pediatrician Participation in Medicaid: 1978 to 1989. *Pediatrics,* v. 85, no. 4, Apr. 1990.

[20]Herdman, Roger, Clyde J. Behney, and Judith L. Wagner. Do Medicaid and Medicare Patients Sue Physicians More Often than Other Patients? U.S. Office of Technology Assessment.

If State law authorizes such providers to practice, State Medicaid programs are required to cover services furnished by a nurse-midwife, a certified pediatric nurse practitioner, or a certified family nurse practitioner, whether or not the provider is under the supervision of, or associated with, a physician or other health care provider. The HHS Office of Inspector General reports that 49 States and the District of Columbia are using certified nurse midwives to deliver Medicaid-covered prenatal care; 42 States use nurse practitioners, and 33 States use physicians' assistants. The States that cover services by alternative providers of prenatal care under Medicaid are shown in table B-6.[21]

---

[21]U.S. Dept. of Health and Human Services. Office of Inspector General. *Medicaid Expansions for Prenatal Care: State and Local Implementation*, OEI-06-90-00160, 1991.

TABLE B-6. States Using Alternative Providers of Prenatal Care
Covered under Medicaid, as of September 1990

State	Certified nurse midwives	Nurse practitioners	Physicians' assistants
Alabama	Yes	No	No
Alaska	Yes	Yes	Yes
Arizona	Yes	Yes	Yes
Arkansas	Yes	No	Yes
California[a]	Yes	Yes	Yes
Colorado	Yes	Yes	Yes
Connecticut	Yes	Yes	Yes
Delaware	Yes	Yes	No
District of Columbia	Yes	No	No
Florida	Yes	Yes	No
Georgia	Yes	Yes	No
Hawaii	Yes	No	No
Idaho	Yes	Yes	Yes
Illinois	Yes	No	No
Indiana	Yes	No	No
Iowa	Yes	Yes	Yes
Kansas	No	Yes	Yes
Kentucky	Yes	Yes	Yes
Louisiana	Yes	Yes	Yes
Maine	Yes	Yes	Yes
Maryland	Yes	Yes	No
Massachusetts	Yes	Yes	No
Michigan	Yes	Yes	Yes
Minnesota	Yes	Yes	Yes
Mississippi	Yes	Yes	No
Missouri	Yes	Yes	No
Montana	Yes	Yes	Yes
Nebraska	Yes	Yes	Yes

See notes at end of table.

TABLE B-6. States Using Alternative Providers of Prenatal Care Covered under Medicaid, as of September 1990--Continued

State	Certified nurse midwives	Nurse practitioners	Physicians' assistants
Nevada	Yes	Yes	No
New Hampshire	Yes	Yes	Yes
New Jersey	Yes	No	No
New Mexico	Yes	Yes	Yes
New York	Yes	Yes	Yes
North Carolina	Yes	Yes	Yes
North Dakota	Yes	Yes	Yes
Ohio	Yes	Yes	Yes
Oklahoma	Yes	Yes	No
Oregon	Yes	Yes	Yes
Pennsylvania	Yes	Yes	Yes
Rhode Island	Yes	Yes	Yes
South Carolina	Yes	Yes	No
South Dakota	Yes	Yes	Yes
Tennessee	Yes	Yes	Yes
Texas	Yes	No	Yes
Utah	Yes	No	Yes
Vermont	Yes	Yes	Yes
Virginia	Yes	Yes	No
Washington	Yes	Yes	Yes
West Virginia	Yes	Yes	Yes
Wisconsin	Yes	Yes	Yes
Wyoming	Yes	Yes	No

ªCalifornia did not respond to the Office of Inspector General survey. Information was obtained by telephone from the California Office of Medicaid in August 1992. It should be noted that in California services provided by certified nurse midwives in independent practice are covered under Medicaid, while Medicaid coverage of services provided by nurse practitioners and physicians' assistants is limited to those operating in a physician group practice, clinic or individual physician practice.

NOTE: States may limit services to those supervised by a physician.

Source: Table prepared by the Congressional Research Service based on information from the Office of Inspector General, DHHS. Data are self-reported from State officials responsible for implementing eligibility expansions for Medicaid-covered prenatal care.

OBRA 89 codified the regulatory requirement that payments must be sufficient to enlist enough providers so that covered services will be available to Medicaid beneficiaries at least to the extent they are available to the general population in a geographic area. States are required to submit to the Secretary their payment rates for pediatric and obstetrical services along with additional data that will assist the Secretary in evaluating the State's compliance with this requirement.

Federally qualified health centers. States are required to cover (and reimburse at reasonable cost) ambulatory services offered by federally qualified health centers.[22] Located in medically underserved areas where they must provide services to all who request them, federally qualified health centers are a major source of perinatal and child health care for the poor.

School-related health services. For several reasons, schools have been suggested as logical sites for the delivery of comprehensive, primary health services for children. Schools are located in rural and urban communities that may have few other health care facilities. They are seen as good sites for permanent records on health status, a relatively inexpensive setting for dental care, and a reasonable place to bring together teams of professionals concerned with improving child health. Finally, schools are where the children are for many hours each week.

School health programs vary widely. Traditionally, school health programs focused on health screening and control of communicable diseases. Since the 1970s, however, comprehensive health centers developed to serve school-aged populations have been providing medical, counseling, and family planning services to young people. In 1991, a total of 327 school-related clinics were identified as operating in the United States. The clinics may be sponsored by public health departments, school systems, hospitals, or other health care providers. It is likely that a large portion of the students receiving services in school-related clinics are uninsured and have no other regular source of medical care.[23]

Medicaid reimbursement may be available to physicians or other practitioners in school-related clinics. In some cases, the clinic is reimbursable as a satellite of a traditional Medicaid provider such as a hospital outpatient department or a community health center. Overall, however, Medicaid does not play a large role in financing these services. In a 1989 survey of 49 school-based clinics, 25 reported using Medicaid as a funding source; only 12 of those used

---

[22]A federally qualified health center is a migrant or community health center which receives a grant under section 329 or 330 of the Public Health Service Act (PHS), a center for health care for the homeless that receives a grant under section 340 of the PHS Act, or a center which has been determined by the Secretary to meet the requirements for such a grant.

[23]Pascale, Alisa. School-Based Clinics: The Facts. Center for Population Options, Washington, June 1990.

Medicaid "frequently."[24] Respondents to a 1991 national survey of school-related clinics said under 8 percent of their operating budgets was from reimbursement for EPSDT and other Medicaid services.[25] Considering that an estimated 30 percent of the children who receive services in school-related clinics are eligible for Medicaid, Medicaid funding for the clinics seems low. However, funding from private insurance and patient fees combined may be even less than from Medicaid. Some clinics do not charge for services, and some report that they do not receive dollars from any source but function entirely on in-kind contributions.[26]

Medicaid policies for reimbursing school-related health services vary by State. The Atlanta school system is a Medicaid provider; California created a provider category for schools to ensure access to Medicaid funds to finance school-based services. Other States may prohibit Medicaid payment for services delivered in schools, or require that a physician be on the premises at all times.[27]

B. Outreach Initiatives

Many women may be unaware that they, or their children, are eligible for health care covered by Medicaid. Outreach is not a covered Medicaid service. However, about 16 States have instituted focused outreach programs using administrative funding or private financial support. Programs may be targeted to special populations such as pregnant teenagers or substance abusers. Some programs use community members to seek out women in need of prenatal care.[28] To heighten awareness of the availability of prenatal care and the benefits of early and continuous care, some States use distinctive logos in client outreach materials and campaigns. Some outreach efforts use toll-free telephone numbers that women can use to identify providers of health care or get information on food assistance, nutrition services, or other community resources.

---

[24]Palfrey, Judith S., et.al. Financing Health Services in School-Based Clinics: Do Nontraditional Programs Tap Traditional Funding Sources? *Journal of Adolescent Health*, v. 12, no. 3, May 1991. p. 233-239.

[25]Waszak, C., and Shara Neidell. School-Based and School-Linked Clinics: Update 1991. Center for Population Options, Washington, 1990.

[26]Ibid.

[27]U.S. Congress. Office of Technology Assessment. *Adolescent Health, Volume I: Summary and Policy Options.* OTA-H-468, April 1991. Washington, 1991.

[28]Hill, Ian T. Improving State Medicaid programs for Pregnant Women and Children. *Health Care Financing Review,* 1990 Annual Supplement.

V. SERVICES AND EXPENDITURES

A. Pregnant Women

A pregnant woman eligible for Medicaid solely because of income level is entitled to services related to the pregnancy and complications of pregnancy, postpartum care for 60 days after the pregnancy ends, and family planning. Under waivers of comparability requirements, a State can offer an enhanced package of services to pregnant women without making the services available to all Medicaid beneficiaries. Additional services commonly include case management, health education, psychosocial assessment, or home visitation services.

Children who obtain poverty-related eligibility under Medicaid are entitled to the full range of Medicaid benefits. In addition, under the early and periodic screening, diagnostic and treatment program (EPSDT) for Medicaid beneficiaries under age 21, children may receive benefits that are not included in a State's plan. A discussion of EPSDT is in the next section of this appendix.

Data are not presently available for assessing the effect of recent Medicaid expansions for pregnant women and children. OBRA 89 amendments to Title V of the Social Security Act, the Maternal and Child Health Services Block Grant program, linked that program's activities to the year 2000 health objectives and provided for consistent planning and uniform reporting among States. New requirements are designed to allow policy makers to monitor progress toward meeting year 2000 objectives, and adjust targets and expenditures as needed. OBRA 89 requires each State to submit an application that contains a needs assessment which identifies the need for preventive and primary care services for pregnant women, mothers, and infants to age 1. OBRA 89 also requires States to submit annual reports that contain detailed information on the status of maternal and child health in the State. Some of the required information is specific to Medicaid benefits for pregnant women and infants.

States have not been able to provide complete information on either their applications or their annual reports. Observers say some States lack the expertise and skills to produce the information while other States lack electronic systems to gather and compile data.

The Health Care Financing Administration (HCFA) is working with the Public Health Service (PHS) to develop a national data system for linking infant birth, death, and Medicaid records for infants up to age 1. Also, HCFA has contracted for research to measure the effectiveness of the expansions using data from the mid-1980s to 1988-1990.[29]

---

[29]U.S. Dept. of Health and Human Services. Office of the Inspector General. Memorandum from Jo Anne B. Barnhart, DHHS Assistant Secretary for Children and Families, to Richard P. Kusserow, Aug. 13, 1991.

B. Children

Children have always made up the largest beneficiary group in the Medicaid program. In FY 1991 over 13 million children accounted for 46 percent of the Medicaid population. Payments for services to these children accounted for 15 percent of Medicaid payments ($11.6 billion). (See figures II-17 and II-15 in *Chapter II, Trends in Medicaid Payments and Beneficiaries*.) Most children require preventive care and episodic treatment for minor acute illnesses. Consequently, they use ambulatory services more than other services. However, inpatient hospital services, though used by a small portion of children, account for the largest share of Medicaid expenditures for children. Per capita payments for inpatient services are higher than for ambulatory services. Inpatient expenditures for infants may be higher than for older children due to extended hospital stays for some and income eligibility standards up to 185 percent of the poverty line in some States. Figure B-2 compares payments for children's use of selected Medicaid noninstitutional services to payments for those services to other beneficiary groups. Table B-7 shows the Medicaid payments for the same services for each of the beneficiary groups.

FIGURE B-2. Medicaid Payments for Selected Noninstitutional Services, by Eligibility Status, 1991

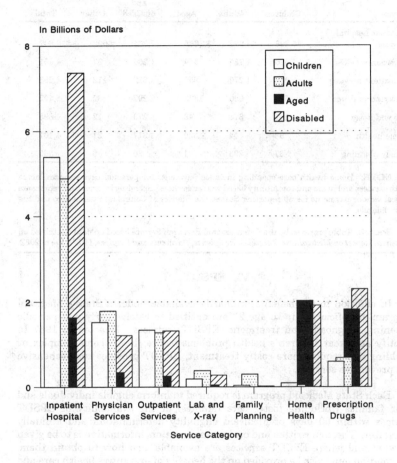

In Billions of Dollars

Legend:
□ Children
▦ Adults
■ Aged
▨ Disabled

Service categories: Inpatient Hospital, Physician Services, Outpatient Services, Lab and X-ray, Family Planning, Home Health, Prescription Drugs

Service Category

Source: Figure prepared by Congressional Research Service based on data from HCFA.

TABLE B-7. Total (Federal and State) Medical Vendor Payments
for Selected Noninstitutional Services, by Eligibility Status, 1991

| Service | Payments (in millions) | | | | | |
	Children	Adults	Aged	Blind and disabled	Other	Total
Inpatient hospital services	$5,396	$4,895	$1,635	$7,364	$602	$19,892
Physician services	1,520	1,785	344	1,206	97	4,951
Outpatient services	1,334	1,270	255	1,312	112	4,283
Prescription drugs	590	680	1823	2,297	32	5,422
Lab and x-ray	187	378	48	273	12	898
Home health	93	44	2,026	1,917	21	4,101
Family planning	37	296	1	20	6	360

NOTE: Home health care spending includes payments for personal care services, home health services and home and community based waiver services. Spending information represents medical vendor payments for 50 reporting States, the District of Columbia, Puerto Rico and the Virgin Islands.

Source: Table prepared by the Congressional Research Service based on data contained on *Statistical Report on Medical Care Eligibles, Recipients, Payments and Services*, HCFA Form 2082.

VI. EPSDT

In addition to the benefits ordinarily available under a State's Medicaid program, beneficiaries up to age 21 are entitled to receive early and periodic screening, diagnostic and treatment (EPSDT) services. Enacted in 1967 to identify and treat children's health problems before they become complex or disabling and require more costly treatment, EPSDT provides comprehensive and preventive services.

Each State Medicaid program is required to inform eligible individuals and their families (including foster care families) of the availability of EPSDT services within 60 days of Medicaid eligibility determination and annually thereafter. Through written and oral communication, information is to be given on what and where EPSDT services are available, and how to obtain them. Information must also be provided on the benefits of preventive health care and the availability of necessary transportation and scheduling assistance.

EPSDT is defined in Medicaid statute as four basic services: (1) screening, (2) vision, (3) dental, and (4) hearing services which are provided periodically according to standards of professional practice. Screening services include the following:

- comprehensive health (physical and mental) and developmental history;

- a comprehensive unclothed physical exam;

- appropriate immunizations according to age and health history;

- laboratory tests including lead blood levels as appropriate; and

- health education including anticipatory guidance.

Children who are found in screening to have conditions which need treatment, must be referred for treatment. In FY 1991, Federal and State payments for EPSDT services totalled nearly $356 million. EPSDT data do not reflect all examinations received by children enrolled in Medicaid as all States may reimburse for some health supervision services that are not billed as EPSDT services.

OBRA 89 changed several EPSDT provisions effective April 1, 1990. These changes expand the number of screens a child may receive before age 21, the intervals at which screens occur, the eligible providers who may perform an EPSDT screen, and the range of treatment services available under EPSDT. The law also changes the EPSDT reporting requirements for States. Each year, States must report to the Secretary the number of children provided full or partial screens, the number referred for corrective treatment, the number of children receiving dental services, and the State's results in achieving the participation goals which the law requires that the Secretary set annually for each State. Several implementation issues have arisen as a result of the legislation.

A. Participation Goals

OBRA 89 directed the Secretary to set annual EPSDT participation goals for each State by July 1 of each year. The goal set by the Secretary is for each State, by 1995, to provide 80 percent of the annual screening services recommended for each age group (under 1, 1-5, 6-14, and 15-20) by the American Academy of Pediatrics. In the interval, each State is expected to reduce the difference between current performance and the 80 percent goal by one-fifth each year from FY 1991 through FY 1995. For any State already at the 80 percent mark, no higher goals have been set. HCFA's proxy measures of States' FY 1989 EPSDT participation rates ranging from 7 percent to 96 percent are shown on table B-8 along with the interval goals for each State. HCFA assumes that children in continuing care arrangements have been fully screened.

To assess each State's performance in providing screening, dental, hearing, and vision services, HCFA changed EPSDT report forms effective April 1, 1990. States are required to report annually by April 1 of each year. Summaries of the first reports from the new forms were not available from HCFA in August 1992.

B. Periodicity Schedule

Prior to enactment of the OBRA 89 amendments, each State was required to establish a periodicity schedule for EPSDT screens according to reasonable standards of medical and dental practice. Schedules varied widely by State, ranging from coverage of 4 screens to 30 screens during the first 21 years of a person's life. (The American Academy of Pediatrics recommends 20 screens during the first 21 years.) Many States maintained a single schedule for general health, dental, hearing, and vision check-ups, resulting in schedules which may have been adequate for medical care but too infrequent for dental or other care. OBRA 89 required States to establish distinct periodicity schedules for each of the four major EPSDT service types. A copy of the schedule recommended by HCFA is reproduced below (see table B-9).

TABLE B-8. Early and Periodic Screening, Diagnostic and Treatment Participation Goals, Fiscal Years 1991 to 1995

State	1989 proxy rate[a]	Percentage points needed to reach 1995 goal	Interval participation goals by fiscal year[b]				
			1991	1992	1993	1994	1995
Alabama	40	40	48	56	64	72	80
Alaska	70	10	72	74	76	78	80
Arizona	96	0	96	96	96	96	96
Arkansas	28	52	38	49	59	70	80
California	63	17	66	70	73	77	80
Colorado	94	0	94	94	94	94	94
Connecticut	10	70	24	38	52	66	80
Delaware	7	73	22	36	51	65	80
District of Columbia	24	56	35	46	58	69	80
Florida	67	13	70	72	75	77	80
Georgia	44	36	51	58	66	73	80
Hawaii	28	52	38	49	59	70	80
Idaho	12	68	26	39	53	66	80
Illinois	57	23	62	66	71	75	80
Indiana	9	71	23	37	52	66	80
Iowa	9	71	23	37	52	66	80
Kansas	13	67	26	40	53	67	80
Kentucky	13	67	26	40	53	67	80
Louisiana	33	47	42	52	61	71	80
Maine	55	25	60	65	70	75	80
Maryland	49	31	55	62	68	74	80
Massachusetts	61	19	65	69	72	76	80
Michigan	48	32	54	62	67	74	80
Minnesota	34	46	43	52	62	71	80
Mississippi	33	47	42	52	61	71	80
Missouri	37	43	46	54	63	71	80
Montana	42	38	50	57	65	72	80
Nebraska	57	23	62	66	71	75	80
Nevada	62	18	66	68	73	76	80
New Hampshire	15	65	28	41	54	67	80

See notes at end of table.

TABLE B-8. Early and Periodic Screening, Diagnostic and Treatment
Participation Goals, Fiscal Years 1991 to 1995--Continued

State	1989 proxy rate[a]	Percentage points needed to reach 1995 goal	Interval participation goals by fiscal year[b]				
			1991	1992	1993	1994	1995
New Jersey	11	69	25	39	52	66	80
New Mexico	35	45	44	53	62	71	80
New York	15	65	28	41	54	67	80
North Carolina	54	26	59	64	70	75	80
North Dakota	19	61	31	43	56	68	80
Ohio	49	31	55	61	68	74	80
Oklahoma	7	73	22	36	51	65	80
Oregon	43	37	50	58	65	73	80
Pennsylvania	44	36	51	58	66	73	80
Rhode Island	45	35	52	59	66	73	80
South Carolina	79	1	79	79	80	80	80
South Dakota	21	59	33	45	56	68	80
Tennessee	27	53	38	48	59	69	80
Texas	24	56	35	46	58	69	80
Utah	32	48	42	51	61	70	80
Vermont	68	12	70	73	76	78	80
Virginia	52	28	58	63	69	74	80
Washington	35	45	44	53	62	71	80
West Virginia	56	24	61	66	70	75	80
Wisconsin	47	33	54	60	67	73	80
Wyoming	27	53	38	48	59	69	80
U.S. rate	39	41	47	56	64	72	80

[a]Proxy rate represents the ratio of continuing care enrollees and initial and/or periodic screening examinations to the average number of eligibles for FY 1989.

[b]Interval goals represent an approximate one-fifth increase from proxy rate or prior year's goal up to 80 percent goal for FY 1995.

Source: Table prepared by the Congressional Research Service based on data supplied by the Health Care Financing Administration. FY 1989 proxy rates are based on data submitted by States to HCFA using HCFA Form 420.

TABLE B-9. Early and Periodic Screening, Diagnostic and Treatment Services, Schedule of Treatment

Age of child:[b]	INFANCY						EARLY CHILDHOOD					LATE CHILDHOOD					ADOLESCENCE[a]			
	By 1 mo	2 mos	4 mos	6 mos	9 mos	12 mos	15 mos	18 mos	24 mos	3 yrs	4 yrs	5 yrs	6 yrs	8 yrs	10 yrs	12 yrs	14 yrs	16 yrs	18 yrs	20+ yrs
History:																				
Initial/interval	P	P	P	P	P	P	P	P	P	P	P	P	P	P	P	P	P	P	P	P
Measurements:																				
Height/weight	P	P	P	P	P	P	P	P	P	P	P	P	P	P	P	P	P	P	P	P
Head circum.	P	P	P	P	P	P														
Blood pressure										P	P	P	P	P	P	P	P	P	P	P
Sensory Screening:																				
Vision	S	S	S	S	S	S	S	S	S	S	O	O	O	O	S	O	O	S	O	O
Hearing	S	S	S	S	S	S	S	S	S	S	O	O	S[c]	S[c]	S[c]	O	S	S	S	S
Developmental/behavioral assessment:[d]																				
	P	P	P	P	P	P	P	P	P	P	P	P	P	P	P	P	P	P	P	P
Physical examination:[e]																				
	P	P	P	P	P	P	P	P	P	P	P	P	P	P	P	P	P	P	P	P

See notes at end of table.

TABLE B-9. Early and Periodic Screening, Diagnostic and Treatment Services, Schedule of Treatment—Continued

Age of child:[b]	INFANCY						EARLY CHILDHOOD					LATE CHILDHOOD					ADOLESCENCE[a]			
	By 1 mo	2 mos	4 mos	6 mos	9 mos	12 mos	15 mos	18 mos	24 mos	3 yrs	4 yrs	5 yrs	6 yrs	8 yrs	10 yrs	12 yrs	14 yrs	16 yrs	18 yrs	20+ yrs
Procedures:[f]																				
Hereditary/metabolic screening[fg]	P																			
Immunization[h]		P	P	P			P	P	P							P				
Tuberculin test[i]	Performed sometime during infancy						Performed sometime during early childhood					Performed sometime during late childhood					Performed sometime during adolescence			
Hematocrit or hemoglobin[j]	Performed sometime during infancy						Performed sometime during early childhood					Performed sometime during late childhood					Performed sometime during adolescence			
Urinalysis[j]	Performed sometime during infancy						Performed sometime during early childhood					Performed sometime during late childhood					Performed sometime during adolescence			
Anticipatory guidance:[k]	P	P	P	P	P	P	P	P	P	P	P	P	P	P	P	P	P	P	P	P
Initial dental referral:[l]										P										

See notes at end of table.

TABLE B-9. Early and Periodic Screening, Diagnostic and Treatment Services, Schedule of Treatment--Continued

KEY:

P - Procedure is to be performed.
S - Procedure is based on the subjective judgment of the practitioner from a review of the child's history.
O - Practitioner should perform procedure using some objective criteria, a standard testing method.

[a] Adolescent related issues (e.g., psychosocial, emotional, substance usage, and reproductive health) may necessitate more frequent health supervision.
[b] If a child comes under care for the first time at any point on the schedule, or if any items are not accomplished at the suggested age, the schedule should be brought up to date at the earliest possible time.
[c] At these points, taking a child's history may suffice if a problem is suggested, a standard testing method should be employed.
[d] Performed by taking a history and appropriate physical examination. If suspicion of a problem follows then an objective developmental test should be performed.
[e] At each visit a complete physical examination is essential, with infants totally unclothed, older children undresses and suitably draped.
[f] These procedures may be modified depending upon the child's entry point into the schedule and the child's individual needs.
[g] Metabolic screenings (e.g., thyroid, PKE, galactosemia) should be done according to State law.
[h] Schedule provided in Report of Committee on Infectious Diseases, 1986 Red Book.
[i] For low risk groups, the Committee on Infectious Diseases recommends the following options: 1) no routine testing; or 2) testing at three times: infancy, preschool, and adolescence. For high risk groups, annual TB skin testing is recommended.
[j] One determination is suggested during each time period. Performance of additional tests is left to individual practice experience.
[k] Appropriate discussion and counselling should be an integral part of each visit for care.
[l] Subsequent examinations as prescribed by dentist.

NOTE: Special chemical, immunologic, and endocrine testing are usually carried out upon specific indications. Testing other than newborn (e.g., inborn errors of metabolism, sickle disease, lead) are discretionary with the physician.

Source: U.S. Dept. of Health and Human Services. Health Care Financing Administration. *State Medicaid Manual*, Part 5, Transmittal 3, Apr. 1990.

Under the old law, States had the option of reimbursing for EPSDT screens outside of the periodicity schedule. The law now requires that States reimburse for medically necessary interperiodic services (check-ups, or screens that fall outside the periodicity schedule) to determine the existence of a suspected illness or condition. Some States paid for interperiodic screens as physician or clinic services and did not count or report them as EPSDT services. In early 1991, 39 States covered interperiodic examinations under EPSDT.[30] Instructions from HCFA to States establish that children are to receive interperiodic services for any problem that is suspected, and that they may be referred for services by any health, developmental, or educational professional with whom the child has contact.[31] States are concerned that there may be no limit to the number of screens provided to a child under these rules.

C. Providers of Partial Screens

One of the OBRA 89 changes to EPSDT requires States to permit participation by providers who do not furnish all components of EPSDT services. Previously, in efforts to avoid fragmentation and duplication of services, 41 States restricted EPSDT screening participation to providers who could furnish complete screening services. Screens in these States were typically performed in public health clinics or community health centers. This restriction may have had the effect of limiting children's access to health care. It prohibited some physicians such as pediatricians or family practitioners from participation because they lacked the equipment needed to perform vision or hearing services. Vision or hearing specialists may have been excluded from participation in EPSDT screens because they could not furnish medical and developmental screens. Under the 1989 amendments, a provider qualified to furnish one or more of the EPSDT items or services must be permitted to provide a partial screening service under EPSDT.

It is not yet known to what extent States will separate the items and services in the EPSDT package and establish reimbursement rates and provider qualifications for them. It is conceivable that a health education specialist would provide and bill for the health education component of a screen while a mental health specialist provides and bills for the developmental assessment. States are concerned that duplicate services will result. They are also concerned that specialists may make diagnoses that require extensive, and expensive follow-up treatment that has limited long-term benefit.

---

[30]Fox, Harriette B. and Lori B. Wicks. Memorandum to State Directors of Maternal and Child Health Programs and Programs for Children with Special Health Care Needs, State Medicaid Directors, and Other Interested Parties, Apr. 8, 1991.

[31]U.S. Dept. of Health and Human Services. Health Care Financing Administration. Early and Periodic Screening, Diagnosis, and Treatment (EPSDT). *State Medicaid Manual*, HCFA-Pub. 45-5, Transmittal No. 4, July 1990.

D. Covered Services

Historically, children who needed services or items that were not covered in a State's Medicaid plan were referred to low cost or no cost providers such as maternal and child health services under Title V of the Social Security Act. Alternatively, States were permitted to provide services and items to EPSDT participants without offering comparable benefits to other Medicaid beneficiaries.

In 1989 a significant change to EPSDT was made. States were required to cover any service that is medically necessary to correct or ameliorate a condition detected in an EPSDT screen, regardless of whether the service or item is otherwise included in a State's Medicaid plan. This provision raised some concerns that States would not be able to control EPSDT costs. However, there is nothing in the new EPSDT laws that changes a State's authority to determine medical necessity or to limit the scope, duration, or amount of service.

VII. CHRONICALLY ILL AND DISABLED CHILDREN

A chronic childhood illness or disability is one that lasts a substantial period of time; it might have a limiting effect on a child's daily activities. Based on data from the 1988 National Health Interview Survey on Child Health (NHIS), about 31 percent of American children under 18 years old, about 20 million children, are estimated to have one or more chronic conditions. These conditions range in severity. The most commonly reported conditions were respiratory allergies (including hay fever) and frequent ear infections. Conditions such as diabetes, sickle cell disease, and cerebral palsy affected fewer than two of every thousand children in the United States.[32] The data suggest that two-thirds of all children with chronic conditions are only mildly affected by their conditions while about 2 million children are severely limited and are restricted in their major activities. About 400,000 children are unable to engage in any major childhood activities. Among these are several thousand children who are technology-dependent. These children need ventilator assistance, intravenous drugs, or other medical device to compensate for a loss of vital body function; generally, they also need ongoing nursing care to avert death or further disability.[33] A special class of ventilator-dependent children may be associated with the incidence of chronic lung disease that afflicts very low birthweight infants who have survived.

Children with chronic illnesses tend to use health services at a greater rate than healthy children. They use twice as many physician visits and prescribed medications, four times as many allied health professional services, and six times the number of other services such as physical therapy and social work.

---

[32]Newacheck, Paul W. and William R. Taylor. Childhood Chronic Illness: Prevalence, Severity, and Impact. *American Journal of Public Health*, v. 82, no. 3, Mar. 1992.

[33]Newacheck, Paul A. Chronically Ill Children and Their Health Care Needs. *Caring*, v. 8, no. 5, May 1989.

Chronically ill children are hospitalized more and account for 31 percent of all hospital days for children.[34]

About 65 percent of children with chronic conditions have some form of private health insurance, generally obtained through a parent's employment. However, the expense of care and the nature of the illness may make it difficult for a child with severe or catastrophic illness to get and keep health insurance coverage. Maximum lifetime dollar limits may be reached. Due to pre-existing condition clauses in some insurance policies, a child who is covered at birth by a parent's insurance may be ineligible for coverage when the parent changes employers, or the child may be ineligible for care related to a specific condition. Newacheck reports that approximately 24 percent of chronically ill children are covered by a public program and 80 percent of these children are covered by Medicaid. This researcher further reports that the 1988 NHIS survey data indicate that 59 percent of disabled children with family incomes below the poverty line are covered by Medicaid.[35]

Historically, children with severe chronic conditions have received institutional care. Technological advancement and changes to Medicaid policy in the 1980s have enabled more children to stay at home where they can participate in family, community and school life. Through home and community-based services waivers, States can provide comprehensive services to an expanded group of chronically ill and disabled children.

Non-medical services that impact on development and functioning are often needed by chronically ill children and their families. Such services may include respite care for the family; transportation; help with acquiring and maintaining special equipment; or case management to coordinate and oversee the health and other services.

A. Medicaid Eligibility for Chronically Ill Children

Disabled children or those with chronic conditions may qualify for Medicaid in the same ways that other children do. (See *Chapter III, Eligibility*.) Chronically ill and disabled children may also qualify for Medicaid if they meet the Supplemental Security Income program's (SSI) disability standard as well as the SSI income and resource standards. Under SSI, disability in children is measured by using functional assessments of developmental delay and limitations in age-appropriate activities of daily living, which may include attending school, or engaging in play.[36] In 1992, an SSI recipient may have an income of up to $422 per month and resources of up to $2,000. As of September

---

[34]Ibid.

[35]Ibid.

[36]Effective since June 1990, these disability criteria for children result from the Supreme Court decision in *Zebley v. Sullivan* in Feb. 1990. The *Zebley* ruling invalidated SSI regulations that used a narrower test for determining children's disabilities than that used for adults.

1991, 361,000 blind and disabled persons under age 21 received SSI benefits; 91 percent of these were under age 18.[37]

Most institutionalized or foster children have been able to meet SSI income and resource standards without difficulty. After the first 30 days away from home, only the child's own financial resources are deemed to be available and the child may qualify for Medicaid. When children live at home, however, the entire family's financial resources are deemed to be available for the child's medical care. Because of the deeming rules, some children who could have been cared for at home have had to remain in institutions or lose their SSI (and therefore Medicaid) benefits. In 1981, this situation received national attention when the parent of a hospitalized child, Katie Beckett, appealed to the President of the United States. Federal policy changes in the Tax Equity and Fiscal Responsibility Act of 1982 (TEFRA, P.L. 97-248) now allow States to extend Medicaid to certain disabled children under age 18 who are living at home and would be eligible for SSI if they were institutionalized.

TEFRA option. TEFRA permitted States to extend regular Medicaid coverage to certain disabled children under age 18 who were living at home and would be eligible for SSI (and therefore Medicaid) if they were in a hospital, nursing facility, or intermediate care facility for the mentally retarded. TEFRA permits States to consider only the child's income and resources when determining eligibility. A State that opts to use the TEFRA option is required to determine that (a) the child requires the level of care provided in an institution; (b) it is appropriate to provide such care outside an institution and; (c) the Medicaid cost of care at home is no more than Medicaid would pay for institutional care for the child.

Under the TEFRA option, cost-effectiveness is determined on a case-by-case basis and is a factor in determining eligibility for services under the option. The annual Medicaid costs for each beneficiary must be less than Medicaid would pay if that beneficiary were in an institution. A child whose private insurance covers institutional care would incur no Medicaid costs in an institution. That child would be ineligible for services under Medicaid, for any amount that Medicaid spent on home care would exceed Medicaid's costs for institutional care.

In some States, to enable children to leave institutions and live with their families, private insurers have cooperated to share home care costs with Medicaid. Insurers at risk of providing the full cost of institutional care have an incentive to convert hospital benefits to home health benefits. It is estimated that 4,000 children are served under TEFRA programs in 17 States.

---

[37]Social Security Administration. *Social Security Bulletin*, v. 54, no. 9, Sept. 1991. p. 139.

B. Home and Community-Based Services Waivers

1915(c) waivers. By permitting States to waive certain rules, Medicaid legislation has increased the opportunities for the care of chronically ill and disabled children at home instead of in hospitals or other institutions. Section 2176 of the Omnibus Budget Reconciliation Act of 1981 (P.L. 97-35) authorized Medicaid coverage of home and community-based services waivers (HCBS). This law allows a State to apply for waivers to provide community-based services to individuals who would otherwise require, or who are at risk of institutionalization which could be covered by the State's Medicaid program. Waiver applications which include the type of services to be offered and the number of persons to be served are submitted for initial terms of 3 years and may be renewed for 5-year periods. The total Medicaid costs of providing services to individuals under a waiver may not exceed the costs that Medicaid would pay for those individuals in institutional settings. Cost-effectiveness of a waiver is determined according to a formula established by HCFA, and is verified at the end of each waiver year. (See *Chapter VI, Alternate Delivery Options and Waiver Programs.*)

Waivers may be used to target specific geographic areas of a State or categories of beneficiaries such as ventilator-dependent children or mentally retarded individuals.

Services under 1915(c) waivers may include medical and non-medical support services (other than room and board). Services which may be provided are optional services (e.g. physical therapy) which may not be included in a State's Medicaid plan, as well as services not otherwise available for Medicaid coverage such as structural modifications to a residence.

In addition to offering services not ordinarily covered, States may extend eligibility under 1915(c) waivers to persons who would not otherwise be eligible for Medicaid except in institutions. For institutionalized beneficiaries, some States use an income standard as high as 300 percent of the State's SSI standard. The higher standard may be used to provide home and community-based services for individuals who require an institutional level of care.

A variation of the 1915(c) waiver, called the "model" waiver, was established by HCFA in 1982 to deal with an eligibility problem faced by certain disabled persons, chiefly children.[38] If a child lives at home, the parents' financial resources are deemed to be available for the child's medical care. If the same child is institutionalized, after the first month away from home only the child's own financial resources are deemed to be available for the child's care. The child may then qualify for Medicaid. Because of these "deeming" rules, some children who could have been cared for at home might remain in institutions because, if they were to return home they would lose Medicaid benefits.

---

[38]The impetus for establishing this waiver was the case of Katie Beckett, a disabled child whose parents sought Medicaid coverage of community-based services.

A model waiver allows a State to waive the deeming rule and pay for support services to help families keep children at home. Application procedures for model waivers are similar to those required for regular waivers; the State must show that Medicaid expenditures for the children are no more than if the children were institutionalized. Originally, HCFA set a limit of 50 persons who could be served under a model waiver. However, a provision in the Medicare Catastrophic Coverage Act (P.L. 100-360) raised the limit to 200.

A 1989 survey indicated that waivers are often used to provide appropriate care to chronically ill and disabled children in home or community settings. Because waiver data do not specify ages, it is difficult to determine how many children receive services under waiver programs. Among 42 regular waivers in the States surveyed, the 3 that were solely for disabled children varied considerably. A waiver for medically fragile children in New Mexico covered a broad range of services including case management; re.pite, homemaker, personal care, and psychosocial services; private duty nursing; and physical therapy. A Maryland waiver covered case management, private duty nursing, and durable medical equipment and supplies while a Texas waiver primarily provided respite care. Of 24 model waivers reported in the survey, 8 targeted disabled children; two of those were solely for children with AIDS.[39]

Children may qualify for services under waivers by meeting applicable income and resource standards, the definition of the target group, the level of care specified in the waiver application, and by accessing a vacant waiver slot.

Most States prefer using HCBS waivers to the TEFRA option to provide services to chronically ill and disabled children. Two features of the TEFRA option make some States reluctant to use it. First, there is uncertainty about the number of people who might use the program. A State that has elected the TEFRA option must provide Medicaid coverage to all qualified individuals with no ceiling on the number served. In some States, the potential costs associated with unlimited numbers of disabled children who may use the option could preclude the State from making the option available. With waivers, States are able to select special populations to receive services, and set manageable limits to the number of individuals served.

Second, there is uncertainty about the ability to provide appropriate care. The TEFRA option allows access only to those services included in a State's Medicaid plan with no flexibility to provide additional services. Appropriate services may not be available under Medicaid for a child who needs more than regular benefits. Cost considerations may deter a State Medicaid program from expanding the availability of certain optional services to all beneficiaries. A HCBS waiver may be used to contain costs for a service or set of services, as well as to test services or service limits.

---

[39]National Governors' Association. *Medicaid Home Care Options for Disabled Children*. Washington, 1990. p. 10.

VIII. ADOLESCENT HEALTH[40]

Adolescents have the lowest death rates of all Americans. They also have the lowest number of physician visits and are least likely to be hospitalized. However, adolescents are more likely to be victims of violent crimes and are more likely to die of injuries than younger or older Americans. For children ages 1 to 14, accidents are the leading cause of death. At ages 15 and above, accidents remain the leading cause of death, while homicide and suicide are the second and third ranking causes.[41]

Adolescents suffer from the acute and chronic conditions that affect all age groups, as well as from conditions peculiar to adolescents. Available data indicate that acute respiratory illnesses are the leading cause of school-loss days among adolescents. An estimated 5 to 10 percent of adolescents have a serious chronic physical condition. Health problems peculiar to some adolescents include family and school problems from which high levels of stress, conflict, neglect, or abuse may result in depression and other psychological difficulties that can lead to school dropout and increase risk for a variety of health, economic, and social problems.

There is evidence of a gulf between what adolescents and adults believe are serious health problems. Common health concerns expressed by adolescents are acne which affects 9 percent of adolescents, and menstrual distress which affects 50 percent of adolescent females. Adults are more likely to identify behavioral and lifestyle problems such as use of alcohol, tobacco, or illicit drugs, unprotected sexual intercourse, poor dietary and physical activity habits, and stress with school or family. These problems are associated with alcoholism, cardiovascular disease, high blood pressure, unwanted pregnancy and sexually transmitted diseases including HIV infection, and other conditions which can cause disability or premature death.

Enrollment in Medicaid can affect the utilization of health care by poor adolescents. In 1988, an estimated 4.58 million U.S. adolescents ages 10 through 18 were enrolled in Medicaid at some time during the fiscal year, making up 17.1 percent of Medicaid enrollment. Uncounted additional pregnant or parenting female adolescents were enrolled as adult heads of household. With a required phase-in of Medicaid eligibility for children born after September 30, 1983, all poor adolescents will be eligible for Medicaid in the year 2002.

No records are maintained for Medicaid expenditures explicitly for adolescents. However, from a sample of paid claims, HCFA estimated that of 1988 expenditures of $48.7 billion, the amount spent for adolescents was approximately $3.3 billion, over 6 percent of total expenditures. In FY 1988,

---

[40]This section relies heavily on a report on adolescent health by the U.S. Office of Technology Assessment. The report focuses on 10 to 18 year olds.

[41]U.S. Dept. of Health and Human Services. Public Health Service. *Healthy People 2000: National Health Promotion and Disease Prevention Objectives.* Conference Edition, Apr. 8, 1991.

Medicaid spent about $1.5 billion for services to 10 to 14 year olds, and $1.85 billion for services to 15 to 18 year olds, or $159 per enrollee in the lower age group and $346 per enrollee in the 15 to 18 year old group.

About 1 in 7 adolescents, 4.6 million, have no health insurance. Those who are insured may not be covered for basic dental, hearing, vision, and maternity-related benefits. In addition, limitations on mental health and substance abuse treatment benefits may constitute a barrier to needed services.

IX. DEMONSTRATIONS PROGRAMS

A. Extending Medicaid Coverage to Pregnant Women and Children Not Eligible for Medicaid[42]

Even with recent Medicaid eligibility expansions, many low-income pregnant women and children have no health care coverage. OBRA 89 directed the Secretary of HHS to enter into agreements with several States to conduct demonstrations of extended Medicaid coverage or alternative coverage, to pregnant women, and children under age 20, with family incomes up to 185 percent of the poverty line and who are otherwise ineligible for Medicaid. Under these demonstration projects, premiums are charged to families with incomes above 100 percent of the Federal poverty level; costs of services are matched at a State's usual Federal matching rate for services. Funding was awarded for projects in Florida, Maine, and Michigan.

The Florida project offers commercial insurance through a single school district (Volusia County) for children ages 5 to 19. Known as Healthy Kids, the project is administered by a corporation created by the Florida legislature. Primary and preventive services are provided under a low-option insurance plan, and inpatient hospital services under a high-option plan. The service provider is a health maintenance organization that is reimbursed at Florida's Medicaid rates. A child found eligible for the school lunch program is eligible for Medicaid in this project. Families with incomes between 100 percent and 133 percent of the poverty level are charged $3.00 per month per child. Families with incomes between 133 percent and 185 percent of the poverty level are charged $16 per month per child. As of July 1992, 4,500 of the project's maximum 7,400 were enrolled.

The Maine Health Program has been in existence since October 1990. It helps low-income workers and their dependents to pay premiums, coinsurance and deductibles associated with employer-sponsored health insurance. Under the demonstration project, funds will be used to help cover dependent children and pay for Medicaid benefits not included in employers' plans. It is expected that 3,500 children will be enrolled in the project.

---

[42]U.S. Dept. of Health and Human Services. Health Care Financing Administration. Office of Research and Demonstrations. Detailed project descriptions were provided via telephone communication. July 1992.

In cooperation with a private insurer, the State of Michigan has established the Child Caring Program for primary care, outpatient and preventive services for poor children up to age 18. As of July 1992, the State is waiting for a waiver of Medicaid freedom-of-choice rules so that the children may all be enrolled in a preferred provider organization (PPO).[43] The PPO is to be paid on a capitation basis using contributions from private foundations as the State share of Medicaid reimbursement. Regular Medicaid applications for eligibility will be used for entry in the program.

B. Demonstrations for Medicaid Coverage of HIV-Positive Individuals and Pregnant Women at Risk

OBRA 90 provided for 3-year demonstration projects in 2 States to provide Medicaid coverage and specified additional services to (a) persons testing positive for HIV infection who meet the State's maximum income and resource standards for disabled persons, or (b) pregnant women under age 19 who have multiple medical and psychosocial needs and who are determined to be at risk of HIV infection because of substance abuse. Contrary to the usual response to such provisions, no State applied to carry out a demonstration project. Observers suggested two possible explanations for the lack of interest. States may have been concerned about the ethical considerations of having a control group which would have received no benefits. Also, in a time of fiscal austerity, the need for State matching funds for additional services may have been a disincentive.

X. COORDINATION WITH OTHER PROGRAMS

Three other federally funded programs provide significant support for services to pregnant women and children. The Maternal and Child Health Block Grant program (MCH) authorized by Title V of the Social Security Act, and administered as a Federal/State partnership by the Health Resources and Services Administration of DHHS, provides grants to each State and territory for a variety of health services. The program is permanently authorized at $686 million per year; $649,650,000 was appropriated for the program in FY 1992. Under this program, low-income pregnant women and children may receive preventive and primary health care, health screening, immunizations, and diagnostic, treatment, and rehabilitation services for children with special health care needs.

Some States use MCH block grant funds to provide care to women and children determined to be ineligible for Medicaid. Prior to the OBRA 89 rules for EPSDT, States may have used these funds for children's services not available under the State's Medicaid program.

---

[43]Medicaid statute requires that beneficiaries be able to obtain covered services from any qualified provider willing to accept Medicaid reimbursement. Waiver of the requirement permits States to limit beneficiaries to enrollment in certain care arrangements.

OBRA 89 amended title V to require that States furnish more information in their applications for grant funds and their annual reports. Applications must contain a statewide needs assessment that identifies the need for services to the population groups served by the program. An annual report must contain detailed information concerning the status of maternal and child health in the State. With the 1991 applications and reports, there were problems with responding to some of the data requirements. For example, States were not able to establish the proportion of infants born with fetal alcohol syndrome or drug dependency, or determine the immunization status of 2 year olds. After the new requirements have been fully met, it is expected that information concerning maternal and child health status and services will be more readily available than at present.

The Special Supplemental Food Program for Women, Infants, and Children (WIC) is authorized under section 17 of the Child Nutrition Act of 1966 and administered by the Food and Nutrition Service in the Department of Agriculture. The program provides nutrition services and supplemental foods to low-income pregnant and breastfeeding women, infants, and children to age 5.

Federally qualified health centers (FQHCs) include community and migrant health centers receiving grants under Title III of the Public Health Service (PHS) Act and other centers that meet the requirements for receipt of grants. They are major sources of preventive and primary health care for low-income pregnant women and children. All such centers serve Medicaid beneficiaries. Medicaid law designates FQHCs as sites for optional presumptive eligibility determination as well as for outstationing of eligibility workers. In addition, FQHC facilities may house WIC clinics or provide services for MCH programs. About half of the federally funded centers operate comprehensive perinatal care programs which use case management to provide and coordinate services specifically intended to reduce infant mortality and the incidence of low birthweight.

State Medicaid, MCH, and WIC programs are required to coordinate their operations. Medicaid programs must notify Medicaid beneficiaries who meet WIC categorical requirements of the availability of WIC benefits and refer them to WIC clinics. State MCH programs must identify Medicaid-eligible pregnant women and infants and help them to apply for Medicaid. Through the MCH program, States are required to maintain toll-free telephone lines for access to information about providers of services under title V and Medicaid. In addition to the required information on providers, some States offer information on other services relevant to maternal and child health. In most States, the State MCH program has a role in establishing EPSDT periodicity schedules and standards.

As required by OBRA 89, the DHHS has developed a maternal and child health handbook that is available to pregnant women and families with young children through public programs such as maternal and child health clinics, community and migrant health centers, WIC clinics, and Head Start. The handbook can remind mothers of their children's preventive health needs and encourage them to document illnesses and services.

To raise awareness of potential benefits from various programs, and simplify the application and review processes, the DHHS, with the Department of Agriculture has developed a 4-page model application form that States have the option of using. The form is designed to be used by pregnant women or by children under age 6 to apply simultaneously for benefits under the following programs: Medicaid; the MCH program; community and migrant health center programs; WIC; the Health Care for the Homeless program under section 340 of the PHS Act; and Head Start. It is uncertain whether any States have adopted the form or any part of it. Several States had already developed application forms for simultaneous eligibility determination for two or more of the programs. As of April 1992, other States were working to develop forms. A reproduction of the model form may be found at the end of this appendix.

Maternal and Child Assistance Programs Model Application Form

This model application form can be used to apply for all or any of the following programs:

Medicaid   Community and Migrant Health Centers
Health Care for the Homeless   Head Start
Maternal and Child Health/Health Departments   The WIC Program

If you, or any people living in your household, already receive or do not want to apply for any of these programs, note this on second page.

Please ask for help if there is anything on this form that you do not understand.   **Date form filled out:** _____

General Information

Name of applicant First	Middle		Last		Home phone	Work phone
Home address (Is this a shelter? ☐ yes ☐ no) Street		Apt. #	City	State	Zip	County
Mailing address (if different from above) Street, P.O. Box		Apt. #	City	State	Zip	County
Name of parent/legal guardian (if the applicant is a child) First	Middle		Last		Home phone	Work phone
Address of parent/legal guardian Street, P.O. Box		Apt. #	City	State	Zip	County

Marital status of applicant   Single ☐   Married ☐   Separated ☐   Divorced ☐   Widowed ☐

Do you speak English?   yes ☐   no ☐   If no, what language do you speak?

Medical insurance and other related information

1. Do you or any family members living in your household have medical insurance?
   yes ☐   no ☐

2. Have you or any family members living in your household been to the doctor, clinic, or hospital in the last ___ months?
   yes ☐   no ☐

3. Are you a veteran?
   yes ☐   no ☐

4. Is your spouse a veteran?
   yes ☐   no ☐

List all the people living in your household (related and non-related)

Names Attach extra sheet, If needed	Relationship to the applicant	Date of birth	Receiving AFDC? yes/no	Receiving Food Stamps? yes/no	Receiving Medicaid? yes/no. If yes give Medicaid #.	Applying for all programs?	If no, list program(s) already receiving or not wanted. *
						yes/no	
1.	(self)						
2.							
3.							
4.							
5.							
6.							

* Medicaid, Health Care for the Homeless, Maternal and Child Health/Health Departments, Community and Migrant Health Centers, Head Start, and the WIC Program

Are you pregnant or breastfeeding? yes ☐ no ☐

Have you been pregnant in the last 6 months? yes ☐ no ☐

Is any other person living in your household pregnant or breastfeeding? yes ☐ no ☐ If yes, who:

Has any other person living in your household been pregnant in the last 6 months? yes ☐ no ☐ If yes, who:

List all the income received by people living in your household (related and non-related)

Name of person(s) working or receiving money ** Attach extra sheet, if needed	Who provides the money? Employer, program or person	How Often? Weekly, every 2 weeks, twice a month, monthly	What amount?
1.			
2.			
3.			
4.			
5.			

Do all of the people living in your household share income (buy groceries, pay bills, etc.)? yes ☐ no ☐

If no, list the names of the people who do not share income with you.

** Be sure to include all sources of gross income (before taxes) such as wages, dividends and interest, AFDC, SSI, annuities, pension, disability, child support, alimony, cash gifts, and other unearned income.

List all the resources owned by family members living in your household * (Must be filled out by Medicaid applicants only.)

Types of resources	Whose	Value
1.		
2.		
3.		
4.		
5.		

* Be sure to include all resources such as bank accounts, trust funds, automobiles, house, property, and life insurance.

List the payments made for child care (or care for an adult who cannot care for himself) so that someone in your household can work.

Name of person(s) who works:

Total amount paid: _____   How often? _____

List all the family members living in your household who are applying for Medicaid (Must be filled out by Medicaid applicants only)

Names	Relationship to the applicant	U.S citizen? yes/no	Social Security number	Name of mother of applicant (if known and if applicant is a child)	Name of father of applicant (if known and if applicant is a child)
1.					
2.					
3.					
4.					
5.					

Social Security Number (SSN)
You must give us your SSN in order to receive Medicaid. This is required by section 1137(a)(1) of the Social Security Act and the Medicaid regulations at 42 CFR 435.910. The Medicaid agency will use the SSN to verify your income, eligibility, and the amount of medical assistance payments we will make on your behalf. It is possible that we will also use the SSN to determine another person's right to Medicaid or to comply with federal law requiring that we disclose information from Medicaid records. The information may be matched with the records in other agencies, such as the Social Security Administration or the Internal Revenue Service. These matches may be done by computer or on an individual basis. Also, if you apply for any of the other programs in this joint application, those programs will have access to your SSN and could use it in the administration of the program.

Assignment of Rights for Medical Support and Third Party Payment
Medicaid does not pay medical expenses that a third party is supposed to pay. All persons applying for Medicaid benefits are required to assign to the State Medicaid agency any rights they may have to medical support or other third party payments for medical care. When you sign this application for yourself, or for another person for whom you can legally assign rights, you are assigning the Medicaid agency all of your rights to receive medical support or third party payments for the entire time you are on Medicaid.

Cooperation Requirements
I understand that by applying for Medicaid benefits, I agree to cooperate with the State Medicaid agency in identifying and providing information to help pursue any third party who may be responsible for paying for care and services for me (or for a person(s) on whose behalf I am applying) that are covered by Medicaid, or enabling third party payments to be made for care (or on behalf of another person). If necessary, I also agree to establish paternity for any children for whom I am applying for Medicaid benefits. If I am applying for Medicaid as a low income pregnant woman, or if I have good reason not to cooperate, I may not have to meet these cooperation requirements. If I am eligible to enroll in any insurance or benefit plan offered to me or my spouse by an employer, I may be required to enroll in that insurance. If the State decides that it will cost the same or less than giving me Medicaid, I understand that the State agency will pay for the costs of this coverage.

If after reading and completing this page, you decide that you do not want to apply for Medicaid be sure to note this on the second page in the top box.

Rights and Responsibilities

This form is being submitted as a joint application for one or more of these programs: Medicaid, Health Care for the Homeless, Maternal and Child Health/Health Departments, Community and Migrant Health Centers, Head Start, and the WIC Program.

I understand that this joint application form will be sent to all of the programs that I am applying for.

I agree to the release of personal and financial information from this application form and supporting documents to the agencies that run these programs so that they can evaluate it and verify eligibility. I understand that the agencies that run the programs will determine confidentiality of this information according to the federal laws, 42 CFR 431.300-431.307, the WIC regulations, 7 CFR 246.26(d), and any applicable federal and state laws and regulations.

Officials from the programs that I, or members of my household, have applied for may verify all information on this form.

I understand that if I applied for Medicaid, I must immediately tell the Medicaid agency about any changes in information on this form.

If I or people in my household have applied for WIC, and/or certain other programs, more information will be needed to determine eligibility. I will be contacted for further information as necessary.

I understand my eligibility for any and all programs will not be affected by my race, color, national origin, age, disability, or sex, except where this is restricted by law.

I have the right to appeal any decisions made by a local Medicaid, WIC, or Head Start program. Information on the appeals process can be obtained from these programs.

I understand that anyone who knowingly lies or misrepresents the truth or arranges for someone to knowingly lie or misrepresent the truth is committing a crime which can be punished under federal law, state law, or both. I understand that I may also be liable for repaying in cash the value of the benefits received and may be subject to civil penalties.

I certify under penalty of perjury that everything on this application form is the truth as best I know.

Signature of applicant/parent or legal guardian (if applicant is a child)	Relationship to applicant	Date

Signature of person who completed the form (if different from above)	Relationship to applicant	Date

Optional Information*	Race/Ethnic group	Black** ☐ Hispanic ☐	Asian or Pacific Islander ☐	American Indian or Alaskan Native ☐	White** ☐	Other (specify) ☐
	Sex	Male ☐ Female ☐				
	Have you received your immunization shots?		Yes ☐ No ☐ Don't Know ☐			
	Have your children received their immunization shots?		Yes ☐ No ☐ Don't Know ☐			
	If pregnant, are you seeing a doctor?		Yes ☐ No ☐ Don't Know ☐			

* The applicant does not have to answer these optional questions. The answers will not affect eligibility. The answers will be used only to collect information about people who apply for the programs.
** Not of Hispanic Origin.

For Agency use only

☐ Meets nutritional risk criteria of WIC.

☐ Meets CSHN requirements

☐ Pregnancy verified

Date received by Agency _____

APPENDIX C. MEDICAID, LONG-TERM CARE, AND THE ELDERLY[1]

SUMMARY

Long-term care refers to a broad range of medical, social, personal care, and supportive services needed by individuals who have lost some capacity for self-care because of a chronic illness or condition. Chronic illnesses or conditions often result in both functional impairment and physical dependence on others for an extended period of time. These conditions include heart disease, strokes, arthritis, and Alzheimer's and related dementias. Long-term care services can be provided either in institutions, such as nursing homes, or in home and community-based care settings. Although chronic conditions occur in individuals of all ages, the elderly are the largest group in need of long-term care. It is estimated that the elderly account for two-thirds of the 10.6 million persons of all ages needing long-term care and living in institutions and the community.

Medicaid funds a broad range of long-term care services for the elderly, including nursing home care, home health care, personal care, and various home and community-based services. Long-term care spending, and especially nursing home spending, accounts for the great bulk of Medicaid's spending for the elderly. Two-thirds of total Medicaid spending for the elderly, or $17.1 billion of $25.4 billion, was for nursing home care in FY 1991. Much smaller amounts were spent for various home care services--$2 billion, or 8 percent of total spending for the elderly, in FY 1991. Together these two categories of long-term care spending amounted to three-quarters of total spending for the elderly.

Medicaid's spending for long-term care for the elderly is driven by its coverage of persons who need nursing home care and who are not poor by cash welfare standards but who qualify under options that States may use for covering persons with higher levels of income. States cover these persons either under a medically needy program or a special income rule, referred to as the "300 percent rule." Medically needy programs allow States to cover persons who have incurred medical expenses that deplete their resources and incomes to levels that make them needy according to State-determined standards. Under the 300 percent rule, States are allowed to cover persons needing nursing home care so long as their income does not exceed 300 percent of the basic Supplemental Security Income (SSI) cash welfare payment (in 1992, 300 percent of $422, or $1,266 a month).

Nursing home payments for these two groups combined accounted for nearly 60 percent of total program payments for all elderly beneficiaries. It is

---

[1]This appendix was written by Richard Price.

nursing home spending for the non-poor that largely explains the fact that elderly Medicaid beneficiaries over the years have accounted for a disproportionately large portion of Medicaid payments for services. In FY 1991, elderly beneficiaries represented 12 percent of total Medicaid beneficiaries and their share of program payments amounted to 33 percent of total program payments.

In the absence of coverage for long-term care under Medicare and the relatively limited coverage currently available through private insurance, Medicaid has become the Nation's major public program of coverage for nursing home care. At an average cost of $30,000 a year, nursing home costs can quickly deplete the resources of most elderly individuals, especially after long stays. A number of different State studies have looked at the percentage of Medicaid residents of nursing homes who were not eligible for Medicaid when they were originally admitted. They found that somewhere between 27 and 45 percent of residents "spent down" while in nursing homes.

After relatively modest rates of growth of 6 to 9 percent in the mid-1980s, nursing home spending increased by 14 percent in 1990 and 17 percent in 1991. These increases may be the result of higher reimbursement rates required as the result of the Omnibus Budget Reconciliation Act of 1987 (OBRA 87) nursing home reform revisions as well as court cases that have required States to increase payments to facilities. To control growth in nursing home care (spending for nursing home care for the elderly represents 22 percent of total Medicaid spending), some States have been exploring ways to link private long-term care insurance and Medicaid. Recently, the Health Care Financing Administration (HCFA) approved Medicaid plan amendments from four States that would allow them to establish more liberal asset standards for persons with private insurance coverage. In addition, States may look more closely at current law prohibitions on transferring assets, with increasing anecdotal reports that non-poor elderly persons are using estate planning to avoid applying their wealth to the costs of long-term care services in order to gain Medicaid eligibility sooner than they otherwise would.

I. INTRODUCTION

The phrase "long-term care" refers to a broad range of medical, social, personal care, and supportive services needed by individuals who have lost some capacity for self-care because of a chronic illness or condition. Chronic illnesses or conditions often result in both functional impairment and physical dependence on others for an extended period of time.

The range of chronic illnesses and conditions resulting in the need for supportive long-term care services is extensive. Unlike acute medical illnesses, which occur suddenly and may be resolved in a relatively short period of time, chronic conditions last for an extended period of time and are not typically curable. These conditions include heart disease, strokes, arthritis, Alzheimer's and related dementias, mental retardation, and mental illness. Major subgroups of persons needing long-term care include the elderly and nonelderly disabled, persons with developmental disabilities (primarily persons with mental retardation), and persons with mental illness.

The presence of a chronic illness or condition alone does not necessarily result in a need for long-term care. For many individuals, their illness or condition does not result in a functional impairment or dependence and they are able to go about their daily routines without needing assistance. It is when the illness or condition results in a functional or activity limitation that long-term care services may be required.

The need for long-term care is often measured by assessing limitations in a person's capacity to manage certain functions or activities. For example, a chronic condition may result in dependence in certain functions that are basic and essential for self-care, such as bathing, dressing, eating, toileting, and/or moving from one place to another. These are referred to as limitations in "activities of daily living," or ADLs. Assistance with these ADLs may require hands-on assistance or direction, instruction, or supervision from another individual.

Another set of limitations that reflects lower levels of disability are used to describe difficulties in performing household chores and social tasks. These are referred to as limitations in "instrumental activities of daily living," or IADLs, and include such functions as meal preparation, cleaning, grocery shopping, managing money, and taking medicine.

Limitations in ADLs and IADLs can vary in severity and prevalence. Persons can have limitations in any number of ADLs or IADLs, or both.

Long-term care services are often differentiated by the settings in which they are provided. In general, services are provided either in institutions or in home and community-based care settings. Institutions caring for persons with long-term care needs include nursing facilities, intermediate care facilities for the mentally retarded (ICFs-MR), and inpatient and outpatient facilities for persons with mental illness. Services provided in these institutions range from medical and skilled health care services to assistance with and/or training in personal care functions, as well as socialization and job training for the mentally retarded and mentally ill.

Home and community-based care also includes a broad range of skilled and personal care services, as well as a variety of home management activities, such as chore services, meal preparation, and shopping. For the mentally retarded and mentally ill, home care services can also include assistance in acquiring and improving self-help and socialization skills, as well as prevocational training and other educational services. Home and community-based care can be provided in a person's home or other place of residence, such as a group living arrangement, or at a community center, such as a day care center or senior center.

Medicaid funds a broad range of institutional and home and community-based care services. Table C-1 shows spending for major categories of long-term care services. By far the greatest share of Medicaid spending for long-term care is for institutional care for various covered populations. Medicaid covers care provided in nursing homes for elderly and nonelderly disabled persons, ICFs/MR, and inpatient facilities serving the mentally ill. In FY 1991, spending for care provided in these various institutional settings amounted to about 87 percent of total long-term care spending.

The remaining 13 percent of Medicaid long-term care spending in FY 1991 was for home and community-based care. Categories of these services covered by Medicaid include home health, home and community-based care, and personal care.

TABLE C-1. Federal and State Medicaid Payments for Long-Term Care Services, by Service Category, Fiscal Year 1991

Service category	Payments (in millions)	Percent of total
Nursing homes	$20,823	58.2%
ICFs/MR	8,039	22.5
Inpatient mental health services	2,137	6.0
Home and community-based waivers	1,609	4.5
Personal care services	2,104	5.9
Home health services	1,039	2.9
Total long-term care	35,752	100.0

NOTE: All figures are estimates and subject to data limitations and methods of calculations. Payments are for medical services and exclude any administrative payments.

Source: Table prepared by the Congressional Research Service based on data submitted by the States to HCFA. HCFA Form 64--*Quarterly Medicaid Statement of Expenditures for the Medical Assistance Program.*

In addition, Medicaid spending for long-term care services is a substantial portion of total spending for all covered services. Figure C-1 indicates that long-term care spending amounted to about 41 percent of total Medicaid spending in FY 1991.

FIGURE C-1. Long-Term Care Spending as a Share of Total Medicaid Payments, FY 1991

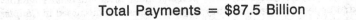

Total Payments = $87.5 Billion

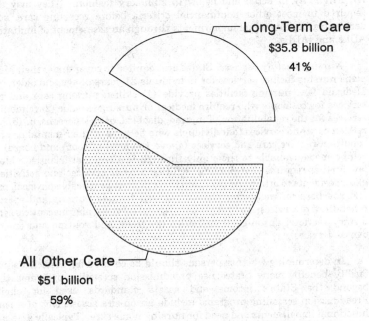

Long-Term Care

$35.8 billion

41%

All Other Care

$51 billion

59%

Source: Figure prepared by Congressional Research Service based on data obtained from the Health Care Financing Administration.

Appendices D and E in this Source Book discuss Medicaid services for the mentally retarded and mentally ill. This chapter will focus on Medicaid and long-term care for the elderly.

II. MEDICAID COVERED LONG-TERM CARE SERVICES FOR THE ELDERLY

Medicaid covers a broad range of long-term care services needed by elderly persons with chronic illnesses and conditions. These include both nursing home care and a variety of home and community-based care services. In order to qualify for coverage of these services, persons must meet financial eligibility criteria that apply to the services they require. These are discussed in *Chapter III, Eligibility* in detail and below in summary fashion. They may also be required to meet other nonfinancial criteria before receiving care, such as demonstrating functional impairments through an assessment of limitations in ADLs and IADLs.

Nursing Facility Services. States are required to cover under their Medicaid plans nursing facility services for individuals 21 years of age and older. Under Medicaid law, nursing facilities provide (1) skilled nursing care and related services for residents who require medical or nursing care, or (2) rehabilitation services for the rehabilitation of injured, disabled, or sick persons, or (3) health-related care and services to individuals who because of their mental or physical condition require care and services (above the level of room and board) which can be made available to them only through institutional facilities. Medicaid law further requires that nursing facilities provide services and activities that allow residents to attain and maintain their highest practicable physical, mental, and psychosocial well-being. These services include nursing and specialized rehabilitative services; medically-related social services; pharmaceutical services; dietary services; an on-going activities program; and routine and emergency dental services.

In determining whether persons should be covered for Medicaid's nursing facility benefit, many States use preadmission screening programs that go beyond the State's income and assets standards used for eligibility. Preadmission screening programs include an on-site assessment of a person's functional impairments and need for nursing home care. Typically assessments include an evaluation of a person's physical and mental health, functional status, and formal (paid services) and informal supports (help from family and friends) needed and available. States generally apply preadmission screening programs to persons already eligible for Medicaid. Certain other States, however, apply them to all persons seeking nursing home placement, regardless of payer status, with the expectation that these persons might become eligible for Medicaid later in their stays.[2] Preadmission screening programs are

---

[2]This discussion is based on findings reported in: Iversen, Laura. *A Description and Analysis of State Pre-Admission Screening Programs.* Excelsior, Interstudy, Center for Aging and Long-Term Care, Mar. 1986; and U.S. Library of Congress. Congressional Research Service. *Medicaid Eligibility for the*
(continued...)

intended to control State spending for nursing home care by ensuring that nursing home beds are reserved for those who need them and by determining whether community care at a lower cost might be an appropriate alternative for meeting the care needs of the individual.

Home Health. States are required to cover home health for any person who is entitled to nursing facility services under the State's Medicaid plan. Medicaid regulations require that these services be provided at the beneficiary's place of residence and be in compliance with a physician's written plan of care that is renewed every 60 days. The regulations require that home health services include nursing care, home health aide services, and medical supplies, equipment, and appliances suitable for use in the home. States may also include physical and occupational therapy, speech pathology, and audiology services as covered home health care if they choose. Medicaid's home health benefit has a skilled medical care orientation and is not intended to provide personal care and other nonmedical supportive assistance that many elderly persons with chronic conditions require in order to remain in the community.

Personal Care. Although personal care services are not specifically included in Medicaid statute as an optional service that States are allowed to provide, the Secretary of the Department of Health and Human Services (DHHS) has authorized in regulations coverage of personal care under a general authority to approve additional medical or remedial services not specified in law. The regulations define personal care as services provided in the individual's home and by a qualified person who is supervised by a registered nurse and who is not a member of the individual's family. Services must be prescribed by a physician according to the beneficiary's plan of treatment. As of October 1, 1991, 28 States covered personal care under their Medicaid plans. Beginning October 1, 1994, Medicaid law will require States to cover personal care for any person entitled to nursing facility services under the State's Medicaid plan.

A recent review of State Medicaid personal care programs found that most offered a basic core of personal care and household services associated with limitations in ADLs and IADLs.[3] Personal care services included bathing, dressing, ambulation, feeding, and grooming. Household services offered by most programs included meal preparation and clean-up, light cleaning, laundry, and shopping. Errands, chores, heavy cleaning, and repairs were less likely to

---

[2](...continued)
Elderly in Need of Long Term Care. CRS Report for Congress No. 87-986 EPW, by Edward Neuschler with the assistance of Claire Gill. Washington, 1987. p. 26-31. Findings are based on a 1986 survey of State preadmission screening programs.

[3]Litvak, Simi, and Jae Kennedy. *The Medicaid Personal Care Services Optional Care Benefit: Policy Issues.* Oakland, World Institute on Disability, June 25, 1991. This discussion is based closely on findings reported in this study. See also: Lewis-Idema, Deborah, Susanna Ginsburg, and Marilyn Falik. *Descriptive Study of Medicaid Personal Care Programs.* Baltimore, The Commonwealth Fund, Commission on Elderly People Living Alone, Jan. 1990.

be provided. About half the programs provided medically-related services, such as injections, medications, respiratory and catheter assistance. Almost three-quarters of the programs reported that they serve people with all disabilities, including those with physical, mental, cognitive, and brain injury impairments. About one-quarter of programs do not serve people with mental disabilities or with cognitive disabilities. Most States with personal care programs assess a person's limitations in ADLs and IADLs and/or minimum number of hours and type of services needed, and require that a minimum level of functional impairment be present for persons to become eligible.

Home and Community-Based Care Waiver Services. States have an option of covering persons needing home and community-based care services, if these persons would otherwise require institutional care that would be covered by Medicaid. These services are provided under waiver programs authorized in section 1915(c) and 1915(d) of Medicaid law. The programs, often referred to as home and community-based care waiver programs, require States to make special application to HCFA for the programs they wish to operate. With approval, States may provide a wide variety of non-medical, social, and supportive services that have been shown to be critical in allowing chronically ill and disabled persons to remain in their homes. These include case management, homemaker/home health aide services, personal care, adult day health, respite, among others.

States are using waiver programs to provide services to a diverse long-term care population, including the elderly, and others who are disabled or who have chronic mental illness, mental retardation and developmental disabilities, and acquired immune deficiency syndrome (AIDS). As of December 1991, almost all States (with the exception of Alaska, Arizona, and the District of Columbia) were using the 1915(c) waiver authority to provide community-based services to these long-term care populations.[4] Forty States operated 53 1915(c) waiver programs serving the aged/disabled, as of December 1991. The aged/disabled represented 73 percent of all persons served in FY 1991, but accounted for only 32 percent of total waiver spending. The mentally retarded/developmentally disabled accounted for 21 percent of total waiver participants, but 64 percent of total spending. One State, Oregon, operated a 1915(d) waiver program for the elderly.[5] Typically States use assessments of ADLs and IADLs to determine

---

[4]Under a separate waiver authority, Arizona began covering home and community-based care, as well as nursing home care, for the elderly on Jan. 1, 1989, as part of a HCFA-approved demonstration program.

[5]The 1915(d) waiver program differs from 1915(c) waivers in two major respects. First, the target population is limited to persons 65 years of age and older who, without home and community-based care, would require nursing home care that would be paid for by Medicaid. Second, the budget neutrality test for 1915(d) waivers is not dependent on a State's supply of nursing home beds, as the 1915(c) program is. Rather it establishes a cap or ceiling on the total amount that States may spend for all long-term care services under Medicaid.

whether an individual's functional impairments would require nursing home placement if home and community-based care services were not available.

A more detailed discussion of home and community-based care waiver programs is contained in *Chapter VI, Alternate Delivery Options and Waiver Programs.*

Optional Home and Community-Based Care Services. States may also provide home and community-based care to elderly persons under a new optional Medicaid benefit called home and community-based care for functionally disabled elderly persons. This benefit requires that eligible persons be 65 years of age or over and be functionally disabled. To be considered functionally disabled, persons must be unable to perform without substantial human assistance at least two of three specified ADLs (toileting, transferring, and eating). Alternatively they may be considered disabled if they require assistance as a result of Alzheimer's disease or cognitive impairments. Services that States may cover under the optional home and community-based care benefit include homemaker/home health aide services, chore services, personal care, nursing care, respite care, adult day care, among others.

This optional benefit is different from others, in that Federal matching payments are capped for FY 1991 to FY 1995. Federal matching payments cannot exceed $40 million for FY 1991; $70 million for FY 1992; $130 million for FY 1993; $160 million for FY 1994; and $180 million for FY 1995. In making allocations to the States, the Secretary is required to take into account the number of persons 65 and older in a State in relation to the number of persons 65 and over nationally, considering, to the maximum extent possible, the number of elderly persons who are low-income. As of July 1992, two States (Texas and Rhode Island) have had Medicaid plan amendments approved to offer home and community-based care under this option.

III. PATTERNS OF MEDICAID PAYMENTS FOR ELDERLY MEDICAID BENEFICIARIES

A. Medicaid Payments for Elderly and Nonelderly Beneficiaries

Table C-2 provides a breakdown of Medicaid spending for various covered services, by elderly and nonelderly beneficiaries. This table indicates that long-term care spending, and especially nursing home spending, accounts for the great bulk of Medicaid's spending for the elderly. Two-thirds of total Medicaid spending for the elderly, or $17.1 billion of $25.4 billion, was for nursing home care in FY 1991. Medicaid spent an additional $2 billion, or 8 percent of total spending for the elderly, for various home care services, including home health, personal care, and home and community-based waiver services. Together these two categories of long-term care spending amounted to three-quarters of total spending for the elderly. The third largest spending category for the elderly is prescription drugs, many of which may be needed for management of chronic illnesses and conditions.

TABLE C-2. Federal and State Medicaid Payments for the Aged and Non-Aged by Service Category, Fiscal Year 1991

(all payment amounts are in millions)

Service category	Aged		Non-aged		Total	
	Payments	Percent of total	Payments	Percent of total	Payments	Percent of total
Total	$25,444		$51,521		$76,964	
Nursing homes	17,121	67.3%	3,578	6.9%	20,699	26.9%
Home care services[a]	2,026	8.0%	2,075	4.0%	4,101	5.3%
Prescription drugs	1,823	7.2%	3,601	7.0%	5,424	7.0%
Inpatient hospital	1,634	6.4%	18,217	35.4%	19,851	25.8%
Inpatient mental health	1,055	4.1%	954	1.9%	2,010	2.6%
ICF/MR	429	1.7%	7,250	14.1%	7,680	10.0%
Physician services	343	1.3%	4,603	8.9%	4,946	6.4%
Outpatient hospital	255	1.0%	4,025	7.8%	4,280	5.6%
Clinic services	137	0.5%	2,071	4.0%	2,208	2.9%
Other practitioner	61	0.2%	376	0.7%	436	0.6%
Dental services	45	0.2%	665	1.3%	709	0.9%
Lab & x-ray	48	0.2%	848	1.6%	896	1.2%
Rural health clinics	2	0.0%	61	0.1%	63	0.1%
Other services[b]	466	1.8%	3,196	6.2%	3,661	4.8%

[a] Home care services in this table include home health, personal care services, and home and community-based waiver services.

[b] Other services include payments for unknown service spending, as well as transportation and other related travel services, physical therapy services, occupational therapy, dentures, hospice services, family planning services and many other services.

Source: Table prepared by the Congressional Research Service based on data contained on *Statistical Report on Medical Care Eligibles, Recipients, Payments, and Services*, HCFA Form 2082.

The distribution of payments for various covered services for the elderly is very different from the distribution for those under 65. Table C-2 and figure C-2 illustrate the differences. For the nonelderly, inpatient hospital care, ICF/MR, and physician services are the three largest spending categories.

FIGURE C-2. Medicaid Payments for Selected Services,
for Aged and Non-Aged Beneficiaries, FY 1991

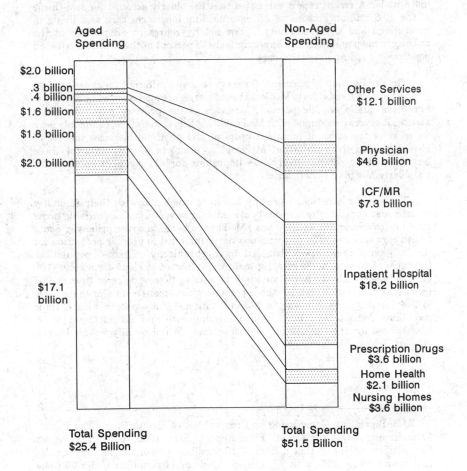

Source: Figure prepared by Congressional Research Service
based on data obtained from the Health Care Financing Administration.

The difference in the distribution of payments for services for elderly and nonelderly beneficiaries reflects a number of factors, including the fact that elderly persons need and use long-term care more often than younger individuals. A recent report estimated that the elderly account for two-thirds of the 10.6 million persons of all ages needing long-term care and living in institutions and the community.[6] The elderly represent 88 percent of the nursing home population and approximately 63 percent of the community-based population needing long-term care.[7]

The distribution of payments for services is also different for these two age groups because most elderly Medicaid beneficiaries are also covered by Medicare. For these dually eligible persons, Medicare is the primary payer for those services it covers in common with Medicaid. Medicare, therefore, commonly pays for most of the costs of inpatient hospital and physician services instead of Medicaid, with the result that Medicaid as a source of payments for these services will be comparatively less important for elderly persons than for nonelderly Medicaid beneficiaries.

The specific benefits covered by Medicare, combined with their eligibility criteria, also explain why Medicaid payments for services, such as nursing home care, are as important as they are. Medicare's benefits cover primarily acute health care services. The program was never intended to provide protection for the long-term care services needed by a chronically impaired population. Coverage of nursing home care, for instance, is limited to short-term stays (100 days per spell of illness) in certain kinds of nursing homes, referred to as skilled nursing facilities, and only for those persons who demonstrate a need for daily skilled nursing care following a hospitalization. Many people with chronic conditions do not need daily skilled nursing care and do not need to be hospitalized for their condition, and, therefore, do not qualify for Medicare's benefit.

---

[6] U.S. Bipartisan Commission on Comprehensive Health Care. The Pepper Commission. *A Call for Action.* Final Report. Sept. 1990. p.91. The Pepper Commission estimated that a total of 10.6 million persons of all ages needed long-term care in 1990, with 7.1 million elderly and 3.5 million under 65 years of age.

[7] The Pepper Commission estimated that the total nursing home population included 1.7 million individuals in 1990, with 1.5 million elderly and 0.2 million nonelderly. The Commission also estimated that the community-based population amounted to 8.9 million persons, with 5.6 million elderly and 3.3 million nonelderly. For a more detailed discussion of the demographic characteristics of the nursing home population according the 1985 National Nursing Home Survey, see: U.S. Library of Congress. Congressional Research Service. *Characteristics of Nursing Home Residents and Proposals for Reforming Coverage of Nursing Home Care.* CRS Report for Congress No. 90-471 EPW, by Richard Price, Richard Rimkunas, and Carol O'Shaughnessy.

Medicaid's nursing facility benefit, on the other hand, is not limited to persons with skilled care needs. It also covers people with health-related needs caused by chronic conditions and illnesses that do not require skilled care to be managed. Nor is Medicaid's coverage limited to a given number of days. As a result of its comparatively broader coverage (not considering for the moment Medicaid's income and assets tests), Medicare's restrictions, and the absence of extensive private insurance coverage at the present time, Medicaid has become the Nation's major program of coverage for nursing home care.

Figure C-3 shows that in 1990, Medicaid spending for nursing home care (including ICFs/MR) amounted to 45 percent of total national spending for this care. By way of contrast, Medicare spending amounted to about 5 percent and private insurance payments to 1 percent of total national spending. Out-of-pocket payments accounted for most of the remaining spending, amounting to 45 percent of total spending. Out-of-pocket spending includes payments from the assets and income of nursing home residents as well as of their relatives.

FIGURE C-3. Sources of Funding for Nursing Home Care, CY 1990

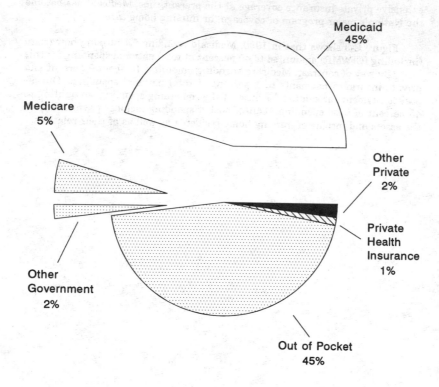

Medicaid
45%

Medicare
5%

Other
Private
2%

Private
Health
Insurance
1%

Other
Government
2%

Out of Pocket
45%

Total Spending = $53.1 Billion

Source: Figure prepared by Congressional Research Service based on data from Office of the Actuary, Division of National Cost Estimates.

B. Medicaid Payments for Elderly Beneficiaries, by Eligibility Status

Elderly persons become eligible for Medicaid-covered benefits in one of three ways.[8] First, there are welfare-related paths to eligibility.

States must generally provide Medicaid coverage to persons receiving Supplemental Security Income (SSI) payments. SSI provides cash assistance to certain "categories" of needy persons, specifically the aged, blind, and disabled, with little or no income and resources. In most States, elderly persons, as one of the groups covered by SSI, can receive SSI--and Medicaid--if their income and assets do not exceed levels specified in SSI law. For single individuals in 1992, these levels are $422 of income per month and $2,000 of resources.

In addition, Medicaid law gives States the option of using an alternative set of eligibility standards that may be more restrictive than SSI policies, but only if those policies were being used for Medicaid eligibility in 1972 when SSI was enacted. Currently 12 States use these alternative eligibility standards and are often referred to as "209(b) States," after the section in the Social Security Amendments of 1972 that authorized this option. See *Chapter III, Eligibility* for a list of these States.

States also have the option of extending Medicaid eligibility to persons who are eligible for State Supplement Payments (SSP). Many States provide these supplemental cash assistance payments because they feel the SSI benefit standard to be insufficient to cover a person's living expenses; in 1992, the SSI benefit for a single individual represented 74 percent of the Federal poverty level. Medicaid allows States to provide automatic coverage to persons receiving SSP on the same basis as they do for persons receiving SSI only.

Elderly persons who become eligible for Medicaid through one of these welfare-related paths are sometimes referred to as the cash categorically needy. They belong to one of the "categories" of persons eligible for SSI and Medicaid, and they receive cash assistance.

Medicaid also allows States to cover persons who are not poor by SSI standards, but who need assistance with medical expenses. One of these groups is known as the medically needy. These are persons who have incomes too high to qualify for SSI, but who have incurred medical expenses that deplete their income and resources to levels that make them needy according to State-determined standards. Persons qualifying for medically needy coverage generally first deplete their resources to the State's eligibility standard--usually $2,000 for an individual--and then continue to incur medical expenses that reduce their income to the level required by the State.

---

[8]Medicaid eligibility policies and the elderly are discussed in greater detail in *Chapter III, Eligibility*. Summary information is presented here.

States are permitted but not required to cover the medically needy under their plans. If they decide to cover the medically needy, they also have the option of including the elderly under their programs. In 1991, 37 States had medically needy programs and 35 elected to extend Medicaid coverage to the elderly. Many elderly persons meet the financial standards for medically needy coverage as the result of needing nursing home care. Not all States, however, cover nursing home care under their medically needy programs. Twenty-nine States with medically needy programs for the elderly included nursing home care as a covered service in 1991.

Under Medicaid law, States may extend coverage to another group of persons who have incomes too high to qualify for SSI or SSP. These persons, however, cannot have income that exceeds a specified level and they must also reside in nursing homes or other medical care institutions. The provision in Medicaid law that allows States to cover these persons is often referred to as the "300 percent rule" because the income level used for coverage cannot exceed 3 times the basic SSI payment level (in 1992, $1,266 per month). States are also permitted to apply the 300 percent rule to persons needing home and community-based care waiver services (since these persons would otherwise require institutional care that Medicaid would cover). Persons qualifying for Medicaid under the 300 percent rule are the largest group of beneficiaries referred to as noncash categorically needy.[9]

Figure C-4 shows the number of elderly Medicaid beneficiaries in each these three groups and payments made on their behalf. A total of 3.34 million elderly persons received Medicaid benefits in FY 1991. Almost half of these were persons receiving cash assistance. The cash categorically needy included 1.49 million elderly, or 45 percent, of total elderly beneficiaries. These are persons who qualify for Medicaid through one of the welfare-related paths to eligibility.

The medically needy and noncash categorically needy represent almost all of the remaining elderly persons receiving benefits in FY 1991.[10] The medically needy included 643,985 persons, or 19 percent of total elderly beneficiaries, and the noncash categorically needy included 953,912 persons, or 29 percent of the total.

---

[9]The noncash categorically needy also include certain persons who were once entitled to SSI, but no longer receiving it, and other groups. See *Chapter III, Eligibility* for additional information.

[10]"Other" in figure C-4 includes those elderly persons who become eligible as "qualified Medicare beneficiaries." A qualified Medicare beneficiary (QMB) is an aged or disabled Medicare beneficiary whose income is at or below 100 percent of poverty, and whose resources are at or below 200 percent of the SSI limit. Medicaid is required to pay Medicare premiums and cost sharing charges for these persons. Medicaid protection is limited to payment of these charges, unless the beneficiary is otherwise eligible for benefits under the program. Persons in this category may actually qualify for Medicaid benefits as cash categorically needy, medically needy, or noncash categorically needy.

Figure C-4 indicates that these latter two groups, which together represent 48 percent of total elderly beneficiaries, accounted for 74 percent of total spending for the elderly in FY 1990. The 45 percent of elderly beneficiaries receiving cash assistance were responsible for only 20 percent of total program payments.

FIGURE C-4. Aged Beneficiaries and Payments for Aged Beneficiaries by Eligibility Status, FY 1991

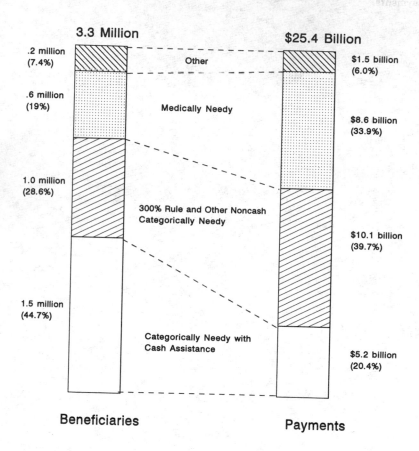

Source: Figure prepared by Congressional Research Service based on data obtained from the Health Care Financing Administration.

Payments for nursing home care explain much of this disparity. The top half of table C-3 shows that comparatively larger numbers of medically needy and noncash categorically needy used nursing facility care than did the cash categorically needy. Approximately 6 of every 10 medically needy beneficiaries and 3 of every 4 noncash categorically needy used nursing home care in FY 1991. Fewer than 1 of every 10 cash categorically needy used nursing home care in that year.

The bottom half of table C-3 shows that nursing facility care had high payment costs per beneficiary, regardless of eligibility status, as compared to most other service categories.

TABLE C-3. Number of Beneficiaries and Payments Per Beneficiary, by Service Category and Eligibility Status for the Aged, Fiscal Year 1991

Number of Beneficiaries

Service category	Categorically needy	Categorically needy with no cash assistance	Medically needy	Other
NF[a]	111,894	700,227	390,725	61,658
Inpatient hospital	350,196	211,104	135,036	63,115
Inpatient mental health	5,347	7,907	6,506	475
ICF/MR	1,795	2,164	1,026	2,684
Physician services	1,083,350	597,016	308,435	195,797
Dental services	99,256	134,625	53,330	20,563
Other practitioners	350,078	242,686	141,656	71,754
Outpatient hospital	539,171	288,626	130,692	90,189
Clinic services	85,416	75,756	34,253	11,849
Home care services	169,632	53,700	64,583	12,304
Lab and x-ray services	395,993	236,967	118,025	71,444
Prescription drugs	1,325,235	814,959	434,179	152,659
Rural health	12,677	4,300	1,419	3,762
Other care	550,996	395,521	265,962	84,505
Any service	1,494,834	953,912	643,985	247,775

See notes at end of table.

TABLE C-3. Number of Beneficiaries and Payments Per Beneficiary, by Service Category and Eligibility Status for the Aged, Fiscal Year 1991--Continued

Payments Per Beneficiary

Service category	Categorically needy	Categorically needy with no cash assistance	Medically needy	Other
NF[a]	$12,842	$11,944	$16,090	$16,764
Inpatient hospital	2,284	1,353	3,233	1,772
Inpatient mental health	63,634	20,238	83,904	17,987
ICF/MR	65,485	43,266	85,737	48,648
Physician services	159	162	137	165
Dental services	194	116	141	117
Other practitioners	70	56	131	54
Outpatient hospital	247	250	233	205
Clinic services	839	416	747	675
Home care services	6,211	3,333	11,577	3,731
Lab and x-ray services	66	50	55	44
Prescription drugs	606	771	673	654
Rural health	85	90	106	81
Other care	346	388	325	408
Any service[b]	3,472	10,594	13,377	6,189

[a]As of Oct. 1, 1990, skilled nursing facility (SNF) and intermediate care facility (ICF) benefits were consolidated into a single benefit called nursing facility (NF) care.

[b]The average payment for beneficiaries using one or more services.

Source: Table prepared by the Congressional Research Service based on data contained on HCFA Form 2082.

The combination of a high proportion of medically needy and noncash categorically needy using nursing facility care and high payment costs for this care results in nursing facility care payments representing a very high percentage of total payments for these two groups. As shown in table C-4, nursing facility payments in FY 1991 amounted to 73 percent of total payments for the medically needy and 83 percent of payments for the noncash categorically needy. Nursing home payments for these two groups combined were so large that they accounted for nearly 60 percent of total program payments for all elderly beneficiaries.

TABLE C-4. Payments by Service Category and
Eligibility Status for the Aged, Fiscal Year 1991
(payments in millions)

Service category	Categorically needy with cash assistance	Categorically needy with no cash assistance	Medically needy	Other
NF[a]	$1,437	$8,363	$6,287	$1,034
Inpatient hospital	800	286	437	112
Inpatient mental health	340	160	546	9
ICF/MR	118	94	88	131
Physician services	172	97	42	32
Dental services	19	16	8	2
Other practitioners	25	14	19	4
Outpatient hospital	133	72	30	18
Clinic services	72	31	26	8
Home care services[b]	1,054	179	748	46
Lab and x-ray services	26	12	6	3
Prescription drugs	803	628	292	100
Rural health[c]	1	0	0	0
Other care	191	153	87	34
All services	5,190	10,106	8,614	1,533

[a]As of Oct. 1, 1990, skilled nursing facility (SNF) and intermediate care facility (ICF) benefits were consolidated into a single benefit called nursing facility (NF) care.

[b]Home care services in this table include home health, personal care services, and home and community-based waiver services.

[c]Payment entries of zero indicate spending in the category is less than $500 thousand.

Source: Table prepared by the Congressional Research Service based on data contained on HCFA Form 2082.

It is nursing home spending for the medically needy and noncash categorically needy that largely explains the fact that elderly Medicaid beneficiaries over the years have accounted for a disproportionately large portion of Medicaid payments for services. In FY 1972, elderly beneficiaries represented 19 percent of total program beneficiaries and accounted for 38 percent of program payments. While the elderly have declined as a proportion of total program beneficiaries since that time, their proportion of total program payments has remained relatively high. In FY 1991, elderly beneficiaries represented 12 percent of total Medicaid beneficiaries and their share of program payments amounted to 33 percent of total program payments.

C. Medicaid Payments for Elderly Beneficiaries, by State

Table C-5 indicates that in each of the States the elderly account for a disproportionately large portion of Medicaid spending. A closer examination of data in this table shows that States actually exhibit a great deal of variation in the proportion of beneficiaries who are elderly, the proportion of program payments made on their behalf, and the magnitude of difference between these two ratios. The percentage of elderly Medicaid beneficiaries in a State's Medicaid program ranged from 6.5 percent in Utah to 19.7 percent in North Dakota. The proportion of total program payments for the elderly ranged from 16.9 percent in Utah to 51.4 percent in New Hampshire. Average payments per elderly beneficiary ranged from $3,426 in Mississippi to $19,278 in Connecticut, with Michigan representing the median value of $6,926. Variation in these ratios can be explained by differences in the scope of benefits covered, reimbursement rates for benefits, and eligibility policies for coverage.

TABLE C-5. State-by-State Comparison of Number of Aged Medicaid
Beneficiaries and Payments for These Beneficiaries,
Fiscal Year 1991

State	Aged beneficiaries		Payments for the aged		
	Number	Percent of total	Payments (in millions)	Percent of total	Payment per beneficiary
Alabama	68,370	17.0	$ 263	32.6	$ 3,841
Alaska	3,368	6.6	34	21.0	9,995
Arizona	0	0.0	0	0.0	0
Arkansas	45,896	16.1	220	31.9	4,788
California	456,700	11.4	1,941	25.6	4,251
Colorado	31,813	14.2	200	29.7	6,279
Connecticut	43,085	15.8	831	51.0	19,278
Delaware	5,038	9.9	57	30.7	11,355
District of Columbia	11,426	11.4	139	31.1	12,136
Florida	174,852	14.0	922	31.3	5,271
Georgia	93,279	12.5	484	26.9	5,190
Hawaii	12,792	14.0	102	42.9	7,974
Idaho	7,586	10.8	64	28.6	8,395
Illinois	91,092	8.0	605	22.2	6,644
Indiana	48,484	11.7	472	28.4	9,743
Iowa	37,013	14.2	219	28.6	5,919
Kansas	24,646	11.8	167	30.2	6,785
Kentucky	57,260	10.9	308	25.6	5,371
Louisiana	90,807	14.2	414	24.0	4,559
Maine	21,600	14.3	212	39.6	9,834
Maryland	43,903	12.1	388	30.0	8,829
Massachusetts	96,198	14.8	1,114	39.4	11,584
Michigan	85,930	7.7	595	23.4	6,926
Minnesota	54,512	12.9	604	38.7	11,089
Mississippi	67,966	14.5	233	30.8	3,426
Missouri	76,579	15.2	427	38.2	5,570
Montana	7,443	11.7	63	32.5	8,434
Nebraska	18,386	13.7	143	36.6	7,751
Nevada	8,303	14.0	49	27.7	5,939
New Hampshire	11,719	19.6	150	51.4	12,829
New Jersey	74,815	12.2	885	32.5	11,835
New Mexico	13,889	8.6	84	24.6	6,062
New York	335,948	13.6	5,739	41.8	17,084
North Carolina	109,796	16.5	581	32.5	5,295
North Dakota	10,343	19.7	90	39.6	8,680
Ohio	117,748	9.1	1,190	32.6	10,102
Oklahoma	53,629	17.6	264	32.4	4,915
Oregon	26,447	10.0	164	24.6	6,188

TABLE C-5. State-by-State Comparison of Number of Aged Medicaid Beneficiaries and Payments for These Beneficiaries, Fiscal Year 1991--Continued

State	Aged beneficiaries		Payments for the aged		
	Number	Percent of total	Payments (in millions)	Percent of total	Payment per beneficiary
Pennsylvania	135,38	10.6	$ 1,137	33.1	$8,397
Rhode Island	30,10	18.4	252	38.3	8,363
South Carolina	55,146	14.7	234	25.7	4,242
South Dakota	9,217	16.1	71	36.4	7,744
Tennessee	89,041	12.8	382	25.7	4,290
Texas	244,136	14.1	1,230	34.8	5,036
Utah	8,412	6.5	53	16.9	6,273
Vermont	10,499	14.9	67	34.1	6,396
Virginia	72,427	16.4	436	35.8	6,025
Washington	47,592	9.4	375	33.1	7,876
West Virginia	29,720	10.5	166	30.6	5,585
Wisconsin	66,001	15.9	596	40.5	9,037
Wyoming	3,044	8.3	28	31.6	9,360
Puerto Rico	0	0.0	0	0.0	0
Virgin Islands	1,125	9.6	1	18.1	676
Reporting States & D.C.	3,339,381	12.5	25,443	33.1	7,619
U.S. Total	3,340,506	11.9	$25,444	33.1	$7,617

NOTE: Spending represents spending by reporting States for medical vendor payments and excludes any administrative spending.

Source: Table prepared by the Congressional Research Service based on data contained on HCFA Form 2082.

Table C-6 provides State level data on long-term care spending for the elderly and the proportion of total Medicaid spending this amount represents. Long-term care payments accounted for 27 percent of total national Medicaid spending, with this proportion ranging from 13.6 percent in Utah to 46.3 percent in New Hampshire. Table C-7 examines the two major components of long-term care spending for the elderly and shows the percentage nursing home payments and home care payments represent of total elderly spending. Nursing facility care accounts for the greatest portion of elderly spending in all States,[11] ranging from 49 percent in New York to 87.8 percent in Wyoming. Home care payments, which include home health, personal care, and home and community-based waiver services, range from less than 0.1 percent in Pennsylvania to 23.2

[11]For FY 1991, Utah incorrectly reported long-term care payments, by type of service. This reporting error has been corrected for subsequent fiscal years.

percent in New York. Variations in payments for nursing home care and home care reflect differences among the States in the supply of nursing home beds, decisions to cover certain optional home care services, such as 1915(c) home and community-based waiver services and personal care, and reimbursement rates for care.

TABLE C-6. Aged Long-Term Care Payments by Service Category and as a Share of Total State Medicaid Payments, FY 1991

State	Nursing home payments (in millions)	Percent	Home care payments (in millions)	Percent	Other long-term care payments (in millions)	Percent	Total long-term care payments (in millions)	Percent
Alabama	$ 186.8	23.2	$18.6	2.3	$ 7.7	1.0	$ 213.2	26.5
Alaska	26.0	16.2	0.3	0.2	0.1	0.1	26.4	16.5
Arizona								
Arkansas	157.0	22.8	16.4	2.4	0.2	0.0	173.6	25.2
California	1221.5	16.1	2.1	0.0	133.7	1.8	1357.3	17.9
Colorado	147.2	21.9	10.6	1.6	1.9	0.3	159.6	23.7
Connecticut	627.9	38.5	67.3	4.1	27.5	1.7	722.7	44.3
Delaware	44.8	24.0	2.8	1.5	1.3	0.7	48.8	26.2
District of Columbia	89.1	20.0	5.6	1.2	21.1	4.7	115.7	26
Florida	665.2	22.6	5.8	0.2	13.1	0.4	684.1	23.2
Georgia	339.8	18.9	24.1	1.3	1.2	0.1	365.0	20.3
Hawaii	78.7	33.2	0.2	0.1	0.1	0.1	79.0	33.3
Idaho	50.1	22.5	3.2	1.4	1.1	0.5	54.4	24.4
Illinois	485.4	17.8	23.0	0.8	4.8	0.2	513.2	18.8
Indiana	386.7	23.3	1.6	0.1	3.2	0.2	391.5	23.6
Iowa	165.0	21.6	4.8	0.6	0.8	0.1	170.6	22.3
Kansas	138.5	25.0	2.2	0.4	4.2	0.8	144.9	26.2
Kentucky	220.6	18.4	14.6	1.2	0.3	0.0	235.5	19.6
Louisiana	267.3	15.5	3.7	0.2	5.5	0.3	276.6	16
Maine	167.7	31.2	7.4	1.4	3.7	0.7	178.9	33.3
Maryland	292.3	22.6	10.3	0.8	7.2	0.6	309.7	24
Massachusetts	818.8	29.0	35.8	1.3	4.4	0.2	859.0	30.4

TABLE C-6. Aged Long-Term Care Payments by Service Category
and as a Share of Total State Medicaid Payments, FY 1991--Continued

State	Nursing home payments		Home care payments		Other long-term care payments		Total long-term care payments	
	(in millions)	Percent	(in millions)	Percent	(in millions)	Percent	(in millions)	Percent
Michigan	$ 458.4	18.1	$ 32.3	1.3	$ 19.8	0.8	$ 510.4	20.1
Minnesota	516.3	33.1	13.5	0.9	13.0	0.8	542.8	34.8
Mississippi	152.7	20.2	0.3	0.0	2.0	0.3	155.1	20.5
Missouri	308.1	27.6	15.6	1.4	5.5	0.5	329.2	29.5
Montana	48.5	25.1	0.2	0.1	0.2	0.1	48.9	25.3
Nebraska	113.8	29.2	2.5	0.6	2.5	0.6	118.8	30.5
Nevada	35.3	19.8	2.4	1.4	0.2	0.1	38.0	21.3
New Hampshire	121.6	41.6	6.6	2.3	7.1	2.4	135.4	46.3
New Jersey	626.5	23.0	48.2	1.8	59.3	2.2	734.1	26.9
New Mexico	67.4	19.7	0.8	0.2	0.2	0.1	68.4	20
New York	2811.4	20.5	1328.7	9.7	870.6	6.3	5010.7	36.5
North Carolina	372.0	20.8	49.7	2.8	21.4	1.2	443.0	24.8
North Dakota	68.5	30.2	5.3	2.3	4.0	1.8	77.9	34.3
Ohio	990.6	27.1	8.4	0.2	12.0	0.3	1011.0	27.7
Oklahoma	183.0	22.5	21.1	2.6	3.5	0.4	207.5	25.5
Oregon	108.3	16.2	23.9	3.6	4.8	0.7	137.0	20.5
Pennsylvania	906.3	26.4	0.5	0.0	82.9	2.4	989.7	28.8
Rhode Island	129.3	19.6	14.7	2.2	2.8	0.4	146.8	22.3
South Carolina	137.7	15.1	17.6	1.9	22.1	2.4	177.5	19.5
South Dakota	54.9	28.0	1.0	0.5	6.0	3.1	62.0	31.6

TABLE C-6. Aged Long-Term Care Payments by Service Category and as a Share of Total State Medicaid Payments, FY 1991--Continued

State	Nursing home payments		Home care payments		Other long-term care payments		Total long-term care payments	
	(in millions)	Percent	(in millions)	Percent	(in millions)	Percent	(in millions)	Percent
Tennessee	$ 305.2	20.5	$ 1.5	0.1	$ 2.8	0.2	$ 309.4	20.8
Texas	801.9	22.7	112.4	3.2	25.9	0.7	940.1	26.6
Utah	0.1	0.0	0.7	0.2	41.4	13.3	42.2	13.6
Vermont	47.4	24.1	2.8	1.4	2.3	1.2	52.5	26.7
Virginia	272.2	22.3	24.8	2.0	18.8	1.5	315.9	25.9
Washington	306.8	27.1	1.8	0.2	0.6	0.1	309.2	27.3
West Virginia	113.8	21.0	0.7	0.1	0.7	0.1	115.3	21.3
Wisconsin	461.4	31.3	27.7	1.9	8.4	0.6	497.5	33.8
Wyoming	25.0	27.8	0.0	0.0	0.4	0.4	25.4	28.2
Puerto Rico	0.0	0.0	0.0	0.0	0.0	0.0	0.0	0
Virgin Islands	0.0	0.0	0.0	0.1	0.0	0.0	0.0	0.1
Reporting States & District of Columbia	17,120.8		2,026.1		1,484.4		20,631.4	
U.S. Total	$17,120.8		$2,026.2		$1,484.4		$20,631.4	

NOTE: Home care payments represent spending in home health, personal care services, and home and community-based care services. Other long-term care services include spending on ICF/MR and IMD services.

Source: Table prepared by the Congressional Research Service based on data contained on HCFA Form 2082.

TABLE C-7. Aged Nursing Home and Home Care Payments as a Percent of all Medicaid Payments for the Aged, by State, FY 1991

State	Nursing home payments		Home care payments	
	(in millions)	Percent	(in millions)	Percent
Alabama	$ 186.8	71.1	$ 18.6	7.1
Alaska	26.0	77.2	0.3	0.9
Arizona	0.0	0.0	0.0	0.0
Arkansas	157.0	71.4	16.4	7.5
California	1,221.5	62.9	2.1	0.1
Colorado	147.2	73.7	10.6	5.3
Connecticut	627.9	75.6	67.3	8.1
Delaware	44.8	78.3	2.8	4.9
District of Columbia	89.1	64.2	5.6	4.0
Florida	665.2	72.2	5.8	0.6
Georgia	339.8	70.2	24.1	5.0
Hawaii	78.7	77.1	0.2	0.2
Idaho	50.1	78.6	3.2	5.0
Illinois	485.4	80.2	23.0	3.8
Indiana	386.7	81.8	1.6	0.3
Iowa	165.0	75.3	4.8	2.2
Kansas	138.5	82.8	2.2	1.3
Kentucky	220.6	71.7	14.6	4.7
Louisiana	267.3	64.6	3.7	0.9
Maine	167.7	79.0	7.4	3.5
Maryland	292.3	75.4	10.3	2.7
Massachusetts	818.8	73.5	35.8	3.2
Michigan	458.4	77.0	32.3	5.4
Minnesota	516.3	85.4	13.5	2.2
Mississippi	152.7	65.6	0.3	0.1
Missouri	308.1	72.2	15.6	3.7
Montana	48.5	77.3	0.2	0.3
Nebraska	113.8	79.8	2.5	1.8
Nevada	35.3	71.7	2.4	4.9
New Hampshire	121.6	80.9	6.6	4.4
New Jersey	626.5	70.8	48.2	5.4
New Mexico	67.4	80.0	0.8	0.9
New York	2,811.4	49.0	1,328.7	23.2
North Carolina	372.0	64.0	49.7	8.5
North Dakota	68.5	76.3	5.3	5.9
Ohio	990.6	83.3	8.4	0.7
Oklahoma	183.0	69.4	21.1	8.0
Oregon	108.3	66.2	23.9	14.6
Pennsylvania	906.3	79.7	0.5	0.0
Rhode Island	129.3	51.3	14.7	5.8
South Carolina	137.7	58.9	17.6	7.5

TABLE C-7. Aged Nursing Home and Home Care Payments as a Percent of all Medicaid Payments for the Aged, by State, FY 1991--Continued

State	Nursing home payments		Home care payments	
	(in millions)	Percent	(in millions)	Percent
South Dakota	$ 54.9	76.9	$ 1.0	1.4
Tennessee	305.2	79.9	1.5	0.4
Texas	801.9	65.2	112.4	9.1
Utah	0.1	0.2	0.7	1.3
Vermont	47.4	70.6	2.8	4.2
Virginia	272.2	62.4	24.8	5.7
Washington	306.8	81.9	1.8	0.5
West Virginia	113.8	68.6	0.7	0.4
Wisconsin	461.4	77.4	27.7	4.6
Wyoming	25.0	87.8	0.0	0.1
Puerto Rico	0.0	0.0	0.0	0.0
Virgin Islands	0.0	0.0	0.0	0.3
Reporting States & D.C.	17,121	67.3	2,026	8.0
U.S. Total	$17,121	67.3	$2,026	8.0

NOTE: Home care payments represent spending on home health, personal care services, and home and community-based care services. Other long-term care services include spending on ICF/MR and IMD services.

Source: Table prepared by the Congressional Research Service based on data contained on HCFA Form 2082.

IV. SPENDING DOWN FOR MEDICAID COVERAGE

A. Spending Down as the Result of
Needing Nursing Home Care

As discussed above, the Medicaid program is the major public source of support for the cost of nursing home care. Its spending for nursing home care is driven largely by its coverage of persons who do not receive cash welfare assistance--the medically needy and persons who become eligible under the 300 percent rule. At an average cost of $30,000 a year, nursing home costs can quickly deplete the resources of an elderly individual, especially after prolonged stays, and these costs also exceed the monthly income of most persons. The depletion of financial resources on the cost of care and the movement from private payment for care to Medicaid coverage is referred to as the "spend-down" process. In 1991, Medicaid nursing home payments for elderly medically needy and 300 percent rule beneficiaries amounted to nearly 60 percent of total Medicaid payments for all services for all elderly beneficiaries.

Spending down under Medicaid is a two-step process. First, persons must meet the resources or assets test. The term "resources" generally refers to liquid assets such as cash on hand, savings and checking accounts, stocks and bonds, etc. In order to become eligible for Medicaid, the value of the individual's available resources must be less than the State-determined dollar standard, usually $2,000 for an individual without a spouse,[12] the level used for the SSI program. Certain items, such as the house, are excluded as countable resources under SSI and Medicaid rules at the point of eligibility determination.

Second, after an individual has depleted virtually all accumulated resources on the cost of care, the Medicaid program considers whether a person satisfies income rules. In States with medically needy programs, persons with incomes above the State's standard must incur medical expenses that deplete their incomes to a specified level. Thus, under the medically needy option, States have no absolute upper limit on income for applicants seeking Medicaid coverage of their care. As long as the applicant's current monthly income is insufficient to cover medical and health-related expenses, including nursing home costs, the applicant can become eligible for Medicaid.

States that do not cover nursing home care under medically needy programs use the 300 percent rule for making persons eligible. In 1991, 17 States used only the 300 percent rule for making persons eligible for institutional care.[13]

---

[12]Medicaid has special rules for protecting resources and income for the community spouse of a nursing home resident. These are referred to as the "spousal impoverishment" protections of Medicaid law, because they are intended to prevent the impoverishment of the spouse remaining in the community. See *Chapter III, Eligibility* for a fuller discussion.

[13]These States were Alabama, Alaska, Arizona, Arkansas, Colorado, Delaware, Florida, Idaho, Iowa, Louisiana, Mississippi, Nevada, New Jersey, New Mexico, South Dakota, Texas, and Wyoming.

This means that persons with income $1 over the State's limit or those who receive cost-of-living adjustments that increase their pension income over the State's limit can not become eligible for Medicaid's coverage of their nursing home expenses, even if the cost of nursing home care far exceeds their income and they have depleted all of their resources on the cost of their care.

Following eligibility, Medicaid then applies post-eligibility rules to determine how much of a beneficiary's income must be applied to the cost of care.[14] Post-eligibility rules require that an individual's payment for care equal total income, minus certain amounts that may be set aside for the personal needs of the beneficiary, the living expenses of a spouse and minor children if those family members have little or no income of their own, and medical care expenses. The State's payment for care equals the difference between its reimbursement rate for the service needed by the eligible individual and the amount the individual must pay as determined under the post-eligibility treatment of income calculation.

Over the past several years, studies have examined existing data bases to develop estimates of the number of nursing home residents who spend down and qualify for Medicaid coverage of their care. They have also focused on the length of time it takes for persons to deplete their resources and become Medicaid eligible. While a number of studies have examined both of these questions in recent years, definitive answers are not yet available, since the ideal data base does not exist.

The ideal data base for measuring spend-down would track all health and long-term care use and expenses associated with these services for a nationally representative cohort of elderly persons over time until their deaths.[15] It would also track sources of payment for care, changes in sources of payment as well as changes in income and assets over time, and the specific point in time when an individual becomes eligible for Medicaid. Existing data bases have a number of limitations. They fail to capture total lifetime use of nursing home care and often have source of payment information for only the most recent admission. State data bases, while tracking nursing home use over a longer period of time and collecting information about multiple admissions, also contain some of these limitations and can not be generalized to the Nation as a whole.

---

[14]The term "spend-down" was originally used to refer to beneficiary contributions to the cost of care from the monthly incomes of medically needy beneficiaries following eligibility. Today the term is generally used to refer to *asset* spend-down that occurs before a person becomes eligible for Medicaid. See: Burwell, Brian. *Middle-Class Welfare: Medicaid Estate Planning for Long-Term Care Coverage.* Lexington, SysteMetrics/McGraw-Hill, Sept. 1991.   p. 3. (Hereafter cited as Burwell, *Middle-Class Welfare*)

[15]Adams, E. Kathleen, Mark Meiners, and Brian Burwell. *A Synthesis and Critique of Studies on Medicaid Asset Spend-Down.* U.S. Dept. of Health and Human Services. Office of the Assistant Secretary for Planning and Evaluation. Jan. 1992. Washington, 1992. p. 5.

A review of existing studies in *A Synthesis and Critique of Studies on Medicaid Asset Spend-Down* by Adams, Meiners and Burwell, found that researchers have generally used two different measures of Medicaid asset spend-down.[16] One measures the percentage of persons originally admitted to nursing homes as private payers who eventually convert to Medicaid prior to final discharge. This method is a measure of the financial risk that a nursing home stay or stays will result in impoverishment and Medicaid eligibility.

A second measure examines the percentage of Medicaid residents of nursing homes who were not eligible for Medicaid when they were originally admitted. This method can be useful for understanding the proportion of State Medicaid expenditures for nursing home care that is accounted for by those who spend-down.

The review of spend-down studies, which use several different national and State-level data bases, found widely varying estimates of spend-down as measured by these two methods. The critical factor explaining differences among these studies is the length of time persons were studied. The proportion of persons spending down during a single stay is much lower than the proportion of persons who spend-down over their entire lifetime, since half or more of persons using nursing home care have multiple stays. In general, studies using national data tend to show lower estimates of spend-down than do State studies that tend to observe people over longer time intervals.

Spend-down rates in studies estimating the percent of nursing home residents entering as private pay patients and converting to Medicaid ranged from 10 to 23 percent. For this method of measuring spend-down, not enough State studies exist to determine the extent to which spend-down rates vary from State to State.

On the other hand, estimates of spend-down as measured by the percentage of Medicaid residents of nursing homes who were not eligible for Medicaid when they were originally admitted vary considerably across States, reflecting variations in Medicaid eligibility policies across the States as well as other factors. Studies measuring spend-down according to this method have found spend-down rates of 27 percent for Michigan, 31 percent for Wisconsin, and 39 to 45 percent for Connecticut.

Tables C-8 and C-9 summarize the findings of the spend-down studies reviewed in *A Synthesis and Critique of Studies on Medicaid Asset Spend-Down.*

---

[16]Ibid.

TABLE C-8. Estimates of the Proportion of Private Pay Admissions to Nursing Homes
Who Eventually Spend-Down to Medicaid

Source	Population	Sample(s)	Estimate	Comments
Arling, et al.	Wisconsin (1988)	Discharge sample	23.0%	Omitted transfers from discharge sample (7%)
Bice	Connecticut (1978-1983)	6 admission cohorts	21.8%	Tail-end of stays and spend-down probabilities estimated by parametric survival models
Bice	Connecticut (1983-1987)	1983-1984 admission cohort	23.0%	Tail-end of stays and spend-down probabilities estimated by parametric survival models
Farbstein, et al.	Connecticut (1985)	Discharge cohort	17.3%	75% of spend-downers had more than one admission
Gruenberg, et al.	Connecticut (1978-1979)	Admission cohort	21.3%	Includes <65 population

TABLE C-8. Estimates of the Proportion of Private Pay Admissions to Nursing Homes Who Eventually Spend-Down to Medicaid--Continued

Source	Population	Sample(s)	Estimate	Comments
Liu and Manton	Connecticut (1977-1986)	Synthetic admission cohort	21.5%	Life table methodologies
Liu, Doty & Manton	United States (1985)	Discharges	10.8%	Payment data in National Nursing Home Survey (NNHS) limited to most recent admission
Rice, Thomas & Weissert	United States (1985)	All users	18.2%	--
Spence & Weiner	United States (1985)	Discharge sample	10.2%	Payment data in NNHS limited to most recent admission
Spillman and Kemper	United States (1985)	Discharge sample	23.0%	Data supplemented by next of kin follow-up survey

Source: U.S. Dept. of Health and Human Services. Office of the Assistant Secretary for Planning and Evaluation. A *Synthesis and Critique of Studies on Medicaid Asset Spend-Down*, by E. Kathleen Adams, Mark Meiners, and Brian Burwell, Jan. 1992. Washington, 1992.

TABLE C-9. Estimates of the Proportion of Medicaid Residents of Nursing Homes Who Were Not Eligible for Medicaid at Admission

Source	Population	Sample(s)	Estimate	Comments
Arling, et al.	Wisconsin (1988)	Discharge sample	30.6%	35% of Medicaid days
Bice	Connecticut (1978-1983)	6 admission cohorts	44.3%	49% of Medicaid days
Bice	Connecticut (1983-1987)	1983-1984 admission cohorts	44.9%	32.4% of Medicaid nursing home expenditures
Burwell, et al.	Michigan (1984)	1984 Medicaid users	27.2%	25% of Medicaid expenditures
Farbstein, et al.	Connecticut (1985)	Discharge cohort	38.9%	Also imputes national estimate of 37.6% from NNHS
Gruenberg, et al.	Connecticut (1978-1979)	Admission cohort	39.3%	41.3% of Medicaid days
Gruenberg, et al.	Connecticut (1985)	Resident sample	39.3%	38.7% of Medicaid expenditures
Liu and Manton	Connecticut (1977-1986)	Synthetic admission cohort	--	27.5% of Medicaid days
Liu, Doty & Manton	United States (1985)	Discharge sample	16.6%	Payment data in NNHS limited to most recent admission
Rice, Thomas & Weissert	United States (1985)	All user sample	16.9%	--
Short, et al.	United States (1987)	Resident sample	18.0%	From 1987 National Medical Expenditure Survey
Spence & Weiner	United States (1985)	Resident sample	14.0%	Payment data in NNHS limited to most recent admission
Spillman and Kemper	United States (1985)	Discharge sample	35.0%	Data supplemented by Next of Kin Follow-up Survey

Source: U.S. Dept. of Health and Human Services. Office of the Assistant Secretary for Planning and Evaluation. *A Synthesis and Critique of Studies on Medicaid Asset Spend-Down*, by E. Kathleen Adams, Mark Meiners, and Brian Burwell, Jan. 1992. Washington, 1992.

Spend-down studies have also examined the length of time it takes for persons to spend-down after nursing home admission. Studies have found that the distribution is bi-modal; that is, a large proportion of persons spend-down in a very short time period, and a sizable minority deplete their assets only after a long period. In all studies, over one-half of those who spend-down do so within a year of nursing home admission. This finding suggests that most people who spend-down have limited assets when they first enter a nursing home.

Certain State studies also show that people who spend-down to Medicaid spend more time on Medicaid in a nursing home after converting to Medicaid coverage than they spend as private payers prior to conversion. The studies show that Medicaid-paid days account for at least 65 to 75 percent of all nursing home days used by those who spend-down. However, the research also shows that, once eligible for Medicaid, people who spend down pay a greater proportion of total nursing home costs, through contributions of their income they are required to make before Medicaid makes its payment, than persons who are eligible for Medicaid at initial admission. As a result, people who spend-down account for a somewhat lower percentage of total Medicaid expenditures than their percentage of Medicaid-covered nursing home days.

B. Spending Down in the Community

Very few studies have examined the likelihood of spending down as the result of needing services other than nursing home care. Persons conceivably could spend-down and qualify for Medicaid because they incur large expenses for home and community-based care, or alternatively, for medical care services or prescription drugs not covered by Medicare. One study analyzed the 1982 and 1984 National Long-Term Care Surveys to compare conversions from non-Medicaid to Medicaid status by persons who used nursing home care and those who did not.[17] The National Long-Term Care Surveys provide information about a nationally representative sample of disabled elderly persons who were originally residing in the community in 1982 and who were followed over a 2-year period.

Analysis of the surveys for spend-down and Medicaid eligibility found that persons using nursing homes at any time during 1982 to 1984 had a higher rate of Medicaid conversion than persons who had never been in nursing homes in the 2-year period. However, more people without nursing home admissions became Medicaid beneficiaries than those with nursing home stays. This reflects the fact that comparatively few people use nursing home care.

The study offers a number of explanations for the conversion from non-Medicaid to Medicaid status in the community during 1982 to 1984. Some persons not on Medicaid in 1982 were actually income-eligible but had not applied for coverage, perhaps because they had not yet incurred uncovered out-of-pocket expenses that would lead them to seek Medicaid coverage. In addition,

---

[17]Liu, Korbin, Pamela Doty, and Kenneth Manton. Medicaid Spend-Down in Nursing Homes. *The Gerontologist*, v. 30, no. 1, 1990. p. 7-15.

some persons not covered by Medicaid in 1982 may have subsequently experienced a decrease in income--perhaps as the result of the loss of pension income following the death of a spouse--that made them Medicaid eligible through welfare-related coverage.

The analysis of the National Long-Term Care Surveys also examined whether Medicaid conversion for those persons living in the community during the 2-year period occurred because persons incurred high out-of-pocket costs for medical expenses not covered by Medicare or high costs for home and community-based long-term care services. The analysis failed to find a distinct relationship between out-of-pocket expenses for community-based long-term care and Medicaid conversion. It did, however, find a direct relationship between out-of-pocket spending for drug costs and the risk of conversion.

Another recent study of first-time elderly Medicaid enrollees in California and Georgia had similar findings.[18] This study, which defined first-time enrollment as the absence of Medicaid enrollment during the 4-year period prior to the study period (1984-1985), found that 81 percent of enrollees in California and 66 percent in Georgia appeared to enroll in Medicaid for reasons unrelated to nursing home use or costs. In addition, only 14 percent in California and 21 percent in Georgia had experienced an acute care stay during the study period. Other expenses, such as prescription drugs or non-health related expenses, or a life change, such as loss of a spouse, were judged more likely to be the cause of new enrollment in Medicaid.

V. PROHIBITIONS ON TRANSFERRING ASSETS WHEN NEEDING LONG-TERM CARE

The Medicaid program is a means-tested program that is intended to provide medical assistance to the poor. Because it also allows States to extend coverage to people with incomes in excess of cash welfare program standards, Medicaid requires these persons first to deplete their assets before they can become eligible. To ensure that these persons actually apply their assets to the cost of their care and do not give them away in order to gain Medicaid eligibility sooner than they otherwise would, Medicaid contains provisions prohibiting the transfer of assets.

Medicaid requires States to prohibit persons seeking Medicaid coverage of their institutional or home and community-based care from transferring resources for less than fair market value during the 30-month period prior to their application for coverage. Spouses of these persons are also prohibited from transferring resources during this same period.

---

[18]Adams, E. Kathleen. *Enrollment in Medicaid by the Elderly: Which Catastrophe?* Report submitted to Health Care Financing Administration under contract No. 500-86-0016. Lexington, SysteMetrics/McGraw-Hill, Mar. 1991, as cited in Adams, et al., *A Synthesis and Critique of Studies on Medicaid Asset Spend-Down.*

If a transfer has occurred, States must establish a period of ineligibility beginning with the month the resources were transferred. The actual length of the period of ineligibility is determined by comparing the cost of care and the value of the assets transferred. The number of months in the period equals 30 months, or a shorter period if fewer months result when the total uncompensated value of the transferred resource is divided by the average monthly cost to a private patient of nursing facility services in the State, or in the community in which the person is institutionalized. For purposes of the prohibition on transfer of assets, resources mean cash or other liquid assets or any real or personal property that an individual (or spouse, if any) owns and could convert to cash to be used for support and maintenance.

The law, however, provides certain exceptions. A Medicaid applicant will not be made ineligible for transfers if:

- the transfer was the applicant's home to: his or her spouse; child under 21; blind or disabled adult child; or sibling who has an equity interest in the home and who was residing in the home for at least a year prior to the individual's admission to the institution; or a son or daughter who was residing in the home for at least 2 years prior to the beneficiary's admission to the nursing home and was providing care that delayed institutionalization of the beneficiary;

- resources were transferred to the community spouse[19] or to the individual's child who is blind or permanently and totally disabled;

- a satisfactory showing is made either that the individual intended to dispose of resources at fair market value or for other valuable consideration or that resources were transferred for a purpose other than to qualify for Medicaid;

- the State determines that the denial of eligibility would work an undue hardship.

Two examples will illustrate how the period of ineligibility is calculated. Mrs. Smith, a widow, transferred her home for less than fair market value to a child on July 1, 1990. She became a resident of a nursing home on November 1, 1990, and was not entitled to Medicaid at the time. On December 7, 1990, while institutionalized, she applied for Medicaid. No exceptions existed which would not require the State to apply the transfer of assets penalty. Since Mrs. Smith was institutionalized and transferred resources for less than fair market value during the 30-month period prior to December 7, 1990, she is subject to a period of ineligibility. The uncompensated value of the home was $90,000 and

---

[19]Spousal impoverishment rules count all resources owned by a couple, whether as an individual or jointly, in the calculation of what amount should be protected for the community spouse.

the average monthly cost of nursing home care to a private patient was $1,500 at the time of application. The $90,000 uncompensated value divided by the average monthly nursing facility rate ($90,000/$1,500) equals 60, the number of months that ineligibility would apply. However, the law limits this period to not more than 30 months. Mrs. Smith remains ineligible for Medicaid coverage of her care from July 1990 through December 1992, or 30 months from the month of transfer and 25 months from the month of application.

Mr. Jones gave $36,000 in stocks to his daughter on July 1, 1990. He was institutionalized on August 1, 1991, and was not entitled to Medicaid. While institutionalized, he applied for Medicaid on September 1, 1991, 14 months after he transferred his stocks. No exceptions existed which would not require the State to apply the transfer of resources penalty. The uncompensated value of the assets was $36,000, and the average monthly cost of nursing home care for a private patient was $1,800. The $36,000 uncompensated value divided by the average monthly nursing facility rate ($36,000/$1,800) equals 20, the number of months that ineligibility would apply. Mr. Jones remains ineligible for Medicaid coverage from July 1990 through February 1992, or 20 months from the date of the transfer and 6 months from the month of his application.

Despite provisions that are intended to ensure that assets are used for the cost of care rather than given away, anecdotal reports and a recent survey of Medicaid officials in six States suggest that non-poor elderly persons are successfully using estate planning to avoid applying their wealth to the costs of long-term care services.

According to reports, a number of different strategies are being used to protect assets.[20] One strategy would have persons convert assets that are counted for purposes of Medicaid eligibility, such as savings accounts or CDs, into exempt assets. The home is the most significant asset that is exempt at the time a person applies for Medicaid. Using cash on hand for a new roof or for remodeling a kitchen or for paying off a mortgage will protect those countable assets from having to be applied to the cost of nursing home care.

Persons can also shelter assets in a trust. A trust allows a person to give ownership of property (personal property, money, real estate) to a trustee who will hold and manage the property for the benefit of that person. Not all trusts, however, will allow persons to shelter assets for purposes of Medicaid eligibility. Medicaid law uses the term "Medicaid qualifying trust" to describe a trust that cannot under any circumstances be used to shelter assets. Medicaid requires that if a trustee has discretion over how the income and principal of a trust is distributed, then the maximum amount that could be made available to the beneficiary must be counted for Medicaid eligibility purposes, regardless of whether the trustee chooses to distribute the amount or not.

---

[20]Budish, Armond, D. *Avoiding the Medicaid Trap: How to Beat the Catastrophic Costs of Nursing Home Care.* New York, Henry Holt and Company, 1989; and Burwell, *Middle-Class Welfare.* This discussion draws heavily on these two works.

How extensively these and many other strategies are being used to protect assets so that Medicaid ends up paying sooner than it otherwise would is unknown. No survey has been conducted to indicate how many people transferred assets or participated in estate planning prior to applying for Medicaid. Nor has research determined what impact estate planning is having on Medicaid expenditures for nursing home care or what impact it will have on future expenditures.

Some argue that the scope of the problem is overstated, since few elderly persons are wealthy enough to be motivated to protect assets.[21] The great bulk of the elderly's assets is in the form of home equity and ignoring home equity sharply reduces their net worth. For instance, the median net worth of the elderly in 1988 was $73,471. Excluding the home, their median net worth was reduced to $23,856, or by 68 percent. In addition, more than two-thirds of impaired elderly persons living in the community are poor or near poor (income less than 150 percent of the Federal poverty level).[22] Studies discussed above also show that large numbers of persons enter nursing homes as private pay and subsequently convert to Medicaid. Moreover, there are disadvantages to sheltering assets in order to gain Medicaid eligibility immediately upon admission to a nursing home. Federal Medicaid law does not require participating nursing homes to accept patients on a first-come first-serve basis. As a result, persons relying on Medicaid at the time of admission may not be able to enter the nursing home of their choosing when they require care.

VI. STATE PLAN AMENDMENTS PROVIDING EXCEPTIONS TO MEDICAID'S RESOURCES REQUIREMENTS FOR PERSONS WITH PRIVATE LONG-TERM CARE INSURANCE

As shown above in figure C-3, nursing home care costs are financed largely by the private out-of-pocket payments of persons needing care and one public program, Medicaid. Nursing home spending for the elderly accounts for 22 percent of total Medicaid payments, and this spending is driven largely by its coverage of people who spend down and deplete their resources on the cost of this care. As a result, some States have been exploring ways to control growth in this spending by linking private long-term care insurance and Medicaid.

During the past several years, the policy debate on long-term care has been occupied largely with the question of what role the public and private sectors should play in any reform of the way these services are currently financed. Private long-term care insurance is generally considered to be the most

---

[21]Hanley, Raymond and Joshua Wiener. A Non-Problem: Scheming Oldsters Bilking Medicaid. *The Philadelphia Inquirer*, May 11, 1992. p. K11; and Wiener, Joshua, Raymond Hanley, and Katherine Harris. Nursing Home Care: Still a Routine Catastrophe. *The Gerontologist*, v. 30, no. 3, 1990. p. 417.

[22]Rowland, Diane. *Help at Home: Long-Term Care Assistance for Impaired Elderly People*. A Report of the Commonwealth Fund Commission on Elderly People Living Alone, May 1989. p. 27.

promising private sector option for providing the elderly additional protection for long-term care expenses.

Long-term care insurance is a relatively new, but rapidly growing, market. In 1986, approximately 30 insurers were selling long-term care insurance policies of some type and an estimated 200,000 persons were covered by these policies. By 1987, a DHHS Task Force on Long-Term Care Insurance found 73 companies writing long-term care insurance policies covering 423,000 persons. By December 1991, the Health Insurance Association of America (HIAA) found that more than 2.4 million policies had been sold, with 135 insurers offering coverage.

Although growth has been considerable in a short period of time, the private insurance industry has approached this potential market with caution. Insurers are concerned about the potential for adverse selection for this product, where only those people who are likely to need care actually buy insurance. In addition, they point to the problem of induced demand for services that can be expected to be generated by the availability of new long-term care insurance. With induced demand, individuals decide to use more services than they otherwise would because they have insurance and/or will shift from families and friends to paid providers for their care. In addition, insurers are concerned that, given the nature of many chronic conditions, people who need long-term care will need it for the remainder of their lives, resulting in an open-ended liability for the insurance company.

As a result of these risks, insurers have designed policies that limit their liability for paying claims. Policies are medically underwritten to exclude persons with certain conditions or illnesses. They contain benefit restrictions that limit access to covered care. Policies also limit the period of coverage they offer, typically to a maximum of 4 or 5 years. In addition, most plans provide indemnity benefits that pay only a fixed amount for each day of covered service. If these amounts are not updated for inflation, the protection offered by the policy can be significantly eroded between the time the policy is bought and the time a person actually needs care. Today policies generally offer some form of inflation adjustment, but only with significant increases in premium costs.

These design features of long-term care insurance raise issues about the quality of coverage offered by policies. The insurance industry has responded to some of these concerns by offering new products that provide broadened coverage and fewer restrictions. In addition, the National Association of Insurance Commissioners (NAIC) has established standards for regulating long-term care insurance. Many States have adopted these standards, but have lagged in adopting NAIC revisions to these standards.

In addition to quality of coverage issues, policymakers are also concerned with the affordability of long-term care insurance. HIAA has reported on the premium costs of policies providing good coverage in December 1991. These policies paid $80 a day for nursing home care and $40 a day for home health care; they had lifetime 5 percent compounded inflation protection, a 20-day deductible period, and a 4-year maximum coverage period. These policies had an average annual premium in December 1991 of $1,781 when purchased at the age of 65 and $5,627 when purchased at the age of 79.

Since 1987, the Robert Wood Johnson Foundation (RWJF) has been interested in exploring the potential role that a public-private insurance partnership could play in financing long-term care. Eight States--California, Connecticut, Indiana, Massachusetts, New Jersey, New York, Oregon, and Wisconsin--were awarded planning grants by RWJF to develop programmatic and empirical experience on how a partnership should be structured. With their grants, States could also work with insurers to develop policies that would provide better coverage for the policyholders and at the same time would be more affordable to a larger segment of the elderly population. States could also establish stronger regulatory controls over long-term care insurance.

During the course of planning grants, States developed different approaches to the partnership. One approach would offer purchasers of policies protection of assets and/or income from Medicaid's spend-down requirements, with the actual amount of protection based on the benefits they received from the insurance policies they bought.[23]

With a Medicaid-private insurance partnership, the States and RWJF intended to provide individuals needing long-term care an alternative to out-of-pocket spending and Medicaid spend-down. They also hoped to reduce reliance of middle-income elderly on Medicaid for their long-term care needs. In so doing, they expected that the partnership would reduce Medicaid spending for nursing home care, since persons with private insurance would conceivably delay that point when they would have to rely on Medicaid to cover their care. The partnership might also discourage persons from sheltering assets because they would have insurance to protect assets from the catastrophic expenses of nursing home care. Finally, insurance under a partnership might become more affordable to more people; with coverage focused on assets protection, policyholders could buy as much or as little insurance as they needed and could afford.

Following completion of the planning phase of the project, States sought waivers from Medicaid requirements in order to operationalize their proposed partnerships. While HCFA has broad authority to waive Medicaid requirements for demonstration projects, the RWJF partnerships would operate for longer periods than allowed under general waiver authority. In the Omnibus Budget Reconciliation Act of 1990 (OBRA 90), Congress considered legislation to authorize waivers for the projects, but the provisions were dropped in conference.

A variety of concerns were expressed about granting waivers to the projects. Wealthier individuals who would never spend-down for Medicaid coverage of their long-term care needs would be able to qualify for protection if they

---

[23]U.S. General Accounting Office. *Long-Term Care Insurance: Proposals to Link Private Insurance and Medicaid Need Close Scrutiny.* GAO/HRD-90-154, Sept. 1990. Washington, 1990. p. 8.

purchased long-term care insurance. Added costs to the program for these persons could be at the expense of expanding coverage for the poor. The demonstration could also end up subsidizing the private insurance industry if Medicaid covered the bulk of nursing home days used by persons with long stays. In addition, to determine whether the partnership reduced Medicaid spending for long-term care, the demonstration would be required to be authorized for 15 to 20 years, and even then adequate data might not be available, since persons purchasing private insurance in the early years of retirement would not generally require services until they were 80 or older.

Between August 1991 and April 1992, HCFA approved Medicaid plan amendments from four RWJF States--California, Connecticut, Indiana, and New York--that in effect operationalize a Medicaid-private long-term care insurance partnership in those States.[24] In general, the plan amendments allow the States to establish more liberal asset standards for persons with private insurance coverage.

California, Connecticut and Indiana will allow individuals with insurance to disregard, for purposes of Medicaid eligibility, assets that are equivalent to the amount of private insurance benefits paid on their behalf for covered services. In other words, each dollar that the insurance policy has paid out is subtracted from the assets the individual still owns and is not required to be spent down. For example, a person living in Connecticut and purchasing a long-term care insurance policy that covers and pays out $50,000 of nursing home benefits will be able to retain those assets and gain Medicaid eligibility for coverage of any additional nursing home care he or she needs. New York requires that qualifying long-term care insurance policies provide coverage for a minimum period of time; they must cover 3 years of nursing home care and 6 years of home care, or a combination of the two. After persons have exhausted their insurance benefits under these policies, they may then retain all resources they own, without applying them to the cost of their care before Medicaid coverage begins. Each of the States also requires insurance policies to meet certain State standards for persons to be eligible for more liberal asset protection.

VII. NURSING HOME REFORM LAW AND MEDICAID PAYMENTS FOR NURSING HOME CARE

OBRA 87 comprehensively revised the statutory authority that applies to nursing homes participating in Medicaid. This revision, often referred to as nursing home reform law, responded to general congressional concern about the quality of nursing home care paid for by the Medicaid and Medicare programs, as well as findings and recommendations of a 1986 Institute of Medicine (IOM) report. In its review of nursing home care and Federal regulation of these providers, the IOM had found the quality of care provided by many nursing homes to be unsatisfactory. It recommended that more effective government

---

[24]These plan amendments were authorized pursuant to section 1902(r)(2) which specifies that States may not impose more restrictive eligibility criteria for the medically needy than for the categorically needy.

regulation, including a stronger Federal role, would substantially improve the quality of life for nursing home residents.

The nursing home reform law eliminated the Medicaid program's previous distinction between skilled nursing facilities (SNF) and intermediate care facilities (ICF). It established a single category of nursing home provider, called "nursing facility" (NF), and a single nursing home benefit. The revised law establishes requirements in three major areas: (1) requirements that must be met by NFs in order to participate in the program; (2) the survey and certification process that States must use for determining whether nursing homes comply with these requirements; and (3) sanctions and enforcement actions that the States and HCFA may impose against noncompliant nursing homes. Each of these sections of nursing home reform law is described in greater detail in *Chapter VII, Administration*.

Effective October 1, 1990, OBRA 87 established requirements for providing care that NFs must comply with in order to participate and receive reimbursement under the program. These standards address such issues as the scope of services a NF must provide, levels of staffing in the facility and the qualifications of staff, residents' rights, and the physical environment of the facility.

For example, NFs must conduct, shortly after admission, a comprehensive assessment of each resident's functional capacity, and must periodically update the assessment during the resident's stay. This assessment must be used to develop a written plan of care for the resident, and facilities must provide the services and activities needed according to this plan for the resident to attain or maintain his or her highest practicable physical, mental, and psychosocial well-being.

NFs must provide 24-hour licensed nursing care sufficient to meet the nursing needs of residents and must use a registered nurse at least 8 consecutive hours a day 7 days a week (although States may waive both the registered nurse requirement and the licensed nurse requirement under certain circumstances). NFs must use as nurse aides only those persons who have completed an approved training and/or competency evaluation program.

OBRA 87 requires States to take into account in their payments to NFs the costs of complying with these and other new requirements. As of October 30, 1990, HCFA had approved increases in Medicaid nursing home rates ranging from a low of $0.07 per day in Nevada to a high of $4.64 in New Hampshire. Table C-10 shows approved amounts for individual States.

TABLE C-10. Medicaid Nursing Home Reform Per Diem Add-Ons, by State, October 30, 1990

Alabama	$ .69/per diem	Montana	$1.90/per diem
Alaska	$1.29	Nebraska	$2.38
Arizona	Waivered program	Nevada	$ .07
Arkansas	$1.50	New Hampshire	$4.64
California	Disapproved	New Jersey	$ .47
Colorado	Pending	New Mexico	Pending
Connecticut	$1.44	New York	$ .10
Delaware	$1.81	North Carolina	$1.82
Dist. of Columbia	Pending	North Dakota	Pending
Florida	Pending	Ohio	$ .48
Georgia	$1.10	Oklahoma	$2.00
Hawaii	$2.90	Oregon	$1.30
Idaho	$1.87	Pennsylvania	Disapproved
Illinois	$1.52	Rhode Island	$ .44
Indiana	$ .62	South Carolina	Disapproved
Iowa	$3.90	South Dakota	$ .42
Kansas	$ .67	Tennessee	$2.30
Kentucky	$1.16	Texas	$2.33
Louisiana	$1.48	Utah	$4.04
Maine	$1.01	Vermont	$1.06
Maryland	Disapproved	Virginia	$ .60
Massachusetts	$3.72	Washington	$ .95
Michigan	$ .93	West Virginia	Disapproved
Minnesota	$1.01	Wisconsin	$1.10
Mississippi	Withdrawn	Wyoming	$ .83
Missouri	Pending		

Source: Data compiled by the U.S. Dept. of Health and Human Services, Health Care Financing Administration, as of Oct. 30, 1990, and distributed by the American Association of Homes for the Aging.

These payment increases came at a time when nursing homes were increasingly challenging the adequacy of State payment rates for Medicaid beneficiaries. Before 1980, States were required to use Medicare reimbursement principles for hospital and nursing facility services. Under these cost-based principles, institutional providers were reimbursed the actual costs of providing care to Medicaid beneficiaries. In response to concerns from the States about the growth of nursing home spending in their Medicaid budgets, as well as criticisms that cost-based reimbursement provided few incentives for providers to perform efficiently, Congress enacted the "Boren amendment" for nursing facility services in the Omnibus Budget Reconciliation Act of 1980 (OBRA 80).

The Boren amendment freed states from cost-based reimbursement requirements for nursing homes and directed only that payment rates be "reasonable and adequate" to meet the costs of "efficiently and economically operated facilities" in providing care meeting Federal and State quality and safety standards.[25] The law did not define "reasonable and adequate payments" or "efficiently and economically operated facilities." It is generally agreed that the flexibility provided to States under the Boren amendment for reimbursing nursing homes, together with other State policies limiting the growth of the nursing home bed supply, helped States to control nursing home spending in the 1980s.

While the Boren amendment provided States a great deal of flexibility to determine the methods and rates by which they could reimburse nursing homes, it also required that States provide assurances to the Secretary of HHS that their Medicaid rates would be reasonable and adequate. Over time, Medicaid providers began to sue State Medicaid agencies, arguing that States had not met the Boren amendment standards. In 1990, the U.S. Supreme Court confirmed providers' right to seek judicial review of States' assurances of the adequacy of Medicaid rates or adequacy of the rates themselves under the Boren amendment in *Wilder vs. Virginia Hospital Association*.

Table C-11 summarizes information about recent Boren amendment suits filed on behalf of nursing homes, as compiled by the American Health Care Association (AHCA). Many of these cases have alleged that States did not identify objective standards as to what constitutes an efficiently and economically operated facility or establish findings that their rate structures met these standards. In many cases, courts have held State Medicaid plans invalid and ordered States to revise their State plans to demonstrate compliance with the Boren amendment. Often the revised State plans increase payment rates for nursing homes.

---

[25]This discussion draws on material contained in: U.S. Library of Congress. Congressional Research Service. *Medicaid: Recent Trends in Beneficiaries and Spending*. CRS Report for the Congress No. 92-365 EPW, by Kathleen King, Richard Rimkunas, and Dawn Nuschler. Mar. 27, 1992. Washington, 1992.

TABLE C-11. Boren Amendment Suits Filed by Nursing Homes

State	Cases Pending	Cases Resolved
Alaska	--	X
California	--	X (2 cases)
Georgia	X	
Illinois	--	X (2 cases)
Indiana	X	
Kansas	X	X
Massachusetts	X	
Michigan	--	X (2 cases)
Mississippi	--	X
Missouri	X	X
Nebraska	X	
Nevada	--	X
New Jersey	X	
New York	--	X
Ohio	X	
Washington	--	X

Source: Table prepared by the Congressional Research Service based on information from the AHCA, *National Legal Trends Reporter*, June 1991; and telephone conversations with AHCA in June 1992.

What impact Boren amendment suits, increased payments due to nursing home reform law, or State provider taxes discussed in *Chapter VIII, Financing* have had on Medicaid payments for nursing home care is difficult to gauge. However, as table C-12 shows, nursing home payments increased by 14 percent in 1990 and 17 percent in 1991. These increases follow more modest rates of growth of 6 to 9 percent in the earlier years. The much higher rates of growth in the last 2 years are largely the result of an increase in average payments per beneficiary. The number of Medicaid beneficiaries of nursing home care remained relatively unchanged during the period. This suggests that most of the increase in payments is the result of increases in reimbursement rates.

TABLE C-12. Medicaid Payments for Nursing Facility Care, Beneficiaries, and Payments Per Beneficiary, Fiscal Years 1980 to 1991

Year	Payments (in millions)	Rate of change	Beneficiaries (in thousands)	Rate of change	Payments per beneficiary	Rate of change
1980	$7,887		1,396		$5,651	
1981	8,542	8.3%	1,372	-1.7%	6,225	10.2%
1982	9,406	10.1	1,324	-3.5	7,105	14.1
1983	10,002	6.3	1,367	3.2	7,317	3.0
1984	10,633	6.3	1,355	-0.9	7,844	7.2
1985	11,598	9.1	1,376	1.5	8,432	7.5
1986	12,436	7.2	1,399	1.7	8,890	5.4
1987	13,247	6.5	1,421	1.6	9,320	4.8

TABLE C-12. Medicaid Payments for Nursing Facility Care, Beneficiaries, and Payments Per Beneficiary, Fiscal Years 1980 to 1991--Continued

Year	Payments (in millions)	Rate of change	Beneficiaries (in thousands)	Rate of change	Payments per beneficiary	Rate of change
1988	$14,276	7.8%	1,445	1.7%	$ 9,880	6.0%
1989	15,531	8.8	1,452	0.5	10,696	8.3
1990	17,693	13.9	1,461	0.6	12,110	13.2
1991	20,699	17.0	1,490	2.7	13,893	14.8
Average annual rate of change:						
1980 - 1985:		8.0		-0.3		8.3
1985 - 1991:		10.1		1.4		8.6
1989 - 1991:		15.5		1.6		14.0

NOTE: As of Oct. 1, 1990, skilled nursing facility (SNF) and intermediate care facility (ICF) benefits were consolidated into a single benefit called nursing facility (NF) care. The payment and beneficiary totals shown prior to 1991 represent the sum of SNF and ICF beneficiaries and payments reported separately for the year.

Source: Table prepared by the Congressional Research Service based on data contained on HCFA Form 2082.

APPENDIX D. MEDICAID SERVICES FOR PERSONS WITH DEVELOPMENTAL DISABILITIES[1]

I. INTRODUCTION

Persons with developmental disabilities have mental retardation and other related conditions. These persons require special care and services to achieve their potential. The term "developmental disability" is broadly used in the disability field to refer to "persons with mental retardation or related conditions," and will be used as such in this appendix. Persons with mental retardation have significant subaverage intellectual functioning accompanied by deficiencies in skills such as self-care and independent living. Persons with conditions related to mental retardation are those with severe chronic disabilities that result in impaired intellectual functioning or deficiencies in skills similar to the deficiencies experienced by persons with mental retardation. Persons with developmental disabilities may be multiply handicapped with mental and physical impairments; their impairments may range from moderately to profoundly incapacitating.

Most persons with developmental disabilities are able to live in community-based homes with their families or other persons who can offer assistance. These persons can generally participate in daytime activities, including programs that offer training ranging from self-help habilitation programs to prevocational or supported employment programs. However, some persons require more intensive services, and many of these most severely impaired persons are served in residential facilities that offer comprehensive, continual care.

The major source of Federal financing for health care services for persons with developmental disabilities is the Medicaid program. Medicaid can provide coverage for the health and health-related services included under a State's plan to all persons with disabilities who meet eligibility requirements.

Most Medicaid funding for services designed specifically for this population is used in large Medicaid-certified residential institutions known as intermediate care facilities for the mentally retarded (ICFs/MR). These facilities provide 24-hour care and range in size from State or private facilities of 15 beds or fewer

---

[1]This appendix was written by Mary F. Smith.

to very large State-operated institutions of over 1,000 beds.[2] In FY 1991, $7.7 billion of Federal and State Medicaid funds were spent on ICFs/MR.

ICF/MR spending has been an important factor affecting overall Medicaid program spending growth. In the mid to late 1970s it was a major component of the program's growth.[3] More recently, the growth in Medicaid spending has moderated somewhat. Between 1975 and 1991 this service category's average annual rate of growth equalled 20.3 percent. In comparison, total spending for Medicaid grew at an average annual rate of 12.0 percent for this same period.

Medicaid's ICF/MR spending is of considerable concern for those attempting to control the program's costs. In particular, while overall ICF/MR spending has increased, the number of beneficiaries using these services has not. This results in an escalation in the payment per ICF/MR beneficiary for a service category that has always been noted for its high per beneficiary costs. In 1977, Medicaid spent over $10,000 per ICF/MR beneficiary per annum as compared to $750 for all beneficiaries. In 1991, Medicaid spent almost $53 thousand per beneficiary, 19 times the overall per beneficiary amount of $2,752.

Historically, residential services were the primary mode of service for the developmentally disabled, but over the past 10 years community-based services have expanded rapidly. In 1981, the Congress authorized home and community-based waivers that among other things, allowed States to use Medicaid funding for services to persons with chronic disabilities in noninstitutional settings. Individuals who typically would be placed in an ICF/MR became eligible for these waivers in many States. For the developmentally disabled, persons participating in this waiver program would be eligible for Medicaid if they were in an institution and must be likely to need ICF/MR services if the waiver services were not available. Noninstitutional services covered under Medicaid waiver programs include such things as: case management services, home maker services, aide services, and personal care services. In FY 1988, 36 States were utilizing the waiver authority to help the developmentally disabled, and it is estimated that by the end of FY 1992, nearly all States will be providing waiver services. This rapidly growing program component serves an increasing number of persons, from just over 29,000 in FY 1988 to an estimated 69,000 in FY 1992. Federal and State Medicaid funding aimed at the developmentally disabled totaled an estimated $1.1 billion in FY 1991.[4]

---

[2]Standards of care established for ICFs/MR and the Life Safety Code of the National Fire Protection Association make a distinction between ICF/MR facilities of 16 or more residents (large facilities) and facilities of 15 or less residents (small facilities). This appendix will employ this distinction.

[3]See *Chapter II, Trends in Medicaid Payments and Beneficiaries*, for a complete description of the payment and beneficiary trends for the ICF/MR service category.

[4]These estimates are based on an analysis by: Smith, Gary and Robert Gettings. *Medicaid in the Community: The Home and Community-Based*

(continued...)

The additional Medicaid supported services being provided through home and community-based waivers add to an already sizable share of total Medicaid spending dedicated to the developmentally disabled population. In FY 1991, the $7.7 billion spent on ICFs/MR combined with the additional $1.1 billion spent on home and community-based services (HCBS) waivers to account for over 10 percent of all (Federal and State) Medicaid assistance payments. While more than 10 percent of payments are dedicated to this population, the number of Medicaid beneficiaries using these services is relatively small, representing less than 1 percent of overall beneficiaries in 1991.[5]

Medicaid's home and community-based waiver spending is only one component of many community-based services provided to the developmentally disabled. However, most community-based residential and day training programs for persons with developmental disabilities are supported with separate non-Medicaid funds. For example, in FY 1988, $4.0 billion in State funding was used for community residential services, case management, respite care, daytime training programs, and other services required to enable persons with developmental disabilities to live and function in community settings. Additional Federal support for the developmentally disabled comes in the form of Supplemental Security Income (SSI) payments, Social Security disability assistance, and through federally supported education programs.

Many persons have advocated that additional Federal funding is needed for community services to meet the needs of persons cared for by families and to assist those being transferred out of large institutions. There are rising expectations on the part of parents that most of these disabled persons are capable of living in the community with some degree of independent functioning. Some advocacy groups have sought to have more Medicaid funding made available for community services and to limit Medicaid funds for the larger institutions. However, these efforts have been resisted by other advocacy groups who oppose restrictions on institutional funding and by those with concerns regarding the potential costs of using Medicaid funding for community services for this population.

Legislative efforts to expand community services under Medicaid have resulted in the 1990 authorization of a new limited option in which eight States will provide "community-supported living arrangement services" to persons with developmental disabilities. Expenditures for this program are limited to $5 million in Federal funding for FY 1991, and increase in annual steps to $35

---

[4](...continued)
Services (HCBS) Waiver and Community Supported Living Arrangements (CSLA) Programs. National Association of State Mental Retardation Program Directors, Mar. 1992. (Hereafter cited as Smith and Gettings, *Medicaid in the Community*) The estimates are somewhat different from those provided in Chapter VI, *Alternate Delivery Options and Waiver Programs.*

[5]It should be noted that this comparison does not include Medicaid payments for other covered services that the developmentally disabled might also use.

million in Federal funding for FY 1995, with such sums as may be provided by Congress for fiscal years thereafter.

This appendix will discuss the service needs of persons with developmental disabilities, the types of Medicaid and other services provided, costs and trends related to these services, and issues associated with service delivery to this population.

II. BACKGROUND

A. Target Population

The American Association on Mental Retardation defines mental retardation as follows:[6]

Mental retardation refers to significant subaverage general intellectual functioning resulting in or associated with concurrent impairments in adaptive behavior and manifested during the developmental period.

Significant subaverage intellectual functioning is defined as an I.Q. of 70 or less, and impairments in adaptive behavior are inabilities to perform personal and interpersonal functions at levels appropriate to the age of the individual.[7] The developmental period is childhood and adolescence.[8]

Medicaid regulations define "persons with related conditions" as individuals who have a severe, chronic disability that is attributable to cerebral palsy or epilepsy or any other condition, other than mental illness, that results in impairment of general intellectual functioning or adaptive behavior similar to that of persons with mental retardation.[9] Persons with related conditions must require treatment or services similar to services required by persons with mental

---

[6]Grossman, H. In *Scheerenberger: Classification in Mental Retardation.* American Association on Mental Deficiency. (Currently called the American Association on Mental Retardation.) Washington, 1983.

[7]Ibid., p. 13. Persons with mental retardation are classified according to degree of intellectual impairment as measured by I.Q.: mild mental retardation, I.Q. of 50-55 to 70; moderate mental retardation, I.Q. of 35-40 to 50-55; severe mental retardation, I.Q. of 20-25 to 35-40; profound mental retardation, I.Q. below 20 or 25.

[8]Whereas mental retardation is diagnosed as a failure in intellectual development that results in limited competence, mental illnesses are psychiatric disorders affecting emotions and include neuroses, psychoses, and organic dysfunctions. Both mental retardation and mental illness can result in incompetent behavior if the impairments are severe. An individual can have a dual diagnosis of both mental retardation and mental illness, but one impairment is generally specified as the primary diagnosis.

[9]*Federal Register*, v. 51, no. 102, May 28, 1986. p. 19181.

retardation. The regulation specifies that the disability must be manifest prior to age 22, be likely to continue indefinitely, and result in substantial functional limitations in 3 or more areas of major life activity: self-care, understanding and use of language, learning, mobility, self-direction, or a capacity for independent living. As stated in the regulation, this definition is based on the definition of "developmental disability" as set forth under the Developmental Disabilities Assistance and Bill of Rights Act.

Persons with developmental disabilities are limited in personal and interpersonal functions, also referred to as behavioral deficits, deficits in adaptive behavior, or functional limitations. These terms refer to the inability to perform activities such as feeding, toileting, bathing, or dressing oneself; speaking or understanding verbal communication; interacting cooperatively with others; learning in school; and living independently. These terms also include inabilities to engage in regular employment; to use public transportation; and to shop or manage money independently. A person is functionally impaired to the extent that he or she is unable to perform the usual activities appropriate for his or her age group.

The actual number of persons with developmental disabilities is not known. One study based on 1984 data established a range of three estimates.[10] This study focused on work limitation of noninstitutionalized persons age 16 to 72. Estimates of the number of persons with developmental disabilities ranged from 1.3 million to 4.6 million, depending on the degree of work limitation. Under this approach, the "narrow definition" resulted in an estimate of 1,284,000 persons with developmental disabilities. This definition stated that a person was developmentally disabled if his or her health or condition had always prevented the person from working at a job or business. The "middle definition" resulted in an estimate of 1,744,000 persons with developmental disabilities. This definition added those persons currently unable to work whose work limitation began prior to working age (they may have attempted work or worked in a supported or sheltered setting), and those persons who had mental retardation resulting in a need for assistance with activities of daily living. The "broad definition" resulted in an estimate of 4,615,000 persons with developmental disabilities. This definition added those persons currently able to work, but who reported a work limitation that began prior to their reaching working age.

Another estimate included children and institutionalized persons, and indicated that the total number of persons with developmental disabilities may be 1.9 million.[11] According to this estimate, in 1985 there were approximately

---

[10]Thornton, Craig. *Characteristics of Persons with Developmental Disabilities: Evidence from the Survey of Income and Program Participation.* Mathematica Policy Research, Inc., New Jersey, Jan. 1990.

[11]Data compiled by K. Charlie Lakin, Center for Residential and Community Services, University of Minnesota. Statistics on the noninstitutionalized population are drawn from Data on the Disabled from the National Health

(continued...)

304,000 institutionalized persons (of whom 49,000 were estimated to be under age 18).[12] Noninstitutionalized persons were estimated to total 1,641,000 (of whom approximately 769,000 were under age 18).

B. Causes of Developmental Disabilities

Developmental disabilities are caused by a variety of factors, including genetic anomalies, birth trauma, head injury (including child abuse), diseases of the central nervous system, and adverse prenatal influences. Adverse prenatal influences relate to conditions of pregnant women that affect the fetus, including drug or alcohol abuse, the acquired immune deficiency syndrome (AIDS), infections, and poor nutrition, many of which tend to be associated with lower socio-economic status.

The total number of persons with developmental disabilities is affected by advances in medical care and life-saving devices, which may be having a dual effect on the incidence of these disabilities. (Data are not available to show the numerical effects of these influences.) For example, prenatal care for pregnant women can reduce the incidence of low birth weight newborns, who are at risk for mental retardation. Intensive care for premature infants allows some newborns to survive who would have died in the past; however, some of these infants are left with severe disabilities that require life-long care and treatment. Also, amniocentesis allows parents to know the disability status of their unborn children, and this offers parents information that may affect their choice regarding termination of pregnancy. Some persons become disabled due to accidents such as near drowning or automobile collisions. In these cases, lifesaving techniques and seat belts save lives and prevent some injuries; and some persons who would have died are left with severe brain injury.

C. Medicaid Eligibility for Persons With Developmental Disabilities

Most persons with developmental disabilities are eligible for Medicaid as a result of their eligibility for Supplemental Security Income (SSI) as disabled

---

[11](...continued)
Interview Survey, 1983-1985 by Mitchell LaPlante. Washington, D.C. U.S. Dept. of Education. Data on those in institutions for persons with mental retardation/developmental disabilities were drawn from the database of the Center for Residential and Community Services, University of Minnesota for 1986. Data on persons with developmental disabilities who were in nursing homes were taken from the 1985 National Nursing Home Survey by the Center for Residential and Community Services, University of Minnesota.

[12]Of the 304,000 persons estimated to be in public residential institutions, approximately 83 percent were in facilities for persons with developmental disabilities, 16 percent were in nursing homes, and 1 percent represented persons with mental retardation served in psychiatric facilities.

persons.[13] These persons generally are not only substantially mentally impaired (usually with an I.Q. of 50 or below), but are also functionally disabled and are unable to perform the usual daily activities appropriate for persons in their age group. Generally, persons with developmental disabilities are eligible for Medicaid services if they meet the definition of disability and if they meet SSI income and resource eligibility requirements. (See *Chapter III, Eligibility*.)[14]

In determining eligibility for a child under age 21, the income and resources of the parents are considered available, or "deemed," to the child if the child is living in the same household as the parents. A child in an ICF/MR or other Medicaid institution is not considered to be living with the parents after one month of institutionalization. Subsequently, only the income actually contributed by the parents of the institutionalized child is considered. Medicaid law also authorizes a waiver of the deeming rule for certain disabled children living at home if the child would be eligible for Medicaid if institutionalized, and if other conditions are met. (See the section in *Chapter III, Eligibility* on optional coverage of noninstitutionalized disabled children.)

D. Services Needed

Many persons with developmental disabilities are multiply handicapped and may have cerebral palsy, epilepsy, or other impairments which affect the central nervous system. Some individuals with the most severe impairments, including many who are profoundly retarded, are medically fragile and require frequent medical and nursing care to sustain life.

The need for supportive services for persons with developmental disabilities is due to their inability to function independently in activities of daily life that might include self-care, sensory and motor skills, use of language, and management of finances. These are persons who are likely to have limited language development, limited housekeeping and vocational abilities, and may exhibit antisocial behavior.[15] Persons with developmental disabilities who have

---

[13]The Supplemental Security Income program is authorized under title XVI of the Social Security Act.

[14]Medicaid-eligible persons with developmental disabilities have covered medical services paid for like any other eligible person. Since there is no separate eligibility category for persons with developmental disabilities, total program expenditures for health services for these persons cannot be isolated from expenditures for other Medicaid clients. However, data for ICF/MR services and limited community care for persons with developmental disabilities are available and will be discussed later.

[15]This listing is intended to include examples of the major types of impaired functioning that may be exhibited by persons with developmental disabilities, but it is not intended to imply that all such persons exhibit all these behaviors. Also, many persons with developmental disabilities have improved their level of
(continued...)

substantial behavioral deficits require supervised living arrangements and daytime services. These persons can receive services in institutional or community-based settings, depending on service availability and family preference.

Daytime services include supervised activities such as habilitation services, generally defined as training in the skills of daily living, self-help, and socialization skills. Habilitation services can also include prevocational or vocational training, or supported employment. Prevocational training includes skills such as paying attention to a task and maintaining time schedules, which are necessary to prepare to learn job skills. Vocational training includes skills needed to perform a job. Supported employment services include special assistance to allow a severely disabled person to enter and maintain employment in work settings with nondisabled persons.

Daytime programs can also include day activity centers (which do not stress productive economic output), and sheltered workshops (in which subminimum wages are paid according to the productivity of disabled persons). Respite care is also provided to give the family caring for a disabled person time for rest, recreation, and other activities. Services covered under Medicaid are discussed below.

E. History

Historically, many persons with developmental disabilities were placed in large custodial institutions which were generally located in rural, isolated settings. Community involvement of these institutionalized persons was not generally accepted practice. Prior to the 1950s, these institutions were virtually the only place that services were available for persons with developmental disabilities. Many families were encouraged by their physicians to institutionalize severely disabled newborns at birth. Conditions in these institutions were generally harsh, treatment programs were limited, and the institutions were crowded. Such facilities served as custodial settings where many people remained for years.[16]

In the 1950s, parents of children with mental retardation began to organize and to encourage the development of community services so that their children could receive specialized developmental services while living at home. These parents also worked to bring about improvements in institutions. In 1962, a panel of experts appointed by President Kennedy recommended that

---

[15](...continued)
functioning due to modern training techniques and behavior modification designed to ameliorate or modify antisocial behavior.

[16]For further information on conditions in early institutions, see U.S. General Accounting Office. Summary of a Report. Returning the Mentally Disabled to the Community: Government Needs to do More; Report to the Congress by the Comptroller General of the United States. HRD-76-152A, Jan. 7, 1977. Washington, 1977.

institutional care for persons with mental retardation be restricted to those whose specific needs could best be met with this type of service. This panel also recommended that local communities, in cooperation with Federal and State agencies, undertake the development of community services for persons with mental retardation. Abuse and neglect of institutionalized persons were reported in the press, and during the 1960s and 1970s efforts were made to improve conditions in institutions, expand alternatives to institutionalization, and move residents from institutional to community settings. Prior to the 1970s, virtually all public services for persons with developmental disabilities were supported with State funds and were delivered in large State residential institutions.

Several pieces of legislation have been enacted by Congress to provide services and protection for persons with developmental disabilities. Among these was the 1971 authorization of Federal Medicaid funding for care provided in ICFs/MR. To participate in Medicaid and receive ICF/MR funds, an institution must meet Federal standards established under the Medicaid program to ensure appropriate treatment, a safe environment, and qualified staff. The ICF/MR program has served, and continues to serve, as a major incentive for States to improve conditions in their institutions in order to qualify for Federal Medicaid payments.[17] The ICF/MR option was quickly selected as a service category by many States. By 1977, 43 States were covering the service, and by 1990 all States were covering ICF/MR services. Medicaid involvement in institutional services for persons with developmental disabilities provided States an incentive to maintain minimum standards for residential programs, and the availability of ICF/MR funding provided States an alternative to placing persons with developmental disabilities in Medicaid-funded nursing homes.[18]

During the 1970s there was increasing interest in placing individuals with developmental disabilities in community settings. Treatment practices increasingly tended toward the placement of many of these persons in smaller,

---

[17]Other legislation that influences services to persons with developmental disabilities includes: 1) The Developmentally Disabled Assistance and Bill of Rights Act, which requires statewide planning and coordination of services for this population; 2) the Individuals With Disabilities Education Act, which provides early intervention services to infants and toddlers with disabilities, and requires that appropriate educational and supportive services be provided to all children with disabilities; 3) the Civil Rights of Institutionalized Persons Act, which gives the U.S. Attorney General explicit authority to initiate and intervene in litigation involving the constitutional rights of institutionalized persons; and 4) the Americans With Disabilities Act, which provides broad non-discrimination protection for individuals with disabilities in employment, public services, public accommodations, and services operated by private entities, transportation, and telecommunications.

[18]See Lakin, K. Charlie and Margaret Jean Hall. *Medicaid-Financed Residential Care for Persons with Mental Retardation.* Health Care Financing Review, 1990 Annual Supplement. p. 150. (Hereafter cited as Lakin and Hall, *Medicaid-Financed Residential Care for Persons with Mental Retardation*)

less restricted community-based settings integrated in typical neighborhoods. During the late 1970s some States focused on obtaining ICF/MR certification for these smaller community-based settings.

The Omnibus Budget Reconciliation Act of 1981 authorized the Secretary to waive certain Medicaid program requirements to allow States to serve persons with developmental disabilities in home and community-based settings.[19] In addition to providing State selected community services to other Medicaid eligibles, the waiver programs provide community-based services to persons with developmental disabilities who would otherwise remain in, or be at risk of being placed in, an ICF/MR in the absence of alternative services. This program has grown from the participation of two States serving a total of 1,381 persons in FY 1982 to an estimated 48 States serving 68,848 persons in FY 1992.

Also in 1981, the Health Care Financing Administration (HCFA) issued guidelines for ICF/MR facilities serving 15 or fewer persons. These guidelines clarified Medicaid's role and established certification criteria for ICF/MR funding for these smaller facilities.

Over the past 20 years, services have been developed in many communities to help families provide care for persons who might otherwise require institutionalization and to provide community living arrangements for persons coming out of institutions. Over this period there has been a steady decline in the number of persons with developmental disabilities served in public residential institutions, as shown in figure D-1. This decline resulted in a 56 percent reduction in the average daily institutionalized population from an all time high of 194,650 in FY 1967 to 86,219 in FY 1990. These numbers include only those persons served in large public residential facilities, and do not include persons served in private residential facilities or smaller group homes. Figure D-1 does not differentiate between those facilities that are certified as ICFs/MR and those that are not.[20] This decrease in the population of State institutions reflects the trend away from the use of large residential facilities to smaller residences and community-based services.

---

[19]In establishing the waiver program Congress did not authorize States to provide home and community-based waiver services as a mandatory or optional service that would be matched with Federal Medicaid matching funds. Rather, States must seek Federal approval for a waiver to provide these services. See *Chapter VI, Alternate Delivery Options and Waiver Programs* for a full description and explanation of home and community-based waivers.

[20]Information on the share of institutionalized residents in ICF/MR certified facilities is provided later in the chapter. In June of 1989, roughly 9 out of every 10 residents of large facilities (16 beds or more) were in ICF/MR certified facilities, but only 23 percent of those in small facilities were in certified facilities.

FIGURE D-1. Average Daily Population of Public Residential Facilities for the Mentally Retarded, 1955 - 1990

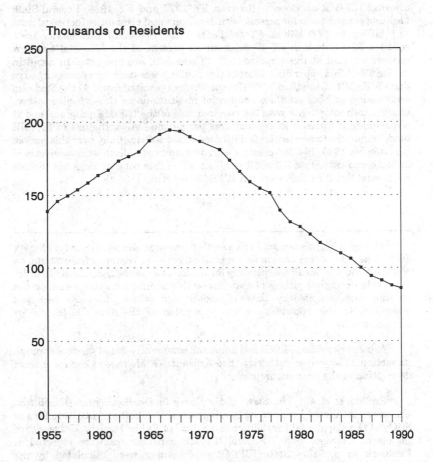

Note: Figure portrays trend in large public residential facilities. Not all of these facilities will be certified to provide ICF/MR services.
Source: Based on data from K. Charlie Lakin.

F. Medicaid Services[21]

1. ICF/MR and Waiver Services

Since the 1970s, Medicaid has become a major funding source for services for persons with developmental disabilities, and in FY 1990 all States were covering ICF/MR services.[22] Between FY 1977 and FY 1988, Federal-State Medicaid expenditures for persons with developmental disabilities increased from $1.1 billion to $7.0 billion. Total Federal and State ICF/MR service costs equalled $6.0 billion in FY 1988, about 85 percent of the Medicaid total for services directed at this population.[23] (These data are presented in detail in section IV of this appendix.) Most of this funding was used for services in large State ICFs/MR. Growth in ICF/MR expenditures resulted from: 1) the Medicaid certification of beds in State residential institutions as those facilities were brought into compliance with the requirements of the ICF/MR program, and 2) a concomitant increase in expenditures per person. Also, the use of ICF/MR funds in non-State residential facilities increased substantially over this period. On June 30, 1990, 144,288 persons with developmental disabilities were served in State and non-State ICFs/MR of all sizes.[24] (This number does not include residential facilities that were not ICF/MR-certified.)

---

[21]The spending discussion in this section provides Medicaid spending for FY 1988. The data source used in this exposition provides complete information on Medicaid and non-Medicaid spending for the developmentally disabled. In order to provide a complete picture of spending on this population this appendix relies on this data compiled by David Braddock and others. See the technical addendum to this appendix for an explanation of the data source and its limitations.

[22]Arizona provides ICF/MR and home and community-based services through its section 1115 waiver authority. See *Appendix G, Managed Care* for a short description of the Arizona program.

[23]Braddock, et al. *The State of the States in Developmental Disabilities*. University Affiliated Program in Developmental Disabilities. Institute for the Study of Developmental Disabilities and School of Public Health. University of Illinois at Chicago, 1990. Federal ICF/MR expenditures were reported at Braddock at p. 513. State ICF/MR expenditures were calculated by the Congressional Research Service (CRS) based on Federal financial participation rates and Federal ICF/MR expenditures reported in Part 2 of Braddock.

[24]Most persons in the ICF/MR program are served in State-operated facilities. In addition, persons are served in ICFs/MR that are operated privately, and a small, but undetermined, number of persons are served in county-operated ICFs/MR. County and private facilities are monitored by State agencies. In this appendix, private and county ICFs/MR are called non-State ICFs/MR. ICF/MR data for June 30, 1990 are unpublished data from K. Charlie Lakin, Center for Residential Services and Community Living, University of Minnesota.

In addition to those served in ICFs/MR, in FY 1988, an estimated 29,243 persons with developmental disabilities were receiving services under the home and community-based waiver program in 39 States at a cost of $454 million.[25] (See *Chapter VI, Alternate Delivery Options and Waiver Programs*.) Waiver services are designed for persons who would require institutionalization in the absence of the waiver program. States must assure that the estimated average per capita expenditure for medical assistance in any fiscal year for those receiving waivered services will not exceed the average per capita expenditure that the State estimates would have incurred in that year for that population if the waiver had not been granted. That is, the services offered under the waiver may not cost more than services that would have been required had the individuals received services in an ICF/MR. Unlike ICF/MR services, waiver authority is not permanent and requires periodic renewal.

2. Other Optional Services

In FY 1988, States used several Medicaid optional care authorities to help fund services for persons with developmental disabilities. (Figure D-2 refers to these programs collectively as "day programs.") Medicaid funding was used for adult day treatment programs for approximately 50,000 persons with developmental disabilities in 19 States in FY 1988. These are optional services that some States included in their Medicaid State plans under clinic or rehabilitative services. The Federal-State Medicaid expenditure for these optional "day program" services was $491 million in FY 1988. These programs provided rehabilitative and developmental training services to persons living in ICFs/MR, other group residences, or family homes. In addition, Medicaid funded targeted case management services for the developmentally disabled in 22 States in FY 1988. Another optional service, personal care services, may be provided in an individual's home if the services are prescribed by a physician, supervised by a registered nurse, and delivered by a qualified individual who is not a member of the recipient's family. Twenty-five States were offering personal care services in FY 1988.

3. Community-Supported Living Arrangements

The Omnibus Budget Reconciliation Act of 1990, P.L. 101-508, authorized a new limited option under the Medicaid program to permit from two to eight States to provide "community-supported living arrangements services" (CSLA) for individuals with developmental disabilities (section 1930 of title XIX).[26] The service is limited to developmentally disabled individuals without regard to whether such individuals are at risk of institutionalization. The developmentally disabled individual must reside in his or her own home or in

---

[25]Smith and Gettings, *Medicaid in the Community*. In FY 1991, 46 States used community-based waiver services with an estimated 47,684 persons using the services at a cost of $1.1 billion in Medicaid spending.

[26]Effective Oct. 1991, the following States are participating in this program: California, Colorado, Florida, Illinois, Maryland, Michigan, Rhode Island, Wisconsin.

the family or legal guardian's home in which no more than three other individuals receiving these services reside. The purpose of the program is to assist these persons in the activities of daily living necessary to permit them to live in a family home or integrated community-based environment. Federal Medicaid expenditures for this program are limited to $10 million for FY 1992 and increase in annual steps to $35 million for FY 1995, with such sums as may be authorized by Congress for fiscal years thereafter.

G. State Services (Non-Medicaid)

Many people with developmental disabilities are not served through ICF/MR or other optional services. In FY 1988, separate State programs served an undetermined number of these persons at a total cost to the States of $4.0 billion. Most of the State-funded services consist of daytime services for disabled persons living with their families and residential services delivered in small group homes in the community (that are not ICFs/MR). The reason that many small State-funded group homes are not certified as ICFs/MR is that the level of care and the life safety requirements under the ICF/MR program would require increased expenditures. For group homes serving mildly and moderately retarded persons, these expenditures are often considered by States to be unnecessary. However, as severely and profoundly retarded persons are increasingly served in group homes, ICF/MR certification of these homes is increasing.

III. MEDICAID SERVICES AND STANDARDS OF CARE

A. Institutional Services Covered Under Medicaid for Persons With Developmental Disabilities

1. Services in ICFs/MR

ICF/MR funds are used for residential services in facilities ranging in size from small public or private residences of 15 beds or fewer to very large State-operated institutions of over 1,000 beds. Both large and small facilities are operated by States and by the private sector. Medicaid law has been interpreted by the Department of Health and Human Services (DHHS) to authorize the Secretary to make payments to private as well as public institutions that are certified according to ICF/MR standards. In 1990, 54 percent of the ICF/MR population was served in large State institutions, but only 3 percent was served in small State facilities. Large and small non-State facilities were used approximately equally by the remaining 43 percent of the ICF/MR population.

Institutional services delivered in ICFs/MR include medical and nursing services, physical and occupational therapy, psychological services, recreational services, social services, speech and audiology services, and other health and rehabilitative treatment and services. Medicaid law specifies that ICF/MR services may include services in a public institution (or distinct part thereof) for the mentally retarded or persons with related conditions if, among other things: 1) the primary purpose of the institution (or distinct part thereof) is to provide health or rehabilitative services for these persons and the institution meets such standards as may be prescribed by the Secretary; and 2) the individual is receiving active treatment.

The regulation specifies that each client must receive a continuous active treatment program which includes aggressive, consistent training and treatment to advance independent functioning and prevent loss of function already acquired. The active treatment requirement is implemented by means of an individual program plan that specifies client needs and objectives, and each client must receive continuous active treatment necessary to support these objectives. Active treatment is required to ensure that facilities receiving Medicaid funding do not merely provide custodial care, but deliver treatment to promote individual functioning. However, controversy has arisen regarding this requirement, because the requirement has been found in some cases to be open-ended, to promote unnecessary and ineffective treatment, and to unnecessarily increase the cost of services.[27] Because there is mounting concern about Medicaid spending growth, some State officials are concerned that the costs associated with the active treatment requirement may limit funds that can be spent on individuals in smaller more community-based settings.[28]

In 1991, roughly 146,000 persons relied on ICF/MR services at a cost of about $7.7 billion in total Medicaid funds.[29] Figure D-2 portrays the spending and beneficiary trend for ICF/MR services over the last 16 years. Based on HCFA data, the number of ICF/MR beneficiaries peaked in 1983, and has declined somewhat since. Spending, however, has continued to increase. During the late 1970s ICF/MR increases dominated Medicaid spending growth. In 1975 ICF/MR spending represented about 3 percent of overall Medicaid spending. By 1980 the service category represented over 8.5 percent. ICF/MR spending continued to outpace other Medicaid spending through 1983. By 1983 this service category represented 12.6 percent of all Medicaid vendor payments. However, in the last 3 years ICF/MR payment growth has been eclipsed by other spending. Between 1988 and 1991 ICF/MR spending represents a declining share of Medicaid payments. In 1991, ICF/MR payments embodied 10 percent

---

[27]Telephone communication with Robert M. Gettings, Executive Director, National Association of State Mental Retardation Program Directors, Inc., Apr. 30, 1992.

[28]See Lakin and Hall, *Medicaid-Financed Residential Care for Persons with Mental Retardation*, p. 157.

[29]The spending and beneficiary trend provided in this section is based on information provided to the Health Care Financing Administration by the States using HCFA Form 2082. *Chapter X, Medicaid Payment and Beneficiary Information, Fiscal Year 1991* provides a description of this data set. The information reported by the States using this form differs somewhat from that reported by Braddock, et al. For instance, the HCFA Form 2082 collects information for the Federal fiscal year, while Braddock's information reflects State fiscal year. This Form 2082 data provides a more timely discussion of overall ICF/MR spending, but lacks much of the detail of the Braddock data set.

of this spending. But this comparison needs to be kept in perspective. ICF/MR spending has increased at an 8.4 percent per annum rate over the last 3 years, despite declines in the number of Medicaid beneficiaries served in these institutions.

FIGURE D-2. Medicaid Beneficiaries Using ICF/MR Services, Fiscal Years 1975 - 1991

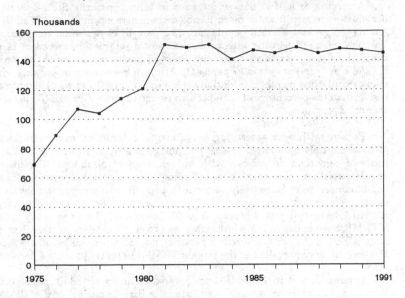

Source: Figure prepared by Congressional Research Service based on data from HCFA Form 2082.

Medicaid Payments for ICF/MR Services, Fiscal Years 1975 - 1991

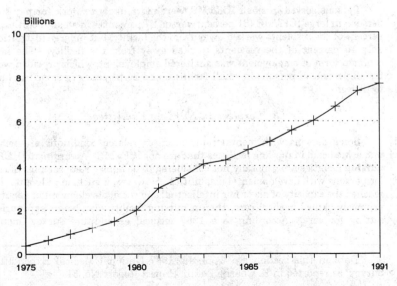

Source: Figure prepared by Congressional Research Service based on data from HCFA Form 2082.

2. Characteristics of Persons Served in ICFs/MR

According to a 1987 survey, persons in large, primarily State-operated, ICFs/MR were significantly more disabled than persons in small ICFs/MR.[30] Among the general ICF/MR population, 99.5 percent have mental retardation. The percentage of persons with profound mental retardation served in large institutions was over three times the share of such persons served in small ICFs/MR (55 percent versus 17 percent). Also, the percentage of persons with mild or borderline mental retardation served in small facilities was 150 percent higher than the percentage of such persons served in large ICFs/MR (30 percent versus 12 percent).

Persons with more severe degrees of mental retardation were more likely to have multiple handicaps. These persons generally require more intensive levels of care than do persons with milder levels of disability. Conditions associated with mental retardation, including epilepsy, cerebral palsy, deafness, and blindness, were more likely to occur in persons with more severe levels of mental retardation. For example, 37 percent of the persons served in large ICFs/MR have epilepsy, whereas only 21 percent of the persons in small ICFs/MR have epilepsy. Cerebral palsy was more than twice as prevalent in large ICFs/MR (15 percent versus 7 percent), and blindness and deafness were 150 percent more prevalent in the large ICFs/MR (10 percent versus 4 percent).

Persons served in ICFs/MR were overwhelmingly an adult population. Persons age 21 years or younger constituted less than 14 percent of the ICF/MR population. Between 1982 and 1987, the number of persons age 21 and under was reduced by one-half as fewer and fewer children were placed in institutional settings before adulthood. Seventy-eight percent of the ICF/MR population was age 22 to 54. Persons over age 54 tended to be placed in nursing homes.

Persons served in small ICFs/MR were more likely to work for pay than persons in large ICFs/MR (61 percent versus 27 percent). In small facilities, 53 percent of the residents worked away from the facility, but in large institutions only 10 percent of the residents worked away from the facility. The most common form of employment was sheltered employment, which provided work for 48 percent of persons in small facilities and 20 percent of persons in large facilities.

3. Services in Nursing Facilities

Some persons with mental retardation or related conditions are served under Medicaid in nursing facilities that are not ICFs/MR. According to HCFA, nursing facilities are generally not considered to be appropriate settings of care for persons with developmental disabilities. However, if such an individual has reached the capacity of his or her intellectual and social development or requires primarily skilled medical care, then a nursing facility may be an appropriate setting for care. According to a 1987 medical expenditure survey, mental

---

[30]Data in this section are from the 1987 National Medical Expenditure Survey, as reported in K. Charlie Lakin, Project Report No. 31.

retardation and other developmental disabilities were the primary diagnoses for 57,849 nursing home residents.[31] This was approximately 4 percent of all nursing home residents. Almost 33,000 additional persons had a diagnosis of a developmental disability, but had a primary diagnosis of a medical or mental health condition, i.e., they were in the nursing home for reasons other than their developmental disability. Approximately 43 percent of all persons with developmental disabilities served in nursing homes were age 65 and older, according to this survey.

The Omnibus Budget Reconciliation Act of 1987 (OBRA 87), P.L. 100-203, addressed the issue of inappropriate placements in nursing facilities of persons with developmental disabilities. Effective January 1, 1989, States were required to have in effect a preadmission screening program to determine whether placement in a nursing facility is appropriate for persons with developmental disabilities. Medicaid reimbursement is not to be made if such placement is found inappropriate. If such placement is found appropriate, States are to determine whether the individual requires active treatment for his or her developmental disability. By April 1, 1990, States were required to have reviewed all persons with developmental disabilities already in nursing facilities to determine whether continued placement is appropriate, and to arrange for discharge and active treatment for persons found to be inappropriately placed.[32]

The requirement regarding inappropriate placements can also be satisfied if, by October 1, 1991, States assured the Secretary that all persons with developmental disabilities found not to require the level of services in a nursing facility would be discharged by April 1, 1994. Several States took advantage of this provision.

B. Home and Community-Based Services Funded Under Medicaid

Medicaid law authorizes the Secretary of HHS to waive certain Medicaid requirements to allow States to provide a broad range of home and community-based services to individuals who would otherwise require institutional care (section 1915(c)). Home and community-based services available under this waiver may include case management, homemaker/home health aide services, personal care, adult day health, habilitation services, respite care, and other services requested by the State and approved by the Secretary. Supported employment services are authorized for persons previously institutionalized in an ICF/MR or nursing facility. Other services have included home modifications, non-medical transportation, nutrition counseling, and

---

[31]Ibid., p. 68.

[32]To assist States with the transfer to the waiver program of clients placed inappropriately in nursing homes, OBRA 87 provided that ICF/MR costs, not the generally lower nursing home costs, could be used in calculating per client expenditures in determining costs that would have been incurred in the absence of a waiver.

congregate and home-delivered meals. (See *Chapter VI, Alternate Delivery Options and Waiver Programs* for a description of the requirements associated with these waivers.)

The statute generally leaves the definition of waivered services to State discretion. However, to clarify congressional intent with respect to habilitation services for persons who were previously institutionalized in a Medicaid facility, P.L. 99-272, the Consolidated Omnibus Budget Reconciliation Act of 1985 (COBRA 85), stated that such services include: 1) services designed to assist individuals in acquiring, retaining, and improving the self-help, socialization, and adaptive skills necessary to reside successfully in home and community-based settings, and 2) prevocational, educational, and supported employment services. Habilitation services provided under the waiver authority cannot include special education or rehabilitation services available to the individual under other Federal programs.

A State's application for a waiver must include assurances that the provision of waiver services will not increase the Federal Medicaid expenditures that the State would have experienced in the absence of a waiver (i.e., budget neutrality). States have met this requirement by assuring that existing ICF/MR capacity can be reduced (that people would be deinstitutionalized and not replaced) and/or that new ICF/MR beds that would otherwise have been opened will not be needed because people will be provided community services under the waiver rather than ICF/MR services.

The number of persons participating in the home and community-based waiver program has increased substantially over the past several years, from approximately 29,000 persons in 36 States during FY 1988 to an estimate of nearly 69,000 in 48 States during in FY 1992.[33] During this period, Federal-State Medicaid expenditures under the waiver increased from $447 million in FY 1988 to an estimated $1.1 billion in FY 1992. (See figure D-3.)

The dramatic increase since FY 1988 is due to an increasing number of participants in existing programs and the addition of 12 States offering home and community-based services. This growth was due to ongoing efforts of States to move persons from ICFs/MR to community-based care, to expansion of programs to include consumers already living in the community; and a requirement that alternative services be made available to persons with developmental disabilities who were inappropriately placed in nursing facilities.

---

[33]Data estimates and issues in this section are taken from Smith and Gettings, *Medicaid in the Community*.

FIGURE D-3.
Home and Community-Based Waiver Beneficiaries and Payments
for Persons with Developmental Disabilities, 1982-1992

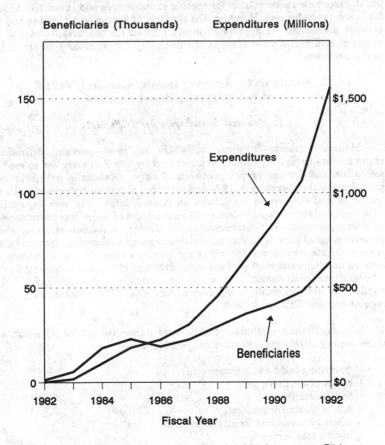

Beneficiaries (Thousands)   Expenditures (Millions)

NOTE: Spending is for home and community-based regular and model waiver programs. Total excludes beneficiaries and expenditures in Arizona.
Source: Figure prepared by Congressional Research Service based on data from Smith and Gettings.

In addition to the home and community-based waiver, which is only for persons at risk of institutionalization, the newly-authorized community-supported living arrangements limited option described above has the potential to expand community-based services to persons who are not at risk of institutionalization. This new program also does not require budget neutrality, i.e., it has a new authorization for specific expenditures and is not tied to level Medicaid expenditures. However, the number of States participating and the amount authorized for appropriation are limited for the first 5 years of the program, and States must apply to the Secretary for permission to participate in the program.

C. Standards for Assuring Quality Care in ICFs/MR and in Community-Based Services

1. Federal Standards for ICFs/MR

Medicaid statute requires ICFs/MR to meet certain definitional requirements as well as standards prescribed by the Secretary for safety and sanitation and for the proper provision of care. Standards were originally published by the Secretary in 1974 and were not significantly revised until the publication of the revised regulations on June 3, 1988. The new regulations were designed to increase the focus on the provision of active treatment services to clients, increase self-determination of clients, maintain essential client protections, and provide facility administrators and monitoring agencies with a more accurate mechanism for assessing quality of care. The standards are focused on client and staff performance, although standards regarding facility specifications and health and safety measures are also included. The regulations are applicable to all sizes of facilities. The effective date of the regulations was October 3, 1988.

The regulations establish "conditions of participation" for ICFs/MR, and these are organized into a number of specified areas:

-- governing body and management;
-- client protections;
-- facility staffing;
-- active treatment services;
-- client behavior and facility practices;
-- health care services;
-- physical environment;
-- dietetic services.

Each condition of participation is composed of a number of standards by which quality can be assessed. All conditions of participation must be met, but institutions will not be decertified if some of the standards within those conditions are not met, if the facility submits an acceptable plan of correction for the deficiencies identified.

States must certify that State and non-State ICFs/MR meet the conditions of participation before Federal payments may be made for care provided to eligible persons in these institutions. Medicaid law requires the State Medicaid agency to contract with a State survey agency to determine, through inspection, whether facilities meet the Medicaid requirements. In addition, the Secretary of HHS is authorized to "look behind" a State's survey and make an independent determination regarding a facility's compliance with program requirements. The Secretary's determination overrides the State's findings. A facility's participation in Medicaid can be terminated until the deficiencies have been corrected, or a plan of correction has been approved.

If an ICF/MR is found to be substantially out of compliance with program requirements, and if such noncompliance immediately jeopardizes client health and safety, the State is required to terminate the facility's participation in the ICF/MR program. If noncompliance is determined not to pose an immediate threat to health and safety of the clients, the State may refuse payment for services for new clients admitted to the facility after a determination of noncompliance with ICF/MR requirements. (For further information on enforcement of ICF/MR standards, see *Chapter VII, Administration.*)

2. Standards for Community-Based Services

For home and community-based services provided under waiver programs, regulations issued by HCFA March 13, 1985, require States to provide assurances that necessary safeguards have been taken to protect the health and welfare of the waiver clients. The regulations specify that safeguards include adequate standards for all types of providers that furnish services under the waiver as well as standards for board and care homes where a significant number of SSI recipients are residing or are likely to reside and where home and community-based services may be provided. If the State has licensure or certification requirements for any services or for individuals who furnish these services under the waiver, it must assure HCFA that the standards in the licensure or certification requirements will be met. The preamble to interim regulations on the waiver program pointed out that the regulations do not attempt to define these safeguards or to prescribe how they are to be developed. Rather they leave to the State the responsibility for determining what the necessary safeguards are, to define them or specify how they will be developed and implemented, and to explain how they satisfy the statute. That is, Federal standards under the waiver program are far less definitive than the quality standards for the ICF/MR program.

Quality assurance provisions under the new community-supported living arrangement option also focus on State (rather than Federal) standards for provider certification, but add external monitoring by other providers, family members, consumers, and neighbors. The Medicaid plan for these services is required to be reviewed by the State developmental disabilities councils and protection and advocacy systems, and public hearings are required prior to the implementation of new services. Federal regulations are required only to specify minimum levels of protection for the health and safety of clients. Providers found out of compliance with the regulations face fines of up to $10,000 per day.

IV. MAJOR PUBLIC EXPENDITURES AND SERVICE PATTERNS REGARDING PERSONS WITH DEVELOPMENTAL DISABILITIES[34]

A. Discussion of Major Expenditures: Medicaid and Non-Medicaid

Both Medicaid and non-Medicaid programs support numerous services for persons with developmental disabilities. The Federal and State governments spent over $20.2 billion on benefits and services for individuals with developmental disabilities in FY 1988. These benefits and services include residential services, day treatment and work programs for persons living in the community, and income maintenance programs. The Medicaid program represents the largest single payment source for this population. In FY 1988, Medicaid spending represented almost $7 billion, or 35 percent of the total. The remaining $13 billion was for income support such as SSI and Federal benefits for adults disabled in childhood, for services such as vocational rehabilitation and special education, and for State-supported community-based services.

Medicaid dollars represent the primary funding source for services provided in large residential facilities of 16 beds or more.[35] In FY 1988, $6.1 billion was spent on large residential facilities, and over $5 billion of these funds was provided by Medicaid. In contrast, non-Medicaid spending was the primary funding source for community-based services. Over $14 billion was spent on community-based benefits and services for persons with developmental disabilities in FY 1988. However, most of this spending was for nonhealth-related services. Medicaid contributed about $2 billion for community-based services. Table D-1 provides these estimates.

---

[34]The following section is based on a data series developed by David Braddock, Richard Hemp and others. Detailed accounting of public expenditures for mental retardation and developmental disabilities appears in a monograph series. At the time of this writing the latest available year providing detailed accounting of expenditures by service type was 1988.

[35]Many discussions of beneficiary and spending patterns for persons with developmental disabilities divide the services used by this population into two or more groups: services provided in large institutions of 16 beds or more, services provided in small facilities of 15 beds or fewer, and non-residential services such as habilitation services, day training, sheltered work, supported employment, and case management. The discussion in the remainder of this chapter will rely on these categories. Since the services provided to persons in small facilities (15 beds or less) are generally considered community-based, this spending category is often grouped with non-residential services to comprise the category of community-based spending. For Medicaid purposes, however, only non-residential services are considered community-based.

TABLE D-1. Federal and State Spending for Benefits and Services for Persons with Developmental Disabilities by Source of Service and Location of Service, FY 1988

(in millions of dollars)

Funding source	Large institutions[36]	Small facilities and home and community-based services[37]	Total
Medicaid	$5,039	$ 1,928	$ 6,967
Non-Medicaid	1,081	12,119	13,201
Total	6,120	14,047	20,168

NOTE: Non-Medicaid funds include a large amount for Federal income maintenance payments and significant State spending for special education and community-based services. See table D-2 for a detailed breakdown of this spending.

Source: Braddock, et al. *The State of the States in Developmental Disabilities.* Federal ICF/MR expenditures were reported in Braddock at p. 513. State Medicaid matching expenditures were calculated by the Congressional Research Service as the sum of such expenditures by the States and the District of Columbia, which were calculated from the Federal financial participation rates and Federal Medicaid expenditures reported in Part 3 of Braddock.

1. Medicaid Spending

Figure D-4 provides the distribution of Medicaid spending by major service category in FY 1988. The large share of Medicaid funds spent on residential services is apparent in the figure. Nearly 87 percent of the $7 billion Medicaid expenditure was used for residential services. Over 61 percent was spent on large public institutions. Although most Medicaid funding is used in facilities of 16 beds or more, the amount used in large public institutions increased only 9 percent between FY 1986 and FY 1988. Medicaid funds for small facilities and non-residential community-based services increased significantly since FY 1986. Funds used in small private residential facilities increased 36 percent, and the

---

[36]Includes spending in State and non-State ICFs/MR with 16 beds or more.

[37]Includes spending in State and non-State ICFs/MR with 15 beds or fewer, any State or local spending on these facilities in addition to the required Medicaid matching amount, title XX social services block grant funding, SSI and Aid to Families with Dependent Children (AFDC) payments, SSI State supplements, vocational rehabilitation spending, special education spending, and other related Federal and State spending on this population.

amount used on waiver programs and day treatment programs more than doubled between FY 1986 and FY 1988.

Numerous factors affect these funding trends. Medicaid services to persons with developmental disabilities have continued to shift from large State institutions to small community residential facilities and community-based non-residential services. This shift reflects on-going efforts to deinstitutionalize persons and to provide these persons services in community settings generally considered to be more supportive of skill development and community integration. In addition, large numbers of individuals with disabilities who might have been placed in institutions in former times are now provided services in the community, thereby decreasing the need for institutional care. Recent data indicate that the number of persons served in large State ICFs/MR decreased 15 percent between 1986 and 1990, while the number of persons served in small non-State ICFs/MR increased more than 64 percent.[38] The number of persons served under the home and community-based waiver more than doubled over this period.

---

[38]K. Charlie Lakin, Carolyn White, Robert Prouty, Robert Bruiniks, Christina Kimm. *Medicaid Institutional (ICF-MR) and Home and Community-Based Services for Persons with Mental Retardation and Related Conditions.* Report #35 and unpublished data..

FIGURE D-4. Relative Size of (Federal and State) Medicaid Expenditures by Service Category, 1988

Total Payments = $6,967 Million

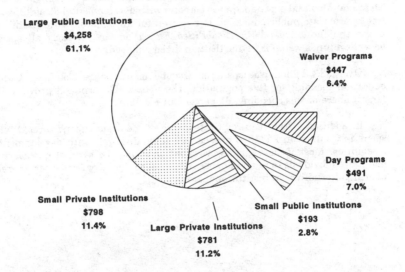

Large Public Institutions
$4,258
61.1%

Waiver Programs
$447
6.4%

Day Programs
$491
7.0%

Small Private Institutions
$798
11.4%

Small Public Institutions
$193
2.8%

Large Private Institutions
$781
11.2%

NOTE: All dollar amounts are in millions.

Source: Figure prepared by Congressional Research Service based on analysis of developmental disabilities data collected by David Braddock, et al. in *The State of the States in Developmental Disabilities*, 1990.

2. Non-Medicaid Spending

There are many non-Medicaid sources of public benefits and services for persons with developmental disabilities. Federal, State, and local payments provide income maintenance, special education, vocational rehabilitation, and other services consisting primarily of State expenditures for community-based services. These funds expand community-based options by providing basic support, small group living arrangements, and daytime training and education programs. Details of this spending are provided in table D-2.

In FY 1988, special education spending for children with developmental disabilities exceeded $5.2 billion, and 91 percent of these funds were State and local spending. Funding for special education represented the single largest State non-Medicaid expenditure for persons with developmental disabilities. A free appropriate public education is required for all children with disabilities under the *Individuals With Disabilities Education Act*. Nearly all special education funds were for noninstitutionalized children.

Over $3.4 billion was spent on income maintenance benefits. Unlike education spending for this population, the Federal Government provides the largest share of this spending, 91 percent in FY 1988.

In addition to the required State share of Medicaid expenditures, States spent $4.0 billion in FY 1988 on services for individuals with developmental disabilities. Most of these funds were spent on supportive services necessary to maintain individuals in family homes and small community residences, thereby offering alternatives to institutionalization.

**TABLE D-2. Federal and State Spending for Benefits and Services
for Persons with Developmental Disabilities, by Source
of Payment and Type of Benefit, FY 1988**
(in millions of dollars)

Payment category	Spending (in millions)	Percent of total
Income maintenance[a]		
Federal	$ 3,109	23.6%
State	316	2.4%
Total	3,425	25.9%
Special education		
Federal	471	3.6%
State	4,767	36.1%
Total	5,238	39.7%
Vocational rehabilitation		
Federal	160	1.2%
State	56	0.4%
Total	216	1.6%
Other services[b]		
Federal	352	2.7%
State	3,969	30.1%
Total	4,321	32.7%
Total		
Federal	4,092	31.0%
State	9,108	69.0%
Total	13,201	100.0%

[a]Spending in this category represents funds for SSI payments, SSI State supplements, and Federal childhood disability benefits for adults disabled in childhood (ADC).

[b]Spending in this category represents any State or local government overmatch payments for ICF/MR services or services provided in a community setting, social service block grant funds (title XX), and other programs used by this population.

Source: Estimates prepared by the Congressional Research Service based on expenditure information in Braddock, et al. *The State of the States in Developmental Disabilities.*

B. Historical Trends: Medicaid Funding for Residential and Community Services for Persons With Developmental Disabilities from FY 1977 through FY 1988

Between FY 1977 and FY 1988, Federal-State Medicaid expenditures for persons with developmental disabilities increased from $1.1 billion to $7.0 billion (See figure D-5). Most of this funding was used for services in large State ICFs/MR. However, the highest rate of growth took place in small private ICFs/MR, due partly to the transfer of persons out of the larger institutions. Federal-State Medicaid waiver expenditures increased from $2.2 million in FY 1982 to $447 million in FY 1988.

FIGURE D-5. Estimated (Federal and State) Medicaid Funding for Services for Persons with Developmental Disabilities, 1977-1988

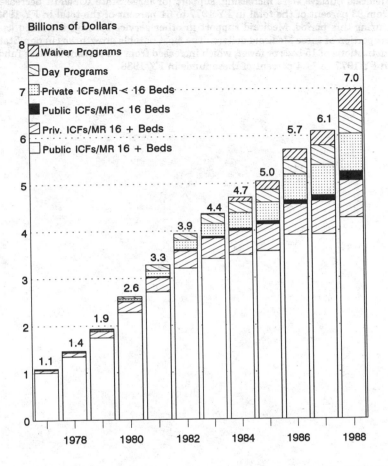

Source: Figure prepared by Congressional Research Service based on analysis of data from the Institute for the Study of Developmental Disabilities, University of Illinois at Chicago.

Figure D-6 shows selected Medicaid expenditures for persons with developmental disabilities by program type as a proportion of all Medicaid dollars spent for these services.[39] This presentation shows that, while overall Medicaid outlays were increasing, support for large State ICFs/MR decreased from 93 percent of the total in FY 1977 to 61 percent of the total in FY 1988. During this period, Medicaid support in other service settings increased as a proportion of these Medicaid dollars. The most notable growth was in non-State institutions of 15 beds or fewer, which increased from 1.6 percent of these funds in FY 1977 to 11.4 percent of these funds in FY 1988.

---

[39]Expenditures are for services specifically for persons with developmental disabilities. This presentation excludes Medicaid funding for other more general health services provided to persons with developmental disabilities.

FIGURE D-6. Allocation of (Federal and State) Medicaid Spending
for Services for Persons with Developmental Disabilities, 1977-1988

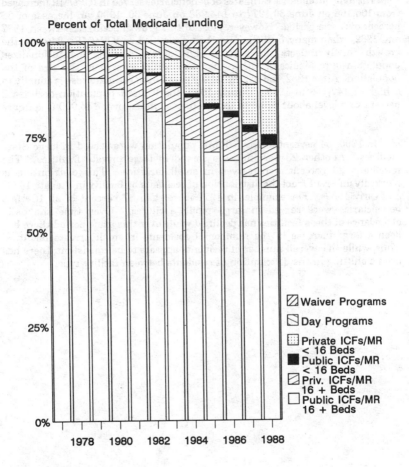

Source: Figure prepared by Congressional Research Service based on analysis of data from the
Institute for the Study of Developmental Disabilities, University of Illinois at Chicago.

C. Factors Affecting Spending Trends: Numbers of ICF/MR Residents and Facilities from FY 1977 through FY 1990[40]

The daily attendance estimates of beneficiaries served in ICFs/MR increased from 106,166 on June 30,1977 to 144,288 on June 30, 1990, an increase of 36 percent over the period. However, most of this growth occurred between 1977 and 1982, when many facilities were being certified as ICFs/MR. That is, the growth chiefly reflects the gradual shift of the existing institutionalized population onto Medicaid, rather than any actual growth in the size of the population. After 1982, the ICF/MR daily population estimate rose gradually to a high of 147,148 in 1989. During 1990, the ICF/MR population declined 2 percent to a level about equal to the 1986 level of just over 144,000 (see figure D-7).

In 1990, 54 percent of the ICF/MR population were served in large State facilities. Another 23 percent were served in large private facilities. The remaining 23 percent were served in small facilities. This distribution is markedly different from the distribution of residents by facility in the late 1970s and early 1980s. For example, in 1977 more than 87 percent of all ICF/MR beneficiaries were served in large public facilities. Over time the daily attendance of these facilities has declined while over this same period there has been a large increase in the number of residents in small private facilities. Thus, while the overall number of residents appears to be consistent, there has been a shifting in the distribution of residents between facility type.

---

[40]The numbers of beneficiaries served in ICFs/MR as reported in this section of the report rely on a survey of the daily populations of ICFs/MR for selected years. As such the estimates will differ from the beneficiary estimates reported by States using the HCFA statistical reporting form 2082 reported elsewhere in this report. Beneficiary estimates as reported on the HCFA Form 2082 represent the number of beneficiaries for which Medicaid paid for services during the fiscal year.

FIGURE D-7. Number of ICF/MR Residents, 1977-1990

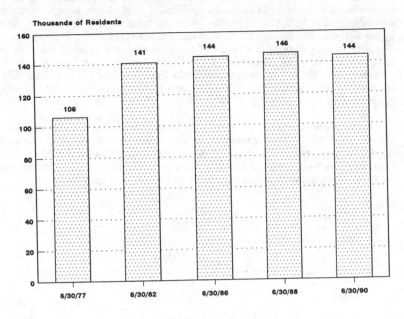

Thousands of Residents

Number of ICF/MR Residents,
by Size and Type of Facility, 1977-1990

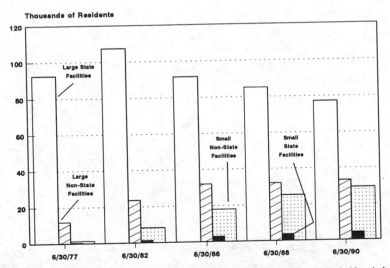

Thousands of Residents

Source: Figure prepared by Congressional Research Service based on data in K. Charlie Lakin, et al.,
ICFs/MR: Program Utilization and Resident Characteristics, and unpublished data.

The trend in the number of ICF/MR facilities between 1977 and 1990 is somewhat different from the resident trend. (See figure D-8.) Like the number of residents, the number of certified ICF/MR facilities has increased. In 1977, there was an estimated 574 facilities, by June of 1990 the number of facilities was estimated to be 5,405. However, while the number of residents increased by 36 percent, the number of facilities increased eight fold. This apparent disparity in growth rates is a result of the increased use of small facilities by this population. The number of large State facilities has remained fairly constant over this period, declining slightly from 292 in 1982 to 268 in 1990. In contrast, the number of small non-State facilities increased significantly, growing from 147 facilities in 1977 to 4,051 in 1990.

Since the number of large State facilities has declined at a slower rate than the decline in the number of residents in these facilities, the result is a smaller number of residents per facility in 1990 compared with the early 1980s. Since these facilities have many fixed costs, a decrease in the residents per facility may be a contributing factor to the high per resident costs of these facilities.

FIGURE D-8. Number of ICF/MR Facilities, 1977-1990

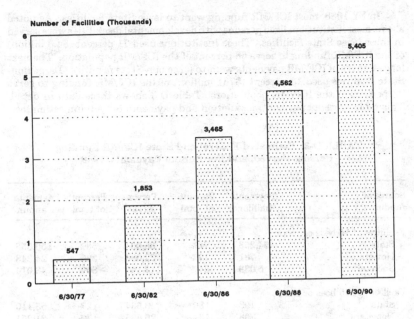

Number of ICF/MR Facilities, by Size and Type of Facility, 1977-1990

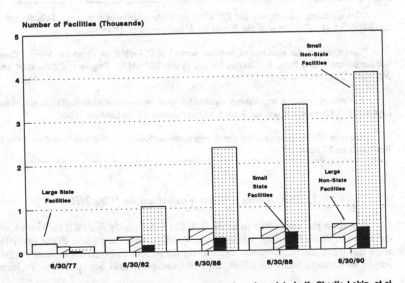

Source: Figure prepared by Congressional Research Service based on data in K. Charlie Lakin, et al., *ICFs/MR: Program Utilization and Resident Characteristics*, and unpublished data.

D. ICF/MR Services, Persons Served, and Estimates of
Per Annum Expenditures

In FY 1988, most ICF/MR funding went to large State facilities. As noted above, most institutionalized persons with developmental disabilities were served in these large State facilities. These institutions used 71 percent ($4.3 billion) of the ICF/MR funding to serve 58 percent of the ICF/MR population. The next largest share of ICF/MR payments went to large non-State facilities. Large non-State facilities used 13 percent ($781 million) of the ICF/MR funding to serve 22 percent of the ICF/MR population. Table D-3 shows these data in detail. This table presents payment, population and payments per annum estimates.

TABLE D-3. Estimated Federal and State ICF/MR Funding, Persons Served, and Per Annum Payments, 1988

Source of funding	Payments[a] (millions)	Percent of total	Persons served[b]	Percent of total	Payments per annum[c]
Facilities of 16 beds or more:					
State	$4,258	71%	85,064	58%	$50,056
Non-state	781	13%	32,083	22%	24,343
Subtotal	5,039	84%	117,147	80%	43,014
Facilities of 15 beds or less:					
State	193	3%	3,634	2%	53,110
Non-state	798	13%	25,535	17%	31,251
Subtotal	991	16%	29,169	20%	33,974
Total	6,029	100%	146,134	100%	41,257

[a]Expenditures shown are for FY 1988 and are estimates based on data found in Braddock, et al. *The State of the States in Developmental Disabilities*.

[b]Estimates of the number of persons served in ICFs/MR on June 30, 1988. These estimates are taken from K. Charlie Lakin, et al. *ICFs/MR: Program Utilization and Resident Characteristics*.

[c]Estimates based on annual payments and June resident estimates. These estimates assume that there is a constant length of stay across all institution types.

Source: Table prepared by the Congressional Research Service based on data in Braddock and Lakin.

1. Discussion of Cost Variation in ICFs/MR

Based on the estimates in table D-3, the most costly ICF/MR services were delivered in State facilities, while services delivered in large non-State facilities were the least costly. Reasons explaining these cost differences include higher employee costs in State facilities, higher fixed costs and depopulation in large

State institutions, the location of the facility, and severity of disability among the client population.

Many large State institutions face fixed institutional costs, such as costs for maintenance, administration, and housekeeping. These fixed costs were generally due to efforts to upgrade the program, physical plant, and staff to comply with ICF/MR standards. Depopulation of large State institutions contributed further to the higher per capita costs in these facilities.

Another factor affecting the higher cost of services in large State ICFs/MR was that these facilities tended to serve persons with the most severe disabilities, who tend to receive very intensive services. Some of these persons also have severe behavior problems, which can further increase the cost of care. Large non-State facilities tended to serve a more mildly disabled population. For example, in FY 1987, 63 percent of the persons served in large State ICFs/MR were profoundly retarded, while only 26 percent of the persons served in large non-State ICFs/MR were profoundly retarded.[41]

Small State facilities, the most expensive service setting, were generally located in urban areas and tended to be newly purchased facilities, while large State facilities had generally been State property for many years and tended to be located in areas outside of large urban centers where real estate values were lower.

V. STATE DATA ON MEDICAID SERVICES FOR PERSONS WITH DEVELOPMENTAL DISABILITIES

A. ICF/MR Residents by Facility Type

States vary greatly in their utilization of ICF/MR funding. Federal Medicaid funding is available to help States provide residential services, and States have discretion regarding whether they use these funds for services in large or small/State or non-State facilities.

The major service mode used by most States on June 30, 1990 was the large State facility, the mode of service for 54 percent of all ICF/MR clients (see table D-4). Only 3 percent of the ICF/MR clients were served in small State facilities. Non-State facilities were used approximately equally, with 23 percent of the clients served in large non-State facilities and 20 percent served in small non-State facilities.

All States served persons in large State facilities, but only 10 States served persons in small State facilities. Large non-State facilities were used in 35 States, and 41 States used small non-State facilities.

---

[41]Data on severity of persons served were obtained by telephone from K. Charlie Lakin on Sept. 23, 1991.

TABLE D-4. Residents in Intermediate Care Facilities for the Mentally Retarded, by Facility Type and Size, June 30, 1990

State	State facilities			Non-State facilities		
	1-15 beds	16 + beds	Total	1-15 beds	16 + beds	Total
Alabama[a]	0	1,298	1,298	31	0	31
Alaska	0	58	58	40	0	40
Arizona	51	65	116	0	40	40
Arkansas	0	1,243	1,243	97	0	97
California	0	6,788	6,788	1,979	2,123	4,102
Colorado[b]	265	429	694	0	280	280
Connecticut	289	867	1,156	271	16	287
Delaware	0	342	342	92	0	92
District of Columbia	0	154	154	458	0	458
Florida	0	1,248	1,248	0	1,931	1,931
Georgia[b]	0	1,822	1,822	0	110	110
Hawaii	0	165	165	55	0	55
Idaho	0	209	209	201	58	259
Illinois	0	4,459	4,459	2,281	4,268	6,549
Indiana[b]	0	1,714	1,714	2,952	264	3,216
Iowa	0	976	976	28	1,508	1,536
Kansas	0	1,017	1,017	285	677	962
Kentucky[b]	0	678	678	0	513	513
Louisiana	30	2,554	2,584	1,714	1,543	3,257
Maine	24	265	289	221	144	365
Maryland	8	1,250	1,258	0	0	0
Massachusetts	232	2,800	3,032	328	328	
Michigan	0	1,044	1,044	2,029	0	2,029
Minnesota	28	1,337	1,365	2,523	1,747	4,270
Mississippi	0	1,131	1,131	0	585	585
Missouri	0	1,666	1,666	192	176	368
Montana	0	235	235	10	0	10
Nebraska	0	472	472	9	250	259
Nevada	0	177	177	15	0	15
New Hampshire	0	36	36	52	25	77
New Jersey[b]	0	3,750	3,750	0	68	68
New Mexico[a]	0	497	497	233	0	233

See notes at end of table.

TABLE D-4. Residents in Intermediate Care Facilities for
the Mentally Retarded, by Facility Type and Size,
June 30,1990--Continued

State	State facilities			Non-State facilities		
	1-15 beds	16 + beds	Total	1-15 beds	16 + beds	Total
New York	2,823	7,208	10,031	5,478	1,452	6,930
North Carolina	0	2,567	2,567	720	512	1,232
North Dakota	0	228	228	443	0	443
Ohio	0	2,515	2,515	1,419	4,057	5,476
Oklahoma[b]	0	994	994	0	1,900	1,900
Oregon	0	804	804	22	140	162
Pennsylvania	0	3,940	3,940	1,135	2,041	3,176
Rhode Island	0	215	215	576	18	594
South Carolina	0	2,251	2,251	886	92	978
South Dakota	0	382	382	186	0	186
Tennessee	0	1,914	1,914	142	200	342
Texas[b]	613	6,576	7,189	1,559	2,514	4,073
Utah	0	452	452	12	525	537
Vermont	0	177	177	54	0	54
Virginia[a]	0	2,669	2,669	141	20	161
Washington	0	1,697	1,697	122	400	522
West Virginia	0	212	212	330	54	384
Wisconsin	0	1,652	1,652	71	3,016	3,087
Wyoming	0	67	67	0	0	0
U.S. Total	4,363	77,266	81,629	29,392	33,267	62,659

[a]Uses 1989 data.
[b]Some statistics for the State are estimates.

Source: Unpublished data provided by K. Charlie Lakin.

B. Per Annum ICF/MR Expenditures by State

States vary significantly in per annum expenditures for ICF/MR services for
FY 1989, ranging from a high of $116,900 per resident per year in Alaska to a
low of $18,399 per resident per year in Wisconsin (see table D-5). The Medicaid
median per annum expenditure was $44,946. Three-fourths of States' per
annum expenditures ranged between $65,000 and $28,000.

The per annum expenditure of a State reflects many variables within the
State ICF/MR program. States with a high cost of living generally pay higher

salaries than States in which the cost of living is relatively low. The per annum cost is dominated by labor costs, i.e., the level of pay of personnel delivering ICF/MR services and the ratio of program personnel to persons served. (Seventy percent of ICF/MR costs are labor and benefits.) As residents are transferred from large State ICFs/MR to community settings, per capita costs in the large State facilities tend to increase due to the need to maintain comprehensive services and extensive overhead for a dwindling and more severely disabled population. Some States have already moved all clients from large State facilities to small non-State facilities or to waiver programs and have closed the large facility, significantly lowering per annum ICF/MR costs.

TABLE D-5. Per Annum Medicaid Payments for ICF/MR Services, States Ranked by FY 1989 Expenditures

State	Payment per annum
Alaska	$116,900
New Hampshire	84,955
Oregon	78,140
New York	76,021
Michigan	66,722
New Jersey	66,424
Maine	65,301
Rhode Island	65,076
Massachusetts	62,650
Connecticut	60,974
Pennsylvania	59,849
North Carolina	57,334
Nevada	56,548
North Dakota	56,244
Iowa	55,198
Vermont	53,771
Washington	53,437
Maryland	52,806
Idaho	52,763
District of Columbia	49,385
Georgia	48,489
Virginia	48,271
Kentucky	45,212
Arkansas	43,904
Montana	43,887
Alabama	43,859
Colorado	42,084
Florida	41,783
Missouri	40,907
Ohio	40,611

TABLE D-5. Per Annum Medicaid Payments for ICF/MR Services,
States Ranked by FY 1989 Expenditures--Continued

State	Payment per annum
Minnesota	40,404
South Dakota	39,760
Nebraska	38,992
Delaware	38,115
Tennessee	37,682
Kansas	35,181
New Mexico	34,534
South Carolina	34,093
California	33,984
Utah	33,421
Texas	32,290
Oklahoma	31,839
Louisiana	28,209
Illinois	28,104
Mississippi	24,491
Hawaii	23,975
West Virginia	19,666
Indiana	18,494
Wisconsin	18,399
U.S. Total	44,946

NOTE: All figures are estimates and subject to the data and methods used in their calculations. Cost data for Arizona ICF/MR services not available for this period.

Source: K. Charlie Lakin, Carolyn White, Robert Prouty, Robert Bruininks, Christina Kimm. *Medicaid Institutional (ICF/MR) and Home and Community-Based Services for Persons with Mental Retardation and Related Conditions*. Report # 35, TABLE 16: Summary Statistics on Expenditures for ICF/MR Care by State an [sic] for Fiscal Year 1989.

C. Percentage of Persons Served in ICF/MR Certified Facilities

States varied significantly in the percentage of persons served in residential settings that were ICF/MR certified on June 30, 1989 (see table D-6). Nationally, 87 percent of the persons served in large facilities were in ICF/MR certified facilities, but only 23 percent of persons served in small facilities were served in ICF/MR certified facilities. In 15 States all persons served in large facilities were in certified facilities, and in 29 States at least 90 percent of all persons served in large facilities were in ICFs/MR. Only seven States serving clients in small facilities had more than half the clients placed in ICF/MR certified facilities.

One explanation for the lower certification rate in small facilities is that some States use family care or small group living arrangements, which would not conform to ICF/MR standards. In addition, the ICF/MR standards require a relatively intense level of care, which is considered inappropriate for the needs of mildly and moderately handicapped persons living in the community.

TABLE D-6. Percent of Residents in Medicaid Certified ICF/MR Facilities by Facility Size and State, June 30,1989

State	Facility size: 1-15 beds	16 + beds	Total	State rank[a]
	Share of Residents in ICF/MR Certified Facilities:			
Alabama	4.0%	92.2%	60.8%	17
Alaska	13.8	100.0	28.0	46
Arizona	2.6	4.7	2.9	50
Arkansas	0.0	100.0	69.4	9
California	9.8	69.8	34.8	41
Colorado	12.3	100.0	36.2	38
Connecticut	14.6	97.9	45.5	27
Delaware	26.5	100.0	64.9	14
District of Columbia	56.6	72.8	60.1	18
Florida	0.0	66.6	37.4	36
Georgia	0.0	83.8	52.8	24
Hawaii	7.9	100.0	22.4	47
Idaho	28.3	76.8	41.7	31
Illinois	39.7	78.0	65.6	11
Indiana	75.5	87.5	80.9	5
Iowa	4.2	80.0	40.1	32
Kansas	12.9	100.0	54.1	23
Kentucky	0.0	94.7	63.2	15
Louisiana	84.9	99.7	95.1	2
Maine	16.3	72.2	32.0	43
Maryland	0.4	94.5	31.4	44
Massachusetts	10.4	92.3	42.8	30
Michigan	28.6	69.5	38.0	35
Minnesota	46.8	96.0	65.4	13
Mississippi	0.0	76.4	65.8	10
Missouri	6.6	58.9	32.8	42
Montana	0.9	100.0	19.1	48
Nebraska	0.5	100.0	30.8	45
Nevada	4.2	100.0	35.2	40
New Hampshire	5.4	88.1	14.0	49
New Jersey	0.0	73.3	44.8	28
New Mexico	33.9	95.3	59.6	19
New York	46.6	99.6	65.5	12
North Carolina	30.2	77.1	59.2	20

See notes at end of table.

TABLE D-6. Percent of Residents in Medicaid Certified ICF/MR Facilities by Facility Size and State, June 30,1989--Continued

State	Facility size: 1-15 beds	16 + beds	Total	State rank[a]
	Share of Residents in ICF/MR Certified Facilities:			
North Dakota	32.9	87.0	42.8	29
Ohio	24.6	89.5	61.1	16
Oklahoma	1.7	100.0	77.9	6
Oregon	1.2	94.7	36.0	39
Pennsylvania	12.2	87.2	47.5	25
Rhode Island	67.4	93.0	72.1	7
South Carolina	54.6	100.0	83.4	4
South Dakota	17.2	100.0	39.7	34
Tennessee	0.7	98.8	55.9	21
Texas	89.0	100.0	98.1	1
Utah	4.8	100.0	54.2	22
Vermont	11.6	100.0	36.5	37
Virginia	23.2	97.4	84.0	3
Washington	4.3	88.9	40.0	33
West Virginia	68.3	72.5	69.9	8
Wisconsin	1.4	99.0	47.1	26
Wyoming	0.0	0.0	0.0	51
U.S. Total	23.0	86.6	53.9	

[a]State ranking based on the share of all residents in Medicaid certified ICFs/MR.

Source: K. Charlie Lakin, Carolyn White, Robert Prouty, Robert Bruiniks, Christina Kimm. *Medicaid Institutional (ICF-MR) and Home and Community-Based Services for Persons with Mental Retardation and Related Conditions.* Report # 35, table 7, 1991.

D. Persons Served in Medicaid Non-Residential Programs

As shown in table D-7, optional Medicaid-funded non-residential community services were distributed unevenly among the States in FY 1988. For example, under the home and community-based services waiver New Jersey served 3,303 persons, Florida served 2,631, and California served 2,500, but 15 States did not offer waiver services. Only 11 States used 1915(c) model waivers for children living at home.[42] Ohio, the State serving the most children under this option, served 134 children. Day programs were used relatively extensively, but Illinois, New York and Ohio served the most individuals. The case management option was also used extensively among States for which data were available.

TABLE D-7. Number of Persons Served by Medicaid Supported Non-Residential Community Services for Persons with Developmental Disabilities, FY 1988

State	Case management	Day programs	Home & community waivers	Model waivers
Alabama	2,000	4,164	1,593	0
Alaska	0	255	0	0
Arizona	42	1,280	0	0
Arkansas	3,588	2,454	0	0
California	79,196	11,945	2,500	0
Colorado	5,771	3,438	1,432	0
Connecticut	9,120	4,754	644	25
Delaware	579	630	130	0
District of Columbia	0	842	0	0
Florida	18,000	17,083	2,631	0
Georgia	0	9,199	0	0
Hawaii	1,034	780	56	0
Idaho	0	3,986	204	1
Illinois	10,829	23,443	637	0
Indiana	16,896	10,263	0	0
Iowa	8,495	3,683	0	8
Kansas	2,812	2,570	242	0
Kentucky	3,541	3,171	659	1
Louisiana	0	3,027	0	0
Maine	1,250	1,764	430	0
Maryland	4,240	6,313	716	0
Massachusetts	14,400	8,500	740	0
Michigan	0	10,000	1,000	34
Minnesota	16,912	12,007	1,644	0
Mississippi	1,500	1,380	0	0

[42]See *Chapter VI, Alternate Delivery Options and Waiver Programs* for a description of the differences between regular home and community-based waiver programs and the model waiver program.

**TABLE D-7. Number of Persons Served by Medicaid Supported
Non-Residential Community Services for Persons with
Developmental Disabilities, FY 1988--Continued**

State	Case management	Day programs	Home & community waivers	Model waivers
Missouri	11,682	4,067	0	0
Montana	2,100	1,325	285	0
Nebraska	2,198	2,144	553	0
Nevada	909	640	147	0
New Hampshire	1,590	1,211	635	0
New Jersey	8,650	6,017	3,303	0
New Mexico	0	832	120	58
New York	62,545	35,580	0	17
North Carolina	369	5,343	375	0
North Dakota	2,634	436	741	0
Ohio	4,482	22,458	0	134
Oklahoma	0	1,588	134	0
Oregon	0	3,022	1,157	0
Pennsylvania	0	0	1,643	0
Rhode Island	0	1,385	520	0
South Carolina	7,619	4,106	0	0
South Dakota	1,427	1,245	704	0
Tennessee	0	3,189	360	50
Texas	7,214	12,846	387	11
Utah	0	1,178	827	0
Vermont	0	670	248	0
Virginia	9,344	3,483	0	0
Washington	14,467	3,528	990	20
West Virginia	124	448	126	0
Wisconsin	10,881	16,778	574	0
Wyoming	0	400	0	0
U.S. Total	348,440	280,850	29,087	359

NOTE: Individual clients may participate in more than one non-residential community service.

Source: Braddock, et al. *The State of the States in Developmental Disabilities.*

E. Per Annum Medicaid Payments for Home and Community-Based Waiver Programs[43]

As shown on table D-8, per annum expenditures for FY 1991 under the home and community-based services waiver program varied from $50,483 in Pennsylvania to $933 in New York. The average per annum cost was $22,329. Because States have discretion regarding the types of services offered under these waivers, there is little comparability among these programs. Also, most persons served under the waivers receive other Medicaid and/or non-Medicaid services, the cost of which is not reflected in table D-8.

States with higher per annum costs tend to have the better established programs and tend to have used the waiver extensively to provide services for persons moved out of large State facilities. States with lower per annum waiver costs tend to be in the earlier stages of implementation in which a broad range of services is not yet offered. The expectation is that interstate differences will narrow as State waiver programs reach maturity.

Per annum waiver and ICF/MR expenditures are not comparable. Persons served under the Medicaid waiver are eligible to receive the full SSI payment and may receive food stamps and other benefits not available to residents of ICFs/MR. (ICF/MR payments include the cost of room and board.) Other differences between ICF/MR and waiver costs include variations in services received (comprehensive ICF/MR services versus optional waiver services), variations in level of disability (ICFs/MR tend to serve persons with more severe disabilities), or other services received by the individual (persons served under the waiver generally receive a variety of other community services). One recent estimate states that, if all comparable costs are taken into account, per capita waiver costs were 20-40 percent lower than average annual per capita ICF/MR services in most States in FY 1990 (Smith, Gettings, p. 13).

---

[43]A major study comparing institutional costs and community residential costs indicated that on average, institutional costs were higher per client day for a group of clients matched for adaptive behavior, age, and medical need. This study found that per diem costs of community residential programs were approximately 70 percent of the cost of institutional services due, in large part, to lower staff salaries and fringe benefits in the community settings. If personnel costs were equal in both settings, per diem rates would be equivalent, according to this study. However, clients in community residential settings received more staff time per client than clients in institutions. (See Conroy, J., and Bradley, V. *The Pennhurst Longitudinal Study: Combined Report of Five Years of Research and Analysis.* Boston, Human Services Research Institute, Mar. 1, 1985. p. 219-244.) Other studies since have corroborated the finding that less is spent by government agencies per person in the community than in institutions for comprehensive care.

TABLE D-8. Estimated Expenditures, and Persons with
Developmental Disabilities in Home and Community-Based
Waiver Programs,[a] FY 1991

State	Expenditures (in thousands)	Participants	Expenditures per annum
Alabama	$12,400	2,000	$ 6,200
Arizona[h]	0	0	0
Arkansas	1,803	196	9,196
California	54,049	3,360	16,086
Colorado	52,714	2,294	22,979
Connecticut	61,575	1,811	34,001
Delaware	4,705	235	20,020
District of Columbia	0	0	0
Florida	18,000	2,631	6,842
Georgia	5,065	178	28,457
Hawaii	3,052	268	11,388
Idaho	2,148	300	7,160
Illinois	16,900	740	22,838
Indiana	360	40	8,998
Iowa	54	15	3,580
Kansas	11,670	416	28,053
Kentucky	16,257	786	20,683
Louisiana	204	40	5,095
Maine	12,500	453	27,594
Maryland	42,979	1,020	42,136
Massachusetts	57,029	1,927	29,594
Michigan	58,635	2,245	26,118
Minnesota	79,344	2,895	27,407
Mississippi	0	0	0
Missouri	28,37	31,671	16,980
Montana	7,693	388	19,826
Nebraska	19,569	705	27,757
Nevada	2,236	172	12,999
New Hampshire	39,200	935	41,925
New Jersey	91,503	3,501	26,136
New Mexico	3,191	267	11,949
New York	140	150	933
North Carolina	12,831	964	13,311
North Dakota	16,33	61,228	13,303

See notes at end of table.

TABLE D-8. Estimated Expenditures, and Persons with Developmental Disabilities in Home and Community-Based Waiver Programs,ª FY 1991--Continued

State	Expenditures (in thousands)	Participants	Expenditures per annum
Ohio	$ 40,912	461	$ 6,628
Oklahoma	11,818	938	12,599
Oregon	40,983	1,430	28,659
Pennsylvania	120,100	2,379	50,483
Rhode Island	14,337	677	21,177
South Carolina	0	0	0
South Dakota	13,334	788	16,921
Tennessee	11,390	687	16,579
Texas	14,368	904	15,894
Utah	20,000	1,415	14,134
Vermont	10,255	353	29,051
Virginia	264	33	8,009
Washington	30,254	1,768	17,112
West Virginia	10,040	415	24,193
Wisconsin	30,132	1,680	17,936
Wyoming	846	140	6,044
Totals	1,064,723	47,684	22,329

ªHome and community-based waiver spending represents spending on regular and model waiver programs in each State with persons with developmental disabilities as a target population.

bArizona provides Medicaid-like services under a different waiver authority. In 1991 the Arizona Health Care Cost Containment System provided acute care and home and community-based waiver services to 4,700 persons costing in excess of $80 million at a per beneficiary cost of $17,043.

Source: Table prepared by the Congressional Research Service based on data contained in Gary Smith and Robert Gettings. *Medicaid in the Community: The HCBS Waiver and CSLA Programs.* National Association of State Mental Retardation Program Directors, Mar. 1992.

F. Notes on Expenditure Data Found in Table D-1

Data on Federal expenditures were obtained from David Braddock, et al, The State of the States in Developmental Disabilities, University Affiliated Program in Developmental Disabilities, Institute for the Study of Developmental Disabilities and School of Public Health, University of Illinois at Chicago, 1990, p. 513. All estimates were prepared by the Congressional Research Service. Federal Medicaid ICF/MR program expenditures for community services were calculated as the sum of Federal ICF/MR program expenditures for State and non-State facilities of less than 16 beds. State Medicaid expenditures are based on the Federal financial participation rates (adjusted Federal Medical Assistance Percentages) and Federal Medicaid expenditures reported in Part 2 of Braddock.

All Federal expenditures under the Medicaid waiver programs reported by Braddock et al. have been assigned to the community services category, as are matching State expenditures. While Federal and State matching expenditures for Medicaid day programs have been assigned to community services, an undetermined share of these expenditures may finance services provided in non-State institutions of 16 or more beds.

State non-Medicaid expenditures used to fund services provided in public institutions of 16 or more beds are calculated as the difference between total State expenditures on these institutions and the amount calculated to be State Medicaid matching expenditures for these institutions. State expenditures not used to finance services provided in public institutions of 16 or more beds are calculated as total State expenditures for services other than those provided in public institutions of 16 or more beds, less the State SSI supplement and all State Medicaid matching expenditures. This amount is assigned to community services. An undetermined share of these expenditures may be used to finance provision of services in private institutions of 16 or more beds.

APPENDIX E. MEDICAID SERVICES FOR
THE MENTALLY ILL[1]

I. INTRODUCTION

Medicaid is an important source of funding for the treatment of mental illness, including long-term serious mental illness and short-term acute problems. In FY 1991, over $2.0 billion in combined Federal-State Medicaid funds went to mental institutions, while additional funds were spent on services for mental illness in ordinary hospitals and nursing homes and in the community.[2] However, the population of individuals with mental illness has never emerged, as has the population of individuals with mental retardation, as a distinct population served by the Medicaid program. Medicaid provides some services to some segments of the mentally ill population under certain conditions.

The limitations on Medicaid's role are due in part to specific policy decisions made in the early years of the program and in part to the nature of the mentally ill population. This population is heterogeneous and ill-defined, with widely differing problems and needs. Before discussing Medicaid's role, then, it is necessary to define the population under consideration.

II. BACKGROUND

A. Defining the Population of Individuals with Mental Illness

Broadly speaking, the "population of individuals with mental illness" at any given time consists of all persons who have been or could be diagnosed as suffering from one of a variety of defined mental disorders. Some of these persons are experiencing moderate problems that are of recent origin and that may never recur. Others have severe problems that have continued over a long period and that may be expected to continue in the future. This latter group, categorized until recently as the "chronically mentally ill," but now most commonly referred to as the "seriously mentally ill," may be thought of as constituting a distinct population and are what are usually meant when people speak of the mentally ill. As used in this appendix, the term mentally ill will generally be used to mean the population of individuals with serious mental illness, and will exclude persons whose primary diagnosis is mental retardation.

---

[1]This appendix was written by Edward Klebe.

[2]Medicaid data do not distinguish expenditures for treatment of mental as opposed to physical problems by providers other than mental institutions.

Even the definition of serious mental illness has been the subject of some disagreement. Historically, the definition was based primarily on psychiatric diagnosis. Gradually this definition has been refined to include psychiatric disabilities. It has become recognized that the population of individuals with serious illness is a heterogeneous group with different diagnoses, levels of disability, and duration of disability, and therefore, different service needs. According to a September 1992 publication containing estimates of serious mental illness in the adult household population, the National Institute of Mental Health (NIMH) is currently developing a more precise definition to encompass the diversity of the population.[3]

In 1989, NIMH collaborated with the National Center for Health Statistics (NCHS) on a special supplement to the National Health Interview Survey to update earlier estimates on the number of persons with serious mental illness in the household population of the United States. The results of the survey indicate that there are approximately 3.3 million persons 18 years of age or older in the civilian noninstitutionalized population of the United States who had a serious mental illness in the 12 months previous to the survey, a rate of 18.2 adults per 1,000 population. Approximately 2.6 million, or 78.8 percent of these adults, have one or more specific limitations in work, school, personal care, social functioning, concentrating, or coping with day-to-day stress attributable to serious mental illness.

The survey estimates that approximately 1.4 million adults between the ages of 18 and 69 are currently unable to work (829,000) or limited in work (529,000) because of their serious mental illness, and over 82 percent of these adults have had this work limitation for a year or longer. Among the 390,000 adults 70 years of age and over with serious mental illness, about 85 percent had current limitations in one or more of the specific activities described above, and approximately 80 percent had been so limited for a year or longer.

The NIMH/NCHS survey further reports that the findings of the survey suggest that the entire adult population of persons with serious mental illness can be conservatively estimated to include 4 to 5 million adult Americans, or 2.1 percent to 2.6 percent of the adult population. In addition to the household population, it is estimated the 200,000 persons with serious mental illness are homeless on any given day. An additional 1 million to 1.1 million are residents of nursing homes, approximately 50,000 to 60,000 are patients of mental hospitals, and approximately 50,000 are inmates of State prisons.[4]

In recent years those persons with serious mental illness who are homeless have been a population of particular concern. Some have estimated that 20 to 40 percent of the homeless population suffer from such serious mental illnesses

---

[3]Barker, P. R., R. W. Manderscheid, G. E. Hendershot, et al. *Serious Mental Illness and Disability in the Adult Household Population: United States, 1989.* Advance Data from Vital and Health Statistics, no. 218. Hyattsville, Md.: National Center for Health Statistics, Sept. 16, 1992. p. 1.

[4]Ibid., p. 2 and 8.

as schizophrenia, manic-depressive illness, or severe depression. As estimates of the total number of homeless persons range from one-quarter of a million to 5 million,[5] it is difficult to provide a reasonable estimate of the number of homeless mentally ill persons. Although "deinstitutionalization," the discharge of mentally ill persons from State mental institutions, has sometimes been referred to as a major factor in homelessness, recent examinations suggest that relatively few of the homeless are actually former residents of mental hospitals. Some observers now speak instead of "noninstitutionalization," the failure to provide residential treatment to persons who need it.[6]

B. Medicaid Eligibility for the Mentally Ill

Medicaid has no special eligibility rules or conditions for mentally ill persons. Those in the community may qualify by receiving Supplemental Security Income (SSI) disability benefits or by meeting medically needy standards in the States with medically needy programs. Those in institutions may qualify because they have no financial resources or because they "spend down," and thereby meet eligibility standards after contributing to the cost of their own care. As with other beneficiaries, persons in institutions must also meet the categorical requirements for eligibility. (See *Chapter III, Eligibility* for further information.)

1. SSI Disabled and Others

The number of mentally ill Medicaid beneficiaries living in the community cannot be firmly established. The Social Security Administration estimates that 2.49 million persons were receiving SSI disability payments in December 1990. Of the 1.95 million for whom diagnoses were available, 26.4 percent, or about 514,087, had a primary disability of mental disorder (other than mental retardation).[7] As only about 4 percent of all SSI disability beneficiaries are in institutions at any given time, the vast majority of these mentally ill SSI beneficiaries must have been living in the community or in settings such as board and care homes or halfway houses. Most of these persons would automatically have qualified for Medicaid. Additional mentally ill persons may qualify for Medicaid through other assistance categories.

---

[5]U.S. Library of Congress. Congressional Research Service. *Homelessness: Issues and Legislation in the 102nd Congress.* CRS Issue Brief No. IB88070, by Ruth Ellen Wasem. (Regularly updated)

[6]Levitan, Sar. A., and Susan Schillmoeller. *The Paradox of Homelessness in America.* Washington, George Washington University. Center for Social Policy Studies, Jan. 1991. p. 18.

[7]Social Security Administration. Social Security Bulletin. Annual Statistical Supplement, 1991. SSA Publication No. 13-11700. Washington, 1991. p. 301. The estimate omits the 213,000 SSI disability recipients who were transferred from the predecessor Aid to the Permanently and Totally Disabled (APTD) program in 1973 and who were still receiving benefits in 1990. Diagnoses are for the most part not available for these recipients.

2. Institutions

According to the Health Care Financing Administration (HCFA), the number of persons receiving Medicaid-covered services in mental institutions during FY 1991 was 64,890 (see table E-2). Data from the 1985 National Nursing Home Survey indicated that 149,811 mentally ill persons were receiving Medicaid nursing home services during that year. No more recent data on persons receiving Medicaid nursing home services are available. (Further details on the institutional population appear in section III of this appendix.)

As will be discussed further in section III of this appendix, Medicaid does not cover services in mental institutions for persons between age 21 and 65. A person in this age group who is in an excluded institution may not receive Medicaid benefits, regardless of his or her financial needs. This means that some persons eligible for Medicaid in the community lose eligibility when they enter an institution. If they then return to the community, there may be delays or problems in restoring eligibility. As a result, some persons may fail to receive outpatient follow-up care.

3. Homeless

Congress has taken some steps to facilitate Medicaid eligibility for the homeless. The Omnibus Budget Reconciliation Act of 1986 (OBRA 86, P.L. 99-509) provided that eligibility could not be denied on the grounds that an applicant had no fixed address. The Omnibus Budget Reconciliation Act of 1987 (OBRA 87, P.L. 100-203) required States to develop systems to ensure that homeless Medicaid beneficiaries receive Medicaid identification cards.

C. Types of Services for Mental Illness

Federal and State Medicaid policies have distinguished among three classes of services for mental illness, each subject to its own rules:

- Services provided by a distinct set of *mental health providers*, such as institutions for mental diseases (IMDs), inpatient psychiatric hospitals, mental health clinics, and mental health providers such as clinical psychologists;

- *Mental health services* furnished by types of providers who also treat physical problems; the State might, for example, define a service called "psychotherapy," which could be furnished by any participating physician;

- General health services that happen in some cases to be furnished to a patient with a *diagnosis of mental illness*. If a patient is admitted to an acute general hospital with a psychiatric diagnosis, the patient is receiving ordinary inpatient hospital services, not inpatient psychiatric hospital services.

The boundaries between the three classes of services have not always been clear; the distinctions may seem almost semantic. As will be seen, however, the use of these distinctions is a central theme in Medicaid policy regarding services for the mentally ill. The assignment of any particular service to one of the three groups may determine whether it will be covered under Medicaid and how it will be reimbursed.

This appendix provides a brief overview of Medicaid's role in two areas: the financing of long-term care in institutions, and the provision of short-term care through community-based providers. The discussion concludes with a look at efforts to improve the coordination of services for the seriously mentally ill in the community.

It should be noted that some of the statistics cited in this appendix relating to treatment of mental illness include treatment for alcoholism or drug abuse. So far as possible, services for the mentally retarded have been excluded. These services are discussed in *Appendix D, Medicaid Services for Persons with Developmental Disabilities*.

III. INSTITUTIONAL SERVICES

State Medicaid programs may, at their option, cover services in two types of institutional mental health providers: "institutions for mental diseases," or IMDs, and inpatient psychiatric hospitals. Services in IMDs, which are facilities with more than 16 beds that primarily serve patients with mental diseases, may be covered only for beneficiaries aged 65 and older. Services in inpatient psychiatric hospitals may be covered only for beneficiaries age 21 and under. Beneficiaries who are under 21 at the time they enter such a facility may continue receiving care until they reach 22. Table E-1 shows the number of States providing each type of service as of October 1, 1991. Table E-2 shows, by State, beneficiaries and payments for each type of service in FY 1991.

The effect of the rules for the two types of institutional mental health providers is to exclude Medicaid coverage of services in mental institutions for persons between 21 and 65 years old. This exclusion is sometimes described as representing a broad policy decision that the Federal Government would not assume overall responsibility for the care of the mentally ill, but would leave this responsibility with the States. However, the legislative history of the Act does not conclusively indicate that the exclusion stems from any abstract principles about appropriate Federal and State roles.

Optional Medicaid coverage of services in mental institutions for persons over age 65 was included in the original 1965 Medicaid legislation, reversing an exclusion of coverage for such services in the precursor Kerr-Mills program of medical assistance for the low-income aged. The option of covering services for persons aged 21 and under in psychiatric hospitals was provided by the Social Security Amendments of 1972. The new coverage, which did not appear in the House bill, was added by the Senate Finance Committee. The Committee report declared that helping mentally ill children become functional members of society was an appropriate use of Medicaid funds, and indicated that further study was

918

necessary to resolve the question of whether it would also be appropriate to extend Medicaid coverage to institutional services for persons aged 21 to 65.

As of 1972, the issue of the Federal role in the treatment of the mentally ill was still open. At the same time, there was increasing congressional concern that the cost of the Medicaid program had far exceeded the original 1965 projections. Medicaid legislation in the years following 1972 focused more on cost containment. The continued exclusion of those between 21 and 65 may therefore represent a response to budgetary constraints, rather than a deliberate policy.

The mentally ill aged between 21 and 65 could receive Medicaid services in facilities that did not specialize in mental health care, such as ordinary nursing homes. Concerns about the adequacy of the care received by the mentally ill in these facilities, and about the difficulties in distinguishing between IMDs and nursing homes that happen to have mentally ill residents, have emerged as major issues in Medicaid policy for the mentally ill. Some observers have noted also that the availability of Federal financial participation for nursing facility coverage for individuals between the ages of 21 and 65 has created a fiscal incentive for the States to institutionalize such individuals.

TABLE E-1. State Coverage of Mental Health Services, as of October 1, 1991

Institutions for mental diseases for persons over age 65			Inpatient psychiatric hospitals for persons under age 21
Inpatient hospital and nursing facility for persons over age 65	Inpatient hospital only for persons over age 65	Nursing facility only for persons over age 65	
		Alabama	Alabama
	Alaska		Alaska
Arkansas			Arkansas
California			California
Colorado			Colorado
Connecticut			Connecticut
	Delaware		
District of Columbia			District of Columbia

See notes at end of table.

TABLE E-1. State Coverage of Mental Health Services, as of October 1, 1991--
Continued

| Institutions for mental diseases for persons over age 65 | | | |
Inpatient hospital and nursing facility for persons over age 65	Inpatient hospital only for persons over age 65	Nursing facility only for persons over age 65	Inpatient psychiatric hospitals for persons under age 21
	Florida		
			Hawaii
		Idaho	
Illinois			Illinois
	Indiana		Indiana
	Iowa		Iowa
Kansas			Kansas
Kentucky			Kentucky
	Louisiana		Louisiana
	Maine		Maine
Maryland			Maryland
Massachusetts			Massachusetts
Michigan			Michigan
Minnesota			Minnesota
	Missouri		Missouri
Montana			Montana
Nebraska			Nebraska
Nevada			Nevada[a]
New Hampshire			New Hampshire
New Jersey			New Jersey

See notes at end of table.

TABLE E-1. State Coverage of Mental Health Services, as of October 1, 1991--
Continued

Institutions for mental diseases for persons over age 65			Inpatient psychiatric hospitals for persons under age 21
Inpatient hospital and nursing facility for persons over age 65	Inpatient hospital only for persons over age 65	Nursing facility only for persons over age 65	
		New Mexico	
	New York		New York
North Carolina			North Carolina
	North Dakota		North Dakota
		Ohio	
	Oklahoma		Oklahoma
	Oregon		Oregon
Pennsylvania			Pennsylvania
Rhode Island			Rhode Island
South Carolina			South Carolina
		South Dakota	
Tennessee			Tennessee
Utah			Utah
Vermont			Vermont
Virginia			
Washington			Washington
			West Virginia
Wisconsin			Wisconsin
	Wyoming		
Total States providing mental health services:			
27	13	4	39

[a]Inpatient psychiatric services for persons under age 21 added in FY 1992.

Source: Health Care Financing Administration. Medicaid Services, State by State. HCFA Pub. No. 02155-92, Baltimore, Md., Oct. 1991.

TABLE E-2. Medicaid Beneficiaries and Payments for Institutional Mental Health Services Fiscal Year 1991

State	Institutions for mental disease for persons 65 years old and older				Inpatient psychiatric services for those age 21 and under		Total	
	Inpatient hospitals		Nursing facilities					
	Patients	Payments (in $1,000)	Patients	Payments (in $1,000)	Patients	Payments (in $1,000)	Patients	Payments (in $1,000)
Alabama	0	$0	323	$5,934	212	$4,846	535	$10,781
Alaska	9	140	6	1	533	6,370	548	6,511
Arizona	0	0	0	0	0	0	0	0
Arkansas	35	23	0	0	1,055	15,603	1,090	15,626
California	112	1,267	77	3,528	551	10,078	740	14,873
Colorado	327	1,459	0	0	877	16,192	1,204	17,651
Connecticut	295	16,787	0	0	903	25,304	1,198	42,090
Delaware	0	0	0	0	0	0	0	0
District of Columbia	345	19,037	0	0	202	2,954	547	21,991
Florida	274	11,688	0	0	0	0	274	11,688
Georgia	0	0	0	0	0	0	0	0
Hawaii	0	0	0	0	0	0	0	0
Idaho	0	0	26	855	0	0	26	855
Illinois	256	2,917	0	0	1,197	15,783	1,453	18,700

TABLE E-2. Medicaid Beneficiaries and Payments for Institutional Mental Health Services Fiscal Year 1991-Continued

State	Institutions for mental disease for persons 65 years old and older				Inpatient psychiatric services for those age 21 and under		Total	
	Inpatient hospitals		Nursing facilities					
	Patients	Payments (in $1,000)	Patients	Payments (in $1,000)	Patients	Payments (in $1,000)	Patients	Payments (in $1,000)
Indiana	131	1,896	0	0	1,977	49,357	2,108	51,253
Iowa	105	701	0	0	421	3,377	526	4,078
Kansas	79	1,870	0	0	772	18,284	851	20,153
Kentucky	192	298	0	0	2,216	27,015	2,408	27,313
Louisiana	10	121	0	0	1,072	48,991	1,082	49,113
Maine	5	3	0	0	478	9,462	483	9,465
Maryland	277	7,110	40	2,122	1,542	38,181	1,859	47,412
Massachusetts	36	1,510	0	0	1,671	40,017	1,707	41,526
Michigan	365	14,219	64	1,590	2,915	56,683	3,344	72,491
Minnesota	226	12,929	0	0	206	8,325	432	21,253
Mississippi	0	0	0	0	130	2,175	130	2,175
Missouri	212	3,375	0	0	222	3,897	434	7,272
Montana	0	0	0	0	543	8,813	543	8,813

TABLE E-2. Medicaid Beneficiaries and Payments for Institutional Mental Health Services
Fiscal Year 1991–Continued

| State | Institutions for mental disease for persons 65 years old and older | | | | Inpatient psychiatric services for those age 21 and under | | Total | |
| | Inpatient hospitals | | Nursing facilities | | | | | |
	Patients	Payments (in $1,000)	Patients	Payments (in $1,000)	Patients	Payments (in $1,000)	Patients	Payments (in $1,000)
Nebraska	55	1,552	0	0	283	4,759	338	6,311
Nevada	85	392	0	0	0	0	85	392
New Hampshire	116	10	126	7,030	0	0	242	7,040
New Jersey	449	25,505	112	3,776	598	21,350	1,159	50,630
New Mexico	0	0	0	0	267	4,812	267	4,812
New York	8,310	791,752	0	0	7,934	243,809	16,244	1,035,560
North Carolina	848	16,261	0	0	1,567	20,862	2,415	37,123
North Dakota	62	1,725	0	0	98	1,638	160	3,362
Ohio	9	32	0	0	46	192	55	223
Oklahoma	65	948	0	0	2,182	44,243	2,247	45,190
Oregon	94	3,987	0	0	230	8,709	324	12,647
Pennsylvania	1,323	54,844	0	0	3,028	67,547	4,351	122,391
Rhode Island	87	3,973	0	0	130	3,714	217	7,687

TABLE E-2. Medicaid Beneficiaries and Payments for Institutional Mental Health Services
Fiscal Year 1991--Continued

| State | Institutions for mental disease for persons 65 years old and older | | | | Inpatient psychiatric services for those age 21 and under | | Total | |
| | Inpatient hospitals | | Nursing facilities | | | | | |
	Patients	Payments (in $1,000)	Patients	Payments (in $1,000)	Patients	Payments (in $1,000)	Patients	Payments (in $1,000)
South Carolina	314	7,705	486	11,508	335	5,371	1,135	24,585
South Dakota	0	0	124	4,223	0	0	124	4,223
Tennessee	357	237	83	873	3,278	23,493	3,718	24,603
Texas	0	0	0	0	0	0	0	0
Utah	66	57	4,342	41,659	1	1	4,409	41,717
Vermont	10	27	8	566	11	92	29	685
Virginia	151	207	460	15,054	0	0	611	15,261
Washington	428	2,643	0	0	0	0	428	2,643
West Virginia	0	0	0	0	408	6,443	408	6,443
Wisconsin	483	6,059	0	0	1,913	26,611	2,396	32,670
Wyoming	6	365	0	0	0	0	6	365
Puerto Rico	0	0	0	0	0	0	0	0

TABLE E-2. Medicaid Beneficiaries and Payments for Institutional Mental Health Services
Fiscal Year 1991–Continued

| State | Institutions for mental disease for persons 65 years old and older | | | | Inpatient psychiatric services for those age 21 and under | | Total | |
| | Inpatient hospitals | | Nursing facilities | | | | | |
	Patients	Payments (in $1,000)	Patients	Payments (in $1,000)	Patients	Payments (in $1,000)	Patients	Payments (in $1,000)
Virgin Islands	0	0	0	0	0	0	0	0
TOTAL	16,609	1,015,579	6,277	98,717	42,064	895,803	64,890	2,009,647

Source: Table prepared by the Congressional Research Service based on data contained in the Health Care Financing Administration: *Statistical Report on Medical Care, Eligibles, Recipients, Payments, and Services, HCFA Form 2082.*

A. Institutions for Mental Disease

IMD services may be provided at the inpatient hospital or nursing facility (NF) level. Until 1988, the Medicaid statute did not make clear what distinguished an IMD from an ordinary hospital or an NF. The Medicare Catastrophic Coverage Act of 1988 (P.L. 10-360), defined an IMD as "a hospital, nursing facility, or other institution of more than 16 beds, that is primarily engaged in providing diagnosis, treatment or care of persons with mental diseases, including medical attention, nursing care, and related services." This definition follows the one already contained in Medicaid regulations, with one addition, the lower limit of 16 beds. This limit means that persons between 21 and 65 in group homes and other small residential facilities may receive Medicaid benefits for physician, clinic, or other services they may require, but Medicaid will not pay the costs of room and board in the facility. Under the IMD exclusion, no Federal financial participation is available for **any** services delivered to individuals in facilities with more than 16 beds.

Medicaid regulations indicate that the classification of an institution as an IMD, rather than as an ordinary provider, "is determined by its overall character as that of a facility established and maintained primarily for the care and treatment of individuals with mental diseases, whether or not it is licensed as such." (42 CFR 435.1009) As will be discussed in section C, the determination of a facility's "overall character" has been a source of controversy between the Federal Government and the States.

B. Psychiatric Hospitals

The definition of an inpatient psychiatric hospital is more clear-cut than the definition of an IMD. A psychiatric hospital must meet Medicare conditions of participation. Prior to 1984, this meant that it had to be specifically certified as a psychiatric facility by the Joint Commission on Accreditation of Hospitals. The requirement was deleted from Medicare law by the Deficit Reduction Act of 1984 (P.L. 98-369), but has been retained in Medicaid regulations. Beneficiaries receiving inpatient psychiatric hospital services must be undergoing active treatment, in accordance with an individual plan of care, intended to "improve the recipient's condition or prevent further regression so that the services will no longer be needed." (42 CFR 441.150) The nature of the care may therefore be different from that provided in IMDs, some of whose patients might receive essentially custodial care.

C. Services for Mental Illness in Other Types of Facilities

Beneficiaries between age 21 and 65 may receive services for mental illness in hospitals and nursing facilities, but only if those facilities are not IMDs or psychiatric hospitals. A beneficiary in this age group could be admitted to an acute general hospital with a diagnosis of mental illness, or could enter a nursing home that was not classified as an IMD. The distinction between an NF that is an IMD and a facility that merely happens to be treating a number of mentally ill patients has been a source of contention between HCFA and the States. HCFA has contended that Medicaid programs are reimbursing, as NF services, care that is actually being furnished by IMDs. As a result, HCFA has argued that some States have improperly claimed Federal funds for IMD services provided to beneficiaries between ages 21 and 65. The dispute has centered on the issue of determining whether the "overall character" of a facility is that of an IMD.

The dispute has its roots in the earliest years of the Medicaid program. Medicaid was enacted in 1965, during the same period that saw the beginning of a national movement to deinstitutionalize serious mentally ill persons from public mental hospitals to be treated in the community. The number of patients in State mental institutions went from 559,000 in 1955 to 107,000 in 1986. [8] [9] Although there is a common perception that the patients released from mental institutions went directly into the community, some did not. Instead, they were "transinstitutionalized," transferred from State hospitals to nursing homes. One study estimated that 25 percent of the total growth in the nursing home industry between 1960 and 1970 was attributable to the substitution of nursing home services for services in mental hospitals. [10] Many of the patients shifted during this period may have been aged; a 1971 study reported that 40 percent of persons over age 65 discharged from State mental hospitals in 1969 were transferred to nursing homes. [11] However, some observers have noted that States would also have had a financial incentive to transfer younger patients from State hospitals, where Medicaid funds were unavailable, to non-IMD nursing homes, where the same patients could receive Medicaid coverage.

Although the era of "transinstitutionalization" is over, a considerable number of mentally ill persons are being treated in nursing homes. A report from the National Medical Expenditure Survey by the Agency for Health Care Policy and Research indicates that, of the 1.5 million nursing home residents in the U.S. in 1987, an estimated 59.1 percent had some form of mental disorder including dementia. Of the total, 28.7 percent had dementia only, including

---

[8]Morrissey, Joseph P., Michael J. Witkin, Ronald W. Manderscheid, and Helen E. Bethel. Trends by State in the Capacity and Volume of Inpatient Services, State and County Mental Hospitals, United States, 1976-1980. Mental Health Service System Reports, Rockville, Md., 1986. DHHS Pub. No. (ADM)86-1460. p. 2.

[9]Witkin, Michael J., Joanne E. Atay, Adele S. Fell, and Ronald W. Manderscheid. Specialty Mental Health System Characteristics, in NIMH, Mental Health, United States, 1990. Rockville, Md., 1990. DHHS Pub. No. (ADM)90-1708. p. 35.

[10]Hawes, Catherine, and Charles D. Phillips. *The Changing Structure of the Nursing Home Industry and the Impact of Ownership on Quality, Cost, and Access.* [In] For Profit Enterprise in Health Care, Institute of Medicine, National Academy of Science, Bradford Gray ed., Washington, 1986. p. 492-541.

[11]Intergovernmental Health Policy Project. Report on Issues of Policy: The Mentally Ill in Nursing Homes. State Health Reports; Mental Health, Alcoholism, and Drug Abuse, no. 25, July 1986. p. 2.

chronic or organic brain syndrome, and 13.7 percent had dementia in combination with one or more other mental disorders. A total of 15.5 percent had a mental disorder or disorders but no dementia. According to this survey, more than two-thirds (68.4 percent) of all nursing home residents in 1987 had one or more psychiatric symptoms, including dullness, withdrawal, impatience, delusions, and hallucinations. Almost two-thirds (64.3 percent) of residents exhibited at least one symptom of depression and nearly 30 percent experienced psychotic symptoms.[12]

Table E-3 gives data on the primary diagnoses of Medicaid and non-Medicaid population in nursing homes in 1985, as estimated from the 1985 National Nursing Home Survey. Overall, 29 percent of nursing home residents under age 65, and 17 percent of those over 65, had a primary diagnosis of mental illness. Among the residents under 65, Medicaid beneficiaries were less likely than other residents to have a diagnosis of mental illness; the reverse was true for those over 65. Among the mentally ill residents over 65, 77 percent had a primary diagnosis of dementia, which includes Alzheimer's disease and other conditions that result from physical damage to or deterioration of the brain. (The survey sample of mentally ill residents below age 65 was too small to permit reliable estimates of the percentage with dementia.)

[12]Lair, Tamra J., and Doris Cadigan Lefkowitz. *Mental Health and Functioning Status of Residents of Nursing and Personal Care Homes.* Rockville, Md., Sept. 1990, DHHS Pub. No. (PHS) 90-3470. p. 9-11.

TABLE E-3. Nursing Home Residents, by Primary Diagnosis and Source of Payment, 1985

Residents	Source of payment			
	Medicaid SNF	Medicaid ICF	Other	Total
Total residents under age 65	38,895	63,094	70,739	172,728
Mental illness, all types	9,271	14,816	26,454	50,041
Percent	23.8%	22.7%	37.4%	29.0%
Total residents age 65 and over	235,686	464,213	616,883	1,316,782
Dementia	41,410	57,390	74,841	173,641
Percent	17.6%	12.4%	12.1%	13.2%
Other mental illness	6,358	20,886	23,136	50,560
Percent	2.8%	4.5%	3.8%	3.8%
Mental illness, all types	47,948	78,276	97,977	224,201
Percent	20.3%	16.9%	15.9%	17.0%

NOTE: Classification of residents is based on all source of payments regardless of dollar amount. Residents may (and often do) have more than a single source of payment. A few residents reporting having both Medicaid SNF and ICF payments; these were recorded in the Medicaid SNF column. At the time this survey was performed Medicaid made a distinction between ICF and SNF facilities; this is no longer the case. Residents classified as "other" relied solely on sources other than Medicaid.

All residents with a primary diagnosis in ICD-9 codes 290 through 317 are included in this table. Those with ICD-9 codes 290-294 (inclusive) and 310.9 were classed as having dementia.

Source: All figures are estimates prepared by the Congressional Research Service. All estimates are based on data contained in the 1985 National Nursing Home Survey.

The presence of large numbers of mentally ill Medicaid beneficiaries in facilities classified as ordinary nursing homes has raised two major issues. The first is whether some facilities that are actually IMDs have been classified as NFs, possibly in order to circumvent the exclusion of Medicaid coverage for persons aged 21 to 65 in IMDs. The second, complementary question is whether mentally ill persons in facilities that do not specialize in the treatment of mental illness are receiving the care they need.

1. Classification of IMDs

In guidelines issued in 1982, HCFA established a number of criteria for classifying a facility as an IMD, including: whether the facility was licensed for or specialized in psychiatric care, the proportion of the facility's patients who were mentally ill or who had come to the facility directly from State mental institutions, and the average age of the patients (a young population was taken to indicate that the facility was treating mental rather than physical problems). Beginning in 1982, HCFA determined that some NFs in a number of States were IMDs. Resulting disallowances of Federal funding were appealed by several of the States.

In general, the most important issue in the appeals was the extent to which HCFA could properly classify a facility as an IMD on the basis of patient diagnosis, as opposed to the nature of the services provided.[13] The results, in a series of Federal cases, have been inconclusive, partly because several of the cases involved facilities that were clearly specializing in the treatment of mental disorders.[14]

In revised guidelines issued in 1986, HCFA continued to take the position that a preponderance of patients with a diagnosis of mental illness may be an important criterion, if not the only criterion, in determining whether a facility is an IMD. Moreover, the guidelines indicate that patients with both physical and mental problems may be considered as mentally ill if the mental problem alone would require institutionalization, even in the absence of the physical problem. This means that patients who entered the home for some other reason and who suffered mental deterioration could be considered as mentally ill for the purpose of an IMD determination.

Under this approach, substantial numbers of NFs with an aged population could potentially be considered as IMDs. While this would not necessarily affect reimbursement for patients over age 65 who are eligible for IMD services, Federal funds could be denied for any younger Medicaid patients in the same facilities. In addition, funds could conceivably be denied retroactively for all patients in such facilities in the States which have never formally exercised the option of covering IMD services at the NF level.

Further legislative or administrative action on the exclusion of IMD coverage under Medicaid likely await the publication of a study ordered by the

---

[13]The one case that reached the Supreme Court turned on another issue, whether HCFA could ever, on any basis, determine that an NF was an IMD. The Court held that it could. *Connecticut Department of Income Maintenance v. Heckler*, 105 S. Ct. 2210 (1985).

[14]See Intergovernmental Health Policy Project, p. 6-9, for a review of this litigation.

Congress in 1989. Section 6408 of the Omnibus Budget Reconciliation Act of 1989, P.L. 101-239, orders the Secretary to conduct a study of:

- the implementation, under current Medicaid provisions, regulations, guidelines, and regulatory practices, of the exclusion of coverage of services to certain individuals residing in IMDs; and

- the costs of providing services under Medicaid in public subacute psychiatric facilities which provide services to certain individuals who would otherwise require acute hospitalization.

The provision requires the Secretary to submit a report to the Congress no later than October 1, 1990, including recommendations on:

- modifications in such provisions, regulations, guidelines, and practices, if any, that may be appropriate to accommodate changes that may have occurred since 1972 in the delivery of psychiatric and other mental health services on an inpatient basis to such individuals; and

- the continued coverage of services provided in subacute psychiatric facilities under Medicaid.

A HCFA spokesman stated in September 1992 that the report on the IMD exclusion had passed HCFA review and was in review at the Office of the Secretary.

2. Prevention of Inappropriate Institutionalization

The States's potential defense in the IMD dispute--that the patients in ordinary nursing facilities are not receiving the type of care characteristic of IMDs--has given rise to an opposite concern: that some of the mentally ill patients may not be receiving active treatment and may be inappropriately placed. Similar concerns have been raised about the mentally retarded. A 1987 General Accounting Office (GAO) study of mentally retarded patients in nursing homes in three States found that many patients were receiving no treatment and that their ability to benefit from treatment had not been assessed.[15]

Concern about the treatment of both the mentally ill and the mentally retarded is reflected in the nursing home reform measures included in the Omnibus Budget Reconciliation Act of 1987 (OBRA 87, P.L. 100-203). Under its provisions, States are now required to have screening and evaluation programs for the mentally ill (as well as for the mentally retarded) in nursing homes, as follows:

---

[15]U.S. Congress. General Accounting Office. *Medicaid: Addressing the Needs of Mentally Retarded Nursing Home Residents*. Report to the Secretary of Health and Human Services. Washington, Apr. 1987. [GAO/HRD-87-77].

- By January 1, 1989, each State was required to have in effect a preadmission program to determine whether the placement of any new mentally ill or mentally retarded patient in an NF is appropriate, or whether the patient would be more appropriately cared for in some other setting. Federal funds would be denied for placements found to be inappropriate;

- By April 1, 1990, each State must have completed a review of all current mentally ill or mentally retarded NF patients to determine whether continued care at the current level is appropriate. For those inappropriately placed, the State must arrange for safe and orderly discharge and active treatment.

Under the law, an individual is considered mentally ill if he or she has a primary or secondary diagnosis of mental disorder and does not have a primary diagnosis of Alzheimer's disease or other forms of dementia. As noted above, an estimated 77 percent of mentally ill nursing home residents aged 65 and over, and an unknown proportion of younger mentally ill residents, have a primary diagnosis of dementia and would therefore not be subject to review. On the other hand, many residents whose primary problems are physical may still have a secondary diagnosis of mental disorder (such as senility or memory loss) and would be reviewed.

The preadmission screening and annual resident review requirements mandated by OBRA 87 are often referred to as PASARR requirements. OBRA 87 required the Secretary to develop by October 1, 1988, minimum criteria as to whether a mentally ill or mentally retarded individual required the level of care provided by a nursing home. The Secretary was also required by that date to develop minimum criteria for States' appeals processes for persons adversely affected by screening decisions. PASARR became effective January 1, 1989, regardless of whether the Secretary had issued guidance to the States or not.

Nursing home groups and advocates of the mentally ill and the mentally retarded have expressed concern from the start with HCFA's implementation of the requirements. During 1988, only drafts of program guidelines were available to the States for implementing their own programs for screening the mentally ill and the mentally retarded. In May 1989, HCFA issued interim guidelines to the States to use for screening and review, but indicated that it intended to use the formal rulemaking process, with a comment period, before making the guidelines' criteria binding on the States.

Numerous comments have been made. Nursing home groups pointed out that HCFA's various drafts differed in their definitions of mental illness and, by implication, who should be screened for the appropriateness of nursing home care. The drafts also had different definitions of active treatment and the services to be provided by the States for those who require this level of care. These groups also expressed a concern that they would once again have to redesign screening programs when the criteria were published as regulations. Nursing home groups also objected to the application of these requirements to all persons, regardless of whether they are private payers, Medicare beneficiaries, or Medicaid-eligible individuals, so long as they are applying for admission to, or residing in, a Medicaid-certified nursing home. For lack of timely guidance and other reasons, two nursing home industry associations, the American Association of Homes for the Aging and the American Health Care Association, on April 11, 1989, entered into a suit against the Secretary of HHS, to stop implementation of the preadmission screening requirements. They subsequently dropped the case a year later following the promulgation of proposed PASARR regulations on March 23, 1991.

In addition to these implementation issues, nursing home groups and advocates for the elderly, mentally ill, and mentally retarded have also been concerned about those persons who are deflected from nursing home care in the preadmission screening process and whether they are directed to other appropriate sources of care. OBRA 87 did not address this issue, except for requiring an appeals process for those adversely affected in the screening. For those who are actually discharged, there is also concern about whether they receive the active treatment and other services they might need. In many cases, such persons will not be eligible for Medicaid services, and States alone are responsible for paying for the costs of their care. These issues reflect ongoing problems in providing and paying for care for the seriously mentally ill and mentally retarded.

The Congress in 1989 considered a number of issues related to PASARR, but the OBRA 89 legislation, P.L. 101-239, included only one related provision. This provision required the Secretary to issue proposed regulations on PASARR requirements not later than 90 days after enactment of OBRA 89.[16] On March 23, 1990, the proposed rule for the PASARR requirements was published in the *Federal Register*. Final regulations were published November 30, 1992, with few changes from the original 1990 proposed rule. The regulations take effect January 29, 1993.

The Omnibus Budget Reconciliation Act of 1990 (OBRA 90), P.L. 101-964, included some amendments to the PASARR requirements that were designed to clarify their structure and operation. The OBRA 90 amendment:

- Narrows the definition of "mental illness" to focus on persons with chronic and acute illness inappropriately placed in nursing facilities and exclude those with minor mental disorders;

- Requires State authorities, in addition to determining if persons with mental illness require nursing home services, to

---

[16]U.S. Congress. Congressional Research Service. *Medicare and Medicaid Nursing Home Reform Provisions in the Omnibus Budget Reconciliation Act of 1987, P.L. 100-203.* CRS Report for Congress No. 90-80 EPW, by Richard Price. Washington, Aug. 10, 1989, (revised Jan. 16, 1990). p. 11-14. The preceding paragraphs on the implementation of PASARR use this document as source.

determine if they require "specialized services," instead of "active treatment," as originally required;

- Clarifies the responsibilities of States and nursing facilities for provision of services to persons with mental disabilities;

- Prohibits State authorities from delegating authority to nursing homes for PASARR determinations;

- Clarifies the principle that no Federal Medicaid matching funds are available for nursing facility care furnished to any person who does not require the level of services provided by such a facility;

- Creates two exceptions to the preadmission screening component of the PASARR requirements for (a) residents who are readmitted to the nursing facility after a hospital stay, and (b) persons who seek admission to a nursing facility directly from a hospital and expect to stay for only a short time;

- In response to the delay in publishing PASARR final regulations before the effective date of the requirements, prohibits any compliance action that made a good faith action to comply with the requirements before the effective date;

- Provides for revision of alternative disposition plans after HCFA approval; and

- Requires States to report annually to the Secretary on the number and disposition of nursing facility residents covered under the State alternative disposition plan.[17] The HCFA Program *Memorandum* instructing States on the required annual alternative disposition plan was issued in September 1992. The first annual report is due from States by November 16, 1992, and by February 15 for years thereafter.

IV. ACUTE CARE SERVICES

Medicaid programs also furnish mental health care as part of the general coverage of services rendered by physicians, clinics, hospitals, and other providers. The distinctions noted earlier, between mental health providers, mental health services, and ordinary services for a diagnosis of mental illness, have affected Medicaid policies relating to short-term, as well as long-term, care.

---

[17]Mental Health Law Project. *Changes in the Nursing Home Preadmission Screening and Annual Resident Review Process for Older People with Mental Disabilities.* Mental Disability Law and the Elderly, issue paper no. 1. Washington, Jan. 1991.

As was discussed in *Chapter IV, Services*, there is a general requirement that States may not vary the amount, duration, or scope of Medicaid services on the basis of diagnosis. This has meant that a Medicaid program could not, for example, limit stays in acute general hospitals for patients with a psychiatric diagnosis, unless similar limits were applied to stays for all diagnoses.

States may, however, define distinct types of providers that furnish only mental health care services. These could include specialized mental health care clinics or such providers as clinical psychologists or psychiatric social workers. Coverage of these provider types may then be subject to special coverage limits, or the State may decline to cover any services rendered by these types of providers.

Some States have also defined distinct mental health services delivered by broader classes of providers. The States may, for example, distinguish between an ordinary physician office visit and a "psychotherapy visit," and limit coverage of the latter. A 1989 survey found that 25 States had imposed some restrictions on mental health visits by physicians and psychiatrists, and 22 States had imposed some restrictions on outpatient mental health services in general and psychiatric hospital clinics.[18]   Limits ranged from requirements that preauthorization be obtained before furnishing certain psychiatric services to absolute restrictions on the number of visits or the dollar amounts that would be reimbursed in a given time period. Another limit on practitioner services in general is the generally low rate of reimbursement for services, which along with the limits related to prior authorization and number of visits helps to limit use of noninstitutional mental health services.

A. Physician and Other Practitioner Services

In most States, Medicaid beneficiaries may obtain services from psychiatrists under the same rules that apply when they obtain services from physicians in other specialties. Beneficiaries may also receive some mental health care from physicians who are not psychiatrists. Table E-4 provides a State-by-State listing of State restrictions of psychiatrist visits based on a 1989 survey.

---

[18]Fox, Harriette B., Lori N. Wicks, Margaret A. McManus, and Rebecca W. Kelly. *Medicaid Financing for Mental Health and Substance Abuse Services for Children and Adolescents*. Draft Report prepared for U.S. Department of Health and Human Services. Alcohol, Drug Abuse, and Mental Health Administration. May 1990. p. 39-44. (Hereafter cited as Fox, Wicks, McManus, and Kelly, *Medicaid Financing for Mental Health*)

**TABLE E-4. State Restrictions on Psychiatrist Visits,
June 30, 1989**

State	Psychiatrist visit/dollar limit	Prior authorization requirements	Psychiatrist-supervised services	
			Practitioner assisting physician	Practitioner working autonomously
Alabama	None	No	Yes	Yes
Alaska	None	No	Yes	Yes
Arkansas	None	No	Yes	No
California	None	Yes	No	No
Colorado	None	No	Yes	Yes
Connecticut	None	Yes	Yes	Yes
Delaware	None	No	No	No
District of Columbia	None	Yes	Yes	No
Florida	None	No	No	No
Georgia	24 hours/yr	No	No	Yes
Hawaii	None	Yes	Yes	No
Idaho	Varies	No	No	No
Illinois	None	No	No	No
Indiana	None	Yes	Yes	Yes
Iowa	None	No	Yes	No
Kansas	Varies[a]	No	Yes	Yes
Kentucky	None	No	Yes	Yes
Louisiana	None	No	Yes	No
Maine	1 hr/day, 5 hrs./week	No	No	No
Maryland	None	No	Yes	Yes
Massachusetts	None	Yes	No	No
Michigan	None	No	No	Yes
Minnesota	Varies[b]	No	Yes	Yes

See notes at end of table.

TABLE E-4. State Restrictions on Psychiatrist Visits, June 30, 1989--Continued

State	Psychiatrist visit/dollar limit	Prior authorization requirements	Psychiatrist-supervised services	
			Practitioner assisting physician	Practitioner working autonomously
Mississippi	Varies[b]	No	Yes	Yes
Missouri	None	Yes	No	No
Montana	None	No	Yes	No
Nebraska	None	No	No	Yes
Nevada	None	Yes	No	Yes
New Hampshire	None	No	Yes	Yes
New Jersey	None	Yes	Yes	Yes
New Mexico	Varies[c]	No	No	No
New York	None	No	Yes	Yes
North Carolina	None	Yes	No	Yes
North Dakota	None	No	Yes	Yes
Ohio	None	Yes	Yes	Yes
Oklahoma	None	No	No	No
Oregon	None	No	No	No
Pennsylvania	None	No	No	No
Rhode Island	None	No	Yes	No
South Carolina	Varies	No	No	No
South Dakota	None	Yes	Yes	Yes
Tennessee	None	No	Yes	Yes
Texas	$313/yr.	No	No	Yes
Utah	None	Yes	No	No
Vermont	None	Yes	Yes	No

See notes at end of table.

TABLE E-4. State Restrictions on Psychiatrist Visits, June 30, 1989--Continued

State	Psychiatrist visit/dollar limit	Prior authorization requirements	Psychiatrist-supervised services	
			Practitioner assisting physician	Practitioner working autonomously
Virginia	52 visits/yr. for 1st yr. then 26 visits/yr.	Yes	Yes	Yes
Washington	None	Yes	No	No
West Virginia	None	Yes	Yes	Yes
Wisconsin	None	Yes	Yes	Yes
Wyoming	None	No	Yes	Yes
Total States with restrictions	10	18	29	27

[a]Visit limit varies with intervention. There is a 200 visit limit per lifetime for all outpatient mental health visits.

[b]Varies with intervention for all outpatient mental health visits.

[c]A lifetime limit for all outpatient mental health visits varies with diagnosis.

Source: Fox, Harriette B., Lori N. Wicks, Margaret A. McManus and Rebecca W. Kelly. Information obtained from telephone interviews with State Medicaid agencies during the spring and summer of 1989. Reported in *Medicaid Financing for Mental Health and Substance Abuse Services for Children and Adolescents*. Draft report prepared for U.S. Dept. of Health and Human Services. Alcohol, Drug Abuse, and Mental Health Administration. May 1990.

TABLE E-5. State Coverage of Other Licensed Practitioner Services, June 30, 1989

State	Psychologists	Social workers	Coverage limits	Prior authorization requirement
Alabama	No			
Alaska	No			
Arkansas	No			
California	Yes	No	2 visits/mo.	Yes
Colorado	Yes	No	None	No
Connecticut	Yes	No	None	Yes
Delaware	No			
District of Columbia	No			
Florida	No			
Georgia	No			
Hawaii	Yes	No	None	Yes
Idaho	Yes	No	45 visits/yr.	no
Illinois	No			
Indiana	Yes	No	None	Yes
Iowa	Yes	No	40 visits/yr.	No
Kansas	Yes	No	Varies[a]	No
Kentucky	No			
Louisiana	No			
Maine	Yes	No	1 hr./day, 5 hr./week	No
Maryland	No			
Massachusetts	Yes	Yes	None	No
Michigan	No			
Minnesota	Yes	No	Varies	No
Mississippi	No			
Missouri	No			

See notes at end of table.

TABLE E-5. State Coverage of Other Licensed Practitioner Services,
June 30, 1989--Continued

State	Psychologists	Social workers	Coverage limits	Prior authorization requirement
Montana	Yes	Yes	22 visits/yr.	No
Nebraska	No			
Nevada	Yes	No	None	Yes
New Hampshire[b]	Yes	No	12 visits/yr.	No
New Jersey	Yes	No	None	Yes
New Mexico	Yes	No	Lifetime limit	Yes
New York	Yes	No	None	No
North Carolina	No			
North Dakota	No			
Ohio	Yes	No	Varies	No
Oklahoma	No			
Oregon	Yes[c]	No	None	Yes
Pennsylvania	No			
Rhode Island	No			
South Carolina	No			
South Dakota	No			
Tennessee	No			
Texas	No			
Utah	Yes	No	None	Yes
Vermont	Yes	No	None	Yes
Virginia	Yes	No	52 visits/yr. for first yr. then 25 visits/yr.	Yes

See notes at end of table.

TABLE E-5. State Coverage of Other Licensed Practitioner Services,
June 30, 1989--Continued

	Psychologists	Social workers	Coverage limits	Prior authorization requirement
Washington	Yes[c]	No	1 evaluation per yr.	No
West Virginia	Yes	No	None	Yes
Wisconsin	Yes	No	None	Yes
Wyoming	No			
Total States with restrictions	25	2	12	13

[a]Visit limit varies with intervention. There is a 200 visit limit per lifetime for all outpatient mental health visits.

[b]New Hampshire reimburses community health centers under this category.

[c]Limit psychologists' services to testing and evaluation.

Source: Fox, Harriette B., Lori N. Wicks, Margaret A. McManus and Rebecca W. Kelly. Information obtained from telephone interviews with State Medicaid agencies during the spring and summer of 1989. Reported in *Medicaid Financing for Mental Health and Substance Abuse Services for Children and Adolescents*. Draft report prepared for U.S. Dept. of Health and Human Services. Alcohol, Drug Abuse, and Mental Health Administration. May 1990.

Only a minority of States cover the services of other types of mental health professionals. Clinical psychologists were covered in 25 States in 1989, but only two covered such other types of professionals as social workers.[19] The coverage rules depend in part on which types of professionals are permitted to practice independently under State law. Other States may pay for services furnished by psychologists or other mental health professionals if they are providing services under the direct supervision of a physician, either in the physician's office or in a clinic setting.

Psychiatrists have been less willing than any other group of physicians to accept Medicaid patients. A 1984 study indicates that, in 1977-78, only 57.8 percent of psychiatrists participated in the Medicaid program compared to 77.5 percent of primary care physicians, 73.4 percent of medical specialists, and 82.9 percent of surgical specialists.[20] In a 1990 survey for the Physician Payment Review Commission, the National Governors' Association found that two States cited difficulties with participation of psychiatrists in their Medicaid programs. Florida cited low participation of child psychiatrists and Maryland noted low participation of psychiatrists in general.[21]

Even more than other kinds of physicians, psychiatrists may be deterred from participating by States' reimbursement and coverage policies. A 1991 report from the Physician Payment Review Commission indicates that State payments for individual psychotherapy in 1989 ranged from $18 to $86 for a 45-50-minute session, with a median payment of $42.[22] This range of fees is substantially lower than the fees charged by psychiatrists for 45-50 minutes of psychotherapy, as reported in a survey published by *Medical Economics* magazine in 1990. According to this survey, only 4 percent of psychiatrists report charging less than $80 for a session of individual psychotherapy in an office or hospital. Charges for office psychotherapy range up to $150 or more with the median charge of $101. Hospital psychotherapy charges range up to $175 or more, with the median at $120.[23]

---

[19]Ibid., p. 54-55.

[20]Mitchell, Janet B. and Rachel Schurman. *Access to Private Obstetrics/Gynecology Services under Medicaid.* Medical Care, v. 22, no. 11, Nov. 1984. p. 1028 (Data based on HCFA/NORC physician surveys, 1977-8)

[21]Physician Payment Review Commission. Annual Report to Congress, 1991. Washington, 1991. p. 277.

[22]Physician Payment Review Commission. Physician Payment Under Medicaid. Report no. 91-4. Washington, 1991. p. 27 and 73.

[23] Kirchner, Merian. *Where Do Your Fees Fit In?* Medical Economics, v. 67, no. 19, Oct. 1, 1990. p. 105.

B. Mental Health Clinics and Other Outpatient Services

According to a 1989 survey, 38 States cover mental health clinic services provided in community mental health centers. These clinic providers may include State or county facilities, often funded through the Federal Alcohol, Drug Abuse, and Mental Health Services Block Grant.[24] The survey also showed that 24 States also covered services provided in private mental health clinics.[25] Direct patient services in mental health clinics are generally provided by nonphysician mental health professionals, such as psychologists or social workers. In many States a physician is expected to oversee the activities of the direct providers, developing a treatment plan or periodically reviewing the care being furnished.

Forty-one States cover mental health services furnished in general hospital outpatient departments; 18 States cover outpatient mental health services in a psychiatric hospital.[26] In a number of States, outpatient mental health services may include "partial hospitalization" or "psychiatric day care" programs. These provide services in a structured setting for part of the day for patients living in the community. Some States cover comparable programs furnished by mental health clinics.

---

[24]Fox, Wicks, McManus, and Kelly, *Medicaid Financing for Mental Health*, p. 49-50. It should be noted that the Federally Qualified Health Center (FQHC) benefit, enacted after this survey was completed, includes the Health Care for the Homeless program, authorized under section 340 of the PHS Act, some of the grantees of which offer mental health services.

[25]OBRA 87 provided that States could cover, as clinic services, services provided by clinic personnel outside the actual clinic facility. This provision permits clinics to furnish offsite care to homeless chronically mentally ill patients in shelters or other locations.

[26]Fox, Wicks, McManus, and Kelly, *Medicaid Financing for Mental Health*, p. 42-44.

TABLE E-6. State Coverage of Mental Health Clinics, June 30, 1989

State	Community mental health centers	Private mental health centers	Day treatment	Other services[a]	Coverage limits	Prior authorization requirement
Alabama	Yes	No	Yes	Yes	30 visits/yr	No
Alaska	Yes	No	Yes	Yes	None	No
Arkansas	Yes	Yes	Yes	Yes	Varies	Yes
California	Yes	Yes	Yes	Yes	None	Yes
Colorado	Yes	No	Yes	Yes	1 visit/day	No
Connecticut	Yes	Yes	Yes	Yes	None	Yes
Delaware	No					
District of Columbia	Yes	Yes	Yes	Yes	None	Yes
Florida	No					
Georgia	Yes	Yes	Yes	Yes	Varies	No
Hawaii[b]	yes	Yes	No	No	48 visits/yr.; 1/day	No

See notes at end of table.

TABLE E-6. State Coverage of Mental Health Clinics, June 30, 1989--Continued

State	Community mental health centers	Private mental health centers	Day treatment	Other services[a]	Coverage limits	Prior authorization requirement
Idaho	Yes	Yes	Yes	Yes	45 visits/yr.	No
Illinois	No					
Indiana[b]	Yes	Yes	No	Yes	Varies	Yes
Iowa[b]	Yes	Yes	Yes	Yes	Varies	Yes
Kansas	Yes	No	Yes	Yes	Varies[c]	No
Kentucky	No					
Louisiana	Yes	Yes	No	Yes	None	No
Maine	No					
Maryland	Yes	Yes	Yes	Yes	1 visit/day	No
Massachusetts	Yes	Yes	Yes	Yes	None	Yes
Michigan	Yes	No	Yes	No	1 visit/day[d]	No
Minnesota	Yes	No	No	Yes	Varies	No

See notes at end of table.

TABLE E-6. State Coverage of Mental Health Clinics, June 30, 1989--Continued

State	Community mental health centers	Private mental health centers	Day treatment	Other services[a]	Coverage limits	Prior authorization requirement
Mississippi	No					
Missouri	Yes	No	No	Yes	None	No
Montana	Yes	Yes	Yes	Yes	None	No
Nebraska	Yes	Yes	Yes	Yes	None	Yes
Nevada	Yes	No	No	Yes	None	No
New Hampshire	No					
New Jersey	Yes	Yes	Yes	Yes	1 visit/day	Yes
New Mexico	No					
New York	Yes	Yes	Yes	Yes	None	No
North Carolina	Yes	Yes	Yes	Yes	None	No
North Dakota	Yes	Yes	Yes	Yes	Varies	No
Ohio	Yes	No	Yes	Yes	None	No

See notes at end of table.

TABLE E-6. State Coverage of Mental Health Clinics, June 30, 1989--Continued

State	Community mental health centers	Private mental health centers	Day treatment	Other services[a]	Coverage limits	Prior authorization requirement
Oklahoma	Yes	Yes	Yes	Yes	Varies	No
Oregon	No					
Pennsylvania	Yes	Yes	Yes	Yes	1 visit/day[d]	No
Rhode Island	No					
South Carolina	Yes	No	Yes	Yes	None	No
South Dakota[b]	Yes	Yes	Yes	Yes	None	No
Tennessee	Yes	No	Yes	Yes	None	No
Texas	No					
Utah	Yes	No	Yes	Yes	Varies	No
Vermont	Yes	Yes	Yes	Yes	Varies	Yes

See notes at end of table.

TABLE E-6. State Coverage of Mental Health Clinics, June 30, 1989--Continued

State	Community mental health centers	Private mental health centers	Day treatment	Other services[a]	Coverage limits	Prior authorization requirement
Virginia	Yes	No	No	Yes	52 visits/yr. for first yr.then 26 visits/yr.	Yes
Washington[b]	Yes	No	Yes	Yes	None	No
West Virginia	Yes	Yes	Yes	Yes	Varies	Yes
Wisconsin	No					
Wyoming	Yes	Yes	Yes	Yes	None	No
Total States with coverage/ restrictions	38	24	31	36	20	12

See notes at end of table.

TABLE E-6. State Coverage of Mental Health Clinics, June 30, 1989--Continued

[a]"Other services" includes medication management and collateral contacts. All States include individual, group and family therapy.

[b]Clinic service benefits in these States apply to all clinic services generally; they are not specific to mental health services.

[c]Visit limit varies with intervention. There is a 200-visit limit per lifetime for all outpatient mental health visits.

[d]In addition, these States have an annual limit that varies with service or intervention.

Source: Fox, Harriette B., Lori N. Wicks, Margaret A. McManus, and Rebecca W. Kelly. Information obtained from telephone interview with State Medicaid agencies during the spring and summer of 1989. Reported in *Medicaid Financing for Mental Health and Substance Abuse Services for Children and Adolescents.* Draft report prepared for U.S. Dept. of Health and Human Services. Alcohol, Drug Abuse and Mental Health Administration. May 1990.

TABLE E-7. State Coverage of Outpatient Mental Health Services in General and Psychiatric Hospitals, June 30, 1989

| State | Mental health visits | | | | Partial hospitalization | | |
	General hospitals	Psychiatric hospitals	Coverage limits	Prior authorization requirement	Available for severely emotionally disturbed youth	Coverage limits	Prior authorization requirement
Alabama	No						
Alaska	Yes	No	None	No			
Arkansas	Yes	No	12 visits/yr.	No			
California	Yes	Yes	None	Yes	No	None	Yes
Colorado	Yes	Yes	1 hour/day	No	Yes	None	No
Connecticut	Yes	Yes	None	Yes	Yes	None	Yes
Delaware	Yes	No	None	No	Yes	None	No
District of Columbia	Yes	Yes	2 visit/day	Yes	No		
Florida	Yes	No	$1,000/yr. for all outpatient hospital	No	No		
Georgia	Yes	No	None	No	No		
Hawaii	Yes	No	None	Yes	No		

TABLE E-7. State Coverage of Outpatient Mental Health Services in General and Psychiatric Hospitals, June 30, 1989--Continued

State	Mental health visits				Partial hospitalization		
	General hospitals	Psychiatric hospitals	Coverage limits	Prior authorization requirement	Available for severely emotionally disturbed youth	Coverage limits	Prior authorization requirement
Idaho	Yes	Yes	45 hrs./yr. for all outpatient hospital	No	No		
Illinois	Yes	No	None	No	No		
Indiana	No	No	None	No	No		
Iowa	Yes	Yes	None	Yes	No		
Kansas	Yes	Yes	Varies	No	Yes	1,560 hrs. per year	Yes
Kentucky	Yes	No	None	No	No		
Louisiana	Yes	No	None	No	No		
Maine	Yes	No	None	No	Yes	None	No
Maryland	Yes	Yes	None	No	Yes	None	No
Massachusetts	Yes	Yes	None	Yes	Yes	6 hrs./day	No
Michigan	No				Yes	None	Yes

TABLE E-7. State Coverage of Outpatient Mental Health Services in General and Psychiatric Hospitals, June 30, 1989--Continued

State	Mental health visits				Partial hospitalization		
	General hospitals	Psychiatric hospitals	Coverage limits	Prior authorization requirement	Available for severely emotionally disturbed youth	Coverage limits	Prior authorization requirement
Minnesota	Yes	No	None	No	Yes	80 days per year	Yes
Mississippi	Yes	No	6 visits/yr. for all outpatient hospital	No	No		
Missouri	Yes	Yes	None	No	No		
Montana	Yes	No	None	No	No		
Nebraska	Yes	Yes	None	Yes	Yes	None	No
Nevada	Yes	No	None	Yes	No		
New Hampshire	Yes	No	12 visits/yr. for all outpatient mental health	No	No		
New Jersey	Yes	Yes	None	Yes	Yes	None	Yes

TABLE E-7. State Coverage of Outpatient Mental Health Services in General and Psychiatric Hospitals, June 30, 1989--Continued

State	Mental health visits				Partial hospitalization		
	General hospitals	Psychiatric hospitals	Coverage limits	Prior authorization requirement	Available for severely emotionally disturbed youth	Coverage limits	Prior authorization requirement
New Mexico	Yes	No	Lifetime limit	Yes	No		
New York	Yes	Yes	None	No	Yes	None	Yes
North Carolina	Yes	Yes	24 visits/yr. for all outpatient hospital, clinic, and physician	Yes	Yes	24 visits/yr. for all outpatient hospital, clinic, and physician	Yes
North Dakota	Yes	Yes	None	No	No		
Ohio	Yes	No	10 visits/month	Yes	No		
Oklahoma	Yes	No	1 visit/day for all outpatient hospital	No	No		
Oregon	No						

TABLE E-7. State Coverage of Outpatient Mental Health Services in General and Psychiatric Hospitals, June 30, 1989--Continued

State	Mental health visits				Partial hospitalization		
	General hospitals	Psychiatric hospitals	Coverage limits	Prior authorization requirement	Available for severely emotionally disturbed youth	Coverage limits	Prior authorization requirement
Pennsylvania	Yes	Yes	Varies	Yes	Yes	720 hours per year	No
Rhode Island	Yes	No	None	No	No		
South Carolina	Yes	No	None	No	No		
South Dakota	Yes	No	None	No	No		
Tennessee	Yes	No	30 visits/yr. for all outpatient hospital	No	No		
Texas	Yes	No	$313/year	No	No		
Utah	No						
Vermont	Yes	Yes	None	No	No		
Virginia	No			No			
Washington	No						

TABLE E-7. State Coverage of Outpatient Mental Health Services in General and Psychiatric Hospitals, June 30, 1989--Continued

State	Mental health visits				Partial hospitalization		
	General hospitals	Psychiatric hospitals	Coverage limits	Prior authorization requirement	Available for severely emotionally disturbed youth	Coverage limits	Prior authorization requirement
West Virginia	No						
Wisconsin	Yes	Yes	None	Yes	Yes	None	yes
Wyoming	No						
Total States with coverage/restrictions	41	18	15	14	16	5	9

Source: Fox, Harriette B., Lori N. Wicks, Margaret A. McManus, and Rebecca W. Kelly. Information obtained from telephone interview with State Medicaid agencies during the spring and summer of 1989. Reported in *Medicaid Financing for Mental Health and Substance Abuse Services for Children and Adolescents.* Draft report prepared for U.S. Dept. of Health and Human Services. Alcohol, Drug Abuse and Mental Health Administration. May 1990.

Despite the limitations on Medicaid coverage of outpatient mental health care services, it has been found that Medicaid beneficiaries are more likely to obtain mental health care than other low-income persons without Medicaid or even than higher-income persons.[27]   Table E-8 shows the probability of obtaining any health care, and any mental health care, during a year for three groups: low-income persons with and without Medicaid and higher-income persons.

TABLE E-8. Probability of Use of Ambulatory Health and Mental Health Services, Persons Under 65 by Poverty Status and Medicaid Coverage, 1980

Poverty and Medicaid status	Probability of	
	Ambulatory health use	Mental health use
Total	0.776	0.045
Poor or near poor:		
Medicaid, enrolled all year	0.779	0.079
Non-Medicaid	0.716	0.046
Non-poor, non-Medicaid	0.791	0.038

Source: Taube, Carl A., and Agnes Rupp. *The Effect of Medicaid Access to Ambulatory Mental Health Care for the Poor and Near-Poor Under 65.* Medical Care, v. 24, no. 8, Aug. 1986. p. 677.

The three groups were about equally likely to have received some health care services during the year. However, Medicaid beneficiaries were nearly twice as likely to have received mental health care during the year than persons classified as "non-poor," and about 70 percent more likely than other poor or near-poor persons. The authors speculate that the non-poor were deterred from obtaining mental health services because private health insurance may limit or exclude coverage of these services.

Another study, by Shapiro et al., attempted to measure the relative need for mental health care of the poor and near-poor, with and without Medicaid coverage, and the non-poor (table E-9). Medicaid beneficiaries who also receive public assistance were nearly three times as likely as the non-poor to need mental health care. (The measurement of need considered both actual use of mental health services and manifestations of emotional problems not accompanied by use of such services.) The study also found, however, that Medicaid beneficiaries were somewhat more likely to have their needs met. This

---

[27]Taube, Carl A., and Agnes Rupp. *The Effect of Medicaid on Access to Ambulatory Mental Health for the Poor and Near-Poor Under 65.* Medical Care 24:8, Aug. 1986. p. 677-86.

was especially true of those receiving public assistance; 38.3 percent were found to have unmet need, compared to 47.4 percent of the non-poor.

TABLE E-9. Need for Mental Health Care and Unmet Need by Poverty Status

Poverty and cash assistance status	Percent with need for care	Percent of those who need care, but need it unmet
All persons	13.6%	47.4%
Medicaid:		
With public assistance	33.8	38.3
Without public assistance	23.8	46.8
Poor and near poor without Medicaid	13.1	55.6
Non-poor	11.4	47.4

NOTE: Poor and near poor includes persons with income not more than 150 percent of poverty.

Source: Shapiro, Sam, et al. *Measuring Need for Mental Health Services in a General Population.* Medical Care, v. 23, no. 9, Sept. 1985. p. 1039.

C. Hospital Inpatient Services

Short-term acute care for mental illness is an important component of Medicaid inpatient hospital expenditures in some States. These services may be provided in a general hospital, whether or not the hospital has distinct psychiatric wards or units. Under Medicaid rules, however, even short-term services in a facility or part of a facility specifically licensed as a psychiatric hospital would not constitute ordinary hospital care and would be subject to the coverage limitations for IMD or psychiatric hospital services.

Table E-10 shows the results of a detailed HCFA analysis of 1982 Medicaid payment records from three States, California, Michigan, and New York. Within this three State sample, there is considerable variation in the proportion of expenditures and utilization devoted to care of psychiatric diagnoses. Mental disorders accounted for just 3 percent of hospital costs in California, but nearly 20 percent in New York. In the absence of detailed data from other States, there is no way of knowing whether New York or California is more nearly representative of the national experience.[28]

TABLE E-10. Medicaid Inpatient Services for Mental Disorders and for all Diagnoses, California, New York, and Michigan, 1982

	California	Michigan	New York
Total discharges	628,455	199,070	493,340
Discharges for mental disorders	18,511	10,509	42,908
Percent, mental disorders	3.0%	5,3%	8.7%
Total days (est.)	3,959,267	1,413,397	3,897,386
Days for mental disorders (est.)	207,323	171,296	862,450
Percent, mental disorders	5.2	12.1	22.1
Total payments (thousands of dollars):			
All diagnoses	1,547,694	350,830	1.206,876
Mental disorders	47,521	30,845	236,647
Percent, mental disorders	3,1	8.8	19.6
Average payment per day (est.):			
All diagnoses	$391	$248	$310
Mental disorders	$229	$180	$274

NOTE: Days and per diem payments are estimated using unpublished data on discharges, total payments, and average length of stay. Data includes stays in inpatient psychiatric hospitals.

Source: Pine, P., Embry Howell and William Buczko. *Hospital Utilization and Expenditures for Medicaid Enrollees by Major Diagnosis Group.* Health Care Financing Review, v. 9, no. 1, fall 1987. p. 91, 96.

---

[28]It should be noted that the data include discharges from inpatient psychiatric hospitals for beneficiaries under age 22. As the national total of beneficiaries receiving these services in FY 1982 was only 23,362, the impact on the discharge totals reported here is likely to be minimal. Data on IMD services are not included. The data are drawn from the Medicaid "tape-to-tape" project, in which five States have furnished complete computer data on all Medicaid transactions to HCFA for statistical analysis (the researchers were unable to use data from two of the five States). Other States provide only summary statistical reports, such as the HCFA-2082 reports from which many of the statistics in this report are drawn.

Two patterns hold across all three States. First, each day of care for a person with a diagnosis of mental disorder is less expensive than a day of care for other diagnoses. This is presumably because psychiatric patients receive fewer of the ancillary services, such as diagnostic tests, that increase the charges for other kinds of patients. Second, patients with a diagnosis of mental disorder stay in the hospital significantly longer than other kinds of patients.

However, several studies have found that Medicaid beneficiaries treated for mental disorders have shorter hospital stays than comparable patients covered by other insurers. Frank and Lave found that Medicaid stays were especially short in States that had general limits on the number of inpatient days covered, per admission or per year. Coverage limits also had some impact on the chances of a patient's being discharged to another facility, rather than to the community.[29]

A 1986 analysis of 1970-77 data found that differences between Medicaid and private patients, both in length of stay and in likelihood of discharge to another facility, remained even after correction for the severity of the patients' problems at the time of admission.[30] The author suggests that the higher number of discharges to other facilities could indicate that the outreach and treatment services that would permit discharge to the community are harder to arrange for Medicaid beneficiaries.

V. STRUCTURED CARE SYSTEMS FOR MENTAL ILLNESS

A number of observers have suggested that Medicaid and other public mental health policies have resulted in discontinuous and uncoordinated care for the seriously mentally ill. Coverage limits may result in some beneficiaries being shifted from one treatment setting to another--from outpatient services to an inpatient hospital, from a general hospital to a State institution, from the State facility to a nursing home or back to the community. States have experimented with a variety of systems meant to improve the management of Medicaid mental health services.

A. Case Management Programs

Case management services are services that help eligible individuals gain access to necessary medical, social, education, and other services. Three States, Minnesota, South Carolina, and Utah, are currently using the section 2175 waiver authority established by OBRA 81 for case management programs to serve the mentally ill and related populations. Section 2175, as described in

---

[29]Frank, Richard, and Judith Lave. *The Impact of Medicaid Benefit Design on Length of Hospital Stay and Patient Transfer.* Hospital and Community Psychiatry, 36:7 (July 1985). p. 749-753.

[30]Wallen, Jacqueline. *Case Mix and Treatment Patterns of Medicaid and Privately Insured Psychiatric Patients in Short-Term General Hospitals.* Hospital Cost and Utilization Project Research Note 9, DHHS Publication No. (PHS) 87-3402. 1986.

Chapter VI, Alternate Delivery Options and Waiver Programs, permits a State to obtain waivers of the Medicaid "freedom-of-choice" requirement and other rules in order to require selected groups of beneficiaries to participate in a primary care case management system, under which all of a patient's treatment must be provided or authorized by a single physician or other primary care provider. These programs are designed to reduce unnecessary duplication of services and provide care more efficiently. Minnesota has implemented a case management program for chemical and substance abuse patients, and South Carolina for mental health patients. Utah has initiated a mental health capitation program.

B. Home and Community-Based Services Waivers

States have used the OBRA 81 section 2176 waiver authority to develop home and community-based services programs for the seriously mentally ill who would otherwise qualify for institutional services under Medicaid. Section 2176 waivers, also referred to as section 1915(c) waivers, allow a State to develop a coordinated care system to this population that are not available to other Medicaid beneficiaries. Only one State, Vermont, currently operates a program specifically targeted at the mentally ill. Oregon provides services to mentally ill persons through a combined waiver.

C. Targeted Case Management

The Consolidated Omnibus Budget Reconciliation Act of 1985 (COBRA, P.L. 99-272), authorized States, without a waiver, to provide case management services to target groups of Medicaid beneficiaries, such as disabled persons, pregnant women, or young children. As of March 1992, 28 States had approved or pending targeted case management services for chronically mentally ill persons: Alabama, Georgia, Hawaii, Idaho, Illinois, Kansas, Kentucky, Louisiana, Maine, Massachusetts, Montana, Nevada, New Hampshire, New Jersey, New York, North Carolina, North Dakota, Ohio, Oklahoma, Pennsylvania, Rhode Island, South Carolina, Tennessee, Texas, Utah, Vermont, Virginia, and West Virginia.[31]

D. Program for the Chronically Mentally Ill

Finally, OBRA 87 authorized special waivers of Medicaid rules to facilitate a set of demonstration projects being conducted by State and local governments under a Program on Chronic Mental Illness, funded by the Robert Wood Johnson (RWJ) Foundation and cosponsored by the U.S. Department of Housing and Urban Development (HUD). The basic premise of the program has been that a central mental health authority is the cornerstone of improved systems of care. To be eligible for participation in the program, each city had to develop a service system incorporating a central authority and four other features:

---

[31]Health Care Financing Administration. Medicaid: spDATA System. Characteristics of Medicaid State Programs. HCFA Pub. No. 02178, May 1992. Table 3-5.2.

continuity of care, a full range of services, a housing plan, and new sources of financing.

In November 1986, projects were established in nine cities: Austin, Texas; Baltimore; Charlotte, North Carolina; Cincinnati, Columbus, and Toledo, Ohio; Denver; Honolulu; and Philadelphia. Each recipient received a $2.5 million grant over a 5-year period and a $1 million low-interest housing development loan. In addition, HUD provided 125 Section 8 housing certificates for rent subsidies to each of the selected cities.[32]

The RWJ Foundation chose the University of Maryland Mental Health Policy Studies Program to make an independent evaluation of the program, funded jointly by the foundation, NIMH, and a consortium of other Federal agencies. The evaluation effort will comprise five groups of interrelated studies: a site-level study, a community care study, housing studies, financing studies, and disability and vocational rehabilitation studies. The financing studies have two principal components; one focuses on costs and patterns of care for individuals with chronic mental illness enrolled in Medicaid, and the other concerns the impact local mental health authorities have on the flow of funds, on economic relationships with providers, and on financial incentives.

The Medicaid analyses are designed to assess the impact of the program on utilization and cost for the mentally ill population and on indicators of outcome. Utilization and cost data will be compiled from Medicaid management information systems in Ohio and Maryland for mentally ill Medicaid beneficiaries who meet certain diagnostic and utilization criteria. The analysis will address the experience of Medicaid beneficiaries with mental illness who are living in the four Ohio and Maryland program sites compared with mentally ill Medicaid recipients living in the two States but outside the demonstration cities.[33]

VI. DISPROPORTIONATE SHARE PAYMENTS FOR MENTAL HEALTH SERVICES

A number of States are applying for Federal matching funds under Medicaid disproportionate share provisions to help pay for certain mental health services. According to an October 1991 report from the Intergovernmental Health Policy Project (IHPP), at least 30 States have submitted State plan amendments to provide disproportionate share payments for State and private psychiatric facilities which serve a high proportion of Medicaid and/or low-income patients. This comes as a result of amendments to the Medicaid law in OBRA 87, which required States to make extra payments to hospitals serving

---

[32]Shore, Miles F., and Martin D. Cohen. *The Robert Wood Johnson Foundation on Chronic Mental Illness: An Overview.* Hospital and Community Psychiatry, 41:11 (Nov. 1990). p. 1212-1216.

[33]Goldman, Howard H., and others. *Design for the National Evaluation of the Robert Wood Johnson Foundation Program on Chronic Mental Illness.* Hospital and Community Psychiatry, 41:11 (Nov. 1990). p. 1217-1221.

a disproportionate share of Medicaid and low-income patients according to criteria established in the 1987 Act.[34]

A hospital is eligible for additional payments as a disproportionate share hospital if: (1) its Medicaid utilization rate is more than one standard deviation above the mean Medicaid utilization rate for all Medicaid participating hospitals in the State; or (2) its low-income utilization rate is at least 25 percent. States may also establish additional criteria. The legislation allows "specialty" hospitals to be designated as disproportionate-share facilities, and some States have established this category for their State psychiatric hospitals. Because most of these facilities are considered IMDs under Medicaid, services for patients aged 22 to 64 are unreimbursable under the program. Under the new provisions, most of the patients at these facilities, although not eligible for Medicaid, are indigent with no source of payment for services; thus the low-income utilization rate for the facility usually far exceeds the 25 percent criterion under the law.

According to the IHPP report, some States are making additional payments for Medicaid eligible individuals under age 22 and over age 65 being treated in psychiatric facilities. The additional Federal matching funds resulting from these payments may help finance the indigent care provided to all age groups in State facilities. Treatment for such patients, without these payments, would be the total responsibility of the State.

New Hampshire is one of the early States to take advantage of the change in the disproportionate-share policy to apply for and receive additional Federal matching funds for its State psychiatric facility. The State's psychiatric facility qualified for disproportionate share payments because of the high percentage of low-income patients (87.5 percent of the patients admitted either have Medicaid eligibility, or have no insurance or other fee-paying capability). New Hampshire received approximately $7.5 million in 1991 disproportionate-share matching payments from the Federal Government.

Kansas, another State to increase disproportionate share payments under this program, received $27 million in FY 1991 in resulting Federal matching payments, and expects to receive $103 million in FY 1992. Between 50 and 80 percent of the patients in the State's four psychiatric hospitals have no means to pay for their care.

Other States that have received Federal matching for disproportionate-share payments for their psychiatric facilities include New York, Tennessee, Louisiana, and Michigan. Other States, Delaware, Pennsylvania, and Texas, were in the process of submitting State plan amendments to HCFA or awaiting approval of such proposals at the time of the IHPP report.

---

[34]Bergman, Gail Toff. *States Seek Disproportional Share Payments to Help Maintain Medicaid Programs.* Intergovernmental Health Policy Project State ADM Reports, Oct. 1991. p. 1, 2, 5-7. This report is used as the source for this section of this appendix.

APPENDIX F. MEDICAID SERVICES FOR SUBSTANCE ABUSE TREATMENT[1]

I. INTRODUCTION

Medicaid provides a limited source of funding for treatment of substance abuse, including alcohol abuse and alcoholism and drug abuse. Neither the Medicaid statute nor the regulations governing the program specify treatment for substance abuse as a particular service that is reimbursed under the program. States providing treatment for substance abuse to Medicaid-eligible populations can often be reimbursed if the treatment is provided under a Medicaid service category that qualifies for Federal matching funds.

If alcohol or drug detoxification treatment, for instance, which is not listed as a reimbursable service, is provided as part of inpatient hospital treatment, it is reimbursable under Medicaid in most States. Similarly, emergency hospitalization for a drug overdose would generally be covered. Other aspects of substance abuse treatment, such as physician examination at admission to treatment, psychiatrists' or clinical psychologists' counseling and related services, and prescription of methadone for treatment of opiate addiction, may also be covered. Such common treatment modes for substance abuse as non-medical residential treatment or counseling by other than physicians or psychologists, however, are generally not eligible for reimbursement.

Some States, such as Illinois, Minnesota, New York, North Carolina, Ohio, Oregon, Pennsylvania, and Wisconsin, according to a recent survey, have well-developed, and well-coordinated substance abuse treatment programs for their Medicaid populations, but other States cover such treatment for this population in a limited way only.[2] Determining which treatment services for substance abuse can be reimbursed under Medicaid is complicated both by questions of personal eligibility of the persons needing services and by the Medicaid program characteristics of the State in which such a person resides. The Health Care Financing Administration (HCFA) does not collect data on the type and amount of Medicaid-reimbursable substance abuse services provided by the States.

---

[1]This appendix was written by Edward Klebe.

[2]Solloway, Michele R. A 50-State Survey of Medicaid Coverage of Substance Abuse Services: Executive Summary. Prepared by the Intergovernmental Health Policy Project for the Robert Wood Johnson Foundation. Feb. 1992. Washington, 1992. p. 18. (Hereafter cited as *A 50-State Survey of Medicaid Coverage*)

This appendix discusses Medicaid's role in substance abuse treatment. After a discussion of the prevalence of substance abuse in the United States and the population in need of treatment services, there is a description of the various treatment modes currently in use for substance abuse. Then there is a discussion of Medicaid coverage for substance abuse treatment in general. The appendix concludes with discussions of the special problems of substance abuse among pregnant and postpartum women and among children and adolescents, with descriptions of Medicaid treatment services available for these populations.

II. BACKGROUND

A. Defining and Counting the Population of Substance Abusers

1. Population of Substance Abusers

There is no easy way to enumerate the population at need for treatment for substance abuse. The Alcohol, Drug Abuse, and Mental Health Administration (ADAMHA)[3] of the Department of Health and Human Services (DHHS) over the years has financed and published several national surveys that measure the extent of alcohol and illicit drug use in the United States. Probably the most widely-cited of these surveys is the National Household Survey on Drug Abuse. The 1991 edition of the Household Survey is the 11th in a series of national surveys first carried out in 1971 to measure the prevalence of drug use among the American household population aged 12 and over. For this survey, a national probability sample of households in the United States is selected from 125 primary sampling units. The 1991 sample for the first time includes persons living in some group quarters or institutions, such as civilians living on military installations, college dormitories, and homeless shelters, but did not include transient populations such as the homeless not in shelters. The 1991 Household Survey is based on 32,594 interviews.[4]

The Household Survey reports estimates of illicit drug, alcohol, and tobacco use in three categories: "current" use (within the past 30 days); "past year" use; and lifetime use. Starting in 1985, the survey also began to report on frequency of use in the past year for marijuana and cocaine, including data on those using

---

[3]P.L. 102-321, the ADAMHA Reorganization Act, signed into law on July 10, 1992, changed the name and mission of ADAMHA. The legislation transferred the three research institutes of the agency--the National Institute on Alcohol Abuse and Alcoholism (NIAAA), the National Institute on Drug Abuse (NIDA), and the National Institute of Mental Health (NIMH)--to the National Institutes of Health, and changed ADAMHA to a services-oriented agency named the Substance Abuse and Mental Health Services Administration (SAMHSA) as of Oct. 1, 1992.

[4]U.S. Dept. of Health and Human Services. National Institute on Drug Abuse. *National Household Survey on Drug Abuse: 1991 Population Estimates.* NIDA, DHHS Publication No. (ADM) 92-1887, 1991. Maryland, 1991. (Hereafter cited as NIDA, *National Household Survey on Drug Abuse, 1991*)

such drugs "12 or more times" and "once a week or more." The 1991 National Household Survey found that 6.2 percent of the household population aged 12 and over (12.6 million persons) were "current" users of illicit drugs, including marijuana, nonmedical use of psychotherapeutics, inhalants, cocaine, hallucinogens, and heroin. This was a decrease of 3 percent from the 13 million "current" users in the 1990 survey, and a decrease of 45.2 percent from the estimated 23 million "current" users in the 1985 survey. (See figure F-1.)

FIGURE F-1. Trend in Current Use of Illicit Drugs, 1985, 1990, and 1991

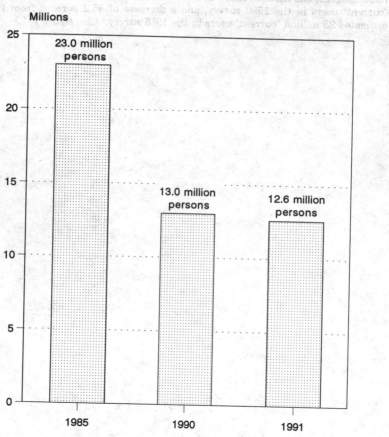

Millions

23.0 million persons

13.0 million persons

12.6 million persons

1985

1990

1991

Source: Figure prepared by Congressional Research Service based on estimates and data from ADAMHA.

Recent trends in cocaine use do not follow the overall pattern of illicit drug use. According to the Household Survey, the proportion of the population who had used cocaine in the past year decreased from 4.1 percent in 1988 to 3.1 percent in 1990, and then stayed at 3.1 percent in 1991. A similar trend appeared for those using cocaine during the past month, declining from 1.5 percent in 1988 to 0.8 percent in 1990, and then increasing to 0.9 percent in 1991. These small increases can be attributed to increases within one age group--the age 35 and older age group. Past year use of cocaine by this age group remained stable at 0.9 percent in 1988 and 1990, while other age groups were experiencing decreases, before increasing to 1.6 percent in 1991.[5]

There has been criticism about the limitations of the Household Survey as an accurate measure of the Nation's drug abuse problem. One of the major limitations of the survey is that it does not include certain populations that do not live in households, that are likely to have high incidence of drug addiction. These include homeless persons not living in shelters, persons in drug treatment facilities, and persons in State and Federal prisons. Some observers feel that the exclusion of these populations results in an underestimation of the scope of drug use, particularly hard-core drug addiction, in the United States. Others cite the nature of the Household Survey itself as a factor that may result in underestimates of the drug problem. The use of self-reports of an illicit activity may result in significant underreporting.

A 1990 Senate Judiciary Committee estimate of hard-core cocaine addicts in the United States in 1988 came up with a total that was more than twice the Household Survey estimate for that year. This estimate included, in addition to the Household Survey estimate of 860,000 cocaine addicts, estimates of cocaine addicts in the drug treatment system, in correctional systems, and in the homeless population. With adjustments to eliminate overlap among the four groups, the Judiciary Committee report estimated that there were nearly 2.2 million hard-core cocaine addicts in the United States in 1988.[6]

There are other surveys and studies that provide indicators of drug and alcohol use in the United States. ADAMHA, through its National Institute on Drug Abuse (NIDA), has also funded an annual study entitled "Monitoring the Future: A Continuing Study of the Lifestyles and Values of Youth," conducted by the University of Michigan's Institute for Social Research. This survey,

---

[5]U.S. Dept. of Health and Human Services. National Institute on Drug Abuse. *National Household Survey on Drug Abuse: 1988 Population Estimates.* NIDA, DHHS Publication No. (ADM) 89-1963, 1988. Maryland, 1989. (Hereafter cited as *NIDA, National Household Survey on Drug Abuse, 1988*)

National Institute on Drug Abuse. *National Household Survey on Drug Abuse: 1990 Population Estimates.* NIDA, DHHS Publication No. (ADM) 91-1732, 1990. Maryland, 1990.

[6]U.S. Congress. Senate. Committee on the Judiciary. Hard-Core Cocaine Addicts: Measuring--and Fighting--the Epidemic. 101st Cong., 2d Sess., May 10, 1990. Washington, GPO, 1990. p. 5-6.

better known as the High School Senior Survey, has studied a sample of high school seniors on their drug use and related attitudes annually since 1975, with follow-ups of selected numbers through college into young adulthood, for current, annual, and lifetime use of illicit drugs, alcohol, and tobacco. As with the National Household Survey, the High School Senior Survey in recent years has reported decreases in illicit drug and alcohol use among its survey population. As with the Household Survey, a limitation of the High School Senior Survey that may lead to underreporting is that it does not include high school dropouts, a group that may likely have higher rates of illicit drug use than those who remain in school.

Another NIDA-sponsored survey appears to contradict the reported decreases in illicit drug use in the Household Survey and the High School Senior Survey, at least for 1991. The Drug Abuse Warning Network (DAWN) monitors the number and pattern of drug-related health emergencies and drug-related deaths in major metropolitan areas across the country. Initiated in 1972, DAWN collects two basic types of information: drug-related deaths reported by medical examiners (87 medical examiners in 27 metropolitan areas in 1989) and drug-related visits to hospital emergency rooms (700 emergency rooms in 21 metropolitan areas in 1989). The DAWN survey has been especially crucial in showing the steep increases in the use of cocaine since the appearance of crack in the mid-1980s. In 1985, the DAWN emergency rooms reported 10,248 cocaine-related cases; by 1988, the number of cocaine "mentions" had increased by more than 400 percent to 42,512 "mentions." Similarly, the number of cocaine-related deaths reported by DAWN medical examiners increased by more than 300 percent from 717 in 1985 to 2,496 in 1989.

Starting in 1990, the DAWN survey started reporting weighted estimates for substance abuse related emergency room episodes for the total coterminous United States (excluding Alaska and Hawaii). DAWN data for 1989 and 1990 showed a decline in the numbers of visits to emergency rooms between the 2 years for illicit drugs in general and for cocaine in particular, apparently confirming a leveling off in the cocaine epidemic reported by the Household and High School Senior Surveys. The DAWN emergency rooms reported a 13 percent decline in drug abuse episodes in 1990 from the previous year. Emergency room mentions of cocaine dropped over the same period by 27 percent.[7] The preliminary DAWN data for 1991, however, show significant increases in illicit drug episodes in each of the first 3 quarters of the year. Although drug abuse-related emergency room visits declined in the final quarter of 1991, the large increases in the first 3 quarters produced a statistically significant 7.3 percent increase for the year. Cocaine-related emergencies

---

[7]U.S. Dept. of Health and Human Services. National Institute on Drug Abuse. *Press Release: DAWN*. Report for third quarter of 1991. Washington, May 12, 1992.

showed a 29.3 percent increase in 1991, and heroin-related emergencies increased by 9.7 percent for the year.[8]

The reduction of drug-related emergency room visits is one of the objectives related to substance abuse that were developed in conjunction with the *Healthy People 2000* national health promotion and disease prevention objectives published in 1991 by DHHS.[9] The report proposed to reduce such visits by 20 percent by the year 2000. The data above indicate that progress in achieving this objective may be slow in coming. Efforts to meet other objectives have met with some success. A February 1992 progress review noted that alcohol-related motor vehicle deaths had fallen significantly from a rate of 9.8 per 100,000 at the 1987 baseline to 8.9 per 100,000 in 1990; the target for 2000 is 8.5 per 100,000. The cirrhosis death rate also showed a significant decline from a 1987 baseline of 9.1 per 100,000 to a 1990 rate of 8.3 per 100,000; the target for 2000 is 6.0 per 100,000. In contrast, the rates of drug-related deaths increased from 3.8 per 100,000 in 1987 to 4.1 in 1989, the most recent years for which data are available; the year 2000 target is 3.0.[10]

2. Estimates of Population in Need of Substance Abuse Treatment

These and other surveys are used to estimate the extent of illicit drug and alcohol abuse in the United States, but estimating the number of persons in need of treatment for such abuse or addiction is more difficult. The Household Survey and other surveys of substance abuse have been used to provide such an estimate of the need for service. The Institute of Medicine (IOM) of the National Academy of Sciences, for a 1990 report on treating drug problems, used the 1988 National Household Survey, along with a number of surveys and studies of criminal justice populations conducted or sponsored by the Bureau of Justice Statistics and the National Institute of Justice, as well as several studies of the homeless population, to develop estimates of the need for treatment.

The IOM study concluded that, of the estimated 14.5 million persons in the 1988 Household Survey who used an illicit drug at least once in the month before the survey, 1.5 million could be categorized as having a clear need for treatment. Another 3.1 million persons had a probable need for treatment, and 2.9 million had a possible need. The IOM study estimated that there were 320,000 persons in correctional institutions and 730,000 persons in the

---

[8]The National Report on Substance Abuse. *DAWN: Drug-Related ER Visits Drop 7.1 Percent in Last Quarter of 1991*. Buraff Publications, v. 6, no. 19, Sept. 11, 1992. Washington, 1992. p. 4-5.

[9]U.S. Dept. of Health and Human Services. *Healthy People 2000: National Health Promotion and Disease Prevention Objectives*. DHHS Publication No. (PHS)91-50212. Washington, 1991.

[10]U.S. Dept. of Health and Human Services. Public Health Service. *A Public Health Service Progress Report on Healthy People 2000: Alcohol and Other Drugs*. Washington, 1992. (Hereafter cited as *Healthy People 2000*)

community under supervision of the criminal justice system (parolees and probationers) who needed treatment for drug abuse. The final two groups in the IOM study are the homeless population, estimated to include 170,000 in need of treatment, and pregnant women who are using drugs, estimated at about 105,000 in need of treatment. After deducting the 470,000 persons it estimates as the number of parolees and probationers, homeless persons, and pregnant women who are also part of the household population, the IOM concludes that a total of 5,455,000 persons in the United States needed treatment for drug abuse on a typical day at the time of the 1988 Household Survey. Of this total, according to the IOM study, about 1.5 million in the household population clearly needed treatment for illicit drug abuse or addiction, and 3.1 million probably did.[11]

Similar estimates of the number of persons needing treatment for alcohol abuse or alcoholism are not available, although the National Institute of Alcohol Abuse and Alcoholism (NIAAA) has estimated that about 10 percent of the adult population of the United States are either nondependent problem drinkers (4 percent), or alcohol dependent (6 percent). This works out to a total of 18 million adults who experience serious alcohol-related problems. Nondependent problem drinkers or alcohol abusers are persons who experience a variety of social and medical problems as a result of high-risk drinking but who are not dependent on alcohol. Alcohol-dependent persons--alcoholics--not only experience adverse consequences from single bouts of drinking and social and medical consequences from chronic high-risk alcohol use. They also experience physical and psychological dependence on alcohol that results in impaired ability to control drinking behavior.[12] NIAAA also estimates that 4.6 million adolescents under age 18 have significant alcohol-related problems.

Among those persons in need of substance abuse treatment, there are some population groups which have particular difficulty in obtaining such treatment services. As noted in *Healthy People 2000,* access to treatment services is often limited by structural, economic, linguistic, and cultural barriers. People with low incomes, for instance, faced with the limited coverage for such services in both private and public financing programs, have difficulty in paying for substance abuse treatment services out of their own resources. Women, especially pregnant women or women with young children, have limited access to programs to treat their drug or alcohol problems. Adolescents with substance abuse problems cannot be treated adequately in most existing programs designed for adults and require treatment programs tailored to their specific needs. Non-

---

[11]Gerstein, Dean R., and Henrick J. Harwood, eds. Treating Drug Problems: A Study of the Evolution, Effectiveness, and Financing of Public and Private Drug Treatment Systems. Washington, National Academy Press, v. 1, 1990. p. 76-88. (Hereafter cited as Gerstein and Harwood, *Treating Drug Problems*)

[12]U.S. Dept. of Health and Human Services. National Institute on Alcohol Abuse and Alcoholism. *Seventh Special Report to the U.S. Congress on Alcohol and Health from the Secretary of Health and Human Services.* DHHS Publication No. (ADM) 90-1656, Jan. 1990. Washington, 1990. p. 1-2. (Hereafter cited as NIAAA, *Seventh Special Report*)

white and non-English speaking populations require treatment programs that take into account specific cultural influences on alcohol and other drug use and that impose no language barriers. A large number of inmates in correctional institutions have varying degrees of alcohol and drug abuse problems. According to *Healthy People 2000*, treatment programs in such facilities are generally underfunded and understaffed, and when offenders are released, the probability is great that their untreated substance abuse problems will reemerge along with criminal behavior.[13]

Healthy People 2000 includes in its objectives the establishment and monitoring in the 50 States of comprehensive plans to ensure success to alcohol and drug treatment programs for traditionally underserved people. The 1992 progress report on the alcohol and other drugs objectives for the year 2000 notes that no data are available to report on any progress on achieving this and other services-related objectives.

III. SUBSTANCE ABUSE TREATMENT SERVICES

Treatment services for alcohol and drug abuse are provided in a variety of settings and modalities. Some forms of treatment are aimed at illicit drug abusers only, such as in the case of methadone maintenance for heroin addicts, and others are used for alcohol abuse only, such as treatment involving the use of the sensitizing drug disulfiram (Antabuse). Aside from such exceptions, however, similar modalities of treatment are used for both alcohol or drug abuse, and often in the same setting. In addition, increasingly larger numbers of persons are treated for polydrug abuse--abuse of more than one substance, including illicit drugs and alcohol, at the same time.

Treatment can be provided on an inpatient basis, in such settings as detoxification and rehabilitation units in general hospitals, treatment units in public and private psychiatric hospitals, and free-standing treatment facilities. Substance abuse treatment may also be provided in an outpatient setting, in the office of a private physician or other treatment professional, in treatment units of community facilities such as community mental health centers or hospitals, or in free-standing outpatient substance abuse treatment facilities. It is not at all unusual for a drug or alcohol abuser to go through many different types and settings of treatment before achieving long-term success in becoming alcohol- or drug-free.

Substance abuse treatment commonly begins with a period of detoxification, which is followed by a more extensive course of treatment designed to prevent relapse. Such treatment modalities include methadone maintenance for opiate addiction, as well as inpatient chemical dependency treatment, therapeutic communities, and outpatient drug-free programs for all types of alcohol and drug abuse.

---

[13]*Healthy People 2000*, p. 173.

A. Detoxification

Substance abuse treatment often starts with a short-term program of detoxification, which involves the process of clearing the patient's system of the physical remnants of the drug or alcohol. Detoxification is sometimes necessary in helping patients with the problems of the immediate withdrawal from drug or alcohol use so that they can proceed to the treatment and related services that will help them stay off. Detoxification can be provided on an inpatient basis in a hospital or other residential facility or in an outpatient program. Although many substance abusers do not receive any treatment services beyond it, detoxification is not a treatment for the substance abuse dependence as such. For those who choose and are able to proceed to further care following detoxification, a variety of program modalities are available to prevent relapse and enable patients to remain alcohol-or drug-free.

B. Methadone Maintenance

Methadone maintenance is a treatment designed to help persons addicted to heroin and other opium-derivative drugs. Methadone may be used to ease withdrawal symptoms during detoxification, but, with its ability to control the craving for heroin in the addict, its main purpose is in long-term substitution for heroin. Its main benefits are that it is taken orally, removing the dangers of intravenous injection that accompany heroin addiction, and that it is effective for a 24-hour period, making it conducive to a daily maintenance regime. Methadone maintenance programs are administered by licensed programs regulated by detailed Federal regulations under the Food and Drug Administration (21 CFR 291.505). These regulations provide that methadone can be provided only in conjunction with provision of appropriate social and medical services.

C. Inpatient Chemical Dependency Treatment

Chemical dependency treatment programs are based in hospitals, psychiatric facilities, and specialized free-standing facilities. They are sometimes known as the Minnesota Model (after the Willmar State Hospital in Minnesota, where the model was developed in the 1950s), the 28-day program, or the 12-step program. Such programs generally extend for 3 to 4 weeks (28 days), and feature a variety of treatment, counseling, and other techniques. These programs initially focused on individuals with alcohol problems and the use of the 12-step approach of Alcoholics Anonymous (AA). The chemical dependency approach has been expanded in recent years to include treatment of illicit drug dependence as well, particularly addiction to cocaine. The 12-step approach utilizes what has been described as a spiritual or moral approach to helping alcohol and drug abusers change their patterns of behavior. The steps include the admission of addiction, acknowledgement of one's impotence to stop it without the help of a higher power, and the need to confront the harm one has done.[14]

---

[14]Office of National Drug Control Policy. *Understanding Drug Treatment*. White Paper, June 1990. Washington, 1990. p. 16. (Hereafter cited as Office of National Drug Control Policy, *Understanding Drug Treatment*)

D. Therapeutic Communities

The therapeutic community approach is a residential drug-free program. One of the earliest models of this approach was the Synanon program in California in the late 1950s, which was developed initially to rehabilitate "hardcore" heroin addicts, particularly those with records of criminal behavior or social pathology. Therapeutic communities are designed to get patients to face the fact that they are addicted to drugs, and then to foster change in their personalities so they can live without drugs.[15] They are full-time, drug-free residential programs which provide a highly-structured, nonpermissive program of treatment. Therapy in a therapeutic community is generally a long-term course of treatment, ranging in length of stay from 6 months to 2 years. Treatment in a therapeutic community is provided typically by treatment professionals and by former addicts, and features peer support and confrontation, individual and group counseling, and educational and job training activities when appropriate.

E. Outpatient Non-Methadone Programs

Outpatient programs that do not use methadone vary widely in duration, goals, and content. Some use medications, such as Naltrexone, a nonaddicting narcotic antagonist, for the treatment of heroin addiction or other drugs in the treatment of cocaine addiction. Others are drug-free and make extensive use of counseling as the major form of therapy. Outpatient treatment programs, which operate out of hospitals or other treatment facilities or as free-standing facilities, began as a response to a need for community-based crisis centers for addicts. Some outpatient programs operate largely as drop-in "crisis" centers, while others are more structured. Other day treatment programs operate almost as outpatient therapeutic communities, with daily sessions of counseling and therapy. Most fall somewhere in between the two extremes, with regular, perhaps weekly or twice weekly, sessions. Outpatient programs offer a variety of therapeutic methods, such as individual and group therapy, family therapy, as well as specific training in relapse prevention. As with the therapeutic community approach, many outpatient programs make extensive use of former addicts as staff counselors and therapists.

F. Treatment Effectiveness

Research into the effectiveness of substance abuse treatment can be described as inconclusive. Treatment research carried out during the past 2 decades on various treatment settings and modalities has shown at least limited effectiveness for most if not all types and settings of treatment of alcohol and drug abuse. In a 1990 review of research on drug abuse treatment, Anglin and Hser summarize the findings of research on the efficacy of drug abuse treatment as follows:

---

[15]Office of National Drug Control Policy, *Understanding Drug Treatment*, p. 14.

There is no simple cure for drug dependence; once drug dependence has developed, the problem can persist as a chronic condition, and relapse is often the rule. The majority of clients in most treatment programs have traditionally been, and remain, opiate abusers, and evaluation studies are mostly based on opiate users in methadone maintenance programs. Although cocaine abuse has become one of the Nation's major drug problems, adequate data on the long-term processes and consequences of cocaine abuse have yet to be collected. However, findings regarding other drug dependencies and other modalities are typically consistent with those reported for methadone maintenance.

Anglin and Hser found that efforts to identify factors that consistently predict post-treatment abstinence or relapse patterns have not produced definitive findings. All major treatment modalities can be shown to have some positive effects on the clients in the criteria of drug use, criminality, employment, and other aspects of social functioning. For most types of programs, the more time clients spend in treatment, the more positive are their long-term outcomes. A significant proportion of those seeking treatment do not stay in treatment for more than a few weeks. Dropouts are high for all modalities except some methadone maintenance programs. Typically, an intact marriage, a job, shorter drug use history, low levels of psychiatric dysfunctioning, and a history of minimal criminality predict a better outcome in most programs. Demographics are related to likelihood of entering treatment but are only moderately associated with outcome. Program characteristics, such as quality of staff, breadth of services, and morale, are often significant determinants of outcome.[16]

IV. SUBSTANCE ABUSE TREATMENT STATISTICS

The National Association of State Alcohol and Drug Abuse Directors (NASADAD) annually surveys State Alcohol and Drug Abuse Agencies for client and fiscal data from substance abuse treatment programs. The survey includes only those treatment programs which receive some funds administered by a State agency. For FY 1990, the most recent year for which data have been published, 47 States, the District of Columbia, Guam, and Puerto Rico provided statistics on alcohol and other drug client treatment admissions for the year. The total number of reported treatment admissions during the year was more than 1.9 million--nearly 1.25 million for alcohol treatment (65.3 percent), and nearly 663 thousand for other drug treatment (34.7 percent).

Of the total admissions, 56 percent (1.08 million) were for ambulatory care treatment programs, including 73,331 for outpatient detoxification and 1,005,025 for outpatient treatment programs. The survey reported that 25 percent of total admissions (472,302) were for inpatient detoxification, 84.5 thousand in hospital inpatient settings and 387.8 thousand in free-standing residential facilities.

---

[16]Anglin, M. Douglas, and Yih-Ing Hser. *Treatment of Drug Abuse*. In Tonry, Michael, and James Q. Wilson, eds. *Drugs and Crime*. Chicago, University of Chicago Press, 1990. p. 393-397.

Fifteen percent of all admissions (292,481) were to residential rehabilitation programs, including 17.6 thousand to hospital treatment programs (other than detoxification), 173.8 thousand to short-term (30 days or fewer) residential programs, and 101.1 thousand to long-term (over 30 days) residential programs. (See figure F-2.) Among these treatment totals, the survey reported nearly 110 thousand admissions during the year to methadone treatment programs.[17]

---

[17]Butynski, William et al. *State Resources and Services Related to Alcohol and Other Drug Abuse Problems, Fiscal Year 1990.* National Association of State Alcohol and Drug Abuse Directors, Inc., Nov. 1991. Washington, 1991. p. 17-20.

FIGURE F-2. Distribution of Treatment Admissions, by Location of Treatment, FY 1990

Ambulatory Care
Treatment
1.1 million
56%

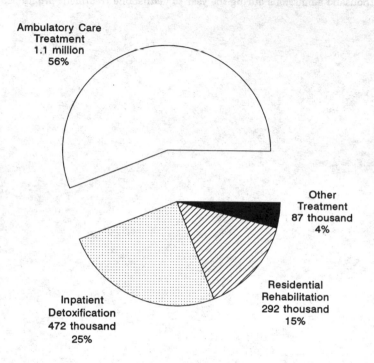

Other
Treatment
87 thousand
4%

Residential
Rehabilitation
292 thousand
15%

Inpatient
Detoxification
472 thousand
25%

NOTE: Statistics are for 47 States, the District of Columbia, Guam and Puerto Rico.
Source: Figure prepared by Congressional Research Service based on data from
the National Association of State Alcohol and Drug Abuse Directors.

The NASADAD survey also includes information on expenditures in the States for alcohol and other drug services. Forty-eight States, the District of Columbia, Guam, and Puerto Rico provided data on total expenditures by source of funding and types of program activity--treatment, prevention, and other activity for FY 1990. As with the other data in the NASADAD survey, the data on expenditures do not include information on those programs that did not receive any funding from the State alcohol and drug agency (e.g., most, if not all, private, for-profit programs; some private, not-for-profit programs; and some public programs). As a result, the overall expenditure estimates are conservative and, to varying degrees, underestimate expenditures by other departments of State government, by Federal agencies such as the Department of Veterans Affairs, and private, non-State agency-supported alcohol and other drug abuse treatment and prevention programs.

In FY 1990, according to the NASADAD survey, a total of over $2.9 billion was spent for alcohol and other drug services in those programs receiving at least some State-administered funds. Of the total, States spent $2.1 billion (72.3 percent) for treatment activities, over $429 million (14.7 percent) for prevention activities, and the remaining $377.9 million (13 percent) for other activities, such as capital construction, research, administration, and training. The total expenditure of $2.9 billion includes nearly $1.1 billion (37.8 percent) from State alcohol and drug agency sources, $285.7 million (9.8 percent) from other State agency sources, $645.5 million from the Alcohol, Drug Abuse, and Mental Health Services Block Grant and related grants from ADAMHA, $199.2 million (6.8 percent) from other Federal sources, $223.3 million (7.7 percent) from county or local agency sources, and $457.6 million (15.7 percent) from other sources (e.g., reimbursements from private health insurance, client fees, court fines or assessments for treatment imposed on intoxicated drivers).[18] (See figure F-3.)

---

[18]NASADAD FY 1990 State Report, p. 5-8. According to the publication's glossary of terms, "other Federal sources" includes all Federal funds used for support of alcohol and/or drug treatment or prevention services other than the block grant, and could include the Federal share of Medicaid. "Other State sources" would include the State share of Medicaid funds provided for treatment services unless the Medicaid share is provided by the State Alcohol and/or Drug Agency's State appropriation. According to NASADAD sources, it is not possible to determine the specific amounts of Medicaid dollars in either of these totals.

FIGURE F-3. Expenditures Reported for State Supported Alcohol
and Other Drug Abuse Services by Funding Source, FY 1990

Total Expenditures = $2.9 Billion

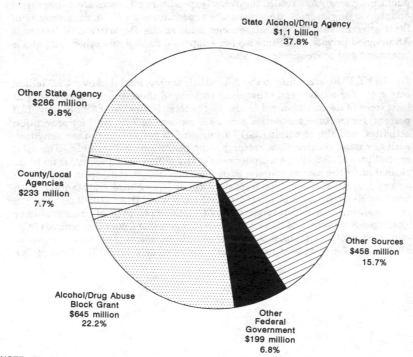

State Alcohol/Drug Agency
$1.1 billion
37.8%

Other State Agency
$286 million
9.8%

County/Local
Agencies
$233 million
7.7%

Other Sources
$458 million
15.7%

Alcohol/Drug Abuse
Block Grant
$645 million
22.2%

Other
Federal
Government
$199 million
6.8%

NOTE: The "Other Sources" category includes funding from sources such as client fees,
court fines and reimbursements from private health insurance. "Other Federal Government"
could include Federal Medicaid funds. "Other State Agency" could include State Medicaid
funds.
Source: Figure prepared by Congressional Research Service based on data from the National
Association of State Alcohol and Drug Abuse Directors. Data are included for "only those
programs which received at least some funds administered by the State Alcohol/Drug Agency
during the State's fiscal year 1990."

V. MEDICAID COVERAGE OF SUBSTANCE ABUSE TREATMENT SERVICES

A. Background

Medicaid does not specifically provide, either in law or regulation, for the coverage of treatment for substance abuse. Such treatment is covered to the extent that it can be covered under an approved Medicaid category. The program is used in varying degrees to cover substance abuse services under such categories as inpatient hospital services, hospital outpatient services, physician-supervised services, clinic services, licensed practitioners' services, and rehabilitative services.

Over the years, HCFA had provided guidance to State Medicaid agencies on whether substance abuse treatment services were reimbursable under the Medicaid program. Such guidance was provided on a case-by-case basis, whenever a State requested it. In 1990, HCFA provided two statements of Medicaid policy regarding reimbursement for substance abuse treatment. The first was in a May 23, 1990, letter from HCFA Administrator Gail Wilensky to Senator Daniel P. Moynihan to clarify what coverage exists under Medicaid for treatment of addiction to crack cocaine. Later in the year, in an August 2 guidance sent to State Medicaid directors, the Medicaid Bureau of HCFA reviewed the ways that Medicaid benefits relate to the treatment of drug addiction and related problems. A provision in the Omnibus Budget Reconciliation Act of 1990 (OBRA 90) then codified to a certain extent the HCFA policy regarding Medicaid reimbursement for substance abuse treatment as stated in the two documents--that nothing shall be excluded from Federal financial participation solely because it is provided as a treatment service for alcoholism or drug dependency.

The Wilensky letter to Senator Moynihan states that, "To the extent individuals are eligible for Medicaid and need inpatient hospital care, it is covered under the Medicaid program. For mandatory Medicaid benefits, such as inpatient hospital services, regulations explicitly prohibit States from using a recipient's diagnosis, type of illness, or condition as the basis for arbitrary limiting or denying coverage."[19] (*Chapter IV, Services* provides State level information on optional services covered in State Medicaid plans.)

The August 1990 guidance to State Medicaid directors from the Medicaid Bureau reviewed the ways Medicaid program benefits can help persons with drug addiction and related problems. According to this communication, "a number of primary care services may be used, including physicians' services, clinic services, and pharmaceuticals (e.g., methadone)."[20] Additionally,

---

[19]Wilensky, Gail. Statement by Senator Moynihan. *Congressional Record*, Daily Edition, v. 136, June 12, 1990. p. S 7805.

[20]U.S. General Accounting Office. *Substance Abuse Treatment: Medicaid Allows Some Services but Generally Limits Coverage*. Report No. GAO/HRD-91-
(continued...)

addiction-related services may be provided by home health agencies, under home and community-based services waivers (section 1915(c)), and as part of the Early and Periodic Screening, Diagnostic and Treatment (EPSDT) services. According to the HCFA guidance, a number of States have used freedom-of-choice waivers or exceptions to their State plans to implement managed care programs targeted to substance abuse. Case management may be used to coordinate the needed services, and special day treatment programs may be established that combine needed therapy, counseling and other services.

Inpatient hospital benefits may be used for such services as acute treatment of symptoms, detoxification, and drug-related medical complications. Rehabilitation services may be provided in such settings as outpatient programs in hospitals and clinics, and inpatient programs located in nursing facilities, psychiatric hospitals, and special units in general hospitals. Rehabilitation services may also be provided in settings that are not Medicaid participating facilities.

An amendment to the Medicaid Act enacted as part of OBRA 90 set in law the Medicaid policy described in the two communications. The Senate Finance Committee, which originated the amendment, noted in its report on the legislation the "confusion among States about whether substance abuse treatment may be covered" and cited the August 1990 guidance to the States which clarified "that any of the Medicaid services that States may offer may be used to treat substance abuse." The new statutory language, added to the end of section 1905(a) of the Act, states: "No service (including counseling) shall be excluded from the definition of 'medical assistance' solely because it is provided as a treatment service for alcoholism or drug dependency." That is, States can receive Federal Medicaid matching payments for these services.

The statutory restriction described in *Appendix E, Medicaid Services for the Mentally Ill* that precludes the payment for services to individuals between the ages of 22 and 65 in Institutions for Mental Diseases (IMDs) can affect some inpatient programs for treating substance abuse. The Medicaid program, using the International Classification of Diseases, Clinical Modification (ICD-9-CM), classifies alcohol and drug abuse as mental disorders. Consequently, facilities that exclusively treat psychiatric or substance abuse disorders are considered by Medicaid as IMDs. The Medicaid Bureau's guidance to the States notes that these restrictions do not apply to any facility with fewer than 17 beds, and suggests that it may be advantageous to set up this type of program in smaller facilities, even though room and board payment would not be made unless it is a participating facility. Optional IMD benefits are also available in psychiatric facilities for individuals under age 21 and for individuals age 65 and over regardless of the size of the facility.

It is difficult to determine the amount of Medicaid payments for substance abuse treatment and related services. The General Accounting Office (GAO), in

---

[20](...continued)
92, June 1991. Washington, 1991. p. 16-17. (Hereafter cited as GAO Report, *Substance Abuse Treatment*)

a 1991 report, found that HCFA and the States were unable to document Medicaid substance abuse treatment expenditures because there is not a separate category for substance abuse treatment on States' Medicaid expenditure reports. Expenditures are reported by type of Medicaid service, such as inpatient hospital, physician, rehabilitative, or clinical services, not by condition diagnosis, such as substance abuse.[21]

B. State Summaries

In its 1991 review, GAO visited nine State Medicaid offices and substance abuse agencies (Alabama, California, Florida, Georgia, Massachusetts, Minnesota, New York, Oregon, and Texas) to determine the types of substance abuse services available under Medicaid. They found, as table F-1 shows, that some States had made little use of Medicaid options for substance abuse treatment, while others offered a wide variety of services.

[21]GAO Report, *Substance Abuse Treatment*, p. 8.

TABLE F-1. Summary of Substance Abuse Treatments Available Under Medicaid and Offered by States GAO Visited, 1991

Type of Medicaid service	Examples of available treatments	Available in these States
Inpatient hospital	Detoxification, any acute treatment of symptoms, or treatment for complications	Alabama, Florida, Georgia, Massachusetts, New York, Texas, California, Oregon
Outpatient hospital	Detoxification, counseling, or methadone maintenance	Massachusetts, New York, California, Georgia
EPSDT	Any treatment to correct physical or mental problems found during EPSDT screening	All nine States
Physician services	Detoxification, counseling, psychotherapy, or methadone maintenance	Alabama, California, Florida, Georgia, New York
Home health services	Services for treating addiction	None
Other medical/remedial care	Counseling	Georgia, Oregon
Clinic services	Detoxification, counseling, psychotherapy, methadone maintenance	Alabama, California, Georgia, Massachusetts, New York
Drug services	Methadone	None

TABLE F-1. Summary of Substance Abuse Treatments Available Under Medicaid and Offered by States GAO Visited, 1991--Continued

Type of Medicaid service	Examples of available treatments	Available in these States
Other preventive and rehabilitative care	Counseling, psychotherapy, and day treatment services	Oregon, Florida, Minnesota
Inpatient psychiatric services in an IMD for individuals over 65	Residential services, psychiatric counseling, methadone maintenance, or other psychiatric services	Florida, New York
Inpatient psychiatric services in an IMD for individuals under 21	Residential services, psychiatric counseling, methadone maintenance, or other psychiatric services	Alabama, Massachusetts, New York, Oregon
Other medical or remedial care	Any other services authorized by the Secretary of HHS	None
Home or community-based services (waivers only)	Case management, home health, personal care, adult day health services, or respite care services	None
Waivers or exceptions	Managed-care programs	None
Targeted case-management services	Any service that will assist a recipient in gaining access to needed services	Georgia

Source: U.S. General Accounting Office. *Substance Abuse Treatment: Medicaid Allows Some Services But Generally Limits Coverage.* GAO-HRD-91-92, June 1991. Washington, 1991. p. 16 and 17.

According to the GAO survey, the nine States they visited varied in coverage limits of substance abuse treatment under Medicaid. Massachusetts, for instance, limited counseling to 24 visits per year, while Florida had no such limitations. Alabama restricted all outpatient counseling treatment to a mental health clinic, while Georgia had no such location restriction. Seven States did not allow inpatient rehabilitation following detoxification, and all nine States either denied or limited inpatient hospital treatment for substance abuse treatment.

State Medicaid officials in five States indicated to the GAO researchers that they planned new initiatives to implement additional substance abuse services reimbursable under Medicaid. Alabama planned to offer expanded comprehensive treatment under the rehabilitation option. Massachusetts indicated that it was working with other agencies on substance abuse shelters and trying to get day treatments covered. New York was planning to offer case management of pregnant women in 11 specific neighborhoods, coordinating services from 16 agencies. Oregon was planning initiatives for drug users, such as treatment on demand for pregnant women and adolescents, the provision of services for the deaf and hearing impaired, and special services for some ethnic groups. Texas had submitted a State plan amendment to offer treatment when substance abuse is detected during early and periodic screening.[22]

Until recently there was not available any general review of all States' coverage of substance abuse treatment under Medicaid, except for a survey of Medicaid substance abuse services for children and adolescents which will be cited later in this appendix. In February of 1992, the Intergovernmental Health Policy Project (IHPP) published the results of a 50-State survey of Medicaid substance abuse services. The report includes the results of a survey conducted by questionnaire sent to State Medicaid agencies in 1990, which provides more extensive information than has previously been available on States' coverage of substance abuse services under Medicaid. According to this survey, Arizona, Kentucky, New Hampshire, and South Dakota do not offer substance abuse services under their Medicaid programs, but most other States provide at least some (if limited) services and represent an array of service or program alternatives.[23]

Alaska, for instance, provides crisis intervention services and methadone maintenance therapy as part of rehabilitation but only when chemical dependency is identified as a dual or secondary diagnosis. Colorado provides emergency admission for detoxification; Idaho will reimburse inpatient hospitalization for acute withdrawal and detoxification. Arkansas' services are for the most part restricted to hospital settings, including inpatient hospital facilities, inpatient psychiatric facilities for clients under age 21, inpatient care for clients over 65 in IMDs, and outpatient hospital-based clinics. The

---

[22]GAO Report, *Substance Abuse Treatment*, p. 6-7.

[23]Solloway, *A 50-State Survey of Medicaid Coverage*, p. 13-29. This section of the appendix describing State coverages of services uses this document and the State Profiles that accompany it as sources.

exceptions to the hospital setting-only requirement in Arkansas are physician services, which may be provided in private offices, and counseling services, which are restricted to public health clinics. South Carolina has a limited set of services for substance abuse, including: assessment counseling (diagnosis and evaluation); individual, group, family and family unit counseling; intensive outpatient care; crisis management, targeted case management; medical assessment; and medical reevaluation.

A number of States use the rehabilitative services optional benefit to provide substance abuse treatment clients. Alabama, for example, uses this category to provide an array of services, including intake evaluation; medical assessment and treatment; crisis intervention; counseling and therapy (individual, family, group); medication administration and monitoring; treatment plan review; day treatment; and in-home intervention. Kansas and Ohio offer similar services under the rehabilitative services benefit. Kansas further includes screening services and day treatment, while Ohio includes case management services. Iowa uses this benefit to reimburse up to 28 days of outpatient substance abuse treatment.

California uses the clinic services benefit to cover outpatient heroin detoxification on a fee-for-service basis. It also uses clinic services to provide a variety of substance abuse services through county Alcohol and Drug Programs (ADP), which are operated through an interagency agreement with the State's Department of Alcohol and Drug Programs. Services include: methadone maintenance; drug-free treatment; naltrexone treatment; and day-habilitative programs to maintain drug-free status. Hawaii uses the benefit categories of physician and non-physician services to provide diagnosis and referral; individual and group counseling; and prescription drugs. Montana uses four benefit categories--physician services, clinic services, outpatient hospital services, and non-physician services--to provide substance abuse services to Medicaid recipients.

Several States have developed special programs under Medicaid waiver options or targeted case management services for specific populations, such as those with acquired immune deficiency syndrome (AIDS) or those who are human immunodeficiency virus (HIV) positive (California); high-risk children (Wisconsin) and adolescents (Ohio); pregnant women and drug-dependent babies (Pennsylvania); and Medicaid clients participating in jobs programs (Ohio). Some of these programs, such as those for AIDS/HIV and high-risk, low-income pregnant women, may contain components that deal with substance abuse services, but that may or may not be specifically designed to treat chemical dependency.

The IHPP survey found that a number of States have developed coordinated substance treatment programs to serve their Medicaid populations. States such as California, Illinois, Maryland, New Jersey, New York, North Carolina, Ohio, Oregon, Pennsylvania, and Wisconsin, for instance, have developed linkages between their Medicaid programs and their substance abuse treatment programs, which are usually located in a different State agency. The State of Minnesota has a consolidated program in which Medicaid funds, along with State appropriations, other Federal funds, county funds, and client fees, finance a public substance abuse program that serves Medicaid clients and those who are not Medicaid-eligible. The funds finance the State's "Consolidated Chemical Dependency Treatment Fund," which is designed to operate like an insurance policy for the State's poorest citizens in need of substance abuse treatment.

C. Discussion

The IOM, in its 1990 report on treating drug problems, characterized the general level of coverage provided by States. It found that States that provided Medicaid support to substance abuse treatment providers commonly reimbursed such services as physician examinations at admission to treatment (but generally at a rate equal to a conventional outpatient office visit rather than a multiphasic examination appropriate for an individual potentially severely compromised by drug abuse or dependence), methadone prescription (but generally at a rate that does not cover the cost of meeting Federal regulations to run a lawful maintenance clinic), and services of psychiatrists or licensed clinical psychologists (but not other counseling professionals). Emergency hospitalization for drug overdoses is generally covered, but, according to the IOM survey, treatment in residential programs is rarely reimbursed.[24]

One of the reasons for such limitations in Medicaid coverage for substance abuse treatment is that the Medicaid program was designed originally to cover health care services provided through a "medical model." Of the various modes of substance abuse treatment, only detoxification and methadone maintenance, and those hospital-based programs that provide treatment by or under the direction of a physician, fit comfortably into a medical model. Treatment programs such as therapeutic communities and most outpatient programs in which treatment is provided through peer counseling, group meetings, and the use of such nonmedical personnel as former addicts, would not be considered as medical in nature and would not be reimbursable under Medicaid.

Substance abuse treatment provided in nonhospital residential treatment, such as therapeutic communities and other residential treatment programs, rarely receives Medicaid reimbursement because a significant portion of the costs of these programs is often the room and board costs for their patients, and Medicaid does not reimburse for room and board costs for nonhospital programs.[25] The consistent comment of the States responding to the IHPP survey was that the reimbursement restrictions on IMD services and residential treatment prohibit cost-effective provision of substance abuse services under Medicaid.[26]

---

[24]Gerstein and Harwood, *Treating Drug Problems*, p. 271.

[25]Gates, David. An Overview of Federal Funding Programs for the Prevention and Treatment of Alcoholism and Drug Dependency. *National Health Law Program*, Jan. 1991. Washington, 1991. p. 6-18.

[26]Solloway, *A 50-State Survey of Medicaid Coverage*, p. 14.

VI. SUBSTANCE ABUSE TREATMENT SERVICES FOR PREGNANT AND POSTPARTUM WOMEN

A. Background

Women of child-bearing age have become increasingly vulnerable to substance abuse problems in the United States in recent years. This has become particularly evident since the appearance and spread of "crack" cocaine in the mid-1980s. Young women have been identified as one of the fastest growing crack user groups. The 1988 National Household Survey on Drug Abuse indicated that 14.1 percent of women between the ages of 18 and 25, and 9.6 percent of the women between the ages of 26 and 34 were currently using at least one illicit drug, that is, they reported using drugs within the last month. The 1991 Household Survey found decreases in reported drug use among these groups--13.4 percent of women between the ages of 18 and 25 and 6.6 percent of women between ages 26 and 34 had used an illicit drug during the previous month.[27]

A 1988 survey found that 11 percent of women presenting for prenatal and related childbirth services at 36 hospitals across the Nation admitted to illicit drug use during pregnancy; projected nationwide, this means that 375,000 infants born each year are exposed to drugs in utero. The Inspector General of the Department of Health and Human Services estimated in a 1990 report that 100,000 infants a year are born to women who use drugs during pregnancy. Other surveys estimated that up to 739,000 infants each year are exposed to illicit drugs.[28] The IOM, in its 1990 study on drug abuse treatment, estimated that 105,000 pregnant women a year need treatment for substance abuse.[29]

Alcohol and illicit drug use during pregnancy can lead to medical and other complications for both mother and infant. Among the common medical complications that can be attributed to alcohol or drug use during pregnancy, in addition to miscarriage and premature delivery, are such disorders as anemia, bacteremia, cardiac disease, hepatitis, pneumonia, urinary tract infections, and various sexually transmitted diseases. The use of alcohol during pregnancy can cause serious problems for the mother, including miscarriage or stillbirth, or premature delivery. Many chronic substance abusers often use both illicit drugs and alcohol, increasing the hazards for their health.

Drug and alcohol use during pregnancy can cause short- and long-term difficulties for the fetus as well. Research suggests that prenatal exposure to cocaine and to other illicit drugs can lead to such immediate problems as

---

[27]NIDA, *National Household Survey on Drug Abuse*, 1988, p. 17; and NIDA, *National Household Survey on Drug Abuse*, 1991, p. 19.

[28]Chasnoff, Ira J. Drugs, Alcohol, Pregnancy, and the Neonate: Pay Now or Pay Later. *Journal of the American Medical Association*, v. 266, no. 11, Sept. 18, 1991. p. 1567.

[29]Gerstein and Harwood, *Treating Drug Problems*, p. 234.

premature birth, low birthweight, birth defects, and respiratory and neurological problems. Cocaine-exposed children also appear to have a higher rate of sudden infant death syndrome (SIDS). Early studies on maternal cocaine use during pregnancy also indicated that so-called cocaine babies would pose behavioral problems and experience difficulties in learning that would cause significant societal problems once they reached school age in large numbers.[30]

More recent research reports, however, indicate that maternal cocaine use during pregnancy may not lead to lasting harm in the children born to such pregnancies. Methodologic problems that raise critical questions about the findings of such research have been found. Current researchers state that they do not underestimate the potential impact of the use of cocaine by pregnant women, but feel that early studies failed to take into account other factors that may have contributed to the medical and developmental problems suffered by these children. They suggest that the various problems previously associated with intrauterine cocaine exposure may be more accurately attributed to a combination of factors, such as premature birth, sexually transmitted diseases, the effects of poverty and poor medical treatment, lifestyle, and maternal exposure to alcohol, tobacco, and other drugs during pregnancy. These researchers emphasize that the children born under these conditions are not necessarily permanently disabled and do benefit from comprehensive services, such as adequate nutrition, health care, and early developmental intervention programs. They recommend for the mothers drug treatment, health care, and family support services, emphasizing the importance of coordination of service delivery.[31]

Some researchers feel that maternal use of alcohol during pregnancy may pose a greater risk to the fetus than does cocaine. The cluster of symptoms describing a common pattern of birth defects observed in children born to alcoholic mothers was first reported in 1973 and labeled Fetal Alcohol Syndrome (FAS). The defects of FAS include prenatal and postnatal growth retardation, craniofacial anomalies, central nervous system dysfunction, and major organ

---

[30]Chasnoff, Ira J., et al. Cocaine Use in Pregnancy. *New England Journal of Medicine*, v. 313, no. 11, Sept. 12, 1985. p. 666-669.

Chasnoff, Ira J., et al. Temporal Patterns of Cocaine Use in Pregnancy: Perinatal Outcome. *Journal of the American Medical Association*, v. 261, no. 12, Mar. 24/31, 1989. p. 1741.

Zuckerman, Barry, et al. Effects of Maternal Marijuana and Cocaine Use on Fetal Growth. *New England Journal of Medicine*, v. 320, no. 12, Mar. 23, 1989. p. 762-768.

[31]Mayes, Linda C., et al. The Problem of Prenatal Cocaine Exposure: A Rush to Judgment. *Journal of the American Medical Association*, v. 267, no. 3, Jan. 15, 1992. p. 406-408.

Viadero, Debra. New Research Finds Little Lasting Harm for 'Crack' Children. *Education Week*, Jan. 29, 1992. p. 1,10.

system malformations. When only some of these defects are present, the child may be described as suffering from suspected fetal alcohol effects, or FAE. Estimates of the incidence of FAS range for one to three cases per 1,000 live births; the incidence of FAE is estimated to be approximately three times higher.[32]

B. Coverage of Treatment Services for Pregnant Substance Abusers

Many of the women who are substance abusers are persons with sufficiently low income that, if they are not already eligible for Medicaid services, are likely to be eligible for maternal and child health services under the program. When pregnant, they and their children may be eligible to receive such services related to the pregnancy as prenatal care, delivery, and post partum care. Services under Medicaid may be delivered as soon as the pregnancy is verified and continues until the end of the month in which the 60-day post partum period ends to ensure that adequate postnatal care is provided.

In addition to such childbirth-related medical services, pregnant women may also be eligible for Medicaid coverage of substance treatment, as discussed in the main body of this appendix. It should be noted that because Medicaid covers all pregnant women up to 133 percent of poverty, and in nearly half of the States up to 185 percent, the program has the potential to be a major funding source for substance abuse treatment services for this population. According to HCFA, however, the extent of Medicaid payments specifically related to substance abuse treatment services is currently not well known, and can be expected to vary widely among States. The agency has research underway through a cooperative agreement with the Bigel Institute for Health Policy of Brandeis University to estimate costs to Medicaid for alternative levels of treatment services to pregnant, substance-abusing women. Results of the research are expected by the end of 1992.[33]

Despite the obvious need of pregnant substance abusers for such services, there is evidence that many drug treatment programs do not adequately serve this population. Women substance abusers have always faced difficulties in obtaining treatment services, but women who are also pregnant or have children face even more extensive barriers. Many drug treatment programs have traditionally been unwilling to provide services to pregnant women. One researcher surveyed treatment programs in New York City and found that 54 percent categorically excluded pregnant women. In addition, availability of treatment services was limited by restrictions on method of payment accepted by the program or by the specific substance abuse that would be treated. Sixty-

---

[32]NIAAA, *Seventh Special Report*, p. 139-140.

[33]U.S. Dept. of Health and Human Services. Health Care Financing Administration. *Improving Access to Care for Pregnant Substance Abusers*. Special Solicitation to State Medicaid Agencies on Availability of Funds for Demonstration Project Grant Funds, Dec. 1990; and telephone communication with HCFA personnel.

seven percent of the programs surveyed rejected pregnant Medicaid patients and only 13 percent would accept pregnant Medicaid patients addicted to crack.[34]

HCFA in December of 1990 announced a program of five demonstration projects to help improve access to early medical and substance abuse treatment services, and other relevant services to address the varied needs of Medicaid-eligible, pregnant substance abusing women and their infants. The demonstration is being implemented in geographically dispersed areas with demonstrated substance abuse problems and large numbers of Medicaid-eligible females of child-bearing age. The five projects will provide for the modification of services and/or payment approaches under Medicaid to promote access to comprehensive services for pregnant substance abusers and their infants. Projects may offer services to Medicaid-eligible, pregnant substance abusers between the ages of 22 and 65 who are patients in IMDs. Medicaid payment for services provided in IMDs within this age range is currently precluded by law. The demonstration is being funded at a level of $6 million to administer and monitor the five projects. Funding will be available for up to a 12-month developmental period, 3 years of service delivery, and a 6-month phase-out period.

The five project awards, announced in September of 1991, went to develop programs in Baltimore, Maryland; Boston and Holyoke, Massachusetts; New York City and three New York upstate areas; Edisto Health District, South Carolina; and Yakima County, Washington. The applicants selected for funding, according to HCFA, presented strong perinatal and substance abuse treatment systems, viable research designs, rich sources of data, and other innovative components, including creative and culturally sensitive methods of outreach. The successful applications commonly included case-finding, case management, provider training, community outreach, and other ancillary services, such as parenting education, nutrition counseling, and transportation. Three of the projects proposed providing services in an IMD setting. The demonstration projects will be evaluated under a separate contract with the results available at the end of the 4½ year grant period, in 1996 or 1997.

Since 1989, ADAMHA, through its Office for Substance Abuse Prevention (OSAP), has supported a demonstration grant program, authorized under title V of the Public Health Service (PHS) Act, for substance abuse prevention and treatment for pregnant and postpartum women. In addition, the Alcohol, Drug Abuse, and Mental Health Services Block Grant, originally authorized in 1981 under title XIX of the PHS Act, has included a provision requiring States to use 10 percent of their allotments for substance abuse programs and services designed for women (especially pregnant women and women with dependent children) and demonstration projects for the provision of residential treatment services to pregnant women. The ADAMHA Reorganization Act passed in July 1992, P.L. 102-321, authorized new grant programs for substance abuse treatment for pregnant and postpartum women. A new section 508 of the PHS Act authorizes grants, cooperative agreement, and contracts to establish and

---

[34]Chavkin, Wendy. Drug Addiction and Pregnancy: Policy Crossroads. *American Journal of Public Health*, v. 80, no. 4, Apr. 1990. p. 485.

support residential treatment programs for such women, including child care and other related services. A new section 509 of the Act authorizes grants to establish projects for the outpatient treatment of substance abuse among pregnant and postpartum women and their infants.

The 1992 ADAMHA legislation also split the block grant into two separate block grants--a substance abuse block grant and a mental health services block grant. The new substance abuse block grant authority under title XIX, as amended, contains specific authorities to ensure the availability of treatment services for pregnant women and women with children. The block grant authority requires each State to use not less than 5 percent of its allocation in each of FY 1993 and 1994 to increase, relative to the previous year, the availability of such treatment services, either by establishing new programs or expanding the capacity of existing programs. For subsequent years, States are required to spend at least as much as it spent in FY 1994 for treatment services for this population. The legislation also requires that each entity providing treatment services under this provision must make available, either directly or through arrangements with other entities, prenatal services or childcare services to women receiving such services. States will be required, under the block grant authority, to ensure that each pregnant woman in the State who seeks or is referred for and would benefit from substance abuse treatment services is given preference in admissions to treatment facilities receiving funds under the block grant.

VII. CHILDREN AND ADOLESCENTS WITH SUBSTANCE ABUSE PROBLEMS

A. Background

The 1991 National Household Survey on Drug Abuse reported that 20.1 percent of the U.S. population aged 12-17 (4 million persons) had ever used an illicit drug, 14.8 percent (nearly 3 million persons) had used such a drug during the previous year, and 6.8 percent (1.37 million persons) had used an illicit drug during the previous month.[35] The report of the National High School Senior Drug Abuse Survey, conducted annually for NIDA by the University of Michigan's Institute for Social Research, showed that 44 percent of the class of 1991 had used an illicit drug sometime during their lifetimes; 88 percent had used alcohol. The report also showed that 16.4 percent of the class of 1991 had used an illicit drug during the 30 days prior to the survey; 54 percent had used alcohol in that period. These measures do not necessarily indicate a need for treatment services, although the findings from the survey that 3.6 percent of high school seniors in the class of 1991 reported using alcohol daily during the previous 30 days and that 29.8 percent reported engaging in binge drinking (5 drinks or more in a row) during the previous 2 weeks do represent a disturbing level of abuse.[36]

---

[35]NIDA, *National Household Survey on Drug Abuse, 1991*, p. 19.

[36]National Institute on Drug Abuse. *Press Release: 1991 National High School Senior Drug Abuse Survey*, Jan. 27, 1992. Washington, 1992.

The 1990 IOM study on treating drug problems estimated that, of the 4.6 million persons with a clear and probable need for drug treatment, 9 percent, or about 396,000 persons, were youths under the age of 18.[37] In a 1991 study on adolescent health, the Office of Technology Assessment (OTA) estimated that nearly 272,000 adolescents a year are treated for substance abuse--157,000 for drugs and 115,000 for alcohol.[38]

B. Medicaid Treatment Services for Children and Adolescents

Substance abuse treatment services for children and adolescents are provided in the same modalities described above--detoxification, and the treatment and rehabilitation services provided in inpatient and residential, as well as outpatient settings. Medicaid has the potential for reimbursing a variety of such services through both mandatory and optional services, including the mandatory services required under EPSDT. (See table F-2.)

A survey of State Medicaid coverage of substance abuse services for children and adolescents conducted for a report for ADAMHA found that States make only limited use of both mandatory and optional benefit coverage for reimbursement of such services.[39] Of the mandatory benefits, for instance, inpatient hospital services were provided without limits in about half the States. Coverage in all but two States included substance abuse treatment in inpatient units, although reimbursement in 30 States was limited to detoxification. Twenty-two States impose limits on inpatient substance abuse services, either limits of days per admission or days per year, while 19 States impose prior authorization requirements on stays for substance abuse treatment. (See table F-3.)

The survey found that outpatient hospital services for substance abuse were provided without limits in about half the States. A total of 31 States covered outpatient substance abuse services provided by general acute care hospitals. Only 14 of these also allowed psychiatric hospitals to enroll as providers of outpatient substance abuse services. Ten States restricted coverage for hospital outpatient services for substance abuse. In five of these States, the limit extended to include all outpatient hospital services and, in some instances, physicians' and clinic services as well. In the other five States, coverage limits varied from $313 annually to as much as 3 hours per day. Coverage included partial hospitalization for substance-abusing children in six States; two States

---

[37]Gerstein and Harwood, *Treating Drug Problems*, p. 80.

[38]U.S. Congress. Office of Technology Assessment. *Adolescent Health, Volume II: Background and the Effectiveness of Selected Prevention and Treatment Services.* Washington, GPO, Nov. 1991. p. II-547.

[39]Fox, Harriette B. et al. *Medicaid Financing for Mental Health and Substance Abuse Services for Children and Adolescents.* Draft report prepared for the Alcohol, Drug Abuse, and Mental Health Administration. Washington, May 1990.

required prior authorization of the service, but only one imposed a limit on the amount of partial hospitalization (24 hours a year). (See table F-4.)

Physician services were provided without limits in nearly two-thirds of States, which, however, sometimes placed greater restrictions on psychiatrists' services than on the services of other physicians. Benefits in over half the States included services furnished by practitioners working autonomously but supervised by nurse practitioners and clinical social workers. (See table F-4.)

At the time of the survey in 1989, States, for the most part, had not used the EPSDT program's potential for providing specialized screening or augmented diagnostic and treatment benefits to children with substance abuse problems. Most States (43) reported that they would pay for laboratory tests under EPSDT to confirm substance abuse where suspected by the screening provider, but no State had established referral protocols for further evaluation and treatment of children suspected of having a substance abuse problem.

The survey also discovered that only a few States used such optional services as clinic services, rehabilitative services, inpatient psychiatric facility services, and targeted case management services, for children's substance abuse treatment services. Substance abuse clinic services, for instance, were covered in only 11 States. While all but one of these States provided potentially unlimited coverage, 5 of the 11 covered treatment services for drug abuse only and the other 6 reimbursed alcohol abuse and drug abuse treatment. (See table F-5.)

TABLE F-2. Potential for Financing Substance Abuse Prevention and Treatment Services for Children and Adolescents under Medicaid

Service	Mandatory Medicaid service (including mandatory EPSDT service)[a]	Optional Medicaid service (including mandatory EPSDT service)[a]
Early identification	Outpatient hospital, physician and physician-supervised, and EPSDT services	Clinic, rehabilitative, licensed psychologist and social worker, and screening services
Assessment and diagnosis	EPSDT diagnostic services	Diagnostic services
Case management	None	Targeted case management
Outpatient treatment	Outpatient hospital and physician-supervised services	Clinic, rehabilitative, and licensed psychologist and social worker services
Residential treatment services (excluding room and board)	Some components under physician and physician-supervised services	Rehabilitative services (and some components under clinic, personal care and licensed psychologist and social worker services)
Inpatient hospital	Inpatient hospital services (and some components under physician services)	Psychiatric facilities for individuals under 21
Detoxification	Inpatient hospital, outpatient hospital, and physician and physician-supervised services	Psychiatric facilities for individuals under 21 and rehabilitative services

[a]OBRA 89 made all federally allowable services mandatory when medically necessary to correct or ameliorate a physical or mental problem discovered during an EPSDT screening examination.

Source: Adapted from a table in Fox et al. U.S. Dept. of Health and Human Services. *Medicaid Financing for Mental Health and Substance Abuse Services for Children and Adolescents.* Report prepared for ADAMHA, May 1990. Washington, 1990.

TABLE F-3. State Coverage of Inpatient Substance Abuse Services in General Hospitals, as of June 30, 1989

State	Includes substance abuse treatment	Day limit for inpatient substance abuse services	Prior authorization required
Alabama	Yes	12 days/year	No
Alaska	Detox only	None	Yes
Arkansas	Yes	35 days/year	Yes
California	Detox only	None	Yes
Colorado	Yes	None	Yes
Connecticut	Yes	None	Yes
Delaware	No	NA	NA
District of Columbia	Detox only	21 days/year	No
Florida	Detox only	45 days/year	No
Georgia	Detox only	Varies with diagnosis	No
Hawaii	Detox only	None	Yes
Idaho	Detox only	None	No
Illinois	Detox only	5 days/admission	No
Indiana	Detox only	None	Yes

See notes at end of table.

TABLE F-3. State Coverage of Inpatient Substance Abuse Services in General Hospitals, as of June 30, 1989--Continued

State	Includes substance abuse treatment	Day limit for inpatient substance abuse services	Prior authorization required
Iowa	Yes	None	No
Kansas	Yes	3 admissions/lifetime	Yes
Kentucky	Detox only	14 days/year	Yes
Louisiana	Yes	15 days/year	No
Maine	Yes	None	No
Maryland	Detox only	None	No
Massachusetts	Methadone only	28 days/6 months	No
Michigan	Detox only	None	No
Minnesota	Yes	None	Yes
Mississippi	Yes	15 days/year	Yes
Missouri	Yes	Varies with diagnosis	No
Montana	Detox only	None	Yes
Nebraska	Detox only	5 days/admission	Yes

See notes at end of table.

TABLE F-3. State Coverage of Inpatient Substance Abuse Services in General Hospitals, as of June 30, 1989--Continued

State	Includes substance abuse treatment	Day limit for inpatient substance abuse services	Prior authorization required
Nevada	Detox only	4 days/admission	Yes
New Hampshire	Detox only	None	No
New Jersey	Detox only	None	No
New York[a]	Detox and rehab/Detox only	None	No
North Carolina	Yes	None	Yes
Ohio	Detox only	None	No
Oklahoma	Yes	60 days/year	No
Oregon	Detox only	5 days/admission	Yes
Pennsylvania	Detox only	None	No
Rhode Island	Yes	None	No
South Carolina	Detox only	None	No
South Dakota	Detox only	5 days/admission	No
Tennessee	Detox only	None	Yes
Texas	Detox only	6 days/admission	No

See notes at end of table.

TABLE F-3. State Coverage of Inpatient Substance Abuse Services
in General Hospitals, as of June 30, 1989--Continued

State	Includes substance abuse treatment	Day limit for inpatient substance abuse services	Prior authorization required
Utah	Detox only	21 days/admission	No
Vermont	Yes	None	No
Virginia	No	NA	NA
Washington	Detox only	3 days/admission	No
West Virginia	Detox only	3 days/admission	No
Wisconsin	Yes	None	Yes
Wyoming	Detox only	None	Yes
TOTAL	48	21	19

ªNew York has separate policies for alcohol and drug abuse reimbursement. In cases in which both policies apply, the alcohol policy is listed first, followed by the drug policy.

Source: Fox et al. U.S. Dept. of Health and Human Services. *Medicaid Financing for Mental Health and Substance Abuse Services for Children and Adolescents.* Report prepared for ADAMHA, May 1990. Washington, 1990.

TABLE F-4. State Coverage of Outpatient Substance Abuse Treatment Services in General and Psychiatric Hospitals, as of June 30, 1989

State	General hospitals	Psychiatric hospitals	Coverage limits	Prior authorization required	Available for youth	Coverage limits	Prior authorization required
Arkansas	Yes	No	12 visits/ year for all outpatient hospital	No	No	NA	NA
California	Yes	Yes	None	No	No	NA	NA
Colorado	Yes	Yes	None	No	No	NA	NA
Connecticut	Yes	Yes	None	Yes	Yes	None	Yes
Delaware	Yes	No	None	No	Yes	None	No
Georgia	Yes	No	None	No	No	NA	NA
Hawaii	Yes	No	None	Yes	No	NA	NA
Idaho	No	Yes	None	No	No	NA	NA
Illinois	Yes	No	3 hours/day	No	No	NA	NA
Indiana	Yes	Yes	None	Yes	No	NA	NA
Iowa	Yes	Yes	25 visits/year	Yes	No	NA	NA
Kentucky	Yes[a]	No	None	No	No	NA	NA

See notes at end of table.

TABLE F-4. State Coverage of Outpatient Substance Abuse Treatment Services in General and Psychiatric Hospitals, as of June 30, 1989--Continued

State	General hospitals	Psychiatric hospitals	Coverage limits	Prior authorization required	Available for youth	Coverage limits	Prior authorization required
Louisiana	Yes	No	None	No	No	NA	NA
Maine	Yes	No	None	No	Yes	None	No
Maryland	Yes	Yes	None	No	No	NA	NA
Massachusetts	Yes	Yes	None	No	No	NA	NA
Mississippi	Yes	No	6 visits/year for all outpatient hospital	No	No	NA	NA
Missouri	Yes	Yes	None	No	No	NA	NA
Montana	Yes	No	None	No	No	NA	NA
Nevada	Yes	No	NA	NA	No	NA	NA
New Hampshire	No	No	NA	NA	No	NA	NA
New Jersey	Yes	Yes	None	No	Yes	None	Yes

See notes at end of table.

TABLE F-4. State Coverage of Outpatient Substance Abuse Treatment Services in General and Psychiatric Hospitals, as of June 30, 1989--Continued

State	General hospitals	Psychiatric hospitals	Coverage limits	Prior authorization required	Available for youth	Coverage limits	Prior authorization required
New York[b]	Yes/ methadone maintenance only	Yes/No	None	No	Yes/No	None	No
North Carolina	Yes	Yes	24 visits/ year for all hospital, clinic, and physician	Yes	Yes	24 visits/ year for all hospital, clinic, and physician	No
North Dakota	Yes	Yes	None	No	No	NA	NA
Ohio	Yes	No	10 visits/month	Yes	No	NA	NA
Oklahoma	Yes	No	1 visit/day for all outpatient hospital	No	No	NA	NA
Pennsylvania	Yes	No	Varies with intervention	No	No	NA	NA
Rhode Island	Yes	No	None	No	No	NA	NA

See notes at end of table.

TABLE F-4. State Coverage of Outpatient Substance Abuse Treatment Services
in General and Psychiatric Hospitals, as of June 30, 1989--Continued

State	General hospitals	Psychiatric hospitals	Coverage limits	Prior authorization required	Available for youth	Coverage limits	Prior authorization required
South Carolina	Yes	No	None	No	No	NA	NA
South Dakota	Yes	No	None	No	No	NA	NA
Tennessee	Yes	No	30 visits/ year for all outpatient hospital	No	No	NA	NA
Texas	Yes	No	$313/ year	No	No	NA	NA
Vermont	No	Yes	None	No	No	NA	NA
TOTAL	31	14	10	7	6	1	2

[a]Substance abuse visits are covered only if another primary diagnosis is present and substance abuse is secondary.

[b]New York has separate policies for alcohol and drug abuse reimbursement. In cases in which both policies apply, the alcohol policy is listed first, followed by the drug policy.

Source: Fox et al. U.S. Dept. of Health and Human Services. *Medicaid Financing for Mental Health and Substance Abuse Services for Children and Adolescents.* Report prepared for ADAMHA, May 1990. Washington, 1990.

TABLE F-5. State Coverage of Substance Abuse Clinic Services, as of June 30, 1989

State	Assessment	Individual, group, and family therapy	Day treatment	Other services[a]	Coverage limits	Prior authorization required
California	Yes	Yes	No	Yes	None	No
Connecticut	Yes	Yes	No	Yes	None	Yes
Delaware	No	No	No	Yes	None	No
Hawaii[b]	Yes	Yes	No	Yes	None	Yes
Illinois	Yes	Yes[c]	Yes	No	None	No
Indiana[b]	Yes	Yes	No	Yes	None	Yes
Iowa[b]	Yes	Yes	Yes	Yes	None	No
Louisiana	Yes	Yes	No	Yes	None	No
Maryland	Yes	Yes	No	Yes	None	No
Nevada	No	No	No	Yes	None	Yes
New Jersey	Yes	Yes	No	Yes	None	No
New York[d]	Yes	Yes/No	Yes/No	Yes	None	No
Pennsylvania	Yes	Yes	No	Yes	Varies with intervention	No
Utah	No	No	No	Yes	None	No
TOTAL	11	11	3	13	1	4

[a]"Other services" include drug maintenance and collateral contacts.
[b]Clinic services in these States apply to all clinic services generally; they are not specific to substance abuse clinics.
[c]Illinois does not cover family therapy.
[d]New York has separate policies for alcohol and drug abuse reimbursement. In cases in which both policies apply, the alcohol policy is listed first, followed by the drug policy.

Source: Fox et al. U.S. Dept. of Health and Human Services. *Medicaid Financing for Mental Health and Substance Abuse Services for Children and Adolescents.* Report prepared for ADAMHA, May 1990. Washington, 1990.

The rehabilitative services benefit was used in 10 States to reimburse substance abuse treatment services for children. Six of these States cover treatment only in freestanding alcohol and drug abuse treatment centers. Three States reimburse for rehabilitation services in a combination of outpatient and residential providers: Florida and Wisconsin reimburse both freestanding clinics and residential programs, and Michigan reimburses hospital outpatient units and residential programs. Minnesota restricts its reimbursement for rehabilitative services to inpatient and residential providers. All 10 States provide coverage for individual, group, and family counseling, while 8 States cover assessment as well. Four States include drug maintenance, while three reimburse crisis intervention. Six States have no coverage limitation for rehabilitative services for substance abuse; the other four impose limits which vary by the type of service provided. Five of the 10 States use the rehabilitative services option to cover day treatment for substance abuse. (See table F-6.)

The inpatient psychiatric services benefit for substance abuse services for individuals under age 21 was provided by 35 States, usually without limits. Most of these States reimbursed only traditional freestanding psychiatric hospitals; only seven States reimbursed services in smaller residential treatment facilities. Treatment of substance abuse problems was included in nearly all States when it was the secondary diagnosis and in over one-third when it was the primary diagnosis. (See table F-7.) The targeted case management benefit was used in only four States (Georgia, North Carolina, West Virginia, and Wisconsin) to serve children with substance abuse problems.

TABLE F-6. State Coverage of Substance Abuse Rehabilitative Services, as of June 30, 1989

State	Assessment	Individual, group, and family therapy	Crisis intervention	Drug maintenance	Other services	Day treatment	Coverage limits	Prior authorization required
Florida	Yes	Yes	No	No	No	Yes	None	No
Illinois	Yes	Yes[a]	No	No	No	Yes	None	No
Maine	Yes	Yes	Yes	No	Yes	No	Varies with intervention	No
Michigan	No	Yes	No	Yes	No	No	None	No
Minnesota	No	Yes	No	No	Yes	No	None	Yes
Mississippi	Yes	Yes	No	Yes	No	Yes	Varies with intervention	Yes
Oregon	Yes	Yes	No	Yes	Yes	No	Varies with intervention	No
Rhode Island	Yes	Yes	No	No	No	No	Varies with intervention	Yes
South Carolina	Yes	Yes	Yes	No	Yes	Yes	None	No
Wisconsin	Yes	Yes	Yes	Yes	No	Yes	None	Yes
TOTAL	8	10	3	4	4	5	4	4

[a]Family therapy is not covered.

Source: Fox et al. U.S. Dept. of Health and Human Services. *Medicaid Financing for Mental Health and Substance Abuse Services for Children and Adolescents.* Report prepared for ADAMHA, May 1990. Washington, 1990.

TABLE F-7. State Coverage of Inpatient Psychiatric Facilities for Individuals Under 21, as of June 30, 1989

State	Psychiatric hospitals	ICFs or SNFs[a]	Residential treatment facilities	Includes substance abuse treatment	Coverage limits	Prior authorization required
Alaska	Yes	No	No	As secondary diagnosis	No	Yes
Arkansas	Yes	No	Yes	As secondary diagnosis	No	Yes
California	Yes	No	No	As secondary diagnosis	No	Yes
Colorado	Yes	No	Yes	As secondary diagnosis	No	Yes
Connecticut	Yes	No	No	As primary diagnosis	No	No
District of Columbia	Yes	No	No	As secondary diagnosis	No	No
Illinois	Yes	No	No	As secondary diagnosis	No	No
Indiana	Yes	No	No	As primary diagnosis	No	Yes
Iowa	Yes	No	Yes	As secondary diagnosis	No	No
Kansas	Yes	Yes	No	As primary diagnosis	No	No
Kentucky	Yes	No	No	As secondary diagnosis	No	No
Louisiana	Yes	No	No	As primary diagnosis	No	No
Maine	Yes	No	No	As primary diagnosis	No	No
Maryland	Yes	No	Yes	As secondary diagnosis	No	No
Massachusetts	Yes	No	No	As primary diagnosis	No	No
Michigan	Yes	Yes	No	As secondary diagnosis	No	Yes

See notes at end of table.

TABLE F-7. State Coverage of Inpatient Psychiatric Facilities for Individuals Under 21, as of June 30, 1989—Continued

State	Psychiatric hospitals	ICFs or SNFs[A]	Residential treatment facilities	Includes substance abuse treatment	Coverage limits	Prior authorization required
Minnesota	Yes	No	No	As secondary diagnosis	No	Yes
Missouri	Yes	No	No	As primary diagnosis	No	No
Montana	Yes	No	No	No	No	Yes
Nebraska	Yes	No	No	As secondary diagnosis	No	Yes
New Jersey	Yes	No	Yes	As secondary diagnosis	No	Yes
New York	Yes	No	No	As secondary diagnosis	No	No
North Carolina	Yes	No	No	As primary diagnosis	No	No
North Dakota	Yes	No	No	As secondary diagnosis	No	No
Ohio	Yes	No	No	As secondary diagnosis	No	No
Oklahoma	Yes	No	Yes	As primary diagnosis	60 days/year	No
Oregon	Yes	No	No	Detox as secondary diagnosis	No	Yes
Pennsylvania	Yes	No	No	As primary diagnosis	No	No
Rhode Island	Yes	Yes	Yes	As primary diagnosis	No	No
South Carolina	Yes	No	No	As secondary diagnosis	No	No
Tennessee	Yes	No	No	As secondary diagnosis	No	Yes
Utah	Yes	No	No	Detox as secondary diagnosis	No	Yes

See notes at end of table.

TABLE F-7. State Coverage of Inpatient Psychiatric Facilities for Individuals Under 21, as of June 30, 1989--Continued

State	Psychiatric hospitals	ICFs or SNFs[a]	Residential treatment facilities	Includes substance abuse treatment	Coverage limits	Prior authorization required
Vermont	Yes	Yes	No	As primary diagnosis	No	Yes
Washington	Yes	No	No	As secondary diagnosis	No	Yes
West Virginia	Yes	No	No	As primary diagnosis	No	Yes
Wisconsin	Yes	No	No	As primary diagnosis	No	Yes
TOTAL	36	4	7	35	1	17

[a]Intermediate care facilities or skilled nursing facilities.

Source: Fox et al. U.S. Dept. of Health and Human Services. *Medicaid Financing for Mental Health and Substance Abuse Services for Children and Adolescents.* Report prepared for ADAMHA, May 1990. Washington, 1990.

APPENDIX G. MANAGED CARE[1]

I. INTRODUCTION

In recent years, States have experimented with managed care programs in the hope of reducing unnecessary utilization of Medicaid services and thus containing costs, while possibly achieving greater coordination and continuity of care. The phrase "managed care" is used in a variety of senses; for the purpose of the following discussion, the term is used to refer to systems in which the overall care of a patient is overseen by a single provider or organization.

The basic model for managed care is the health maintenance organization, or HMO, which receives a fixed periodic payment (known as a capitation payment or premium) for each individual served and accepts financial responsibility for all the covered medical services required by that individual. If the beneficiaries enrolled under the arrangement use more, or more costly, services than anticipated, the HMO may suffer a loss. If the enrollees use fewer services than anticipated, the HMO may realize a profit. The organization is therefore said to be "at risk" for the set of services covered by the contract. The risk arrangement is intended to give the HMO a financial incentive to furnish services more efficiently.

Persons enrolled in the HMO receive all services, except in emergencies, from providers employed by or affiliated with the HMO. Ordinarily, the enrollee has a single primary care physician, who must authorize specialty care and inpatient hospital services. The HMO may pass on to physicians some of its own financial incentives to reduce unnecessary services. In some arrangements the physicians receive a fixed monthly payment for their assigned patients or are partially at risk for the costs of services they order; in others, the physicians may share in profits or losses at the end of a year. Their medical decisions may also be subject to review by the central HMO administration. In addition to reducing the use of services, HMOs may also achieve savings by contracting with low-cost hospitals and other providers, or by negotiating discounts from providers' usual charges.[2]

---

[1]This appendix was written by Mark Merlis.

[2]Some analysts believe that HMOs can also achieve savings through preventive medicine--finding problems early, before they become more serious and expensive to treat. Others believe that these "health maintenance" practices, while they gave HMOs their name, are not a significant factor in HMO savings.

The managed care concept has been of interest to Medicaid programs, as well as to other purchasers of health care, because it appears to offer a way of changing provider and beneficiary behaviors which may have contributed to rising costs in the traditional fee-for-service system. In at least some areas, many Medicaid beneficiaries receive routine health services in hospital outpatient departments and emergency rooms, at greater cost than if they had used office-based physician services. In other areas, "Medicaid mills" provide perfunctory care to large numbers of beneficiaries to generate high fee-for-service revenues. Some beneficiaries engage in "doctor shopping," visiting multiple providers for a single complaint. The providers themselves, paid for each service they perform, may have an incentive to maximize their own services and may have no reason to control the referral services they order. Managed care, it is argued, can provide control over the beneficiaries' behavior and change the incentives for providers. Advocates of managed care also contend that it may improve the coordination and continuity of care.

Critics of managed care programs say that providers may respond to the new incentives, not just by providing care more efficiently, but also by denying needed services. Reports of quality problems and other abuses in some Medicaid managed care experiments have led Congress to place restrictions on the types of organizations that may participate and on the terms under which the programs may operate. In addition, there is a continuing debate over the ability of managed care to produce additional savings for Medicaid programs that are already purchasing many services at below-market rates. Still, 31 States were operating some form of managed care program by 1991.

Many States have contracted with HMOs to furnish services to beneficiaries. Others have developed systems that retain some of the managed care features of HMOs but that do not involve the substantial risks (and hence the need for capital and experienced management) presented by HMOs. Some States have used fee-for-service case management. Individual physicians or groups are paid a fee to manage the care of assigned patients but are not at direct financial risk for the services the patients use. Other States have developed "partial capitation systems." The providers are paid a premium for each enrollee and accept financial risk for a limited group of services, such as all physician and diagnostic services, but are not at risk for the most expensive services, such as hospital inpatient. Finally, some States have experimented with health insuring organizations, or HIOs, which are a cross between HMOs and fee-for-service case management programs, enrolling all the beneficiaries in a given area.

This appendix reviews States' experiences with each of these types of managed care systems and discusses their current status and possible future role in the Medicaid program.

II. HISTORY OF MANAGED CARE UNDER MEDICAID

A. HMO Contracting Before 1981

Some States began contracting with HMOs or similar entities almost immediately after implementing their Medicaid programs.[3] The earliest initiatives were in the States where HMOs were already a relatively familiar concept. In New York City, for example, where municipal employees had long been enrolled in the HMO-like Health Insurance Plan of Greater New York (HIP), membership in HIP was made available to Medicaid beneficiaries as early as 1967. The State of Washington began contracting with Group Health of Puget Sound in 1970, while the various regional operations of Kaiser-Permanente were accepting Medicaid enrollments in three different States by 1972.

The earliest significant commitment to Medicaid prepaid contracting came in California, where concerns about the escalating costs of the Medicaid program had led to stringent cost containment measures, including tight restrictions on physician services, by the early 1970s. Prepaid health plans (PHPs) were promoted as an alternative way of achieving savings. The State entered into numerous prepaid contracts, both with established HMOs and brand-new ones--many of them formed solely to deal with Medicaid. The contractors marketed directly, "door to door," to beneficiaries, and enrollment grew rapidly.

Soon, however, there were reports of abuses in the California prepaid program. Some of the contractors used unscrupulous marketing approaches, telling beneficiaries that the State required them to join an HMO, failing to disclose that HMO members had to use the HMO's own providers, or offering additional benefits which never materialized. Some contractors were reported to have engaged in "skimming," refusing to enroll potentially high-cost beneficiaries. Once beneficiaries had joined an HMO, they had trouble getting out; contractors would delay disenrollment requests or refuse to accept them at all. There were quality of care problems as well--some of the organizations were unable to, or refused to, furnish the full scope of Medicaid benefits. Others were financially unsound, leaving beneficiaries at risk of becoming liable for their own medical bills. Still others were reported to have diverted funds from medical services through contracts with profit-making affiliates.[4]

---

[3]As Chapter VI, *Alternate Delivery Options and Waiver Programs* indicates, States may enter into risk contracts with a variety of organizations that are not technically HMOs and that are known as prepaid health plans or PHPs. In the following discussion, the term HMO will generally be used to include both HMOs and PHPs.

[4]The problems in the California program are detailed in three General Accounting Office reports. U.S. General Accounting Office. *Better Controls Needed for Health Maintenance Organizations Under Medicaid in California.* Report to the Committee on Finance, United States Senate. B-164031(3), Sept. 1974. Washington, 1974; U.S. General Accounting Office. *Deficiencies in*

(continued...)

California responded to these problems by enacting more rigorous requirements for HMOs. Federal demonstration funds were made available to develop a model Medicaid HMO contracting and monitoring system. However, national reports of the abuses in California and of similar problems in some of the other States experimenting with prepayment led to congressional action as well.

The Health Maintenance Organization Amendments of 1976 (Public Law 94-460) included the first specific Federal requirements for Medicaid contracts with HMOs or comparable organizations. Full-service risk contracts could be offered only to federally qualified HMOs, those certified by the Secretary as meeting organizational, financial, and quality standards set forth in Title XIII of the Public Health Service Act. Exceptions were made for certain federally funded community or migrant health centers and for organizations, such as HIP of New York, which had Medicaid contracts prior to 1970. In addition, an HMO which had applied for Federal qualification but which had not yet received a final determination could be deemed "provisionally qualified" by the State, and could continue to contract with Medicaid on that basis until the application was approved or denied.

The 1976 amendments also forestalled further development of Medicaid-only HMOs through a provision that no more than 50 percent of a risk contractor's enrollees could be Medicaid or Medicare beneficiaries. Again, exceptions were made for federally funded centers and pre-1970 contractors. New contractors could take up to 3 years to meet the requirement if they could show that they were making satisfactory progress towards compliance.

The effect of these changes was generally to limit new State prepaid initiatives to established organizations which could complete the protracted and elaborate Federal qualification process, as well as to eliminate some existing contractors unable to meet the Federal standards. Although some States, faced with the rapid increases in Medicaid costs of the late 1970s and early 1980s, were interested in trying prepaid approaches, they found that established HMOs were reluctant to take on a Medicaid contract. A number of factors deterred HMOs from participating:[5]

---

[4](...continued)
Determining Payments to Prepaid Health Plans Under California's Medicaid Program. Report to the Committee on Finance, United States Senate. MWD-76-15, Aug. 1975. Washington, 1975; U.S. General Accounting Office. *Relationships Between Nonprofit Prepaid Health Plans With California Medicaid Contracts and For Profit Entities Affiliated With Them.* HRD-77-4, Nov. 1976. Washington, 1976.

[5]For a summary of the status of Medicaid HMO contracting as of early 1981 and the outstanding problems at that time, see: U.S. Dept. of Health and Human Services. Health Care Financing Administration. *HMOs: Issues and Alternatives for Medicare and Medicaid.* Prepared by Trieger, Sidney, Trudi W. Galblum, and Gerald Riley. HCFA Pub. No. 03107, 1981. Baltimore, 1981.

1013

- There was a widespread perception in the HMO industry that Medicaid beneficiaries were costly and had difficulty adjusting to an HMO environment, tending to continue using emergency rooms and other nonplan providers.

- In the private sector, HMOs were accustomed to marketing to large employer groups through direct presentations, mailings, or other means during periodic open seasons. Medicaid beneficiaries were less accessible; they were never assembled in a single place, as employees are at the worksite, and Federal confidentiality rules prohibited the release of their names to HMOs. Medicaid marketing was a costly, hit-or-miss process, often requiring door-to-door canvassing.

- Beneficiaries often had little incentive to enroll. In the private sector, HMOs competed by offering lower out-of-pocket costs or more benefits than other health plans. Medicaid beneficiaries had virtually no out-of-pocket costs, and some States' Medicaid benefits were so comprehensive that HMOs were unable to develop appealing add-ons.

- While private enrollees generally remained enrolled for a year, between annual open enrollment periods, Medicaid beneficiaries might be enrolled for much briefer periods, either because they withdrew voluntarily or because they became ineligible for Medicaid benefits.

- Some HMOs were concerned that participation in Medicaid would give them a "welfare image," hindering them in private market competition.

- HMOs in some States found Medicaid reimbursement rates unacceptable. Federal regulations require that premiums paid for Medicaid beneficiaries enrolled in an HMO not exceed the average amount that would have been paid for the same group of beneficiaries if they had been treated outside the HMO. Medicaid HMO premiums therefore reflected the discounted prices paid by Medicaid in the fee-for-service sector, although HMOs might have been unable to obtain comparable discounts from hospitals or other providers.

As a result of these barriers, along with the reluctance of many States to experiment with the HMO approach, only 281,926 beneficiaries were enrolled in HMOs in June 1981, little more than 1 percent of the Medicaid population. Of the HMO enrollees, 85 percent were in just four States: California, Maryland, Michigan, and New York.

B. Legislative Changes, 1981-1982

The Omnibus Budget Reconciliation Act of 1981 (OBRA 81, Public Law 97-35) gave States greater flexibility in contracting with HMOs and also allowed States to explore other managed care approaches.

There were four important changes in the Federal Medicaid HMO contracting rules. First, Medicaid contracts were no longer limited to federally qualified HMOs. The State could make its own determination that an organization was qualified, if the HMO demonstrated its capacity to provide covered services and to protect beneficiaries from liability in the event of the organization's insolvency. Second, up to 75 percent of an organization's enrollees could be Medicaid and Medicare beneficiaries, as opposed to the previous 50 percent limit. (This requirement has become known as the "75-25 rule.") Third, States could offer "guaranteed eligibility" to beneficiaries joining federally qualified HMOs. The State could continue paying premiums on an enrollee's behalf for up to 6 months following the date of initial enrollment, even if the enrollee ceased to be eligible for Medicaid benefits during that period. While these three changes expanded States' options, a fourth limited them-- States could not restrict voluntary disenrollment. Beneficiaries had to be permitted to terminate their enrollment in an HMO at any time, with the termination taking effect no later than the end of the month following the month in which the beneficiary requested disenrollment.

The OBRA 81 also established the section 1915(b) freedom-of-choice waiver program, under which States could require beneficiaries to enroll in some form of managed care system. (Details of the section 1915(b) provisions may be found in *Chapter VI, Alternate Delivery Options and Waiver Programs.*)

As enacted, section 1915(b) permitted the Secretary to waive provisions of two parts of the Medicaid law: section 1902 (which included such basic requirements as freedom-of-choice, uniform statewide operation, and comparability of benefits for different types of beneficiaries), and section 1903(m), the section of the Medicaid law that contained the basic rules for prepaid contracts. Several States applied for and obtained waivers of section 1903(m) provisions, allowing them to contract with organizations which did not meet contract eligibility requirements (such as the 75 percent Medicaid/Medicare enrollment limit) or to restrict enrollees' ability to disenroll without cause.

These waivers, in combination with waivers for a primary care case management program, might have permitted a State to require all Medicaid beneficiaries to enroll in a single HMO serving Medicaid patients only. The Tax Equity and Fiscal Responsibility Act of 1982 (TEFRA, Public Law 97-248) repealed the Secretary's authority to waive section 1903(m) requirements in connection with a section 1915(b) waiver program; waivers already granted could continue but could not be renewed after their original 2-year term. The Secretary retained the authority to waive HMO requirements in order to conduct short-term demonstration projects.

C. Recent Developments

The TEFRA change in the Secretary's waiver authority left States with four major managed care options:

1. Promotion of voluntary enrollment in HMOs;

2. Voluntary or mandatory enrollment in fee-for-service or "partial capitation" primary care case management systems;

3. Voluntary or mandatory enrollment in "HIOs," which resembled HMOs, but were not at first subject to 1903(m) requirements, for reasons to be detailed below;

4. Mandatory enrollment in multiple-HMO systems, under which a beneficiary could voluntarily disenroll from one organization but would then be required to join another.

The following section provides an overview of the ways in which States have made use of these basic options. The section concludes with a brief discussion of the "social health maintenance organization" (S/HMO) demonstrations and similar experiments. These programs, targeted at the elderly, are largely a Medicare initiative but have some Medicaid involvement.

1. Voluntary HMO Enrollment

As of June 1990, 880,057 beneficiaries were voluntarily enrolled in HMOs and other comprehensive prepaid health plans, in 23 States. Many mainstream HMOs still hesitate to consider a Medicaid contract, for essentially the same reasons cited in 1981--low reimbursement rates, discontinuous Medicaid eligibility, and marketing problems.[6] Still, States have taken a number of steps to make Medicaid participation more attractive.

In place of direct door-to-door marketing, which was costly and subject to abuse, several States have developed "dual choice" systems, in which beneficiaries are informed of their health care options at the time they apply for Medicaid benefits. Usually these systems involve State representatives, stationed in local social services offices, who describe the differences between the HMO and fee-for-service alternatives. In a few States the HMOs themselves have been given direct access to the social services offices.

Some States have implemented the guaranteed eligibility option described above, which prevents rapid involuntary disenrollment because of loss of

---

[6]See U.S. House. Committee on Energy and Commerce. Subcommittee on Health and the Environment. *Medicaid Budget Initiatives*. Testimony of Barbara Hill. Hearings, Serial No. 101-206, 101st Cong., 2d Sess., Sept. 14, 1990. Washington, GPO, 1990. p. 455-477. (Hereafter cited as House Energy and Commerce Committee, *Medicaid Budget Initiatives*)

eligibility and may promote continuity of care. As a result of a change in the Deficit Reduction Act of 1984 (Public Law 98-369), States are also permitted to restrict voluntary disenrollment without cause for up to 6 months (really 5 months following a 1 month trial period); the option applies to enrollees in federally qualified HMOs, most types of PHPs, and State-qualified HMOs that have a Medicare contract.

Possibly as a result of these initiatives, voluntary HMO enrollment under Medicaid grew 33 percent from December 1987 to June 1990, reaching a total of 880,057 enrollees. However, enrollment remains heavily concentrated in a few States. California and Michigan accounted for 41 percent of total enrollment in June 1990; the same two States were also the major centers of HMO enrollment in 1981. Six more States, Illinois, Ohio, Pennsylvania, Florida, New York, and Maryland, account for another 36 percent of total enrollment. Except for Florida, all of these States were already active in prepaid contracting in the 1970s.

A 1990 survey by the Group Health Association of America, an HMO industry organization, found that only 22 percent of the HMOs responding participated in the Medicaid program. Participation was higher among older and larger organizations and among staff-model HMOs (those that use their own facilities and salaried staff to provide care instead of contracting with independent physicians.)[7]

New Jersey has developed an alternative to State contracting with private HMOs. It has established its own organization, the Garden State Health Plan, to provide services to Medicaid beneficiaries enrolled on a voluntary basis. OBRA 87 exempted this organization from some of the Medicaid HMO rules and allowed New Jersey to offer guaranteed eligibility to enrollees in the plan.

2. *Primary Care Case Management*

The reluctance of private market HMOs to serve a Medicaid clientele, along with the statutory constraints which inhibited the development of HMO-like programs for Medicaid beneficiaries alone, led States to look for other ways of obtaining the perceived advantages of HMO contracting--management of patients and financial incentives to improve efficiency. Operating under a section 1115(a) demonstration waiver, Massachusetts developed the first primary care case management program in 1979.

A beneficiary would select a single primary care provider and would agree to obtain covered services from other providers only with the primary care provider's authorization; the State would deny payment for any unauthorized services except emergency care. The primary care provider would manage the overall care of the patient and attempt to reduce unnecessary referral services

---

[7]Group Health Association of America (GHAA). *HMO Industry Profile: 1991 Edition*, v. 1. Washington, 1990. p. 91; Group Health Association of America. *GHAA Survey of Member Plans With Medicaid Contracts: Findings*, GHAA Research Brief No. 11. Washington, Aug. 1990.

or inpatient hospital admissions. The provider would serve as a "gatekeeper," an intermediary between the patient and the rest of the medical care system. Resulting savings could be shared with the State, perhaps in the form of an incentive payment for reduced hospitalization.

The Massachusetts program encountered start-up problems, especially in the area of data processing, and did not produce clear results in the initial demonstration period. Nevertheless, the concept of primary care case management for Medicaid beneficiaries received considerable attention. As noted earlier, OBRA 81 gave States the option of requiring beneficiaries to participate in a case management program.

Michigan was the first State to take advantage of the new option, obtaining approval for its Physician Primary Sponsor Plan in 1981. This program differed from the Massachusetts prototype in two major ways. First, while Massachusetts used a small number of community health centers or physician group practices as case managers, Michigan used numerous individual physicians, each managing a limited number of cases. Second, enrollment in the Massachusetts program was voluntary; beneficiaries were offered cash incentives to participate. Michigan, using the new freedom-of-choice waiver option, planned to require all Aid to Families with Dependent Children (AFDC) beneficiaries in Wayne County (the Detroit area) to participate, or about 280,000 enrollees.

The Michigan program was slow in starting, chiefly because of problems in matching so many beneficiaries with individual physicians. Many of the enrollees failed to select a physician on their own and were assigned to a provider by the State.[8] By mid-1986, 4 years after project implementation, only an estimated 82,000 beneficiaries had actually been enrolled. As of mid-1991 the program had about 100,000 enrollees (including voluntary enrollees but not counting mandatory enrollees who opted for an HMO instead of the Physician Sponsor Program).

In the years since the Michigan project began, two basic kinds of case management programs have evolved. One model resembles Michigan's--the State contracts with individual physicians, paid on a fee-for-service basis, to oversee beneficiaries' care. The second model uses partial capitation--the primary care provider is paid a fixed premium, out of which it covers the costs of its own services and ambulatory referral care, such as specialty or diagnostic services. The State remains directly responsible for inpatient hospital care. This model was used extensively in Oregon, and has also been tried in parts of California, Michigan, Nevada, and New York.

Most of the fee-for-service case management programs have involved mandatory enrollment. Certain types of beneficiaries are commonly exempt

---

[8]National Governors' Association. Center for Research Policy. *Prepaid and Managed Care Under Medicaid: Characteristics of Current Initiatives.* Prepared by Karen I. Squarrell, Suzanne M. Hansen, and Edward Neuschler. Washington, 1985.

from enrollment, including foster children, persons in institutions, and persons eligible for both Medicare and Medicaid. Five case management programs, in Colorado, Kentucky, Maryland, New Mexico, and Utah, operate on a statewide basis as of 1991, though enrollment is not necessarily mandatory in all parts of the State. The remaining programs are confined to individual counties or metropolitan areas. As table G-1 indicates, the partial capitation programs have tended to rely on voluntary enrollment and have involved a relatively small number of participants.

A number of States have structured special case management programs for populations with specific medical needs. South Carolina developed such a program for high-risk pregnancies, Minnesota for substance abusers, and Maryland for diabetics. Illinois has developed a broader program in part of Chicago, under which a physician can refer Medicaid beneficiaries to a case management organization for ongoing coordination of a variety of chronic conditions, such as asthma, diabetes, or chronic mental illness. Although these programs are operated under section 1915(b) freedom-of-choice waivers and may resemble primary care case management projects in some other respects, their chief aim is to coordinate or facilitate services for the target group, rather than to control unnecessary utilization. For this reason, they are not treated as managed care programs for the purpose of this appendix and have not been included in the enrollment tables.

3. The HIO Experiments

After TEFRA repealed the Secretary's authority to waive HMO rules for States wishing to include full capitation as part of a mandatory primary care case management program, some States began exploring approaches that might be permissible within the framework of existing law. One solution was the "health insuring organization," or HIO.

The first HIOs, operating in Texas and in limited areas of California from the 1970s, functioned basically as fiscal intermediaries, processing provider claims for the Medicaid agency. Unlike other fiscal intermediaries, however, an HIO was not simply a conduit for Medicaid funds. The State paid the HIO a fixed per capita amount for each beneficiary in the area the HIO served, and the HIO was expected to cover all Medicaid claims out of that single fixed amount. Within limits, the HIO could make a profit or suffer a loss. Unlike an HMO, the HIO did not manage the care of patients or require beneficiaries to use a limited group of affiliated providers. Instead, the HIO used cost control methods that, in other States, were practiced directly by the State agency, such as preauthorization of services or post-payment utilization review.

In the early 1980s, however, States worked with the Health Care Financing Administration (HCFA) to find a way of incorporating managed care into the HIO structure. HCFA defined a new type of HIO, which could operate much like an HMO but which differed from HMOs in two respects:

- While an HMO could provide services directly, an HIO had to obtain all services through subcontractors, and no subcontractor could be at risk for both ambulatory and inpatient care.

- An HMO could select its own restricted set of participating providers. An HIO was required to accept any provider who could meet standard conditions of participation established by the HIO and who would agree to standard contractual terms.

The HCFA determined that an organization meeting the HIO definition was not subject to the 1903(m) restrictions on prepaid contracts. This meant that an HIO could be exempted from the 75 percent Medicaid enrollment maximum and that the State could restrict disenrollment from an HIO. In effect, the entire Medicaid population in a given geographic area could be required to enroll in a single entity, so long as beneficiaries remained free to select from among the providers participating in the HIO arrangement.

The first HIO program approved under the new rules was CitiCare in Louisville, Kentucky. All AFDC beneficiaries in the city were enrolled under a single contract with CitiCare, which agreed to accept liability for the full scope of Medicaid services. Each beneficiary chose a primary care provider from among those participating in the program. The physician, group, or clinic selected was paid for its own services and shared in any savings resulting from reductions in referral and hospital inpatient care; some of these providers accepted financial risk for ambulatory referral services.

CitiCare lasted only a year, abandoned in a change of State administrations amid charges of inadequate access to care and excess profits for the contractor administering the program.[9] Still, a number of other States proceeded with their own HIO projects, designed to serve whole cities or counties.

Some people argued that the distinction HCFA created between HIOs and HMOs was fictitious. One type of HMO uses an "individual practice association (IPA)" to furnish services; it contracts with individual physicians to treat HMO enrollees in their own offices, and it may allow any physician in the area to participate. If this organization were to contract with a State as an HMO, it would be subject to the requirement for disenrollment on demand and the 75 percent Medicare-Medicaid enrollment maximum. If it were relabeled an HIO, it would be exempt from these rules. Congress eliminated the distinction in the Consolidated Omnibus Budget Reconciliation Act of 1985 (COBRA, Public Law 99-272); any HIO which accepted risk for a comprehensive range of services was subject to the same rules as an HMO. HIO projects already operational as of January 1, 1986, are permanently exempt from the HMO rules. States may still contract with the earlier type of HIO, which more closely resembles a fiscal intermediary, and which does not provide managed care. States' use of this option is discussed in Chapter VI, *Alternate Delivery Options and Waiver Programs*.

---

[9]Freund, Deborah A., Polly M. Ehrenhaft, and Marie Hackbarth. *Medicaid Reform: Four Studies of Case Management*. Washington, 1984. p. 53-56.

Five exempt pre-1986 managed care HIOs were still operating in 1990--two in California and one each in Minnesota, Pennsylvania, and Washington. The largest was HealthPASS, a mandatory program serving beneficiaries in part of Philadelphia. HealthPASS has had numerous problems since it began operations in 1986. The initial contractor's parent firm went into bankruptcy, leading to delayed provider payments and reports of denial of services to beneficiaries. Federal approval of a successor contractor was later delayed because of questions about the State's method of selecting a bidder.[10] As of June 1990, the program had 77,783 enrollees.

The California HIOs are an outgrowth of an experiment under which public authorities were established in Monterey and Santa Barbara counties to serve area Medicaid beneficiaries. The county authority would be paid a premium by the State for each beneficiary and would in turn contract with physicians, hospitals, and other providers of service. These demonstrations faced financial losses and provider resistance, and the Monterey project was terminated.[11] The Santa Barbara Health Initiative continues in operation, and an additional project has been established in San Mateo County. OBRA 90 authorizes the operation of up to three more county-operated programs in California, so long as they do not enroll more than 10 percent of the State's Medicaid population and meet certain other requirements.

4. Mandatory HMO Enrollment

Although TEFRA restricted the Secretary's ability to waive HMO requirements under the 1915(b) freedom-of-choice waiver authority, the Secretary could still waive these requirements under a different authority. Section 1115(a) of the Social Security Act allows the waiver of nearly all Medicaid requirements for the purpose of conducting a demonstration project. The Secretary used this authority to conduct a number of experiments under which all Medicaid beneficiaries, in a given geographic area or a whole State, were required to enroll in an HMO.

In 1982 Arizona, the only State that had never established a Medicaid program, began an experimental medical assistance program under a section 1115(a) demonstration waiver.[12] The Arizona Health Care Cost Containment System (AHCCCS, pronounced "access") is an acute care medical assistance

---

[10]House Energy and Commerce Committee, *Medicaid Budget Initiatives*, the testimony of Thomas D. Roslewicz, Deputy Inspector General, p. 380-427.

[11]See U.S. Dept. of Health and Human Services. Health Care Financing Administration. *Health Care Financing Extramural Report: Nationwide Evaluation of Medicaid Competition Demonstrations.* HCFA Pub. No. 03236, v. 2, Santa Barbara Health Initiative, and v. 3, Monterey County Health Initiative. Baltimore, 1986.

[12]Much of the following discussion is based on: McCall, Nelda, et al. Evaluation of Arizona Health Care Cost Containment System. *Health Care Financing Review*, v. 9, no. 2, winter 1987. p. 79-90.

program comparable to Medicaid for AFDC and Supplemental Security Income (SSI) recipients, except that it does not offer a fee-for-service option. (Some medically needy persons are also served by AHCCCS, but there is no Federal funding for this component of the program.) In place of the usual open-ended Federal matching funds for service expenditures, AHCCCS receives a Federal per capita payment for each eligible beneficiary. The amount of the payment is negotiated with HCFA in advance. Counties make a contribution equal to a percentage of what they were spending for indigent care before 1982, and the State pays the remaining program costs.

Most beneficiaries are required to join an HMO contracting with AHCCCS (Indians eligible for care through the Indian Health Service are exempt and may receive care on a fee-for-service basis). As of June 1990, 216,202 beneficiaries were enrolled in 18 organizations. A combination of local and statewide contractors ensures that enrollees in most areas have at least two HMOs to choose from. Participants receive the mandatory Medicaid acute care services and some optional benefits.

Initially, long-term care services were excluded, as were mental health services for the chronically mentally ill. The omission of these services, normally mandatory under Medicaid, is one key reason that Arizona's program has not legally amounted to a Medicaid program (another is the use of a fixed per capita Federal payment in place of matching funds). Under a newer component of the AHCCCS demonstration, known as Arizona Long-Term Care System (ALTCS), counties and private contractors are furnishing long-term care on a prepaid basis with Federal financial participation. Mental health services are still omitted.

Management of the AHCCCS program was initially contracted out to a private plan administrator. During the early years of the program, there were administrative cost overruns, accompanied by reports of marketing, financial, and quality problems with some contractors. The State then took over direct management of AHCCCS, establishing a quality assurance system and other administrative controls. A 1985 survey of AHCCCS enrollees and a matched group of beneficiaries in New Mexico found little difference between the two groups in access, use of services, or satisfaction.[13] Although a 1987 GAO report found some continuing problems, chiefly in the area of rate setting,[14] AHCCCS appears to be firmly established and has moved on to develop an

---

[13]McCall, Nelda, E., Deborah Jay, and Richard West. Access and Satisfaction in the Arizona Health Care Cost Containment System. *Health Care Financing Review*, v. 11, no. 1, fall 1989. p. 63-77.

[14]U.S. General Accounting Office. *Medicaid: Lessons Learned From Arizona's Prepaid Program*. Report to the Secretary of Health and Human Services. GAO/HRD-87-14, Mar. 1987. Washington, 1987.

insurance package for small employers.[15] However, the current waivers for AHCCCS expire in September 1993, and the program's status after that date is uncertain.

In 1982, the same year AHCCCS began, the Secretary granted a section 1115(a) waiver to Minnesota to allow mandatory HMO enrollment for beneficiaries in the Minneapolis area (the project did not actually become operational until 1985). This project, originally scheduled to end in 1988, has been extended by Congress three times; most recently, OBRA 90 continued the demonstration through June 30, 1996, and authorized expansion to additional counties. Minnesota's program differs from AHCCCS in several key ways. First, it operates within the Medicaid framework--all required Medicaid services are covered and Federal matching funds are provided in the usual way. Second, Minnesota has contracted chiefly with mainstream HMOs. While some HMOs initially participated in AHCCCS, none of its current contractors meets the requirement that no more than 75 percent of enrollees be Medicare or Medicaid beneficiaries.

In addition to conducting these demonstrations, the Secretary has allowed the use of section 1915(b), the freedom-of-choice waiver authority, to permit mandatory HMO enrollment programs. In three areas in Wisconsin, including Milwaukee and Madison, AFDC beneficiaries must select from among a number of participating HMOs. The beneficiaries may disenroll at 6-month intervals, but only to join another HMO. Similar programs operate in Kansas City, Missouri, and Dayton, Ohio. HCFA has allowed mandatory enrollment arrangements so long as there are multiple HMO choices in the area and beneficiaries are permitted to transfer from one organization to another.

This policy might permit the Arizona and Minnesota programs to convert to ordinary Medicaid status under a section 1915(b) waiver when their current demonstration waivers expire (provided that Arizona's contractors furnish the full scope of mandatory Medicaid services or Arizona provides them through other means). However, none of the current AHCCCS contractors meet the 75 percent Medicare/Medicaid enrollee limit. The Secretary has waived this requirement under the section 1115 demonstration authority, but cannot do so under the 1915(b) authority. Unless AHCCCS's contractors were to enter the private market, then, the program could not operate on other than a demonstration basis.

---

[15]As of June 1991, the program had enrolled 3,093 employees of 939 small businesses. Alpha Center. *Health Care for the Uninsured: Program Update*, no. 12. July 1991.

5. Social/HMOs and Related Initiatives[16]

Beginning in 1980, HCFA, Department of Health and Human Services (DHHS), and private foundations worked to develop new systems for coordinating health care services furnished to the elderly, including Medicare beneficiaries and persons jointly eligible for Medicare and Medicaid. These systems, known as social/health maintenance organizations (S/HMOs), would be modeled after HMOs. However, S/HMOs would assume financial risk for long-term care services, including some nursing home care as well as community-based health and social services, in addition to the acute care services traditionally furnished by HMOs. The S/HMOs would have an incentive to find the most efficient way of treating patients within the entire spectrum of acute and long-term care services. S/HMOs would be funded with a combination of Medicare, Medicaid, and private premiums and would serve a mix of enrollees, from the healthy to the significantly impaired.

Congress mandated a demonstration of the S/HMO concept in the Deficit Reduction Act of 1984 (DEFRA, Public Law 98-369). S/HMO projects began operation in 1985 in four cities: Minneapolis, Minnesota; Brooklyn, New York; Long Beach, California; and Portland, Oregon. The demonstrations were originally supposed to run for 3 years. However, the projects encountered delays in reaching their initial enrollment targets. OBRA 87 extended the demonstration period through September 1992. OBRA 90 extended the projects through December 1995 and mandated the development of 4 additional projects. An interim report on the original projects delivered to Congress in 1988 addressed organizational and start-up issues but did not evaluate the S/HMOs' performance in controlling utilization or costs. A second interim report is due in 1993 and a final report in 1996.

In a parallel development, the Secretary in 1979 approved demonstration waivers for the On Lok program in San Francisco. Like the S/HMOs, On Lok receives premium payments from Medicare and Medicaid and assumes risk for both acute and long-term care. However, On Lok's enrollment is limited to the frail elderly at risk of nursing home care, as opposed to the mix of well and impaired persons enrolled by the S/HMOs. Congress mandated continued waivers for On Lok in the Social Security Amendments of 1983 (Public Law 98-21) and again in COBRA; the COBRA extension continues indefinitely unless On Lok ceases to comply with the conditions of its waivers. OBRA 86 (Public Law 99-509) mandates waivers for up to 10 projects intended to replicate the On Lok program in other areas, in an initiative known as the Program for All-inclusive Care for the Elderly (PACE); OBRA 90 increased the number to 15. As of July 1992, waivers had been granted for 8 PACE sites, in New York City, Rochester, Boston, Milwaukee, Portland, Oregon, El Paso, Columbia, South Carolina, and Denver. Projects are also under development in Chicago, Oakland, Sacramento, and Honolulu.

---

[16]Much of the following discussion is drawn from: U.S. Library of Congress. Congressional Research Service. *Financing and Delivery of Long-term Care Services for the Elderly.* CRS Report for Congress No. 88-379 EPW, by Carol O'Shaughnessy and Richard Price, May 1988. Washington, 1988.

6. Summary of Managed Care Programs

Table G-1 summarizes the Medicaid managed care programs in operation in 1990 (1991 for fee-for-service case management programs). Table G-2 compares 1990 enrollment in these programs with enrollment in similar programs in 1987. Table G-3 gives State-by-State details of fee-for-service case management programs as of June 1991.[17] Table G-4 gives similar data for capitated programs as of June 1990.

---

[17]The figures in table G-3 were supplied directly by State officials and reflect estimates of enrollment in fee-for-service case management programs as of June 1991. An unpublished May 1991 HCFA report shows nearly 1.3 million enrollees in such programs. However, the HCFA estimates reflect expected enrollment if current programs reach their full targeted capacity, rather than actual 1991 enrollment.

**TABLE G-1. Types of Medicaid Managed Care Projects
and Estimated Enrollment, June 1990 or 1991**

	Voluntary		Mandatory		Total
	States	Enrollees	States	Enrollees[a]	Enrollees
Health maintenance organizations (HMOs) and full-risk prepaid health plans (PHPs) (June 1990):	23	880,057	5	412,583	1,292,640
Partial capitation plans (June 1990):	4	17,408	2	103,472	120,880
Health insuring organizations HIOs), managed care type (June 1990):			4	151,578	151,578
Social HMOs (S/HMOs) (June 1990):	4	464			464
On Lok and PACE plans (June 1990):	3	356			356
Prescription drug and dental capitation demonstrations (June 1990):	1	2,096			2,096
Total prepaid programs (June 1990):	26[b]	900,381	9[b]	667,633	1,568,014
Fee-for-service case management, estimates (June 1991):	2	28,500	8	622,000	650,500

[a]Programs that are mandatory for some groups but voluntary for others are included in the mandatory column.

[b]Unduplicated count of States with programs.

Source: Table prepared by the Congressional Research Service (CRS) based on analysis of data from the Health Care Financing Administration. Fee-for-service case management estimates obtained by CRS from individual States.

TABLE G-2. Growth in Medicaid Managed Care Enrollment, 1987 to 1990

	Enrollment, Dec. 1987	Enrollment, June 1990	Percent change
Health maintenance organizations (HMOs) and full-risk prepaid health plans (PHPs)	955,618	1,292,640	35.3%
Partial capitation plans	55,719	120,880	116.9%
Health insuring organizations (HIOs), managed care type	130,685	151,578	16.0%
Social HMOs (S/HMOs)	497	464	-6.6%
On Lok and PACE plans	0	356	NA
Prescription drug and dental capitation demonstrations	0	2,096	NA
Total capitated plans:	1,142,521	1,568,017	37.2%
Fee-for-service case management (estimates as of 1986 and 1991)	408,810[a]	650,500[b]	59.1%

[a]National Governors' Association estimates as of 1986.

[b]Estimates by State officials, June 1991.

Source: Except as noted, Congressional Research Service analysis of data from the Health Care Financing Administration.

TABLE G-3. Fee-for Service Case Management Projects by State, 1991

State	Voluntary or mandatory	Population served	Persons enrolled, 6/91
Colorado	Mandatory statewide	All except foster children and dual Medicare/Medicaid eligibles	100,000 (4/91)[a]
Iowa	Mandatory in 7 counties	AFDC and related groups	40,000[a]
Kansas	Mandatory in 7 most populous counties	All except foster children, dual Medicare/Medicaid eligibles, and persons in institutions	60,000
Kentucky	Mandatory in 111 of 120 counties	AFDC	260,000
Maryland	Voluntary statewide (mandatory phased in starting 12/91)	All except foster children, subsidized adoptions, dual Medicare/Medicaid eligibles	25,000
Michigan	Voluntary in Wayne, Marquette, and Genessee	AFDC, SSI (AFDC mandatory in Wayne only)	100,000[a]
North Carolina	Mandatory in 6 counties	All except mentally ill, OBRA pregnant women	10,000
New Mexico	Mandatory in 3 counties (will be statewide)	All except dual Medicare/Medicaid eligibles and home and community-based service enrollees; exceptions for hardship	10,000
Tennessee	Voluntary in Shelby county	Pediatric only	3,500
Utah	Mandatory in urban areas; voluntary in rural areas	All except persons in institutions	42,000[a]

[a]Fee-for service case management only. Mandated enrollees choosing prepaid program included in prepaid counts, table G-3.

Source: Table prepared by the Congressional Research Service based on communications from State officials.

TABLE G-4. Medicaid Capitation Programs by State, 1990

State	Program type (Number of providers in parentheses)	Voluntary or mandatory	Population served[a]	Enrollees, June 1990[b]
Alabama	HMO (1)	Voluntary	AFDC-SSI	2,637
Arizona	PHPs (18)[c]	Mandatory statewide	AFDC-SSI (13), All (4), AFDC (1)	216,202
California	HMOs (12)	Voluntary	All	242,902
	Partial capitation (11)	Mandatory in parts of Los Angeles, San Diego, and 3 other counties	All	52,809
	Partial capitation (1)	Voluntary	All	1,400
	HIOs (2)	Mandatory in Santa Barbara and San Mateo	All	59,896
	S/HMO (1)	Voluntary	Aged	232
	On Lok	Voluntary	Frail elderly	265
Colorado	HMOs (2)	Voluntary[d]	All	8,651
District of Columbia	HMO (1)	Voluntary	AFDC-SSI	8,681
Florida	HMOs (9)	Voluntary	AFDC-SSI (6), AFDC (2), AFDC-SSI-MN (1)	58,374
Hawaii	HMO (1)	Voluntary	AFDC	2,600
Illinois	HMOs (5)	Voluntary	AFDC	119,271
Indiana	HMO (1)	Voluntary	AFDC	1,065

See notes at end of table.

TABLE G-4. Medicaid Capitation Programs by State, 1990--Continued

State	Program type (Number of providers in parentheses)	Voluntary or mandatory	Population served[a]	Enrollees, June 1990[b]
Iowa	HMO (1)	Voluntary[d]	AFDC	3,587
Maryland	HMOs (2), PHP (1)	Voluntary	All	43,520
Massachusetts	HMOs (18)	Voluntary	AFDC (14), All (4)	37,644
	PACE (1)	Voluntary	Frail elderly	26
Michigan	HMOs (6)	Voluntary[d]	AFDC-SSI	121,635
	Partial capitation (5)	Voluntary[d]	AFDC-SSI	7,062
Minnesota	HMOs (7), PHP (1)	Mandatory in Hennepin and Dakota	AFDC-Aged (4),AFDC (2), AFDC-SSI (1), Aged (1)	20,958
	HIO (1)	Mandatory in Itasca	AFDC-SSI	3,321
	S/HMO (1)	Voluntary	Aged	41
Missouri	HMOs (2), PHPs (2)	Mandatory in Jackson	AFDC	23,947
Nevada	Partial capitation (1)	Voluntary	AFDC	3,699
New Hampshire	HMO (1)	Voluntary	AFDC	743
New Jersey	HMOs (2)[e]	Voluntary	AFDC-SSI (1), AFDC (1)	4,252
New York	HMOs (14), PHPs (3)	Voluntary	All (1), AFDC (13), AFDC-SSI (3)	48,460
	Partial capitation (3)	Voluntary	AFDC-SSI	5,247

See notes at end of table.

TABLE G-4. Medicaid Capitation Programs by State, 1990--Continued

State	Program type (Number of providers in parentheses)	Voluntary or mandatory	Population served[a]	Enrollees, June 1990[b]
New York *(continued)*	S/HMO (1)	Voluntary	Aged	126
North Carolina	HMO (1)	Voluntary	AFDC	728
Ohio	HMOs (3)	Mandatory in Dayton	AFDC	39,228
	HMOs (11)	Voluntary	AFDC	79,064
Oregon	Partial capitation (16)	Mandatory in multiple counties	AFDC	50,663
	PACE (2)	Voluntary	Frail elderly	65
	S/HMO (1)	Voluntary	Aged	65
	PHP (Rx)[f]	Voluntary	AFDC	430
	PHP (Dental)[f]	Voluntary	AFDC	1,666
Pennsylvania	HMOs (5)	Voluntary	AFDC (4), All (1)	58,841
	HIO (1)	Mandatory in South Philadelphia	AFDC	77,783
Rhode Island	HMO (1)	Voluntary	AFDC	442
Tennessee	HMO (1)	Voluntary	AFDC	15,579
Utah	HMOs (2)	Voluntary[d]	All	13,339

See notes at end of table.

TABLE G-4. Medicaid Capitation Programs by State, 1990.--Continued

State	Program type (Number of providers in parentheses)	Voluntary or mandatory	Population served[a]	Enrollees, June 1990[b]
Washington	HMOs (4)	Voluntary	AFDC (3), AFDC-Foster (1)	7,743
	HIO (1)	Mandatory in Kitsap, Mason, Clallam, and Jefferson	AFDC	10,578
Wisconsin	HMOs (8)	Mandatory in Milwaukee and Dane	AFDC	112,248
	HMO (1)	Voluntary	AFDC	299
Total U.S. beneficiaries				1,568,014

[a]Federally funded Medicaid groups only.

[b]Counts in some States may include enrollees funded through non-Medicaid State medical assistance programs (including general assistance and "State-only" programs).

[c]Includes PHPs providing acute care services and those providing long-term care under the newer component of the AHCCCS demonstration.

[d]Enrollees may choose between capitated plan or mandatory fee-for-service case management.

[e]Includes Garden State Health Plan, a State-operated HMO-like entity authorized under OBRA 87.

[f]Projects conducted under a section 1115 demonstration waiver and offering only prescription drugs and dental care.

Program Types:

HMO:	Health Maintenance Organization
PHP:	Prepaid Health Plan
HIO:	Health Insuring Organization
S/HMO:	Social/Health Maintenance Organization
On Lok:	Prepaid Program for the Frail Elderly
PACE:	Program for All-Inclusive Care for the Elderly (programs modelled after On Lok)

Source: Table prepared by the Congressional Research Service based on analysis of data from the Health Care Financing Administration.

III. THE IMPACT OF MANAGED CARE

A. Current Status of Managed Care

Widespread interest in pursuing Medicaid managed care initiatives began in the 1981-83 period, when a combination of rising Medicaid costs, a recession, and the temporary OBRA 81 limits on Federal matching funds combined to place increasing pressure on States to find innovative cost saving approaches. Of the 45 managed care waivers approved by HCFA under section 1915(b) from 1981 through January 1990, nearly half (21) date from those first 3 years.

States' interest in pursuing this approach appeared to wane in the mid-1980s, perhaps because there was a temporary moderation of the fiscal pressure that initially caused States to explore managed care alternatives. The rapid growth in Medicaid expenditures that began in the late 1970s slowed somewhat in the middle 1980s. The 1981 cuts in Federal Medicaid cost-sharing were not renewed after their initial 3-year period. While they lasted, States found other ways to achieve more immediate savings than were available from managed care, including changes in hospital and nursing home reimbursement systems and utilization control measures, such as requirements for preauthorization of inpatient services.

By the end of the decade, however, Medicaid costs were again rising rapidly. States reported spending increases of nearly 13 percent a year in the period FY 1987 to FY 1990. Possible explanations for this growth are explored in *Chapter II, Trends in Medicaid Payments and Beneficiaries*. Some factors, such as growth in the covered population, are specific to Medicaid. But medical costs for all payers grew rapidly in the late 1980s, in part because the cost containment measures adopted earlier in the decade appeared to provide diminishing returns. One result may be that States will join other health care purchasers in looking again at managed care options.

So far, however, most activity continues to be concentrated in the same States that developed managed care programs some years ago. As table G-2 indicates, enrollment in prepaid plans grew 37 percent from 1987 to 1990, while enrollment under fee-for-service case management grew 59 percent from 1986 to 1991. At the same time, the number of States with operational programs of each basic type remained the same. Other States may have been reluctant to undertake the administrative tasks involved or may have found that providers were not interested.

The programs that are operational frequently focus on the AFDC population. Programs serving SSI-related groups may be more difficult to manage, in part because many SSI recipients also have Medicare. It should also be noted that many programs continue to rely on managed care systems established specifically for Medicaid. Of enrollees in full-risk HMOs and PHPs, 28 percent are in organizations that have a waiver of or are not subject to the 75 percent limit on Medicare/Medicaid enrollment. All of the partial capitation plans and HIOs are limited to Medicaid enrollees.

Still, there are States with strong commitments to managed care, and some others may become involved shortly; seven 1915(b) managed care waiver applications filed since 1987 are still pending. How well has managed care worked for the States that have chosen to undertake it? This question breaks down into two issues: whether managed care programs have actually achieved savings, and what impact they have had on access to health services and quality of care.

B. Cost Savings

Managed care systems have been shown to achieve savings, relative to traditional fee-for-service insurance programs, in a number of studies. The best known of these is the Health Insurance Experiment conducted by the RAND Corporation in Seattle in the late 1970s. Families agreeing to participate in the study were randomly assigned to an HMO, the Group Health Cooperative of Puget Sound, or to a comprehensive insurance program. Persons assigned to the HMO used 40 percent fewer inpatient hospital days, and their overall estimated costs were 25 percent lower than those for persons assigned to the conventional insurance plan.[18]

Two factors limit the generalizability of the RAND experiment. First, the study was conducted in the late 1970s; the comparison plan was the passive bill-payer prevalent in the insurance industry in that period, with no utilization control mechanisms. The more recent adoption by conventional plans (and many fee-for-service Medicaid programs) of some of the cost-control measures once associated only with HMOs may mean that the difference in efficiency between the two types of plan has narrowed. Second, the HMO used in the Health Insurance Experiment was a highly structured group-practice plan with many years of operating experience. Much of the growth in the industry in recent years has involved a different type of HMO, the IPA, which contracts with independent physicians who see a mix of HMO enrollees and other kinds of patients. There is evidence that these more loosely structured HMOs have not achieved savings comparable to those observed in the HIE.[19]

In any case, while the RAND study demonstrated the capacity of an HMO to reduce utilization and costs in a controlled, experimental situation, demonstrating cost savings outside the experimental setting has proved more difficult. Reliable evaluations of Medicaid managed care projects are only just beginning to appear.

---

[18]Manning, Willard G., et al. A Controlled Trial of the Effect of a Prepaid Group Practice on Use of Services. *New England Journal of Medicine*, v. 310, no. 23, June 7, 1984. p. 1505-1510.

[19]For a fuller discussion of this issue, see: U.S. Library of Congress. Congressional Research Service. *Controlling Health Care Costs*. CRS Report for Congress No. 90-64 EPW, by Mark Merlis, Jan. 1990. Washington, 1990. p. 24-26.

The issue of cost savings appears fairly simple in HMOs or other prepaid systems. Medicaid programs have generally based the premium rates for HMOs on estimates of what would have been spent for a comparable group of beneficiaries not enrolled in the HMO. A State might, for example, estimate that average costs for an adult AFDC beneficiary outside the HMO are $100 a month; it might then pay the HMO 95 percent of this amount, or $95. If the State's estimates were correct, it would presumably save $5 a month for each enrollee.

This will be true, however, only if the beneficiaries enrolled in the HMO are identical in health status and need for health services to the beneficiaries on whose experience the State's estimate was based. If the persons joining the HMO are unrepresentative of the total population, either sicker or healthier, then the State's savings may be more or less than the apparent $5. The possibility that this will occur is known as "biased selection."[20] The problem of biased selection has been a central issue in discussion of HMOs for many years. Some people say that healthier people join HMOs, because sick people have established ties to their own physicians and don't want to give up their choice of providers. Others say that sicker people join HMOs, because of the ready access to comprehensive health services.

The RAND study cited earlier corrected for this problem by randomly assigning the participants, so that there was no difference between the beneficiaries in the HMO and those in the ordinary insurance plan. The RAND Corporation is currently attempting a new set of randomized assignment experiments for Medicaid beneficiaries in New York and Florida in conjunction with a HCFA initiative, the Program for Prepaid Managed Health Care. (Results were not yet available as of September 1992.) Short of full randomization, two approaches to assessment of cost savings have been used.

The first approach is actually to attempt to measure the differences between beneficiaries joining a managed care program and those remaining in the traditional Medicaid system. One way of doing this is to examine the utilization and costs of the beneficiaries **before** they joined the managed care program, to see if the enrollees used more or fewer services than beneficiaries who didn't join. A study in Michigan in 1977-78 concluded that biased selection had in fact occurred. HMO enrollees were less likely to have used health care services before joining the HMO than comparable beneficiaries who didn't enroll.[21] A more recent study, also in Michigan, examined the fee-for-service

---

[20]Two kinds of biased selection may occur: adverse selection, the enrollment of persons sicker than average, and favorable selection, the enrollment of persons healthier than average.

[21]DesHarnais, Susan I. Enrollment In and Disenrollment From Health Maintenance Organizations by Medicaid Recipients. *Health Care Financing Review*, v. 6, no. 3, spring 1985. p. 39-50. It should be noted that there are also studies of biased selection into managed care systems for groups other than Medicaid, such as Medicare beneficiaries or private employee groups. However,
(continued...)

case management Physician Primary Sponsor Plan. This study adjusted for preenrollment use of services and found substantial cost reductions from the case management approach. Estimated savings in 1984 were 13 percent for all Medicaid beneficiaries enrolled, and 21 percent for those in the AFDC group.[22]

The second approach is to evaluate savings in the systems which mandate enrollment by all beneficiaries in a geographic area. Because everyone, healthy or sick, is enrolled in the system, biased selection ceases to be an issue. It is then possible to compare the beneficiaries' costs and use of services to those of a comparable population in another area where the project is not operating. This approach was used in evaluations of several managed care programs operated under section 1115(a) demonstration waivers as part of a HCFA "Medicaid competition" initiative. The results were inconclusive. The programs evaluated did appear to change patterns of service use; in particular they reduced the use of emergency room services. However, they did not have a significant effect on the use of inpatient care and did not produce demonstrable program savings.[23] The evaluation of Arizona's AHCCCS program also yielded unclear results. Depending on the assumptions used, estimates of overall program savings in the first 5 years of operation ranged from $450,000 to $30.4 million.[24]

While the evidence so far is mixed, some people have argued that in many States managed care may be unable to achieve savings over and above the savings realized from some of the other cost containment approaches adopted in the 1980s. If a Medicaid program is paying below cost for hospital services and uses a strict fee schedule for physicians, or if it uses preauthorization of services and other utilization control measures, can it be expected that an HMO or other managed care program can cut costs even further without endangering quality? In this view, managed care should be regarded as an alternative to other cost containment approaches, rather than as a way of obtaining even further savings. Others argue that there remains considerable inefficiency in

---

[21](...continued)
members of these groups, unlike Medicaid beneficiaries, contribute to the cost of their own care. Their reasons for enrolling may be different from those of Medicaid beneficiaries, and studies of their enrollment tendencies may therefore not be generalizable to Medicaid.

[22]Smith, Vernon. *Facilitating Health Care Coverage for the Working Uninsured: Alternative State Strategies.* Michigan's Physician Primary Sponsor Plan. National Governors' Association, Center for Health Policy Studies. Washington, 1987. p. 93-94.

[23]Freund, Deborah A., et al. Evaluation of the Medicaid Competition Demonstrations. *Health Care Financing Review,* v. 11, no. 2, winter 1989. p. 81-97.

[24]Evaluation of the Arizona Health Care Cost Containment System. *Health Care Financing Review,* v. 10, no. 4, summer 1989. p. 148-150.

the fee-for-service sector and that further evaluation is needed to determine the full savings potential of managed care.

C. Access and Quality

The potential impact of managed care programs on access to health services and quality of care has been the subject of debate ever since HMOs first received wide publicity in the 1970s. If the traditional fee-for-service program encouraged overutilization of services, it was feared, the incentives under managed care to treat patients more efficiently might lead to underutilization and denial of needed treatments. Proponents of managed care responded that satisfactory health care outcomes could be achieved with fewer resources--fewer tests, fewer hospital admissions--than traditional medicine provided. They pointed out that overtreatment, such as unnecessary surgery, also posed dangers to patients.

Attempts to determine whether care in managed programs, especially HMOs, was better or worse than care in the fee-for-service system have produced no consistent results. If a consensus has developed, it is that there are variations in quality among managed care providers, just as there are among providers in the fee-for-service sector. In established HMOs treating the general population, health care outcomes do not appear to differ significantly from those obtained by fee-for-service providers.[25]

There are concerns, however, that Medicaid beneficiaries may not always fare as well in managed care systems as the general population does. As in the area of cost savings, the major study on this subject is a product of the RAND Health Insurance Study, which randomly assigned participants to an HMO and a fee-for-service insurance program. In each group, participants were divided into four subgroups according to income (low or high) and whether they had health problems at the outset of the study. On a variety of health outcome measures, such as blood pressure, serum cholesterol level, and overall physical functioning, three of the four subgroups did about as well in the HMO as in the fee-for-service program. One group, the low-income participants with existing health problems, did worse. Their health status at the conclusion of the study was significantly poorer than that of comparable persons in the fee-for-service program.[26]

The investigators speculate that the low-income enrollees might have had difficulty dealing with the bureaucracy of an HMO, and argue that outreach and social services are needed to help low-income patients use an HMO system. As

---

[25]For a review of the literature on this subject, see: Glenn T. Hammons et al. *Selected Alternatives for Paying Physicians Under the Medicare Program: Effects on the Quality of Care*, RAND Note No. R-3394-OTA. Prepared for the Office of Technology Assessment. Santa Monica, 1986.

[26]Ware, John E. Jr., et al. Comparison of Health Outcomes at a Health Maintenance Organization With Those of Fee-for-Service Care. *Lancet*, May 3, 1986. p. 1017-1022.

they acknowledge, the HMO in the study actually provided such services to its ordinary Medicaid enrollees, but not to the participants in the study. One other feature of the study may limit its applicability to other Medicaid managed care programs. The participants assigned to the non-HMO option had an insurance plan which paid providers' full fees, rather than the reduced reimbursement levels prevailing under Medicaid (see *Appendix H, Medicaid as Health Insurance: Measures of Performance*). The investigators suggest that the non-HMO low-income group might have enjoyed greater access to services than would have been the case under regular Medicaid. The study may, then, somewhat exaggerate the real differences in outcomes for managed care and fee-for-service options under Medicaid. One recent study of pregnancy care in Medicaid capitation programs in California and Missouri found little difference in outcomes for the managed care enrollees and a matched fee-for-service population. Incidence of complications and low birth weight babies were about the same for both groups. (The study notes, however, that neither the capitated nor the fee-for-service group used prenatal care at recommended rates.)[27]

Still, Medicaid managed care programs have repeatedly been subject to allegations of inadequate access and quality, along with marketing and enrollment abuses and other violations. Past problems with programs in California, Kentucky, Arizona, and Pennsylvania have already been mentioned. More recently, concerns have been raised about Illinois' HMO contracting program. In 1990, the General Accounting Office found that the HMOs lacked appropriate internal quality review systems and that the State failed to collect data on enrollee utilization and was slow to follow up on quality of care problems. Earlier, congressional hearings in 1988 heard charges of marketing abuses and inadequate neonatal care in the same program.[28]

Concerns about these allegations, along with reports of similar problems in the Medicare HMO contracting program, have led Congress to enact stricter requirements in OBRA 86, the Medicare Catastrophic Protection Act of 1988 (Public Law 100-360), and OBRA 90. While States have always been required to conduct some form of review of HMO services, they must now contract with a peer review organization (PRO) or other independent accrediting body for an outside assessment of Medicaid prepaid contractors. In addition, HMOs may now be subject to civil monetary penalties if they deny medically necessary care, overcharge beneficiaries, discriminate in enrollment on the basis of health status, or provide false information to the Secretary, the State, or any other individual or entity. (See *Chapter VII, Administration* for further details on

---

[27]Carey, Timothy S., Kathi Weis, and Charles Homer. Prepaid Versus Traditional Medicaid Plans: Lack of Effect on Pregnancy Outcomes and Prenatal Care. *Health Services Research*, v. 26, no. 2, June 1991. p. 165-181.

[28]U.S. General Accounting Office. *Medicaid: Oversight of Health Maintenance Organizations in the Chicago Area.* GAO/HRD-90-81, Aug. 1990. Washington, 1990. (Hereafter cited as GAO, *Medicaid: Oversight of HMOs*); U.S. Congress. House. Committee on Energy and Commerce. Subcommittee on Health and the Environment. *Health Services.* Hearings, Serial No. 100-145, 100th Cong., 2nd Sess. Washington, GPO, 1988.

these provisions.) Finally, OBRA 90 requires that HMOs maintain sufficient patient encounter data to identify the specific physicians treating enrollees.

Finally, OBRA 90 addressed a longstanding debate over Medicare and Medicaid treatment of HMOs that make incentive payments to physicians to limit services provided to enrollees. Incentive plans are a common feature in HMOs: physicians may be paid a bonus for reducing the use of services or may be placed at direct financial risk, through a monthly capitation payment, for the costs of services furnished to the enrollees they treat. Critics of physician incentive plans believe that in some cases physicians may respond to financial pressure, not just by improving efficiency, but also by denying or delaying necessary services. For example, a 1990 GAO report on Medicaid HMO contracts in Illinois expressed concern that the incentive plans used by two Chicago HMOs transferred enough risk to physicians to jeopardize the quality of care.[29] Others note that physician incentive plans have been a common practice in HMOs for many years. They argue that some form of financial incentive is necessary as a corrective to the tendency, under the fee-for-service system, to maximize the quantity of services delivered.

The COBRA barred all physician incentive payments by Medicare and Medicaid contractors, effective April 1989 (changed to April 1990 by OBRA 87 and to April 1991 by OBRA 89). The Secretary was required to recommend alternatives to an absolute prohibition of incentive plans. The Secretary's report indicated that there was insufficient evidence to identify broad classes of incentive plans that might present quality problems and recommended that the Secretary be authorized to regulate plans on a case-by-case basis.

The OBRA 90 replaced the total prohibition of incentives with a prohibition (for both Medicare and Medicaid contractors) of specific payments made to physicians as an inducement to withhold or limit services to specific enrollees. It also provided that, if physicians or physician groups are placed at serious risk for services other than their own, the HMO must offer adequate stop-loss protection (as determined by the Secretary taking into account the size of the group and the number of enrollees served) and must periodically survey enrollees to ensure that they have adequate access and are satisfied with the quality of services.

---

[29] GAO, *Medicaid: Oversight of HMOs*, 1990.

APPENDIX H. MEDICAID AS HEALTH INSURANCE: MEASURES OF PERFORMANCE[1]

I. INTRODUCTION

From 1984 through 1990, Congress repeatedly acted to extend Medicaid eligibility to larger numbers of mothers and children, and it has funded demonstrations to test the possibility of making Medicaid available to low-income persons who are outside the "protected" populations of families with children and the aged, blind, and disabled. Even as the covered population has grown, policy interest has increasingly focused on the adequacy of the coverage Medicaid provides. Does Medicaid assure access to care of high quality, or have the recent eligibility expansions merely enrolled more people in a program that consigns them to second-class care in a two-tier system? This question has taken on increasing urgency as Congress begins to examine alternative proposals for providing universal access to health insurance. Many proposals would continue Medicaid in some form as a way of reaching persons not covered through other means (such as employer-based plans). Supporters of some of these proposals often assume that improvements in Medicaid would be necessary before it would constitute an adequate form of health insurance coverage.

It used to be commonly said that Medicaid was not health insurance at all. At its outset, the program was one of grants to States; it did not confer on beneficiaries the contractual rights enjoyed by subscribers to a health insurance plan. On the other hand, the program has taken on many functions not associated with private health insurance, such as financing medical/social services for the aged and disabled and furnishing more comprehensive preventive services for children than are common under private policies. Still, the program serves as the nearest equivalent to insurance for most of its beneficiaries. They carry a Medicaid card as other persons carry a private health insurance card. Many of the questions being asked about the program might be reduced to one: is the card any good?

Any answer to this question depends on assumptions about what Medicaid or any other health insurance plan is supposed to do. Different people might assign different goals to Medicaid, ranging from the least to the most ambitious:

- Protect against financial loss.
- Provide financial access to care of adequate quality.
- Provide access to "mainstream" medical care.

---

[1]This appendix was written by Mark Merlis and Madeleine Smith.

Medicaid began with the narrowest of these goals. Its key predecessor, the Kerr-Mills program for the elderly, aimed at little more than protecting its enrollees against the loss of a home and a small amount of savings in the event of a catastrophic episode. Medicaid still offers this minimal protection. Financial standards for the program are so restrictive that it may seem meaningless to speak of Medicaid as offering catastrophic protection: if a family has incurred medical bills sufficient to reduce its assets to Medicaid limits, the catastrophe has already happened. However, Medicaid may protect beneficiaries who are already poor from having to spend their limited incomes on medical care.

"Catastrophic costs" are often defined as out-of-pocket spending exceeding a given percentage of family income (such as 5, 10, or 20 percent). Because Medicaid beneficiaries' incomes are so low, these thresholds could be reached with relatively small medical bills. It might be expected that they would suffer proportionately "catastrophic" losses more frequently. A review of data from the 1977 National Medical Care Expenditure Survey suggests that the reverse is true. While Medicaid beneficiaries made up 8.6 percent of the sample population, they accounted for only 3 to 4 percent of the groups with catastrophic costs (depending on the percentage of income threshold defined as catastrophic).[2] While the program has changed considerably since 1977, most of the changes are unlikely to have significantly increased beneficiaries' direct financial liability. Medicaid beneficiaries are not "underinsured" in this narrowest of senses.

Simple financial protection is still a paramount aim for some components of the Medicaid program, such as the recently added coverage of Medicare premiums and cost-sharing for low-income "qualified Medicare beneficiaries." For most of the covered population, however, Medicaid is expected to serve broader goals. At a minimum, the program is designed to secure access to basic medical care. In addition, many analysts contend that Medicaid was intended to bring its beneficiaries into the mainstream of the medical care system. Its success or failure in doing so has emerged as a key measure of program performance. In fact, "mainstreaming" was not a goal of Medicaid at the time of its enactment, although some subsequent measures suggest that Congress has at least implicitly adopted this goal.

For the non-elderly population, Medicaid was initially modeled on a set of "vendor payment" medical care programs, which were funded through the cash assistance programs (Aid to Families with Dependent Children (AFDC) and aid to the aged, blind, and disabled) from 1950 on. Under the pre-Medicaid vendor payment programs, a State could (a) furnish the equivalent of health insurance, paying claims for services obtained by beneficiaries from providers of their choice, or (b) contract with specific providers, such as clinics or hospitals, to serve as the sources of care for public assistance recipients. As enacted in 1965, Medicaid continued to allow States the option of making direct arrangements for beneficiaries' care.

---

[2]Wyszewianski, Leon. Families with Catastrophic Health Care Expenditures. *Health Services Research*, v. 21, Dec. 1986. p. 617-634.

The Social Security Amendments of 1967 (P.L. 90-248) provided that Medicaid beneficiaries had to be permitted to obtain covered services from any qualified provider "who undertakes to provide [the beneficiary] such services." The so-called "freedom-of-choice" requirement meant that States could no longer establish special clinics for welfare clients or require all beneficiaries to use county hospitals. Instead, Medicaid would allow low-income citizens to use providers of their choice, to enter the mainstream of American health care.

Whether they could actually do so depended on whether providers were prepared to participate in the program. There was no guarantee that they would do so, as the House Ways and Means Committee acknowledged in reporting the legislation:

> Under the current provisions of law, there is no requirement on the State that recipients of medical assistance under a State title XIX program shall have freedom in their choice of medical institution or medical practitioner. In order to provide this freedom, a characteristic of our medical care system in this country, a new provision is included in the law to require States to offer this choice...*Inasmuch as States may, under title XIX, set certain standards for the provision of care, and may establish rates for payment, it is possible that some providers of service may still not be willing or considered qualified to provide the services included in the State plan.* This provision does not obligate the State to pay the charges of the provider without reference to its schedule of charges, or its standards of care.[3] [Emphasis added.]

More recent legislation has moved somewhat closer towards endorsement of mainstreaming. The Omnibus Budget Reconciliation Act of 1981 (P.L. 97-35) required States' payment rates for hospital care to be sufficient "to assure that individuals eligible for medical assistance have reasonable access (taking into account geographic location and reasonable travel time) to inpatient hospital services of adequate quality." A similar principle was applied to all providers by the Omnibus Budget Reconciliation Act of 1989 (P.L. 101-239): rates must be "sufficient to enlist enough providers so that care and services are available under the plan at least to the extent that such care and services are available to the general population in the geographic area."[4] Neither of these provisions

---

[3]U.S. Congress. House. Committee on Ways and Means. *Social Security Amendments of 1967.* Report to Accompany H.R. 12080. House Report No. 544, 90th Cong., 1st Sess. Washington, GPO, Aug. 7, 1967. (Jurisdiction over Medicaid was later shifted to the Energy and Commerce Committee.)

[4]At least one court has held that other provisions of the Medicaid law also require that States assure adequate access. In *Clark* v. *Kizer* (758 F. Supp. 572, 1990), the U.S. District Court for the Eastern District of California found that California's low payment rates for dental care had limited access to such care in certain counties. The court held that the State had therefore violated the
(continued...)

suggests that Medicaid must confer access to the **same** providers used by everyone else, or even to providers of equal quality, so long as the services are "adequate." The Omnibus Budget Reconciliation Act of 1990 (P.L. 101-508) goes further, specifying minimum qualifications (beyond mere licensure) for physicians providing pediatric and obstetric care to Medicaid beneficiaries.

Whatever the goal of Medicaid, basic access or mainstreaming, it cannot achieve that goal unless people actually enroll in the program. Numerous factors may prevent otherwise eligible individuals from establishing or continuing their enrollment, including complicated application processes, delays in eligibility determination, and requirements for periodic reapplication. The timing of eligibility can be almost equally important. For example, Medicaid enrollment early in the course of a pregnancy is a key factor in the receipt of timely prenatal care.[5] The option of presumptive eligibility for pregnant women aims to address this problem (see *Chapter III, Eligibility* for a discussion of this option). However, potentially eligible individuals with other problems may also face delays in eligibility and resulting delays in treatment.

While eligibility issues may be fundamental, this appendix will focus on a different and narrower question: how well does Medicaid work for persons who are continuously enrolled? Does the program secure access to care, and does it integrate enrollees into the mainstream medical system?

While there is considerable information with which to begin to answer these questions, some preliminary cautions are in order. First, the rapid pace of change in the Medicaid program--changes in enrollment and reimbursement levels, along with cutbacks in States faced with budget deficits--may mean that even fairly recent evidence is already obsolete. In addition, there is no single Medicaid program. Many access studies focus on one State or part of a State, and may not reflect conditions in other States with different Medicaid policies. Finally, it should be noted that much of the data to be considered in the following discussion has also been reviewed in recent studies by the Physician Payment Review Commission (PPRC) and staff of the Health Care Financing Administration (HCFA).[6] This appendix provides some newer findings and also takes a somewhat different approach to earlier data.

---

[4](...continued)
requirement for statewide operation of the plan, even though the States' payment policies operated uniformly throughout the State.

[5]Howell, Embry M., et al. A Comparison of Medicaid and Non-Medicaid Obstetrical Care in California. *Health Care Financing Review*, v. 12, no. 4, summer 1991. p. 1-15.

[6]Physician Payment Review Commission (PPRC). *Physician Payment Under Medicaid*. Washington, 1991. [PPRC Report No. 91-4] (Hereafter cited as PPRC, *Physician Payment under Medicaid*) Jencks, Stephen F., and M. Beth Benedict. Accessibility and Effectiveness of Care Under Medicaid. *Health Care Financing Review*, 1990 Annual Supplement. p. 47-56. (Hereafter cited as Jencks and Benedict, *Accessibility and Effectiveness*)

II. BASIC FINANCIAL ACCESS TO CARE

Most attempts to measure the success of Medicaid in securing basic access to care have relied on comparisons of medical care utilization rates by Medicaid beneficiaries and persons with private health insurance, on the one hand, or with no coverage at all, on the other. The following discussion summarizes some past comparisons and includes new comparative data based on the 1987 National Medical Expenditure Survey (NMES) conducted by the Agency for Health Care Policy and Research (AHCPR).[7] At least three types of comparisons are possible:

- Were Medicaid beneficiaries more or less likely than other persons to receive any care at all over a given period (or care of a given type, such as prenatal or preventive care)?

- Did Medicaid beneficiaries receive different quantities of service (such as physician visits) from other groups?

- Were Medicaid beneficiaries more or less likely to establish an ongoing relationship with a usual source of medical care, and what was that source?

Health insurance coverage is just one of many factors that help to determine whether and to what extent an individual will receive medical care, including the physical availability of health services, individual propensity to seek medical treatment, and basic need for care.[8] Differences in use of services by Medicaid beneficiaries and other groups might reflect basic differences in population characteristics or other cultural and environmental factors that are not directly related to insurance coverage. Most of the estimates in this section attempt to take at least some of these factors into account, but none can fully isolate financial access from the other determinants of health care utilization. The figures may therefore represent not just Medicaid's performance as a source of health insurance, but also limitations on the extent to which insurance alone can overcome barriers to medical care.

A. Use of Any Medical Care

Not everyone who is enrolled in the Medicaid program actually uses medical services. Most recipients of cash assistance, AFDC or Supplemental Security Income (SSI), receive Medicaid automatically as an adjunct to their cash benefits; they may or may not take advantage of Medicaid to obtain medical care. Persons enrolled in Medicaid under other categories, such as the medically needy or the new coverage groups of pregnant women and children, may be

---

[7]AHCPR is the successor agency to the National Center for Health Services Research, which conducted the original survey.

[8]This framework for analyzing access is derived from Aday, Lu Ann, and Ronald Andersen. *Development of Indices of Access to Medical Care*. Ann Arbor, Health Administration Press, 1975.

more likely to use services, since a need for service is likely to have led to their application for benefits.

The distinction between Medicaid enrollees and persons actually receiving care has often been obscured by the practice of basing Medicaid statistical data on paid claims records, rather than on enrollment records. For example, HCFA's standard counts of Medicaid "recipients" include only persons on whose behalf a medical claim has been paid by a State Medicaid agency. Enrollees (persons who have applied for Medicaid benefits, who have been determined eligible, and who generally receive some form of identification card) are not counted if the State has never actually paid a claim on their behalf. Most statistics thus reflect only users of services; this is true of figures for "beneficiaries" elsewhere in this volume. (On the other hand, counts of persons "covered by Medicaid" in *Appendix A, Medicaid, the Poor, and Health Insurance* represent the entire enrolled population, as estimated from Census Bureau surveys.)

Two sources of data provide information on both enrollees and the subset of enrollees who use services. The first is the HCFA-2082 reports filed by States, which are the source of much of the beneficiary data reported in other chapters. In addition to beneficiary data, the HCFA-2082 forms request a limited amount of information about enrollees. All States except Arizona, Pennsylvania, and Rhode Island provided this information for FY 1990 (Arizona does not file a HCFA-2082 report for its Medicaid-like demonstration program). The second data source is the NMES, a comprehensive survey of medical utilization and costs for 38,446 individuals conducted in 1987. NMES provides a representative sample of the entire U.S. population, and may thus be used to compare Medicaid and non-Medicaid utilization.

**TABLE H-1. Utilization Rate for Selected Medicaid Services,
Fiscal Year 1990[a]**

Age of recipient	Inpatient hospital services	Outpatient hospital services	Physician services	Use of any service[b]
Under 1	34.1	34.7	61.5	82.5
1 to 5	7.1	40.4	61.8	81.4
6 to 14	3.1	27.8	51.1	74.6
15 to 20	18.9	41.2	57.2	80.6
21 to 44	21.3	47.4	63.5	86.1
45 to 64	22.9	49.4	72.4	92.2
65 to 74	20.3	33.3	62.9	90.0
75 to 84	22.8	30.5	65.3	95.9
85 and over	23.6	26.6	64.8	104.6[c]
Total	**15.9**	**38.8**	**60.6**	**84.0**

[a]Utilization rate is based on the ratio of individuals receiving services to the total number of enrollees. Service recipiency is based on payment of a Medicaid claim. In some instances recipient claims will be paid after a recipient is no longer enrolled in the program.

[b]Based on the receipt of any Medicaid covered service, not just hospital or physician services.

[c]In many States the number of recipients 85 years and over exceeds the reported enrollment count for this category. This is probably an artifact of the accounting on Form 2082. That is, recipient payments are being made after these individuals no longer are eligible for Medicaid payments.

NOTE: All figures are estimates prepared by the Congressional Research Service. The estimates are based on State responses on HCFA Form 2082. Estimates are for 47 reporting States and the District of Columbia. Arizona, Pennsylvania, and Rhode Island did not provide information on the form to allow estimates for these States.

Source: Table prepared by the Congressional Research Service based on analysis of HCFA Form 2082.

Table H-1 provides HCFA-2082 data on "participation rates"--the percentage of Medicaid enrollees using specified services--for FY 1990. Medicaid paid for at least some form of service on behalf of 84 percent of enrollees during the year.[9] As the table indicates, participation rates varied with age, both for any services and for specific services. Participation is higher for infants and young children than for older children, of whom over one-fourth receive no services. Participation rates then rise gradually through age 64. For those aged 65 and older, participation appears to drop slightly; this may reflect inconsistencies in State reporting of deductible and coinsurance payments made by Medicaid on behalf of dual Medicare/Medicaid eligibles.

1. Ambulatory Care

Table H-2 provides data on ambulatory care participation, this time drawn from NMES. The tables show, by insurance status, self-reported health status, age, and income, the percentages of persons receiving any outpatient physician service during the year, whether in an office, hospital outpatient department (OPD) or emergency room (ER),[10] home, or other non-inpatient setting.

The Medicaid and private insurance categories include only persons who had just one form of coverage or the other throughout the year; persons in the uninsured category are those who had no coverage at any time during the year. Individuals who had multiple coverages or who changed insurance status or source during the year have been dropped from the sample, as have persons covered by Medicare at any time (with or without coverage). This approach permits a clearer comparison of utilization differences among the three groups, although it also prevents investigation of some other issues, such as the effect of gaining or losing coverage on utilization. It should also be noted that, while the HCFA-2082 reports include persons in institutions, the NMES data set used does not (a separate component of NMES surveyed persons in institutions).

---

[9]Strictly speaking, beneficiaries (persons recorded on the HCFA-2082 as having a claim paid during FY 1990) are not a subset of enrollees (persons listed as eligible for Medicaid during FY 1990). Persons whose eligibility ended in FY 1989 might have late claims processed in FY 1990; persons first enrolled during FY 1990 might not have their first claim paid until FY 1991. Because the Medicaid population was growing during this period, the likely effect is an understatement of participation rates).

[10]NMES does not distinguish between ER visits that did or did not include a physician contact. For the purpose of this analysis, all ER visits are counted as physician contacts. The probable overestimate of physician contacts was deemed preferable to the undercount that would have resulted from omission of ER visits.

TABLE H-2. Percent of Non-Elderly Population with at Least One Ambulatory Contact with a Physician by Insurance and Health Status, 1987[a]

Age and health status	Medicaid	Private insurance	Uninsured
Age 1 - 14:			
Excellent	63.3%	75.6%	53.5%
Good	75.0	76.3	48.2
Fair/Poor	82.9	85.0	(NA)
Age 15 - 44:			
Excellent	73.7	68.1	36.9
Good	75.2	72.2	49.3
Fair/Poor	86.7	81.4	55.6
Age 45 - 64:			
Excellent	(NA)	71.8	45.7[b]
Good	(NA)	77.7	52.7
Fair/Poor	94.2	86.0	66.0
All Individuals:			
Excellent	66.8	71.0	43.3
Good	75.9	74.3	49.5
Fair	86.9	83.0	57.8
Poor	92.7	92.5	79.5[b]

See notes at end of table.

TABLE H-2. Percent of Non-Elderly Population with at Least One Ambulatory Contact with a Physician by Insurance and Health Status, 1987[a]--Continued

Income and health status	Medicaid	Private insurance	Uninsured
Poor (Family income less than poverty threshold):			
Excellent	71.2%	67.6%	39.3%
Good	74.4	64.4	49.4
Fair/Poor	88.9	(NA)	62.2
All Poor	78.1	67.0	50.4
Family income between 1 and 2 times poverty threshold:			
Excellent	64.1	64.4	41.6
Good	76.9	72.4	51.9
Fair/Poor	86.7	78.8	60.0
1 to 1.99 Poverty	73.8	70.0	48.7
Family income greater than or equal to 2 times poverty threshold:			
Excellent	59.9[b]	71.8	47.5
Good	79.9[b]	75.0	47.2
Fair/Poor	(NA)	84.9	57.9
2.0 + Poverty	75.2	74.1	49.0

[a]Share of individuals with one or more physician contact in their home, at the physician's office, in an outpatient setting or a hospital emergency room.

[b]Limited reliability. Use caution in interpreting value.

(NA) - Estimate not available due to small sample size.

NOTE: Analysis is limited to those individuals who did not change insurance status during calendar year.

Source: Table prepared by the Congressional Research Service based on analysis of the 1987 National Medical Expenditure Survey.

In general, persons with Medicaid were at least as likely as those with private health insurance to have at least one physician contact during the year, and much more likely than the uninsured.[11] There were some exceptions to this pattern. Children in "excellent" health who were covered by Medicaid were less likely to have seen a physician than comparable privately insured children.[12] This was true despite the fact that Medicaid includes well-child care as a basic service, while most private policies do not.

When income is considered, Medicaid improved the chances that poor or near-poor persons in "fair" health or better would obtain physician care, relative to the privately insured.[13] The pattern does not hold for persons with incomes above 200 percent of poverty.[14] One possible explanation is that the deductible and coinsurance requirements often imposed by private insurance plans deter lower income people from obtaining care.[15] Medicaid beneficiaries are subject only to nominal cost-sharing or none at all.

The efficacy of Medicaid in improving access to at least some physician contact appears to be confirmed by the 1986 Robert Wood Johnson Foundation Access to Health Care Survey. This survey did not distinguish between Medicaid and other sources of health coverage, but did distinguish between the insured poor (most of whom have Medicaid) and the insured non-poor of working age (most of whom have private insurance). The insured poor were no more likely than the insured non-poor to have gone without a physician visit during the year, and less likely than the non-poor to have gone without a visit if they had one of 11 major illnesses.[16]

---

[11]Differences in percents of persons with one or more contacts were not statistically significant at .05 level for those with Medicaid versus those covered by private insurance, but were significant at the .05 level for Medicaid beneficiaries versus the uninsured in each comparison controlling for health status.

[12]The difference was statistically significant at the .05 level.

[13]The difference was statistically significant at the .05 level for the poor, but not for the near-poor.

[14]The difference for those in fair or better was not statistically significant at the .05 level.

[15]It has been demonstrated that cost-sharing requirements have a greater deterrent effect on low-income persons. See Lohr, Kathleen, et al. Use of Medical Care in the RAND Health Insurance Experiment: Diagnosis and Service-Specific Analyses in a Randomized Controlled Trial. *Medical Care*, v. 24, no. 9, (Supplement) Sept. 1986. p. S74-S77.

[16]Hayward, Rodney A., et al. Inequities in Health Services Among Insured Americans. *New England Journal of Medicine*, v. 318, June 9, 1988. p. 1507-1512.

The picture changes if particular types of care, such as prenatal care or preventive visits, are considered. A General Accounting Office (GAO) study of care delivered in 1986-87 found that only 46 percent of women covered by Medicaid received prenatal care in the first trimester of pregnancy, compared to 84 percent of those with private insurance and 41 percent of those with no coverage at all.[17] This and other studies of access to prenatal care have assigned mothers to the Medicaid category on the basis of their payment status at the time of delivery, and the findings may reflect delayed entry into Medicaid as much as limited access to care. (As noted above, women enrolled longer tend to receive earlier care.)

Only about a third of Medicaid-covered children are known to receive preventive care. In the year ended June 30, 1990, there were an average of 11.2 million Medicaid enrollees under age 21 and potentially eligible for screening examinations under the Early and Periodic Screening, Diagnostic, and Treatment (EPSDT) program. Of these, 4.0 million, or 35 percent received examinations during the year. (These figures may understate participation, as some States may not have collected data on services furnished to children enrolled in health maintenance organizations (HMOs) or similar arrangements.)[18] These figures represent a slight improvement over HCFA-reported data for previous years. An independent study conducted in California found that 40 percent of continuously enrolled children under age 15 and 55 percent of those under age 5 had preventive care visits during 1981. (The study included preventive visits that would not have been counted as EPSDT examinations.)[19] No comparable figures are available for privately insured children; however, few private plans cover services comparable to those offered under EPSDT.

2. Hospital Inpatient Care

Table H-3 provides NMES data on the likelihood, by reported health status and insurance coverage, that an individual had at least one hospital admission during the year. Among persons reporting excellent, good, or fair health, Medicaid beneficiaries were more likely to have had a hospital admission than

---

[17]U.S. General Accounting Office. *Prenatal Care: Medicaid Recipients and Uninsured Women Obtain Insufficient Care.* Report to the Chairman, Subcommittee on Human Resources and Intergovernmental Operations, Committee on Government Operations, House of Representatives. [GAO/HRD-87-137], Sept. 1987. Washington, 1987.

[18]Health Care Financing Administration. *Early and Periodic Screening, Diagnosis, and Treatment (EPSDT) Program Performance Indicators;* Memorandum by William Hiscock, Office of Medicaid Management, Medicaid Bureau, Sept. 5, 1990.

[19]Yudkowsky, Beth K., and Gretchen V. Fleming. Preventive Health Care for Medicaid Children. *Health Care Financing Review,* 1990 Annual Supplement. p. 89-96.

the privately insured.[20] This could be due in part to a greater incidence among the Medicaid enrollees of non-recurring acute events (such as deliveries or injuries) that might not affect self-reported health status. Medicaid beneficiaries reporting poor health were slightly less likely than the privately insured to have been admitted, although the difference was not statistically significant. The uninsured had fewer admissions in all health status categories.[21]

TABLE H-3. Percent of Population with at Least One Hospital Admission by Health Status and Source of Insurance Coverage, 1987[a]

Health status	Medicaid	Private	Uninsured
Percent of individuals with inpatient hospital admission:			
Excellent	6.0%	4.2%	2.1%
Good	9.6	7.0	3.7
Fair	16.4	13.9	7.2
Poor	30.9	33.6	20.6[b]

[a]Share of individuals with an inpatient hospital admission during calendar year 1987.

[b]Limited reliability. Use caution in interpreting numbers.

NOTE: Analysis is limited to those individuals who did not change health insurance status during calendar year. Health status is self-reported by survey respondents.

Source: Table prepared by the Congressional Research Service based on analysis of the 1987 National Medical Expenditure Survey.

Admission rates for Medicaid beneficiaries may be affected by their greater reliance on hospital-based sources of ambulatory care. As will be discussed further below, some studies suggest that beneficiaries treated in OPDs or ERs are more likely to be admitted than beneficiaries with the same conditions treated in physicians' offices or community health centers.

[20]The difference was statistically significant at the .05 level for those in good health, but not for those in excellent or fair health.

[21]The differences were statistically significant at the .05 level for those in excellent, good, or fair health, but not for those in poor health.

B. Quantity of Care

In addition to differences in the likelihood of any medical treatment during the year, there are differences in the quantity of treatment received by patients with different payment sources.

With respect to ambulatory care, available data permit little beyond comparisons of numbers of visits: who was seen more often? Table H-4 provides NMES data, by insurance coverage and reported health status, on the median number of non-inpatient physician contacts for patients who had any such contacts during the year. Medicaid enrollees in excellent or good health had numbers of contacts similar to those for the privately insured. Enrollees in fair health had more contacts than the privately insured, those in poor health slightly fewer.[22] In all four health status categories, the Medicaid enrollees were much closer to the privately insured than to the uninsured.[23] These data confirm the earlier observation by Long, Settle, and Stuart, that Medicaid coverage does not necessarily limit access to ambulatory care; it may affect the site of care, a point to be considered below.[24]

---

[22]The difference in mean contacts for those in fair health was statistically significant at the .10 level; differences in means for other health status categories were not statistically significant.

[23]Mean contacts for the Medicaid and uninsured groups differed significantly in all four status categories.

[24]Long, Stephen H., Russell F. Settle, and Bruce C. Stuart. Reimbursement and Access to Physicians' Services Under Medicaid. *Journal of Health Economics*, v. 5, 1986. p. 235-251.

TABLE H-4. Number of Ambulatory Contact with Physicians for Persons with at Least One Contact, by Insurance Status, and Health Status, 1987[a]

Insurance and health status	Median visits
By coverage type:	
Medicaid	3
Private insurance	3
Uninsured	2
By health status:	
Excellent	2
Good	3
Fair	4
Poor	8
By coverage type and health status:	
Medicaid:	
Excellent	3
Good	3
Fair	5
Poor	8
Private insurance:	
Excellent	2
Good	3
Fair	4
Poor	9
Uninsured:	
Excellent	2
Good	2
Fair	3
Poor	5

[a]Median number of contacts for individuals with one or more physician contact in their home, at the physician's office, in an outpatient setting or a hospital emergency room.

NOTE: Analysis is limited to those individuals who did not change health insurance status during the calendar year. Health status is self-reported by survey respondents.

Source: Table prepared by the Congressional Research Service based on analysis of the 1987 National Medical Expenditure Survey.

Table H-5 provides NMES data on inpatient days per enrollee (by insurance coverage and reported health status) and per user of inpatient services (by insurance coverage only). Medicaid enrollees in excellent, good, or fair health use more days of inpatient care than the privately insured.[25] Much of this difference is attributable to a higher proportion of Medicaid users of inpatient services, as discussed earlier. However, Medicaid users of inpatient care also receive more days of care than users who are privately insured or uninsured.[26]

That the data indicate more days of care for Medicaid users is consistent with earlier findings. A study of 1983 data from Massachusetts found that, after adjustment for age, sex, diagnosis-related group (DRG), and other factors, Medicaid patients had longer hospital stays than those with Blue Cross or those categorized as "self-pay" (often the uninsured). However, they had fewer surgical or other procedures than Blue Cross enrollees, and about the same number as the self-pay group.[27] Another study by the same investigators, this time using 1987 data, did not look specifically at Medicaid status. However, it found that patients who were poor, were less educated, or had a lower occupational status had longer stays and higher charges than other patients, again after adjustment for DRG.[28] The higher charges for low-income patients may indicate that they were more severely ill in ways not captured by the DRG classification system. If this is so, the lower rate of procedures found in the earlier study would suggest that they received different treatment from that provided to privately insured patients. This issue will be considered further below.

The length-of-stay differences themselves could reflect factors other than severity of illness. For example, Medicaid patients may remain in the hospital longer than they need to because of difficulties in arranging home care or finding a nursing home placement.

---

[25]The differences are statistically significant at the .05 level for those in good health and for the total.

[26]The difference between Medicaid and privately insured patients is statistically significant at the .05 level; the difference between Medicaid and the uninsured is not significant.

[27]Weissman, Joel, and Arnold M. Epstein. Case Mix and Resource Utilization by Uninsured Hospital Patients in the Boston Metropolitan Area. *Journal of the American Medical Association*, v. 261, June 23/30, 1989. p. 3572-3576.

[28]Epstein, Arnold M., Robert S. Stern, and Joel S. Weissman. Do the Poor Cost More? A Multihospital Study of Patients' Socioeconomic Status and Use of Hospital Resources. *New England Journal of Medicine*, v. 322,. Apr. 19, 1990. p. 1122-28.

TABLE H-5. Inpatient Hospital Days per Enrollee and per User of Inpatient Services, 1987

	Medicaid	Private	Uninsured
		Days per enrollee	
Health status:			
Excellent	.333	.189	.171
Good	.537	.411	.191
Fair	1.599	.991	.468
Poor	4.569	4.864	1.859
Total*	.954	.390	.281
		Days per user	
Total*	8.3	6.0	7.0

*Total includes persons whose health status was not reported.

NOTE: Analysis is limited to those individuals who did not change health status during calendar year. Health status is self-reported by survey respondents.

Source: Table prepared by the Congressional Research Service based on analysis of the 1987 National Medical Expenditure Survey.

C. Regular Source of Care

A final measure of basic access is the ability of patients to establish an ongoing relationship with a regular source of care. Such a relationship can improve continuity and patient compliance and perhaps the use of preventive services. The NMES survey included questions about respondents' usual sources. Table H-6 gives the results. (Note that, unlike the NMES data shown earlier, this table includes in the "any Medicaid/other public assistance" category persons who were covered both by Medicaid and some other form of insurance.)

Medicaid beneficiaries were less likely than the privately insured, and much less likely than the uninsured, to report that they had no usual source of care. No clear pattern appears in the explanations offered by those who lacked a usual source of care. Medicaid beneficiaries were somewhat less likely to say that they were seldom sick or were new to the area, reasons that might tend to be independent of financial or insurance status. However, they were no more likely than the privately insured to say that their previous source had become unavailable or that they used multiple sources. The Robert Wood Johnson Foundation survey cited earlier found that the insured poor were more likely than the insured near-poor or non-poor to report that there were financial barriers to finding a regular source of care.[29]

Of NMES respondents who reported a usual source of care, only 70 percent of the Medicaid beneficiaries used an office-based physician, compared to 88 percent of the privately insured who had a usual source of care. Medicaid beneficiaries were much more likely to report that they relied on hospital OPDs or ERs, or on other non-office sources such as clinics or community health centers. In addition, they were less likely to have an affiliation with a specific physician at their source of care. This appears to be a function of their greater reliance on non-office sources. Within a given site (office or other), Medicaid beneficiaries were only less likely than other patients to see a specific physician.

---

[29]Hayward, Rodney A., et al. Inequities in Health Services Among Insured Americans. *New England Journal of Medicine*, v. 318, June 9, 1988. p. 1507-1512.

**TABLE H-6. Reported Usual Source of Medical Care
by Health Insurance Coverage**

	Any Medicare	Any Medicaid/ other public assistance	Private insurance only	Uninsured
Usual source of care:				
None	9.3%	13.1%	17.8%	35.1%
Physician's office	81.7	61.3	72.7	48.0
Hospital outpatient dept. or emergency room	5.1	11.7	3.9	7.3
Other non-hospital	3.9	13.9	5.6	9.7
Percent of persons with a usual source of care who see a specific physician, by source:				
Any source	93.8	73.4	85.3	75.0
Physician's office	97.8	88.9	91.9	92.4
Other	57.6	36.6	34.4	24.2
For those without a usual source of care, reasons reported:				
Seldom or never sick	74.3	71.7	80.1	78.1
New to area	10.1	10.9	18.2	15.7
Source no longer available	16.6	9.9	9.9	6.1
Goes to different places	14.2	17.7	19.1	10.3

Source: Cornelius, L. K. Beauregard and J. Cohen. Usual Sources of Medical Care and Their Characteristics. *National Medical Expenditure Survey Research Findings 11.* Maryland, Agency for Health Care Policy and Research, Sept. 1991.

Another recent survey of persons living in low-income areas of Chicago produced similar results. Those with public coverage were more likely than those with private insurance to have a regular source of care; the differences were especially significant among blacks. The author speculates that, as was suggested earlier, cost-sharing requirements may deter utilization by the low-income privately insured. Again, however, the privately insured who had a regular source of care were more likely to see a private physician, while those with public coverage were more likely to use hospitals.[30]

While these survey responses confirm the common perception about Medicaid reliance on hospital-based services, the "usual" source of care is not necessarily the only source of care. Table H-7 shows, for NMES respondents who had any physician visits during the year, the percentage using hospital-based and office-based services. Most beneficiaries received at least some care in physicians' offices or at home. Relatively few received only hospital-based care, although the proportion that did so was much higher than among the privately insured.[31] The other major difference between Medicaid beneficiaries and the privately insured is that the former were generally more likely to use a mix of office and hospital-based care.[32] One possible explanation is limited access to office-based specialists. As will be shown below, primary care physicians are more likely to accept Medicaid patients than specialists are. Medicaid beneficiaries might be able to obtain primary care in office settings, but might have to turn to hospitals for specialty referrals. This explanation appears to be contradicted, however, by the fact that the privately insured reporting poor health are as likely as the Medicaid beneficiaries to have had some hospital contact.

A clear understanding of the differences in utilization patterns would require more information about the nature of visits at office and hospital sites. One case in which visits to different sites might be comparable is that of prenatal care. One comparison has indicated that 28 percent of Medicaid beneficiaries receive prenatal care in OPDs and 32 percent in health departments or other non-office settings, while only 24 percent of the population as a whole receives prenatal care in non-office settings.[33] Even in this instance, there might be some differences in the nature of the care provided; for example, high-risk pregnancies might be more likely to be referred to hospital-based specialists.

---

[30]Lewin-Epstein, Noah. Determinants of Regular Source of Health Care in Black, Mexican, Puerto Rican, and Non-Hispanic White Populations. *Medical Care*, v. 29, June 1991. p. 543-557.

[31]The differences were statistically significant at the .05 level except among those in fair health.

[32]The differences were statistically significant at the .05 level in each health status.

[33]Jencks and Benedict, *Accessibility and Effectiveness*.

TABLE H-7. Sites of Care for Users of Ambulatory Services by Source of Insurance and Health Status, 1987

Health status:	Medicaid	Private	Uninsured
	Percent of individuals receiving care at location:		
Excellent:			
Outpatient/ER only	14.9%	5.4%	12.0%
Office/home only	54.7	74.0	69.7
Both	30.4	20.6	18.3
Any office/home	85.1	94.6	88.0
Any OPD/ER[a]	45.3	26.0	30.3
Good:			
Outpatient/ER only	11.9	5.0	12.9
Office/home only	56.6	69.7	65.6
Both	31.5	25.3	21.5
Any office/home	88.1	95.0	87.1
Any OPD/ER[a]	43.4	30.3	34.4
Fair:			
Outpatient/ER only	8.3	4.2	14.2
Office/home only	42.1	61.8	61.0
Both	49.6	34.0	24.8
Any office/home	91.7	95.8	85.8
Any OPD/ER	57.9	38.2	39.0
Poor:			
Outpatient/ER only	11.2	2.6	11.4[b]
Office/home only	40.5	40.8	39.2[b]
Both	48.3	56.6	49.4[b]
Any office/home	88.8	97.4	88.6[b]
Any OPD/ER[a]	59.5	59.2	60.8[b]

[a]Outpatient or emergency room visits.

[b]Limited reliability. Use caution in interpreting numbers.

NOTE: Analysis is limited to those individuals who did not change insurance status during the year. Health status is self-reported by survey respondents.

Source: Table prepared by the Congressional Research Service based on analysis of the 1987 National Medical Expenditure Survey.

Some recent studies have sought to analyze the content of OPD or ER visits, although the data available (usually from paid claims records) are very limited. One analysis of Illinois Medicaid records attempts to distinguish OPD services that might instead have been obtained from an office-based physician care and others that would be unlikely to be furnished in an office (such as "true" emergency care or dialysis). The study found that use of the first type of service, primary care in an OPD setting, was higher in counties that also had higher use of office-based primary care. The authors contend that Medicaid beneficiaries were not substituting OPD care for office-based care, but were expanding access by using both types of care.[34]

Other analyses have focused on the appropriateness of the care Medicaid beneficiaries receive in emergency rooms. In one study, each ER visit was scored by the examining physician on a scale ranging from "inappropriate" (diaper rash, acne) to "essential" (myocardial infarction, stroke). For "welfare" patients, 61 percent of all visits were scored as inappropriate or marginal, compared to 27 percent for patients in other payment categories. Of visits made during weekday office hours, 80 percent of visits by "welfare" patients were inappropriate or marginal, compared to 35 percent for other patients.[35]

Another study, using Medicaid data from upstate New York, classified any ER visit that did not result in a hospital admission as a "primary care" visit, and found that the incidence of such visits was inversely related to the use of primary care from other sources. The authors contend that the use of ER services would drop if alternative sources of care were available. However, they also note that the tendency to use ERs rises in proportion to the percentage of a county's population receiving Medicaid. They argue that this phenomenon may be tied to cultural or environmental factors.[36] Another possibility is that fewer office-based physicians are available in areas with a high concentration of low-income residents. This issue will be considered further below.

Some people say that the use of hospital-based services cannot be attributed solely to the absence of community alternatives, but may also reflect patterns of care-seeking behavior on the part of the beneficiaries themselves, historical patterns that were established long before the enactment of Medicaid. The possibility of changing such behavior patterns has been an important source of State interest in the managed care alternatives described in *Appendix G, Managed Care*; these programs sometimes aim explicitly at reducing

---

[34]Fossett, James W., Chang H. Choi, and John A. Peterson. Hospital Outpatient Services and Medicaid Patients' Access to Care. *Medical Care*, v. 29, Oct. 1991. p. 964-976.

[35]Dickhudt, John S., Dwenda K. Gjerdingen, and Donald S. Asp. Emergency Room Use and Abuse: How It Varies with Payment Mechanism. *Minnesota Medicine*, v. 70, Oct. 1987. p. 571-574.

[36]de Alteriis, Martin, and Thomas Fanning. A Public Health Model of Medicaid Emergency Room Use. *Health Care Financing Review*, v. 12, spring 1991. p. 15-20.

inappropriate ER utilization, rather than at any broader improvement in coordination of care.

It is not certain, however, that current patterns of care-seeking behavior actually date from before Medicaid. One study found that low-income patients actually shifted regular sources of care between 1963 (pre-Medicaid) and 1970 (post-Medicaid). Those reporting a private physician as the regular source of care dropped from 63 percent to 56 percent, while those using "clinics," including hospital sites and other sources, rose from 17 percent to 24 percent. The authors cite additional evidence from Maryland and from Rochester, New York, showing changes during the early years of Medicaid. Beneficiaries used more physician care and less hospital-based care in 1967 than a few years later.[37] One possible explanation is that some private physicians accepted Medicaid at the very start of the program but rapidly dropped out. However, there do not appear to be any data on provider participation levels in the earliest years of the program.

Whether greater use of hospital-based services is an historical pattern or a more recent development, it is clearly tied to beneficiaries' ability to establish ties with an ongoing source of care. One recent study compared ER use by children with Medicaid or private insurance who did or did not have a regular source of care. Among children with a regular source of care, those covered by Medicaid were just as likely to receive care in the ER as privately insured children. Among those without a regular source, Medicaid-covered children received 28.6 percent of their care in ERs; for comparable privately insured children, the figure was 17.3 percent.[38] This would suggest, not that the ER is the provider of choice, but that Medicaid beneficiaries have greater trouble finding an alternative.

A study of care preceding hospital admissions reinforces this view. Medicaid beneficiaries are much more likely to be admitted through the ER than privately insured persons are. Among both Medicaid and uninsured patients, 66 percent were admitted through the ER, compared to 37 percent of the privately insured and 60 percent of Medicare beneficiaries.[39] This difference may partially reflect differences in severity; more admissions of privately insured patients may be elective, scheduled by a non-hospital provider in advance. Even

---

[37]Orr, Suezanne Tangerose, and C. Alden Miller. Utilization of Health Services by Poor Children Since Advent of Medicaid. *Medical Care*, v. 19, June 1981. p. 583-590.

[38]Orr, Suezanne T., et al. Emergency Room Use by Low Income Children with a Regular Source of Health Care. *Medical Care*, v. 29, Mar. 1991. p. 283-286.

[39]Stern, Robert S., Joel S. Weissman, and Arnold M. Epstein. The Emergency Department as a Pathway to Admission for Poor and High-Cost Patients. *Journal of the American Medical Association*, v. 266, Oct. 23/30, 1991. p. 2238-2243.

this explanation, however, suggests differences in timely access to community-based care.

III. MAINSTREAMING

While cultural patterns and environmental factors may have some effect on where Medicaid beneficiaries obtain care, the greatest attention has been paid to one factor: provider participation. Low Medicaid reimbursement, service limits, and bureaucratic red tape are thought to have led many providers to refuse to accept Medicaid patients or limit the number of such patients they will treat. As a result, in this view, Medicaid has failed to achieve the goal of mainstreaming and has led to the development of a two-tier system of medical care.

This section reviews the evidence on the extent to which providers participate in Medicaid, along with the much more limited evidence on two related questions: are the providers who do accept Medicaid of the same quality as those who do not, and do they render comparable care to their Medicaid and non-Medicaid patients? The discussion will focus on physicians and hospitals, because these are the provider types that have received the greatest study in recent years and that account for the greatest share of Medicaid spending (other than long-term care spending). However, comparable participation issues affect other provider types as well. As noted earlier, for example, low participation rates by dentists have recently been the subject of litigation in California.

A. Provider Participation

While States are obligated to provide adequate access to providers, providers have few reciprocal obligations. Providers are usually free to accept or reject Medicaid patients, or to accept them one day and refuse them the next. There are some exceptions. For example, hospitals, nursing homes, and other facilities constructed with Federal grants under the Hill-Burton Act must agree to participate in Medicaid. Similarly, States that require a certificate of need (CON) before a new hospital or nursing home is built may condition the granting of the CON on an agreement that the facility will accept Medicaid patients. In addition, facilities that accept any Federal funds (such as Medicare) are subject to the Civil Rights Act of 1964. Some courts have held that refusal to accept Medicaid has a disproportionate adverse impact on minorities and is therefore forbidden under title VII of the Act. One analyst has argued that even "neutral" policies that indirectly discourage minority patients (such as a hospital's requirement that all patients have an affiliated private physician) may be prohibited if they serve no significant objective.[40] In general, however, participation in Medicaid has been left to the discretion of providers.

---

[40]Watson, Sidney D. Reinvigorating Title VI: Defending Health Care Discrimination--It Shouldn't Be So Easy. *Fordham Law Review*, v. 58, Apr. 1990. p. 939-978.

1. Physicians

a. Levels of Physician Participation

Evidence on physician participation in Medicaid is fragmentary and frequently anecdotal. States do collect and report to HCFA annual counts of participating physicians. However, a physician is considered as "participating" if he or she submits even a single claim for services to a Medicaid beneficiary during a year; the extent of participation is not measured in the data. In addition, some States' physician counts fail to distinguish between individual practitioners and groups. A multi-specialty group with 100 physicians could be reported as a single physician provider. For these reasons, national data on physician participation in Medicaid are not helpful for analysis of access. Instead it is necessary to rely on published studies of small samples of physicians.

Most studies of Medicaid physician participation have therefore used surveys of the physicians themselves, particularly a series of surveys conducted by the National Opinion Research Center (NORC) under contract to HCFA in 1977-78 and again in 1984-85. Physicians in the NORC/HCFA sample were asked whether they accepted Medicaid payment and what proportion of their practice was made up of Medicaid patients. There have been a few more recent national surveys of practitioners in specific specialties, including pediatricians and obstetricians/gynecologists. However, the NORC/HCFA studies are the most recent to include all types of physicians.

Table H-8 shows the percent of physicians responding to the NORC/HCFA surveys who said they ever accepted Medicaid payment and, for those who accepted Medicaid, the average percentage of their case load that they estimated was made up of Medicaid patients. In every specialty except general surgery, the percentage of physicians reporting that they accepted Medicaid increased (or in the case of internists, held steady) between 1977-78 and 1984-85. However, Medicaid's average percentage of caseload for participating physicians dropped in several specialties, with the sharpest drops reported by internists and surgical specialists.[41] If the two measures, participation and Medicaid share, are combined, reported availability declined for all specialties except pediatrics and obstetrics. The declining Medicaid share in practices that accept Medicaid might in some cases reflect physician's decisions to refuse new Medicaid patients while continuing to treat established patients. (However, Medicaid share could decline if the number of patients with other payment sources increased and the number

---

[41]All the physicians' estimates of the Medicaid share of their practice must be interpreted with caution. A comparison of such estimates, made during a 1979 and 1980 NORC study, with actual patient records during the survey period found that the physicians tended to overstate the Medicaid share of their practices by 40 percent. Kletke, Phillip R., et al. The Extent of Physician Participation in Medicaid: A Comparison of Physician Estimates and Aggregated Patient Records. *Health Services Research*, v. 20, Dec. 1985. p. 503-523.

of Medicaid patients went unchanged, or if the supply of physicians grew more rapidly than the number of Medicaid beneficiaries.)

TABLE H-8. Physician Medicaid Participation Rates by Specialty, 1977-78 and 1984-85

	Percent accepting any Medicaid patients			For those accepting Medicaid, Medicaid as percent of total practice			Combined change in reported participation
	1977-78	1984-85	Percent change	1977-78	1984-85	Percent change	
Pediatrics	76.9	81.4	5.9%	14.1	16.9	19.9%	26.9%
General practice	75.1	86.9	15.7%	13.1	10.6	-19.1%	-6.4%
General surgery	90.3	88.4	-2.1%	13.4	11.7	-12.7%	-14.5%
Internal medicine	79.8	79.9	0.1%	13.2	7.7	-41.7%	-41.6%
Obstetrics/ gynecology	64.4	72.9	13.2%	8.4	10.1	20.2%	36.1%
Other medical specialties	73.4	85.1	15.9%	8.8	7.1	-19.3%	-6.5%
Other surgical specialties	82.9	87.0	4.9%	12.2	7.2	-41.0%	-38.1%

Source: Mitchell, Janet B. and Rachel Schurman. Access to Private Obstetrics/Gynecology Services under Medicaid. *Medical Care,* v. 22, no. 11, Nov. 1984. p. 1028 provides data for the 1977-78 period. Data for 1984-85 are from Physician Payment Review Commission. *Physician Payment Under Medicaid.* PPRC Report No. 91-4, Washington, 1991. p. 24.

More recent surveys indicate declining participation levels in pediatrics and obstetrics as well. A survey by the American Academy of Pediatrics found that, between 1978 and 1989, the percentage of pediatricians who accepted any Medicaid patients dropped from 85 percent to 77 percent. Those accepting only a limited number of Medicaid patients increased from 26 percent to 39.4 percent.[42] In a 1987 survey, the American College of Obstetricians and Gynecologists found that only 63 percent of respondents accepted Medicaid. This confirms the perceptions of State Medicaid directors, as reported in a 1990 survey by the National Governors' Association (NGA) and the Physician Payment Review Commission (PPRC).[43] Obstetrics/gynecology was the specialty most often cited (by 31 of 44 States responding) as having low physician participation. Obstetricians/gynecologists were (after psychiatrists) the least willing to accept Medicaid, even in 1977, before the malpractice crisis which is sometimes said to have affected obstetricians' Medicaid participation (the malpractice issue is discussed further below).

An alternative way of measuring physician participation is to consider the extent to which physicians rely on Medicaid as a revenue source. A recent *Medical Economics* survey, confined to office-based practitioners, reported that Medicaid accounted for an average of 7 percent of gross practice income in 1989, down from 8 percent in both 1981 and 1986. Two specialties, general practice and pediatrics, derived 11 percent of average income from income from Medicaid. Three others were well below average: orthopedic surgery and ophthalmology at 4 percent and plastic surgery at 3 percent.[44] Because of low Medicaid reimbursement rates, these percentages cannot be translated into patient share. They do, however, highlight the fact that different medical specialties are likely to have a different patient mix for reasons related to service coverage or population characteristics, rather than just willingness to accept Medicaid. For example, Medicaid rarely covers cosmetic surgery and would therefore be an insignificant payment source for a plastic surgeon. Ophthalmologists derive much of their income from treatment of cataracts and other problems of the elderly, and thus rely chiefly on Medicare.

In addition to differences by specialty, there appear to be regional differences in physician participation. The American Medical Association found participation in 1988 to be highest in the North Central region and lowest in the Northeast;[45] the *Medical Economics* survey produced similar results. The differences may reflect regional variations in the factors that affect physician participation, such as reimbursement rates.

---

[42]Yudkowsky, Beth K., Jennifer D.C. Cartland, and Samuel S. Flint. Pediatrician Participation in Medicaid: 1978 to 1989. *Pediatrics*, v. 85, no. 4, Apr. 1990. p. 567-577.

[43]PPRC, *Physician Payment Under Medicaid*.

[44]Azevedo, David. Which Third Parties Pay You the Most? *Medical Economics*, Nov. 26, 1990. p. 144-157.

[45]PPRC, *Physician Payment Under Medicaid*, p. 24.

Finally, it is possible that even physicians who accept Medicaid may provide some kinds of service and not others. For example, a psychiatrist might accept a Medicaid patient in group therapy but not provide individual psychotherapy. An obstetrician/gynecologist might cease to accept Medicaid for deliveries while continuing to provide other types of care. Few studies have addressed this possibility. One 1983 survey of physicians in several specialties likely to furnish reproductive health services found that participation rates were roughly equivalent for deliveries and other kinds of reproductive services.[46] That is, the data did not suggest that physicians were curtailing deliveries only.

b. Factors in Physician Participation

The PPRC/NGA survey of State Medicaid directors cited earlier included questions on the factors thought to discourage physician participation. Table H-9 gives the results. Low fees were seen as the most important problem, followed by concerns about malpractice premiums.

The responses of State officials can provide only indirect evidence of the reasons behind physicians' decisions; they might reflect the officials' own opinions or those of specific physicians with whom they have been in contact. Numerous other studies have collected information on physicians' training and attitudes, their practices, and the competitive environments in which they practiced, in order to identify possible factors in physicians' decisions about accepting Medicaid and about the number of patients they would accept.

---

[46]Orr, Margaret T., and Jacqueline D. Forrest. The Availability of Reproductive Health Services from U.S. Private Physicians. *Family Planning Perspectives*, v. 17, Mar./Apr. 1985. p. 63-69. The study included general/family practitioners, general surgeons, and urologists, as well as obstetricians.

TABLE H-9. Ranking of Reasons for Physician Non-Participation in Medicaid, 1990

	Number of States ranking reason:		
Reason	Most important rank (RANK 1-2)	Moderately important rank (RANK 3-5)	Least important rank (RANK 6-7)
Malpractice premiums	20	23	4
Patient compliance	10	27	10
Low fees	38	9	1
Payment delays	6	29	11
Clients sue frequently	2	10	33
Complex billing procedures	14	24	9
Disruptive clients	5	18	23

NOTE: States were asked to rank reasons from 1 to 7, with 1 being most important and 7 being least important. Not all States included all seven reasons in their rankings. Totals add to more than 51 for each column because of grouped rankings.

Source: Physician Payment Review Commission. *Physician Payment Under Medicaid.* PPRC Report No. 91-4. p. 23.

1. Dual Market Model

Many investigators have sought to test a "dual market" model for participation, under which physicians enter the Medicaid market only if there is sufficient competition in the private market.[47] If Medicaid patients were less desirable than other kinds of patients, because of lower reimbursement levels or for other reasons, physicians would take the other patients first. Medicaid participation would increase if physician supply increased. Physicians in a highly competitive situation would have fewer of the more desirable patients to go around and would begin accepting Medicaid. Two kinds of evidence would be needed to support this theory: that Medicaid beneficiaries are less acceptable to providers than other patients, and that competition makes a difference.

---

[47]For a summary of this model, see Perloff, Janet D., Phillip R. Kletke, and Kathryn M. Neckerman. *Medicaid and Pediatric Primary Care.* Baltimore, Johns Hopkins, 1987. p. 17-19. (Hereafter cited as Perloff, Kletke, and Neckerman, *Medicaid and Pediatric Primary Care*)

Patient acceptability. Providers' attitudes towards Medicaid patients may be affected both by payment levels and by other factors, such as administrative burdens.

It has been shown repeatedly that Medicaid reimbursement levels--or, more precisely, the gap between Medicaid reimbursement and what a physician can obtain from other payers--have a significant effect on participation.[48] (See *Chapter V, Reimbursement* for data on individual State payment rates.) Most recently, Joel W. Cohen has shown that Medicaid outpatient use is higher in the States with the lowest Medicaid physician fees, indicating that more beneficiaries are required to turn to alternate sources of care.[49]

Other factors may also work to make Medicaid patients more or less acceptable. Physicians have been found to refuse Medicaid patients because they find dealing with program administration cumbersome or because Medicaid takes too long to pay bills. Participation was higher in States that paid claims promptly or that used independent fiscal agents as intermediaries between providers and the Medicaid agency. A recent report by the Department of Human Services (DHHS) Office of the Inspector General (OIG) found that, while some States were making efforts to reduce Medicaid administrative burdens, some amount of red tape was inevitable given government requirements for financial accountability. In addition, the report noted that further State initiatives might be limited by current budgetary constraints.[50]

Physicians may also be frustrated by Medicaid coverage restrictions or authorization requirements, which may be regarded as interfering with the physician's professional judgment. Finally, there has been speculation that some characteristics of Medicaid beneficiaries may make them less acceptable to some providers. Physicians may find that Medicaid patients take more time and require more support services than others, or that they are less compliant with medical advice.[51]

---

[48]Hadley, Jack. Physician Participation in Medicaid: Evidence from California. *Health Services Research*, v. 14, winter 1979. p. 266-280. (Hereafter cited as Hadley, *Physician Participation in Medicaid*) Mitchell, Janet B., and Rachel Schurman. Access to Private Obstetrics/Gynecology Services under Medicaid. *Medical Care*, v. 22, Nov. 1984. p. 1026-1037.

[49]Cohen, Joel W. Medicaid Policy and the Substitution of Outpatient Care for Physician Care. *Health Services Research*, v. 24, Apr. 1989. p. 33-66.

[50]U.S. Dept. of Health and Human Services. Office of the Inspector General. *Medicaid Hassle: State Responses to Physician Complaints.* OIG Report No. OEI-01-92-00100, Mar. 1992. Washington, 1992.

[51]Davidson, Stephen M. Physician Participation in Medicaid: Background and Issues. *Journal of Health Politics, Policy and Law*, v. 6, winter 1982. p. 703-717. Sloan, Frank, Janet Mitchell, and Jerry Cromwell. Physician Participation in State Medicaid Programs. *Journal of Human Resources*, v. 13,
(continued...)

Competition. The evidence is much less clear on the second major component of the market model, the hypothesis that Medicaid participation would increase if physicians faced heavy competition for other kinds of patients. Studies have repeatedly found that, as the ratio of physicians to the general population in a given county or metropolitan area rises, the extent of Medicaid participation drops.[52] Some analysts suggest that competition reduces physicians' earnings from private insurers and makes them less willing to subsidize unprofitable patients.[53] One recent study has found that use of OPDs rises in areas with a higher concentration of primary care physicians, again perhaps indicating that competition discourages physician participation in Medicaid instead of encouraging it.[54]

However, the few studies which have looked below the county level have also found a strong correlation between a physician's willingness to accept Medicaid patients and the number of Medicaid beneficiaries in the zip code where the physician's practice is located. Taken together, the two findings may suggest that each physician in a highly competitive area does not add a Medicaid component to his or her practice to make up for a declining pool of private patients. Instead, some observers have noted, competition may lead physicians to specialize in one market or the other.[55] The extent to which this specialization may be related to simple geographic distribution, the presence or absence of physicians in areas with a high concentration of Medicaid beneficiaries, has not been systematically studied.

Yet another explanation is suggested by a recent study of the willingness of pediatricians in North Carolina to accept Medicaid patients. Rural physicians and those in areas with a low physician-to-population ratio were much less likely than urban ones to restrict Medicaid access. One factor appears to have been a perception by urban physicians that alternative sources of pediatric care

---

[51](...continued)
1978 Supplement. p. 211-245. (Hereafter cited as Sloan, Mitchell, and Cromwell, *Physician Participation in State Medicaid Programs*)

[52]Mitchell, Janet B. Medicaid Participation by Medical and Surgical Specialists. *Medical Care*, v. 21, Sep. 1983. p. 929-938. (Hereafter cited as Mitchell, *Medicaid Participation by Medical and Surgical Specialists*) Hadley, *Physician Participation in Medicaid*. Perloff, Kletke, and Neckerman, *Medicaid and Pediatric Primary Care*.

[53]Schlesinger, Mark, and Karl Kronebusch. The Failure of Prenatal Care Policy for the Poor. *Health Affairs*, v. 9, winter 1990. p. 91-111. (Hereafter cited as Schlesinger and Kronebusch, *The Failure of Prenatal Care*)

[54]Fossett, James W., Chang H. Choi, and John A. Peterson. Hospital Outpatient Services and Medicaid Patients' Access to Care. *Medical Care*, v. 29, no. 10, Oct. 1991. p. 964-976.

[55]Perloff, Kletke, and Neckerman, *Medicaid and Pediatric Primary Care*, p. 54-57.

were available to Medicaid beneficiaries. Physicians in isolated areas felt a stronger obligation to accept patients regardless of payment source.[56]

2. Malpractice Premiums

Malpractice premiums were cited as the second most important reason for low physician participation in the PPRC/NGA survey of State Medicaid officials; several States also cited a tendency of clients to "sue frequently" as a factor. Concerns about malpractice may have been especially important in limiting participation by obstetricians. Average annual malpractice premiums for obstetricians were $37,000 in 1989, more than twice the average for all physicians; obstetricians were also more than twice as likely than other physicians to have incurred a professional liability claim in 1989.[57] In States where Medicaid fees are low, physicians may feel that Medicaid is contributing less than its fair share of the malpractice premiums.

The perception among physicians that Medicaid beneficiaries are more likely to sue than other patients may also be important, although this view is not supported by the evidence.[58] A GAO study of malpractice claims found that Medicaid patients accounted for 5.8 percent of claims for which a patient insurance source could be identified, less than their share of the population.[59] A more recent study in Maryland produced similar results for physician services in general. For obstetrical services, claims by Medicaid beneficiaries were in proportion to their share of obstetric discharges (21 percent of both).[60] However, if Medicaid payment rates were below a physician's usual charges, a physician might still conclude that the assumed risk per dollar received was greater for Medicaid patients.

Some analysts have suggested that the malpractice issue reflects a basic conflict between the two goals of maintaining the unitary standard of quality assumed by the legal liability system and providing access to care. In this view,

---

[56]Margolis, Peter A., et al. Factors Associated with Pediatricians' Participation in Medicaid in North Carolina. *Journal of the American Medical Association*, v. 267, no. 14, Apr. 8, 1992. p. 1942-1946.

[57]American Medical Association. Center for Health Policy Research. *Socioeconomic Characteristics of Medical Practice: 1990/91*. Chicago, 1991. p. 17-18.

[58]For a review of the evidence, see Institute of Medicine. *Medical Professional Liability and the Delivery of Obstetrical Care*. Washington, National Academy Press, v. 1, 1989. p. 64-65.

[59]U.S. General Accounting Office. *Medical Malpractice. Characteristics of Claims Closed in 1984*. GAO/HRD-87-55, Apr. 1987. Washington, 1987.

[60]Mussman, Mary G., et al. Medical Malpractice Claims Filed by Medicaid and Non-Medicaid Recipients in Maryland. *Journal of the American Medical Association*, v. 265, June 12, 1991. p. 2992-2994.

if providers are expected to choose between providing equally good care to low-income patients at reduced prices and refusing care altogether, their incentive is to do the latter.[61]

3. Other Factors

Some other apparent factors in participation have been identified that do not fit readily into the dual-market model. Characteristics of individual physicians may have an impact. Some studies have found higher participation among physicians who are younger, who are certified by specialty boards, and who believe that society has a responsibility to ensure that medical care is available.[62] One recent study has found a shift in physician attitudes in recent years. A cohort of medical school graduates followed over 25 years is now more likely than at the time of graduation to agree with statements such as "those who accept charity lack dignity" and "for a private practitioner it is important that Medicaid patients be separated from other patients."[63]

Finally, primary care physicians who are graduates of foreign medical schools are somewhat more likely to accept Medicaid patients and significantly more likely to have a high proportion of Medicaid patients. No such correlations were found for foreign medical graduates who were specialists, rather than primary care physicians.[64]

2. Hospitals

Virtually all hospitals (other than Federal facilities or hospital units within prisons and other institutions) participate in Medicaid to some extent. Of nonfederal hospitals responding to the 1984 American Hospital Association (AHA) survey, 98 percent treated at least some Medicaid beneficiaries on an

---

[61]Siciliano, John A. Wealth, Equity, and the Unitary Medical Malpractice Standard. *Virginia Law Review*, v. 77, Apr. 1991. p. 439-487. Siciliano notes that, in other areas of tort law, the consumer is supposed to expect lower quality for lower cost goods. See also Morreim, E. Haavi. Cost Containment and the Standard of Medical Care. *California Law Review*, v. 75, Oct. 1987. p. 1719-1763.

[62]Mitchell, *Medicaid Participation by Medical and Surgical Specialists.* Perloff, Kletke, and Neckerman, *Medicaid and Pediatric Primary Care.*

[63]Barney, Joseph A., et al. The Physician and the Poor: A Study of Expressed Willingness to Serve the Indigent Patient--A Twenty-Five Year Longitudinal Study. *Education*, v. 110, fall 1989. p. 61-69.

[64]Sloan, Mitchell and Cromwell, *Physician Participation in State Medicaid Programs.*

inpatient basis during the year. Among those offering outpatient services, only a handful--12 out of 5,606 respondents--had treated no Medicaid patients.[65]

As with physicians, however, a simple classification of facilities as participating or non-participating gives no indication of the extent to which hospital services are available to beneficiaries. Hospitals may be presented with some cases to whom they cannot refuse services on financial grounds, such as women in labor or other patients in need of urgent care, and still have an overall policy of refusing non-emergency care to patients with insufficient resources. There are widespread allegations that some private hospitals, especially those operated for profit, tend to deny elective care to Medicaid patients because of reimbursement levels they regard as inadequate. In order to examine these allegations, it is necessary to consider relative levels of Medicaid participation, and to take into account factors other than explicit hospital policies that could affect different hospitals' Medicaid caseloads.

a. Hospital Participation Levels

The level of a hospital's participation in Medicaid can be measured in two ways:

- The hospital's share of the total Medicaid patient load. Which hospitals are Medicaid beneficiaries likely to use?

- The Medicaid share of the hospital's total patient load. At which hospitals do Medicaid patients make up a higher proportion of the total patient population?

The Prospective Payment Assessment Commission (ProPAC) has recently analyzed Medicaid participation levels in 1985 and 1989, using data from cost reports submitted by hospitals to Medicare. Table H-10 gives the results. Medicaid discharges as a percentage of all discharges increased from 10 to 12 percent. While Medicaid discharges were increasing, from 2.8 million to 3.4 million, discharges of privately insured patients and Medicare beneficiaries were dropping. The general decline in inpatient hospital use has many causes, such as substitution of outpatient services for inpatient care and the increasing prevalence among insurers of requirements that patients obtain prior authorization before admission to the hospital. Medicaid trends are thus running counter to trends for other insured groups.

Only a small part of the growth in Medicaid admissions is attributable to overall growth in the Medicaid population. The number of Medicaid beneficiaries grew 7.8 percent from 1985 to 1989, while Medicaid discharges grew by 22 percent (subsequent Medicaid population growth has been much higher). However, the newly added beneficiaries may have been more likely to use inpatient care than those already on the program. For example, new enrollments resulting from expanded coverage for pregnant women (and for

---

[65]Except as noted, information from the AHA survey was compiled by the Congressional Research Service from tape data supplied by AHA.

their newborns, who are often separately billed at birth) would be nearly matched by new admissions. One factor that does not appear to have been at work is any growth in multiple admissions for single beneficiaries. On the contrary, the number of Medicaid beneficiaries receiving inpatient care, as measured by the HCFA-2082 report, grew at about the same rate (22 percent from 1985 to 1989) as the number of discharges.[66]

[66]The figures for users of general hospital care in 49 States and the District of Columbia (omitting Arizona and the territories) were 3.36 million in 1985 and 4.10 million in 1989.

TABLE H-10.Medicaid Discharges and Average Length of Stay, by Hospital Group, 1985 and 1989

Hospital group	Total Medicaid discharges		Percent change	Percent of all Medicaid discharges		Medicaid discharges as a percent of all discharges		Average length of stay (days)	
	1985	1989		1985	1989	1985	1989	1985	1989
Total	2,806,960	3,415,641	21.7%	100.0%	100.0%	9.5%	12.0%	5.4	5.6
Urban	2,202,460	2,682,108	21.8	78.5	78.5	9.3	11.5	5.7	5.9
Rural	604,500	733,533	21.3	21.5	21.5	10.4	13.6	4.5	4.5
Major teaching	567,504	620,576	9.4	20.2	18.2	14.8	17.6	6.6	6.7
Other teaching	939,945	1,221,810	30.0	33.5	35.8	9.1	11.8	5.6	5.8
Non-teaching	1,298,125	1,574,028	21.3	46.2	46.1	8.5	10.7	4.8	4.9
Disproportionate share:	1,754,272	2,175,286	24.0	62.5	63.7	14.4	18.4	5.5	5.7
Urban	1,590,256	1,969,186	23.8	56.7	57.7	13.9	17.5	5.7	6.0
Rural	164,016	206,100	25.7	5.8	6.0	15.8	21.8	4.8	4.8
Non-disproportionate share	1,052,560	1,241,016	17.9	37.5	36.3	6.2	7.5	5.0	5.0
Voluntary	1,924,182	2,301,750	19.6	68.6	67.4	9.1	11.2	5.5	5.7
Proprietary	272,356	355,152	30.4	9.7	10.4	7.8	10.2	4.9	5.2
Urban public	414,162	512,381	23.7	14.8	15.0	13.5	17.8	5.8	5.7
Rural public	175,480	201,756	15.0	6.3	5.9	10.6	14.0	4.3	4.4

NOTE: 1985 estimate of Medicaid discharges as a percent of all discharges differs from estimate in the original table. This new estimate was provided by ProPAC.

Source: Prospective Payment Assessment Commission. Medicaid Hospital Payment. Congressional Report C-91-02.

Whatever the reasons for the overall growth in Medicaid inpatient utilization, it did little to modify the distribution of Medicaid patients among classes of hospitals. Medicaid discharges as a percent of all discharges rose for every type of hospital. In both 1985 and 1989, public hospitals, rural hospitals, and teaching hospitals (those with interns and residents) had higher Medicaid patient shares than other facilities. Facilities labelled as "disproportionate share" had the highest Medicaid caseloads. (Note that the data use Medicare's criteria for classifying a facility as disproportionate share, instead of individual States' Medicaid criteria. Since the Medicare classification is itself based directly on Medicaid patient share, to observe that disproportionate share hospitals had high Medicaid shares is redundant.) Data from another source indicate that children's hospitals also have very high Medicaid caseloads. Medicaid beneficiaries accounted for an average of 25.6 percent of discharges from children's hospitals in 1987.[67]

Public hospitals have heavier Medicaid caseloads only in urban areas. Rural public hospitals have almost the same Medicaid patient share as all rural hospitals. That is, ownership has no apparent impact on the extent to which hospitals participate in Medicaid. One possible explanation is that, whether public or private, a hospital in a nonmetropolitan area is more likely to serve as the primary source of care for the area it serves. Some people have suggested that, if a hospital is the only provider of care in an area, it will be more likely to accept all kinds of patients, regardless of insurance source or ability to pay. If, on the other hand, there are many hospitals in an area, some may be tempted to act as "free riders," allowing other hospitals to carry the burden. That is, they will feel more able to deny care to some patients if they can assume that other hospitals are available to those patients.[68] This hypothesis assumes, however, that all the hospitals in a metropolitan area are operating in a single market and that Medicaid beneficiaries are equally likely to seek care at any of the facilities. It is possible that, within a metropolitan area, public hospitals are located in areas with high concentrations of Medicaid beneficiaries and are simply more accessible to them.

In any event, classification of hospitals into broad categories for the purpose of analyzing Medicaid participation has the effect of masking substantial variation at the individual facility level. Figure H-1 shows the 1984 distribution of hospitals by the percentage of their total inpatient days furnished to Medicaid beneficiaries. In each of the three categories (public, private non-profit, and private for-profit), a handful of facilities treat a very high proportion of Medicaid patients, while the rest treat relatively few. The pattern is strongest among for-profit facilities. In 85 percent of the for-profits, Medicaid accounts for less than 10 percent of patient days; Medicaid accounts for 20 percent or more of the days in only 5 percent of the for-profit hospitals. Among

---

[67]National Association of Children's Hospitals and Related Institutions. *Assuring Children's Access to Health Care: Fixing the Medicaid Safety Net.* Alexandria, Va. 1989.

[68]As was noted earlier, a similar explanation has been advanced for higher Medicaid participation rates among rural physicians.

the public hospitals, 45 percent furnished less than 10 percent of total days to Medicaid beneficiaries. Nearly 20 percent of the public hospitals had Medicaid shares of 20 percent or higher.

FIGURE H-1. Medicaid Inpatient Days as a Share of Total Days, by Hospital Ownership, 1984

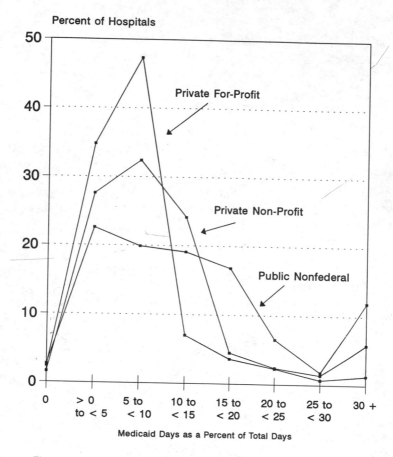

Source: Figure prepared by Congressional Research Service based on data from the American Hospital Association.

The overall growth of Medicaid admissions in recent years might have altered the distribution of patients among individual facilities, or it might instead merely have increased the caseload at the facilities already treating the most Medicaid patients. This cannot be determined from the aggregate ProPAC data, which are the most recent available.

One factor which should be considered before drawing any conclusions from these statistics is the possibility that the national data are affected by regional differences in the numbers of persons covered by Medicaid, differences which happen to correspond to regional patterns of hospital ownership. For-profit hospitals have historically been most prevalent in the South and West. States in these regions, especially those in the South, have also tended to have the most restrictive Medicaid eligibility policies. They are, for example, less likely to have medically needy programs. The effect may be that there are proportionately fewer Medicaid beneficiaries in the areas most likely to be served by for-profit facilities. Recent expansions in Medicaid eligibility in these areas may account for some of the growth in patient share at proprietary hospitals between 1985 and 1989.

National data on hospital participation levels may also conceal variation at the State and local level. One recent study, using 1984 Medicaid claims data, compared the hospitals used by beneficiaries in California and Michigan. In California, Medicaid patients were concentrated in hospitals (chiefly public and teaching hospitals) different from those used by the population as a whole. No similar pattern appeared in Michigan. One partial explanation for the pattern seen in California is the State's program of selective provider contracting, under which beneficiaries are expected to receive most non-emergency care from hospitals chosen by the State through a competitive process. Still, the findings for California more nearly represent the national pattern, while the Michigan experience appears not to.[69]

b. Explaining Levels of Participation

Broadly speaking, there are two possible ways of explaining a particular hospital's relative level of participation in Medicaid. First, the pool of Medicaid beneficiaries seeking treatment at the hospital might be larger or smaller, depending on circumstances which may or may not be under the hospital's control. Second, the hospital could have explicit policies relating to the acceptance or non-acceptance of Medicaid patients.

1. Variations in Medicaid Demand

As was suggested above, some hospitals might have fewer Medicaid patients than others because they were in locations not readily accessible to many Medicaid beneficiaries, or because they did not offer specific kinds of services that Medicaid beneficiaries are likely to require. Within a metropolitan area, for

---

[69]Andrews, Roxanne, et al. Access to Hospital Care for California and Michigan Medicaid Recipients. *Health Care Financing Review*, v. 12, no. 4, summer 1991. p. 99-104.

example, a suburban hospital might be less likely than a hospital in a central city to treat many Medicaid patients. A hospital that failed to offer obstetrical care, which is a major source of Medicaid admissions (see below), might also be expected to see fewer Medicaid patients.

Some observers have argued that these differences among hospitals are themselves market-driven. In deciding about location or about the kinds of services to offer, some hospitals might take into account the potential impact of these decisions on the hospitals' volume of private, Medicare, Medicaid and uninsured patients.

On the issue of location, at least, this view may be an oversimplification. Where hospitals are located today is the product of historic decision making over many years. These decisions were economic in the sense that most hospital construction in recent decades has been in areas of population growth, such as the suburbs, and areas with a strong economic base. Less new construction occurred in areas with declining populations, such as the older central cities, and a weaker economic base. One consequence may have been that many new facilities were located in areas with a lower concentration of Medicaid and uninsured patients. To say this is not to say, however, that the insurance status of the local population was a direct factor in the location decisions.[70]

Decisions about the types of services to offer may be more directly driven by current market factors. Some kinds of services are generally less profitable than others, partly but not entirely because they are more likely to attract Medicaid beneficiaries or uninsured patients. These include, not only obstetrical care, but also outpatient and emergency room services.[71] Unlike decisions about location, hospitals' decisions about services can be changed at any time. Recently, for example, hospitals in some areas have closed existing emergency rooms or have dropped out of trauma networks, reportedly because they were losing money on Medicaid and uninsured patients. According to the American Hospital Association, community hospitals reported 323 fewer State-certified trauma centers in 1988 than in 1987; another 74 were gone by 1989.[72]

---

[70]It is possible that assessment of a hospital's current market plays a more direct role in acquisition, as opposed to construction, decisions. A national proprietary hospital chain considering whether to buy an existing hospital would be expected to consider the hospital's mix of insured and uninsured patients in deciding whether the hospital could be profitable.

[71]Watt, J. Michael, et al. The Effects of Ownership and Multihospital System Membership on Hospital Functional Strategies and Economic Performance. Institute of Medicine, For-Profit Enterprise in Health Care. Washington, 1986. p. 260-289.

[72]American Hospital Association. Hospital Statistics. 1989-90 and 1991 editions. Chicago, 1990 and 1991. Note that some of the drop between 1987 and 1988 may be attributable to a change in the definition of trauma centers.

One other indirect factor in the extent of a hospital's Medicaid participation does not appear to have been investigated. The volume of Medicaid patients admitted to a particular hospital might be related to the practice patterns of the physicians associated with that hospital. For example, if a hospital's admissions came mainly from affiliated office-based practitioners with very limited Medicaid practices, the hospital's Medicaid volume might be relatively small even in the absence of any direct hospital decision to limit Medicaid volume.

Hospitals that have received Hill-Burton Act construction grants and whose affiliated physicians do not treat Medicaid beneficiaries are required by regulations (42 CFR 124.602(d)(2)) to find other ways of insuring that Medicaid beneficiaries have access to their services. For example, they may require staff physicians to accept Medicaid patients or may contract with outside physicians who do treat Medicaid beneficiaries.

2. Hospital Admission Policies

Unlike individual practitioners, most hospitals do not have complete discretion over whom they will and will not treat. The decision making is usually shared between the hospital and its attending physicians, who traditionally control admissions. Hospital administrators who wish to limit their Medicaid patient load may vary in the degree of direct control they are able to exercise over physician admitting decisions. Because open interference in these decisions may be taken as interference with physician prerogatives, some hospitals might seek to influence the flow of admissions in more subtle ways.

One study has attempted to investigate this possibility. Schlesinger et al., drawing on a 1984 American Medical Association (AMA) survey of physicians, explored the physicians' own perceptions of the extent to which the principal hospital they used attempted to discourage the admission of Medicaid and uninsured patients. Table H-11 shows the results, by type of hospital. (It should be noted that the percentages are of responding physicians affiliated with the type of hospital in question, not percentages of hospitals.) The pattern of reported "discouragement" conforms roughly to the pattern of actual Medicaid participation levels, with physicians at for-profit facilities considerably more likely to report that their institutions discouraged Medicaid patients.[73]

[73]Schlesinger, Mark, et al. The Privatization of Health Care and Physicians' Perceptions of Access to Hospital Services. Milbank Quarterly, v. 65, 1987. p. 25-58. (Hereafter cited as Schlesinger, The Privatization of Health Care)

TABLE H-11. Percent of Physicians Reporting that their Primary Hospital Discouraged Admission of Medicaid Patients

Hospital type	Percent
Independent hospitals:	
For-profit	15
Private nonprofit	5
Public	3
Multi-hospital systems:	
For-profit	16
Private nonprofit	6
Public	3

Source: Schlesinger, Mark et al. The Privatization of Health Care and Physicians' Perceptions of Access to Hospital Services. *Milbank Quarterly,* v. 65, no. 1, 1987. pp. 25-58. Table 1, p. 33.

The extent to which some institutions may be deliberately refusing Medicaid admissions, rather than merely discouraging them, is less clear. Several studies in the early 1980s explored the issue of inappropriate hospital transfers: the allegation that some facilities refuse to treat severely ill Medicaid patients, or transfer them as rapidly as possible to other hospitals. The studies found that disproportionate numbers of patients transferred from other hospitals to the emergency rooms of public hospitals were uninsured or covered by Medicaid or other public programs.[74]

"Anti-dumping" provisions in the Consolidated Omnibus Budget Reconciliation Act of 1985 (COBRA, Public Law 99-272) prohibit hospitals participating in Medicare from refusing treatment to or transferring medically unstable patients, unless the transfer is medically necessary or the patient requests transfer. Note that the provision applies only to medically unstable patients. Hospitals may still deny care on financial grounds to patients presenting for elective or non-urgent care. No data are yet available on the extent to which COBRA may have affected hospital acceptance of Medicaid patients.[75]

---

[74]Himmelstein, David U., et al. Patient Transfers: Medical Practice as Social Triage. *American Journal of Public Health,* v. 74, May 1984. p. 494-7. Schiff, Robert L., et al. Transfers to a Public Hospital: A Prospective Study of 467 Patients. *New England Journal of Medicine,* v. 314, Feb. 27, 1986. p. 552-57.

[75]For further information see: U.S. Library of Congress. Congressional Research Services. *Hospital Patient Protection: The Consolidated Omnibus*
(continued...)

3. Impact of Medicaid Policies

The Schlesinger study cited earlier, detailing the extent to which hospitals discouraged physicians from admitting Medicaid patients, found some correlation between State Medicaid policies and hospitals' perceived willingness to accept Medicaid beneficiaries. (However, other factors, such as ownership, were much more important.) Hospitals in States that had shifted from full cost reimbursement to prospective payment for inpatient services were more likely to discourage Medicaid admissions, as were hospitals in States that had established prior authorization requirements for inpatient care.[76] Hospitals in these States were also more likely to discourage admission of uninsured patients, a phenomenon to be discussed further at the end of this section.

Medicaid Hospital Reimbursement. As *Chapter V, Reimbursement* indicates, in 1989 States on average paid hospitals at rates well below their costs for treating Medicaid patients. Much has changed since 1989, including dramatic growth in State-reported expenditures for inpatient services and particularly in payment adjustments to disproportionate share hospitals. Medicaid inpatient spending grew 79 percent between 1989 and 1991. Not all of these increases necessarily resulted in actual increases in hospital revenues. State provider donation and provider-specific tax programs, whether broad-based or more narrowly targeted, had the effect of returning to State treasuries some portion of any increase in hospitals' Medicaid payments. Depending on the size of the donations or taxes involved, the net effect in some States could have been no change in the ratio of a hospital's net Medicaid revenues to its Medicaid costs.

The ProPAC study found that Medicaid patient share at an individual hospital was strongly related to how well Medicaid paid the hospital. Table H-12 shows the distribution of hospitals by Medicaid patient share and Medicaid payments as a percent of costs. Hospitals with the highest Medicaid payments relative to costs were also more likely to have high proportions of Medicaid patients; the lowest paid hospitals had lower proportions of Medicaid patients. This represents a reversal from 1980, when the hospitals with the lowest proportions of Medicaid patients tended to have the highest Medicaid payments. ProPAC suggests that some of the change may be due to the advent of payment adjustments for hospitals treating a disproportionate share of Medicaid and low-income patients. If States are required to make higher payments to the hospitals treating the most Medicaid beneficiaries, it is logical that payments to those hospitals would meet a greater proportion of costs. However, the substantial payment shortfalls at facilities not qualifying for the payment

---

[75](...continued)
Budget Reconciliation Act "Anti-Dumping" Law. CRS Report for Congress No. 90-321 EPW, by Beth C. Fuchs and Joan Sokolovsky. Washington, July 5, 1990.

[76]Schlesinger, *The Privatization of Health Care,* p.41.

adjustments would clearly create incentives to hold steady or further reduce their Medicaid patient share.[77]

TABLE H-12. Distribution of Hospitals by Medicaid Payments as a Share of Costs and Patient Share, 1989[a]

Medicaid payments as a share of costs	>11.2%		Medicaid patient share: 5.6% to 11.2%		< 5.6%		Total
Greater than 90 percent	452	(++)	501	(-)	274	(0)	1,227
62 to 90 percent	572	(0)	1,456	(+)	426	(-)	2,454
Less than 62 percent	203	(-)	497	(-)	527	(++)	1,227
Total	1,227		2,454		1,227		4,908

$X^2 = 411$ p < 0.001

[a]Number of hospitals in patient and payment category.

NOTE: The pluses and minuses indicate whether hospitals are over (+) or under (-) represented in each cell.

Source: Prospective Payment Assessment Commission. *Medicaid Hospital Payment.* Congressional Report C-91-02, Oct. 1991. Table 3-12, p. 79.

Other Medicaid Policies. A second area of Medicaid policy that potentially affects hospital participation is service limitations. As *Chapter IV, Services* indicates, a number of States have fixed limits on the number of inpatient days they will cover. States may also limit coverage of, or offer reduced reimbursement for, "administrative days," the time spent in a hospital by a patient who no longer requires hospital services but who cannot be placed elsewhere. Many States have adopted systems of retrospective utilization review. Payment may be denied if a beneficiary's inpatient stay, or some part of it, is found to be medically unnecessary. All of these practices place hospitals at some risk of furnishing care for which payment may later be unavailable and may have the effect of discouraging participation. Limits on covered days may have an especially strong effect on hospitals' willingness to accept severely ill patients.[78]

Other State policies are aimed directly at deterring avoidable hospital admissions. These include requirements for prior authorization of elective admissions, second surgical opinion programs, or policies intended to encourage

---

[77]As *Chapter V, Reimbursement* suggests, this incentive might not hold if a hospital had low occupancy and Medicaid payments at least met marginal costs.

[78]It should be noted that, in data such as the ProPAC estimates of State reimbursement levels, service limits have the same effect as actual rate reductions. In either case, the State is reducing overall payment for a hospital stay, and both types of reductions are combined into one overall estimate of "shortfall."

the performance of certain kinds of surgery on an outpatient basis. (See *Chapter IV, Services* for a discussion of these policies.) Although comparable policies have increasingly been adopted by other insurers, Medicaid programs were among the first to impose these sorts of controls. While it would seem that policies of this kind would affect all hospitals equally, it is conceivable that some hospitals find them administratively cumbersome or that they have a disproportionate impact on the types of services offered at specific facilities.

B. Quality of Participating Providers

Concern over the failure to mainstream Medicaid beneficiaries does not stem simply from the fact that providers used by Medicaid beneficiaries may not be identical to those used by other patients. Simple geography might often dictate that the providers most accessible to low-income persons would be different from those most convenient to higher-income persons. Quality issues would be raised by these differences if the providers available to beneficiaries, were less accessible or were somehow inferior to those used by other patients, or if whole classes of providers more frequently used by Medicaid beneficiaries (such as OPDs or ERs) were thought to furnish inappropriate or inadequate care. The following discussion considers evidence on each of these points.

Physical Access. The portion of the NMES survey relating to usual sources of care included questions on travel and waiting time. The results are shown in table H-13. Reported travel time to the usual source of care tended to be slightly longer for Medicaid beneficiaries than for the privately insured and somewhat shorter than for Medicare beneficiaries or the uninsured. There were greater differences in waiting time before seeing the provider. Medicaid beneficiaries were more likely than the privately insured to wait 30 minutes or more, and more than twice as likely to wait 60 minutes or more. Even the uninsured were more likely than Medicaid beneficiaries to be seen within 30 minutes. (Note, however, that these experiences are those reported by patients with a usual source of care; waiting times might be different for those without an established provider.)

**TABLE H-13. Reported Travel and Waiting Times for Usual
Source of Care, by Health Insurance Status
(Percent of persons reporting any usual source of care)**

	Any Medicare	Any Medicaid/ other public assistance	Private insurance only	Uninsured
Travel--				
Less than 30 minutes	79.9%	82.5%	86.0%	80.8%
30-59 minutes	16.0	12.6	12.3	15.4
60 minutes or more	4.0	4.9	1.7	3.9
Waiting time--				
Less than 30 minutes	54.6	44.1	61.1	48.6
30-59 minutes	22.4	25.7	22.0	25.5
60 minutes or more	12.4	19.8	8.5	15.5
Unknown	10.5	10.4	8.3	10.4

Source: Cornelius, L.K. Beauregard and J. Cohen. Usual Sources of Medical Care and
Their Characteristics. *National Medical Expenditure Survey Research Findings 11*. Maryland,
Agency for Health Care Policy and Research, Sept. 1991.

Individual Providers. There have long been allegations that some of the
providers most accessible to Medicaid beneficiaries may furnish inadequate care.
Stories of "Medicaid mills," clinics that treat large numbers of beneficiaries in
brief and perfunctory visits, have been told since the beginning of the program
and continue to appear.[79] Beyond such anecdotes, there is no evidence so far
on the relative quality of specific providers treating Medicaid beneficiaries.

One recent study investigated the hospital characteristics associated with
"adverse events" in hospitals in New York City. There were higher rates of
problems due to substandard care or negligence in hospitals with a high
proportion of minority patients, but lower rates in public and teaching hospitals.
Level of Medicaid participation was not measured, and it is not clear which of
the two characteristics (high minority use or public/teaching status) is the better
proxy. However, the study at least suggests an approach for further
investigation of the quality of facilities available to Medicaid beneficiaries.[80]

---

[79]See, for example, U.S. Congress. House. Committee on Government
Operations. Subcommittee on Human Resources and Intergovernmental
Relations. *Quality of Care Provided by Medicaid Physicians in New York*.
Hearings, 101st Cong., 2nd Sess., Mar. 19, 1990. Washington, GPO, 1990.

[80]Brennan, Troyen A., et al. Hospital Characteristics Associated with
Adverse Events and Substandard Care. *Journal of the American Medical
Association*, v. 265, June 26, 1991. p. 3265-69.

Provider Classes. As was noted earlier, the fact that Medicaid patients are more likely to use hospital-based physician services does not necessarily mean that they are receiving less ambulatory care overall. However, there are concerns that use of OPDs results in a lack of continuity, and that an inability to establish ongoing ties with a single physician may produce negative outcomes. For example, a study of the care received by low-income children found that, of those whose usual source of care was an OPD or ER, only one in four had an ongoing tie to a specific physician. (A comparable finding in the NMES data was cited earlier.) However, those who **had** established such a tie received care comparable to that in physicians' offices.[81]

In addition, hospital-based services may be more costly than equivalent services provided by office-based physicians. This point is open to debate, at least with regard to services other than those in emergency rooms. Apparent cost differences may simply reflect the tendency of Medicaid programs to pay office-based physicians according to a fee schedule while paying hospitals (until recently) on a cost basis. It is not clear that the price difference for equivalent services would have been so great if Medicaid had paid office-based physicians' full charges. Beyond the cost of individual visits, however, there may be differences in overall cost of treatment for patients with different sources of care. One comparison of Medicaid users of OPDs and users of physicians' offices in Maryland suggests that the former may have more visits and more inpatient admissions, even after some correction for severity.[82]

C. Content and Outcome of Care

Even when Medicaid beneficiaries receive care from the same sources used by other patients, they may be treated differently. For example, low reimbursement might discourage providers from performing surgery or costly diagnostic tests. In addition, some analysts have suggested that payment status could affect the content of particular physician encounters; for example, some physicians might spend less time with lower-paying patients.[83]

There is some evidence that Medicaid beneficiaries with a given condition are less likely to receive certain procedures than other patients. A Massachusetts study of persons hospitalized with circulatory disorders or chest pain found that those with Medicaid were less likely than the privately insured to receive an angiography or a coronary artery bypass graft, and less than half as likely to receive angioplasty. Even the uninsured had higher rates of angioplasty than Medicaid beneficiaries. A study of cardiac patients in New

---

[81]Kasper, Judith D. The Importance of Type of Usual Source of Care for Children's Physician Access and Expenditures. *Medical Care*, v. 25, May 1987. p. 386-398.

[82]Stuart, Mary et al. Ambulatory Practice Variation in Maryland: Implications for Medicaid Cost Management. *Health Care Financing Review*, 1990 Annual Supplement. p. 57-67.

[83]Schlesinger and Kronebusch, *The Failure of Prenatal Care.*

York State produced similar results.[84] Another study compared treatment of lung cancer patients with private insurance, public insurance (including Medicaid), and no coverage. The privately insured were more likely than the other two groups to receive surgery, radiation, or other active treatment. However, they had no clear advantage in survival rates. The authors suggest that the additional treatment provided to the privately insured may have gone to patients who had little or nothing to gain from it.[85] Finally, a study of the allocation of organ transplants found that privately insured patients were more likely than Medicaid beneficiaries to receive heart transplants even when the procedure had a low chance of success; no similar pattern was found for liver transplants.[86]

A recent study of the treatment of sick newborns in California hospitals in 1987 found that those covered by Medicaid had shorter stays and lower charges than the privately insured, but longer stays and higher charges than comparable uninsured newborns. These differences were not affected by hospital ownership or diagnostic category.[87]

Finally, several studies have compared rates of cesarean section by income or payment source. One study found that higher-income women were more likely to have cesareans even after correction for age and parity of the mother, birthweight of the child, race or ethnic group, and presence or absence of complications.[88] A California study found that Medicaid beneficiaries were less likely to have cesareans than the privately insured and more likely than self-pay or indigent patients. They were also more likely to have cesareans than

---

[84]Wenneker, Mark B., Joel S. Weissman, and Arnold M. Epstein. The Association of Payer with Utilization of Cardiac Procedures in Massachusetts. *Journal of the American Medical Association*, v. 264, Sept. 12, 1990. p. 1255-1260. Hannan, Edward L., et al. Interracial Access to Selected Cardiac Procedures for Patients Hospitalized with Coronary Artery Disease in New York State. *Medical Care*, v. 29, May 1991. p. 430-441.

[85]Greenberg, E.R., et al. Social and Economic Factors in the Choice of Lung Cancer Treatment: A Population-Based Study in Two Rural States. *New England Journal of Medicine*, v. 318, Mar. 10, 1988. p. 612-617.

[86]Friedman, Bernard, Ronald J. Ozminkowski, and Zachary Taylor. Excess Demand and Patient Selection for Heart and Liver Transplantation. Agency for Health Care Policy and Research Pub. No. 92-0025. [Reprint from *Health Economics Worldwide*, 1992.]

[87]Braveman, Paula A., et al. Differences in Hospital Resource Allocation Among Sick Newborns According to Insurance Coverage. *Journal of the American Medical Association*, v. 266, Dec. 18, 1991. p. 3300-3308.

[88]Gould, Jeffrey B., Becky Davey, and Randall S. Stafford. Socioeconomic Differences in Rates of Cesarean Section. *New England Journal of Medicine*, v. 321, July 27, 1989. p. 233-239.

enrollees in the Kaiser Foundation Health Plan, a health maintenance organization.[89]

The lower cesarean rate in Kaiser, which has controls in place intended to limit unnecessary surgery, raises the question of whether the privately insured and Medicaid patients might have received cesareans more often than necessary. A similar question might be raised by the lung cancer study cited above. Because of ongoing uncertainty about the efficacy of different medical procedures, it is difficult to determine the optimum rate of cesareans, radiation therapy, or other treatments. Different benchmarks may be assumed in analyses with different focuses. Studies of geographic variation in surgery rates often assume that patients in the areas with the highest rates are receiving excessive treatment. The reverse is sometimes implied in comparisons of treatment by payment source: utilization rates for the privately insured are assumed to reflect the correct level, while the care provided to Medicaid beneficiaries is deemed insufficient.

The difficulty of deciding just how much care, and of what kind, is appropriate is one of the sources of growing interest in efforts to measure the outcomes of medical care. Congress has responded to this interest by funding an effectiveness research initiative to be carried on by a newly formed agency within DHHS, the Agency for Health Care Policy and Research. Findings from this initiative may eventually provide better measures of the adequacy of the care received by different segments of the population, including Medicaid beneficiaries.

So far, however, there has been little study of outcomes of care under Medicaid. A few studies have found adverse health consequences after beneficiaries lose Medicaid coverage entirely or lose coverage for specific services because of program limits.[90] These studies show that having coverage is better than not having coverage, but do not allow comparison of outcomes for Medicaid beneficiaries and for other insured individuals. One exception is a study showing that children on Medicaid were much more likely than other children to be admitted to hospitals with asthma. Although other factors (such as race) potentially complicated these findings, they may to some extent reflect the consequences of late or inadequate access to ambulatory treatment that might have prevented admission.[91]

The Omnibus Budget Reconciliation Act of 1986 (P.L. 99-509) required HCFA to study the appropriateness, necessity, and effectiveness of selected

---

[89]Stafford, Randall S. Cesarean Section Use and Source of Payment. American Journal of Public Health, v. 80, Mar. 1990. p. 313-15.

[90]See Jencks and Benedict, Accessibility and Effectiveness, for a review of these studies.

[91]Wissow, Lawrence S., et al. Poverty, Race, and Hospitalization for Childhood Asthma. American Journal of Public Health, v. 78, July 1988. p. 777-782.

medical treatments furnished to Medicaid beneficiaries. The final phase of this study, now under way, will provide a large-scale analysis of patient outcomes including direct review of a broad sample of medical records.

One area in which outcomes have received particular attention is that of prenatal care. Expanding access to timely prenatal care has been a major focus of Medicaid policy for some years, and assessment of birth outcomes might seem to be a test of the success of the program. However, some studies have suggested that the connection between the receipt of prenatal care and avoidance of such adverse outcomes as low birthweight is a "tenuous" one.[92] Schlesinger and Kronebusch found that prenatal outreach programs are more effective in reducing the incidence of low birthweight than Medicaid. While Medicaid has improved financial access to medical care, case management systems that refer patients to high-quality providers and to related services such as nutrition programs and substance abuse treatment have a greater impact.[93]

These findings highlight a basic limitation in the measures of program performance outlined at the start of this appendix, including providing basic access or mainstreaming. These measures can test the adequacy of Medicaid as health insurance: whether Medicaid has leveled the playing field, whether it has given its enrollees the same access to medical care that other insured persons enjoy. However, health insurance alone cannot overcome non-financial barriers to care, poverty, and other social factors that play an important role in health outcomes. If the policy goal is to improve those outcomes, measures beyond expansion of health insurance and changes external to the entire medical care system are likely to be necessary.

---

[92]Howell, Embry M., et al. A Comparison of Medicaid and Non-Medicaid Obstetrical Care in California. *Health Care Financing Review*, v. 12, no. 4, summer 1991. p. 1-15.

[93]Schlesinger and Kronebusch, *The Failure of Prenatal Care.*

TECHNICAL APPENDIX ON NATIONAL MEDICAL EXPENDITURE
SURVEY AND SAMPLE SIZE

This technical appendix provides a brief summary of the National Medical Expenditure Survey (NMES) used to produce comparisons in health use patterns among Medicaid beneficiaries, the privately insured, and the uninsured. It describes the NMES survey and the sample from that survey on which the analysis is based.

The 1987 NMES household survey is a national probability sample of the civilian, noninstitutionalized population living in the community. It provides information on the use and financing of health services during calendar year 1987. Survey responses are weighted to provide estimates for the entire U.S. noninstitutionalized population, or 239 million persons.

The survey collects information about health insurance coverage during each of four rounds, and reports coverage status for each round. Current data provides use of health services only on an annual basis. If coverage status changes during the year, for example from Medicaid to uninsured, we are unable to determine from the survey results which health services were used when the person was covered by Medicaid. In addition, some respondents were not eligible for the survey for the full calendar year, because they were born or died during 1987, or because they became institutionalized. To provide a clean basis for comparisons, we deleted some survey respondents from analysis as follows:

- Persons not eligible for the sample for the full year
- Persons covered by Medicare or the Civilian Health and Medical Program of the United States (CHAMPUS)
- Persons with health insurance from more than one source during the year (e.g. persons with Medicaid for part of the year and uninsured for part of the year, or persons with private health insurance for part of the year and Medicaid for part of the year)
- Persons with private, non-group coverage
- Persons age 65 or older.

These deletions produce a study sample size of 154.6 million, or approximately 65 percent of the U.S. population. The numbers of persons in the study sample, by health insurance coverage status, are shown below.

Type of health coverage	Number of persons (in millions)
Medicaid	10.3
Private, group	120.8
Uninsured	23.5
Total	154.6

APPENDIX I. MEDICAID AND HIV DISEASE[1]

I. INTRODUCTION

Medicaid has emerged as the most important single source of coverage for persons with acquired immune deficiency syndrome (AIDS) and may play a growing role in funding treatment for other persons who are infected with the human immunodeficiency virus (HIV) but who have not been diagnosed as having AIDS.

Current estimates suggest that as many as 40 percent of all AIDS patients become eligible for Medicaid benefits at some point in the course of their illness. Medicaid's share of total costs for these patients is somewhat lower, perhaps 30 percent, in part because some persons with AIDS qualify for Medicaid only after having been ill for some time. Medicaid's role in financing health services for persons with AIDS may expand in the future, both because of changes in the nature of the population developing AIDS and because other forms of insurance coverage may become less available to persons with AIDS. The Health Care Financing Administration (HCFA) estimates that Medicaid payments for persons with AIDS will reach $2.1 billion in FY 1992, or about 1.7 percent of the projected $120 billion in total FY 1992 Medicaid spending.

Persons with HIV disease qualify for Medicaid in two basic ways. First, they may become disabled as a result of their illness, deplete their resources, and thus be eligible for Supplemental Security Income (SSI) payments or qualify as medically needy. Second, they may qualify for reasons unrelated to their illness, by meeting the usual categorical and financial tests for Medicaid eligibility. As the incidence of AIDS cases grows among low-income women and minorities, more persons with AIDS are likely to qualify for Medicaid and to receive benefits earlier in the course of their illness.

Congress and the States have taken some measures to increase Medicaid coverage and reimbursement for HIV-related services. Thirteen States have developed home and community-based services programs for persons with AIDS under the section 2176 waiver option; others have developed special programs for HIV-infected children or offer targeted case management services for persons with HIV disease. A majority of States now cover hospice care, and several States have developed special reimbursement rules to improve access to nursing home care for persons with AIDS. One coverage issue, Medicaid payment for HIV-related drugs, was partly resolved by the Omnibus Budget Reconciliation Act of 1990 (OBRA 90, P.L. 101-508)--States may no longer deny coverage for

---

[1]This appendix was written by Mark Merlis.

any drug approved by the Food and Drug Administration (FDA), but they may still refuse payment for drugs in the experimental stage.

This appendix is in four parts. The first explores trends in overall spending for HIV-related health care services and estimates of Medicaid's share of that spending. The second reviews how persons with HIV disease may become eligible for Medicaid and discusses the factors that may lead to a greater role for Medicaid in the future. The third summarizes recent legislative initiatives affecting Medicaid services to persons with HIV disease, while the fourth examines Medicaid coverage of specific HIV-related services.

II. TRENDS IN HIV SPENDING AND MEDICAID SHARE

A. Prevalence of HIV Infection and Disease

The AIDS was first reported in the United States in 1981. As of October 1992, 242,146 cases of AIDS had been reported to the Centers for Disease Control and Prevention (CDC); 66 percent of these persons had died. CDC has estimated that, as of mid-1989, as many as 1 million Americans may have been infected with HIV, which causes AIDS. (This represents a downward revision from previous estimates, which assumed that at least that number had been infected by 1986.) CDC further projects that between 390,000 and 480,000 persons will have been diagnosed as having AIDS by the end of 1993.[2]

Many more infected persons will develop HIV-related illnesses that are not officially categorized as AIDS. The term "AIDS" has been used by CDC only for HIV-infected persons who develop certain specific problems, such as pneumocystis pneumonia, Kaposi's sarcoma (a form of skin cancer), or central nervous system deterioration. Persons who develop other problems not on the official list may be just as ill as those who have AIDS. For this reason, many analysts believe the distinction between AIDS and other HIV-related conditions is artificial and should be abandoned. In this view, AIDS is part of a continuum that ranges from asymptomatic HIV infection at one extreme to terminal illness at the other. Nevertheless, the distinction between AIDS and other HIV disease is still commonly made. For example, the CDC definition is used to determine case load for the purpose of allocating Federal grant funds to States and localities, as well as in establishing individual eligibility for Federal assistance programs. (The debate over the use of the CDC definition for Medicaid purposes is discussed below.)[3]

---

[2]U.S. Dept. of Health and Human Services. Public Health Service. Centers for Disease Control. In HIV Prevalence Estimates and AIDS Case Projections for the United States: Report Based on a Workshop. *Morbidity and Mortality Weekly Report*, v. 39, no. RR-16, Nov. 30, 1990. (Hereinafter cited as DHHS, HIV Prevalence Estimates)

[3]In Oct. 1992, CDC announced plans to broaden the definition of AIDS to include HIV-infected persons who have low levels of certain immune system cells, as well as to include additional conditions to the list of symptoms

(continued...)

B. Costs of Treating HIV Disease

Almost from the beginning of the HIV epidemic, analysts have attempted to measure the costs of treating infected persons and the potential impact of the epidemic on overall health care spending. Most studies to date have focused on costs incurred by persons formally diagnosed as having AIDS. Little is known about expenditures for the much larger population whose HIV disease has not yet progressed to the point of AIDS, or who are currently asymptomatic but are receiving treatments intended to slow the onset of disease.

Early estimates of health care expenditures for a typical patient from AIDS diagnosis to death ranged from $24,000 to $147,000. More recent estimates, based on larger samples, have been in the $40,000 to $75,000 range. However, most of the data used for these estimates are already some years old and may not fully reflect the effects of longer survival times, costly new therapies, or changes in the nature of the population with AIDS (such as the increased number of patients who are women or children) and accompanying changes in the manifestations of the disease. In addition, the estimates include only costs incurred after an individual has been officially diagnosed as having AIDS. One recent attempt to consider these factors has resulted in projections that a person with AIDS will incur costs of $38,300 per year, while costs for an HIV-infected person who has not yet developed AIDS could reach $10,000 per year. This study estimates total costs per person of $102,000 from diagnosis to death.[4]

Uncertainty about case load at any given time and about per capita costs has led to a wide range of estimates of overall AIDS-related spending. The new study cited above projects total lifetime expenditures of $10.3 billion for persons with HIV disease first diagnosed in 1992 and $15.2 billion for those diagnosed in 1995. Other studies have attempted to estimate costs incurred during a single year for all persons with AIDS living in that year. One such estimate, developed in 1986, projected spending of $8-16 billion during 1991, in 1991 dollars; note that this figure excludes treatment prior to a diagnosis of AIDS.[5] The $8 billion projection, extrapolated to later years, continues to form the basis for HCFA estimates of Medicare and Medicaid AIDS spending.

---

[3](...continued)
previously used to identify AIDS. This change is expected to have a significant effect on overall case counts. However, there will still be many people with HIV disease who will not be counted as having AIDS.

[4]Hellinger, Fred J. Forecasts of the Costs of Medical Care for Persons with HIV: 1992-1995. In press, cited in Agency for Health Care Policy and Research. *Research Activities*, no. 155, July 1992.

[5]Coolfont Report: A PHS Plan for Prevention and Control of AIDS and the AIDS Virus. *Public Health Reports*, v. 101, no. 4, July-Aug. 1986. p. 341-348.

C. Medicaid Share of HIV-Related Costs

In addition to the uncertainties about overall costs, there are differing estimates of the shares of those costs borne by public and private payers. Most early studies found that Medicaid was covering 20 to 30 percent of the total costs of AIDS treatment, compared to the 40 to 60 percent of total costs covered by private health insurance.[6] HCFA's Medicaid projections assume that 40 percent of all persons with AIDS receive Medicaid benefits, but that Medicaid pays only 58 percent of the costs for these patients, chiefly because of low reimbursement rates. HCFA therefore estimates that Medicaid will cover 23 percent of total AIDS costs, or $2.1 billion in FY 1992, rising to $3.8 billion by FY 1997.[7]

Other estimates have tended to agree that Medicaid's share of total AIDS spending is less than its share of the AIDS population. While HCFA's estimates assume low reimbursement, there are other possible explanations. For example, many patients may qualify for Medicaid late in the course of their illness, after already having received services covered by another source of coverage or having spent their own resources.

A number of recent studies have suggested that Medicaid's share of the total patient load is rising, while the share covered by private insurance is dropping. Table I-1 shows the results of a comparison of funding sources for AIDS-related hospitalizations in New York, San Francisco, and Los Angeles. Medicaid's share of cases grew sharply in all three cities between 1983 and 1987, while the share of cases paid by private insurance dropped. (New York had a higher share of Medicaid cases than the other two cities in both years, for reasons to be discussed below.)

---

[6]For a review of these studies, see U.S. Congress. Office of Technology Assessment. *The Costs of AIDS and Other HIV Infections: Review of the Estimates.* OTA staff paper. Washington, GPO, 1987.

[7]Unpublished estimates from the Office of the Actuary. The Federal share for FY 1992 is projected to be $1.08 billion, or about 51 percent. This is slightly below the average Federal Medicaid share of 57 percent, because AIDS cases are concentrated in States with the minimum 50 percent Federal matching rate.

**TABLE I-1. Percentage of AIDS Hospitalizations Funded by
Medicaid and Private Insurance, 1983 and 1987**

	1983	1987	Percent change
New York			
Medicaid	39.7%	53.4%	34.5%
Private insurance	43.4%	31.6%	-27.2%
San Francisco			
Medicaid	18.5%	30.0%	62.2%
Private insurance	55.0%	28.8%	-47.6%
Los Angeles			
Medicaid	10.4%	27.8%	167.3%
Private insurance	70.6%	42.5%	-39.8%

Source: Green, Jesse, and Peter S. Arno. The 'Medicaidization' of AIDS.
Journal of the American Medical Association, v. 264, no. 10, Sept. 12, 1990, p.
1261-1266.

Whether the same pattern has been repeated nationally is not yet clear.
The largest studies of AIDS treatment costs to date, surveys of hospitals
conducted by the National Public Health and Hospital Institute in 1985, 1987
and 1988, produced mixed results. Between the first and second surveys
Medicaid's share of AIDS admissions increased, relative to those covered by
private insurance, in some types of hospitals and some regions, while the reverse
occurred in others. The surveys in all 3 years showed much higher proportions
of Medicaid patients overall than have other studies of AIDS spending: 54
percent in 1985, 44 percent in 1987, and 47 percent in 1988. One reason may
be that the surveys focused on public and teaching hospitals, which tend to
serve a disproportionate share of Medicaid patients. (The 1987 survey included
some private nonteaching hospitals; this may partially explain the overall drop
in Medicaid share.) The 1988 survey also included data on admissions for non-
AIDS HIV illness. Medicaid beneficiaries accounted for 49 percent of these
admissions, compared to just 17 percent for the privately insured.[8]

While Medicaid is clearly a major source of funding for AIDS treatment, the
exact share of AIDS costs being borne by Medicaid is still unclear. Even less is
known about costs related to treatment of non-AIDS HIV disease. Still, there

---

[8]Andrulis, Dennis P., Virginia Beers Weslowski, and Larry S. Gage. The
1987 U.S. Hospital AIDS Survey. *Journal of the American Medical Association*,
v. 262, no. 6, Aug. 11, 1989. p. 784-794; Andrulis, Dennis P., Virginia Beers
Weslowski, Elizabeth Hintz, and Audrey Wright Spolarich. Comparisons of
Hospital Care for Patients with AIDS and Other HIV-Related Conditions.
Journal of the American Medical Association, v. 267, no. 18, May 13, 1992. p.
2482-2486.

is widespread agreement that Medicaid's role in HIV funding is likely to grow in the future. In order to understand these predictions, it is necessary to review how persons with HIV disease can become eligible for Medicaid benefits.

III. MEDICAID ELIGIBILITY FOR PERSONS WITH HIV DISEASE

Persons with HIV disease qualify for Medicaid in two basic ways. First, they may become disabled as a result of their illness, deplete their resources, and thus be eligible for SSI payments or qualify as medically needy. Second, they may qualify for reasons unrelated to their illness, by meeting the usual categorical and financial tests for Medicaid eligibility.

A. SSI Disability Coverage

Persons who receive SSI on the basis of disability are generally eligible for Medicaid, with exceptions in certain States discussed in *Chapter III, Eligibility*. In order to receive SSI, a disabled person must meet income and resource standards, must be determined by a physician to meet medical standards of disability, and must not be engaged in substantial gainful activity (earnings from work may not exceed $500 per month). As a result of a Social Security Administration (SSA) ruling, persons with a confirmed diagnosis of AIDS are presumed to have met the disability standard. The "presumptive disability" rule does not confer automatic eligibility on persons with AIDS. They must still meet the financial standards and must not be engaged in "substantial gainful activity" (generally, must not have employment earnings over $500 per month); but they may qualify for benefits more rapidly than other applicants, whose medical disability must be determined on an individual basis.

In applying the presumptive disability rule, the SSA initially used the definition of AIDS established by the CDC. Under this definition, an HIV-positive individual is not considered to have AIDS unless he or she has had certain opportunistic infections or has exhibited other specified symptoms. More recently, SSA has developed a broader listing of HIV-related impairments that can be used to establish presumptive disability for persons who do not have AIDS but are considered equally disabled.

The HIV-infected persons who are not yet symptomatic or who do not have the particular impairments on the SSA list are not presumptively eligible. Some may be ill enough to qualify as disabled for SSI purposes on an individual basis by going through a standard medical review process. Those who are not yet ill may not qualify at all. One consequence is that low-income persons in the early stages of HIV disease may not receive Medicaid coverage for the treatments that could slow the progress of the disease. In addition, the medical review requirement may delay coverage even for persons who are seriously ill.

Table I-2 shows the initial disposition in FY 1986 through FY 1988 of applications for SSI or for Social Security disability insurance (SSDI) on the basis of HIV-related problems. SSDI uses the same disability criteria as SSI, but does not impose income or asset tests. Instead, a disabled person is potentially eligible if he or she is "insured" under the Social Security system by having paid the Social Security payroll tax for the required number of quarters. Some low-income people with sufficient work history may receive both SSI and SSDI.

TABLE I-2. Disposition of Initial Social Security Decisions for Cases with HIV-Related Impairments, Fiscal Years 1986 to 1988

	Allowed in initial decision			Total allowed	Denied	Percent allowed
	DI only	SSI only	SSI and DI			
Impairment:						
AIDS	3,399	2,619	4,416	10,434	384	98.2%
Symptomatic HIV	406	844	918	2,168	1,562	73.5%
Other AIDS-related	4,686	3,564	5,148	13,398	2,738	90.7%
Total	8,491	7,027	10,482	26,000	4,684	91.7%

NOTE: "Other AIDS-related" includes persons who were recorded as having AIDS or HIV, but for whom other problems were listed as the first and second impairments in Social Security records.

Source: Social Security Administration, Office of the Actuary.

As the table shows, a total of 26,000 applicants with an HIV-related impairment were approved for SSDI, SSI, or both in the initial decision on their applications, while 4,684 were denied benefits. (Some of these were later approved on reconsideration or appeal.) The approval rate was much higher for applicants with AIDS than for those with non-AIDS symptomatic HIV disease. Persons whose primary impairment was some problem other than HIV disease, but who also reported HIV, were more likely to be approved than those whose non-AIDS HIV disease was the primary impairment.

The SSA standards governing presumptive SSI eligibility for persons with HIV disease have been challenged in court in at least one State on the grounds that they discriminate against women. The contention is that the listing of impairments reflects the course of HIV disease in men, while women tend to have different symptoms and are therefore excluded. Others have argued that the CDC definition and the somewhat broader SSA listing have more generally failed to keep pace with changing manifestations of HIV disease. In 1989, for example, one in four deaths among persons with symptomatic HIV disease were of persons who did not meet the CDC AIDS definition.[9]

As was noted earlier, CDC has proposed a revision of the AIDS definition to include certain asymptomatic persons with depleted immune systems. SSA will not be bound by this change, but has published proposed rules that would allow consideration of functional impairment, rather than just a particular list of problems or symptoms, in determining whether an individual's illness is

[9]DHHS, HIV Prevalence Estimates, Nov. 30, 1990.

sufficiently severe to warrant presumptive disability.[10] While the replacement of simple decision rules with a fuller evaluation may make more people eligible, some advocates have expressed concerns that it will also lengthen the eligibility determination process.

B. Medically Needy Eligibility

As of January 1991, disabled persons could qualify as medically needy in 35 States.[11] Medically needy disabled persons do not meet the income standards for SSI, and therefore do not receive cash assistance, but do meet the other criteria for SSI eligibility. They may receive Medicaid if they meet the State's asset limits and if their net income, after subtracting incurred medical expenses and certain other disregarded amounts, is below a medically needy standard established by the State. Some persons who lack other insurance coverage may "spend down" to Medicaid eligibility by incurring large medical bills.

One group that may be especially likely to qualify as medically needy are those who are receiving SSDI payments but have not yet become eligible for Medicare benefits. Recipients of SSDI benefits must wait 5 months for those benefits and may receive Medicare only after completing an additional 24-month waiting period, for a total delay of 29 months. Because this is longer than the average life span after a formal diagnosis of AIDS, few SSDI recipients with AIDS ever receive Medicare benefits. (Estimates are that Medicare covers no more than 1 to 3 percent of total costs for the treatment of AIDS.)

As was noted earlier, some persons with low enough SSDI benefits may also qualify for SSI and thus receive Medicaid. This was true for about 55 percent of the successful SSDI applicants in FY 1986-FY 1988. For the rest, however, the SSDI benefits raise their incomes above SSI cash assistance standards. Those who are in States with medically needy programs can spend down to Medicaid eligibility; those in States without such programs may be left with no coverage at all. (Applicants for SSI must also apply for, and if eligible accept, SSDI benefits; thus they cannot forgo the SSDI payment in order to qualify for Medicaid.)

C. Low-Income Persons With HIV Disease

Some persons with HIV disease may be eligible for Medicaid for reasons not directly related to their illness. This may be especially true of intravenous (IV) drug users and their sexual partners and children, who are likely to have low incomes and who may have qualified for Medicaid prior to developing HIV disease on a basis other than disability. These include recipients of Aid to Families with Dependent Children (AFDC) and others qualifying through recent expansions of Medicaid eligibility for low-income mothers and children.

---

[10]*Federal Register*, v. 56, no. 243, Dec. 18, 1991. p. 65702-65714.

[11]See *Chapter III, Eligibility* for a listing of these States.

One recent study of Medicaid enrollees with AIDS in California and New York found that, in an average month in 1986, one third of the beneficiaries in New York had qualified through AFDC or as Ribicoff children, compared to just 4 percent in California.[12] This corresponds to the greater prevalence of AIDS among women and children in New York, which in turn reflects the higher proportion of cases related to drug use. A study of Medicaid spending for persons with AIDS in Michigan confirms that women were more likely than men to be eligible for Medicaid before they were diagnosed as having AIDS.[13]

D. Future Trends

Two major trends are likely to affect the role of Medicaid in financing care for persons with HIV disease. The first is a shift in the epidemic towards populations that are more likely to qualify for Medicaid early in the course of the disease. The second is a possible erosion in private insurance coverage.

The HIV disease is now spreading more rapidly among IV drug users and their sexual partners, and less rapidly among gay and bisexual men. This means that an increasing proportion of AIDS cases will be among the low-income persons who are least likely to have other insurance coverage and most likely to qualify for Medicaid. The shift in risk factors is accompanied by a shift in demographic characteristics. HIV infection is increasingly a problem of minorities and women. CDC estimates that new AIDS cases among blacks and Hispanics will grow 30 to 40 percent faster than among whites in the 5 years ended 1993, while cases among women will grow 30 percent faster than among men.

This shift is significant, because of the strong relationship between demographic characteristics and the likelihood that a person with AIDS will qualify for Medicaid. Table I-3 shows the sources of third-party payment for AIDS hospitalizations in greater New York in 1985. Black and Hispanic men were much more likely to rely on Medicaid than were white men, and much less likely to have Blue Cross or commercial insurance. The pattern was even more pronounced for women with AIDS. (The study did not categorize women by race. However, three out of four women with AIDS are black or Hispanic.)

[12]Ellwood, Marilyn Rymer, Thomas R. Fanning, and Suzanne Dodds. *Medicaid Eligibility Patterns for Persons with AIDS: California and New York, 1983-1987.* Lexington, MA, SysteMetrics/McGraw-Hill, 1991. Prepared for Office of Research, Health Care Financing Administration. Ribicoff children meet the financial standards for AFDC but not the categorical standards. They may include children in foster care, in two-parent families, or in other settings.

[13]Solomon, David J., et al. Analysis of Michigan Medicaid Costs to Treat HIV Infection. *Public Health Reports*, v. 104, no. 5, Sept.-Oct. 1989. p. 416-424.

**TABLE I-3. Source of Payment for AIDS Hospitalizations
in Greater New York by Race, 1985**

	Blue Cross	Commercial insurance	Medicaid	Self-pay	Other
White male	49.6%	16.1%	23.0%	7.4%	3.8%
Black male	19.5	3.9	52.5	15.6	8.4
Hispanic male	17.7	4.5	56.9	11.9	9.0
Other male	30.9	9.6	45.9	7.3	6.2
Female	15.5	1.9	70.2	9.4	3.0
Total	30.9%	8.8%	43.9%	10.5%	5.9%

Source: Table prepared by the Congressional Research Service based on analysis of data from Ball, Judy K., Joyce V. Kelly, and Barbara J. Turner. Third-Party Financing for AIDS Hospitalizations in New York. *AIDS and Public Policy Journal*, v. 5, spring 1990. p. 51-58.

The shift in AIDS case load towards low-income women and minorities who are more likely to qualify for Medicaid before becoming disabled may also mean that Medicaid will pay a greater share of the lifetime costs for each individual. As was noted above, Medicaid's share of total AIDS expenditures is believed to have been less than its share of the AIDS patient population, in part because many persons have qualified for Medicaid after being diagnosed and after having incurred medical expenses paid for by some other carrier. If more patients qualify for Medicaid prior to the onset of the disease or very rapidly thereafter, Medicaid will be covering these patients' costs for the entire course of the illness. The demographic shift in the AIDS population could thus mean, not only that Medicaid will cover a larger portion of the population, but also that Medicaid expenditures for each patient covered will increase.

Even the groups that have in the past been more likely to rely on private insurance coverage may become increasingly dependent on Medicaid. Many private insurers have attempted to limit their potential risk for HIV-related claims. A 1987 Office of Technology Assessment survey of commercial insurers, Blue Cross/Blue Shield plans, and health maintenance organizations found that a majority of all three types of insurers were screening out or restricting coverage for persons with HIV infection who applied for individual health insurance coverage.[14] These policies would not generally affect persons obtaining coverage through their employment; ordinarily, all members of an employer group are automatically eligible for the employer's health benefit program. However, some employers may choose to restrict benefits for specific diseases or conditions. The Supreme Court has let stand a lower court ruling

[14]U.S. Congress. Office of Technology Assessment. *AIDS and health insurance: An OTA survey.* Washington, GPO, 1988. p. 3.

that Federal law does not prohibit a self-insured employer health plan from limiting coverage for HIV disease.[15] In addition, persons obliged to give up working as their disability progresses may lose coverage as well. This problem may have been alleviated to some extent by the continuation coverage provisions of the Consolidated Omnibus Budget Reconciliation Act of 1985 (COBRA, P.L. 99-272), which are discussed below.[16]

While the demographic shift and possible erosion of private coverage suggest a growing role for Medicaid in HIV funding, one offsetting factor could work to restrict Medicaid coverage. As the HIV epidemic shifts from its original epicenters in New York and California, the greatest growth in case load may occur in States with more restrictive Medicaid eligibility and coverage policies. The surveys of public and teaching hospitals cited earlier found significant regional variation in the percentages of persons with AIDS covered by Medicaid. In the Northeast, 54 percent of AIDS patients treated in 1987 were Medicaid-eligible at the time of admission, while 11 percent were classified as "self-pay" or "other," usually indicating a lack of coverage. The situation was reversed in the South. Hospitals there reported that Medicaid covered only 18 percent of all AIDS admissions, while 69 percent were self-pay/other. The authors suggest that the major reason for the disparity is that Medicaid programs in many southern States have more restrictive eligibility standards than those elsewhere; they are, for example, least likely to offer medically needy coverage.

Shifts in the nature of the population with HIV disease may, then, lead to increases in the number of uninsured patients, as well as in the number with Medicaid. In addition, it should again be emphasized that nearly all of the available data reflect eligibility patterns for persons already diagnosed as having AIDS, and not the larger population with HIV infection. As has been suggested, there are barriers to Medicaid coverage for the non-AIDS HIV population, and rates of uninsurance may be even higher among this group. Services for the uninsured are a major focus of the HIV grant programs established by the Ryan White Comprehensive AIDS Resources Emergency Act of 1990 (P.L. 101-381).[17]

---

[15] *McGann vs. H & H Music Co.*, 742 F.Supp. 392 (1990); affirmed CA-5, 1992; Supreme Court declined review Nov. 9, 1992.

[16]One study has documented the loss of private health insurance, most often because of loss of employment, as HIV-positive individuals progress to AIDS. Kass, Nancy E., et al. Loss of Private Health Insurance Among Homosexual Men with AIDS. *Inquiry*, v. 28, fall 1991. p. 249-254. The study was conducted in 1987-1988 and may not reflect the full impact of the COBRA continuation provisions.

[17]The Act authorizes emergency grants to cities with a high caseload or incidence of AIDS for health care delivery programs; providers under these programs are expected to obtain Medicaid reimbursement for eligible persons before turning to grant funds. The Act also authorizes formula grants to States for a variety of HIV-related programs, one of which is treatment of low-income persons.

In summary, it seems likely that Medicaid's share of overall HIV-related spending is rising, although the full extent of this shift is still uncertain. Even if Medicaid's share of spending were to stay constant, actual outlays will rise as the number of affected persons grows. One recent estimate projected that AIDS-related Medicaid spending would reach $2.9 billion in 1992 and $3.7 billion in 1993.[18] These projections, considerably higher than the HCFA estimate cited earlier, do not include any spending for non-AIDS HIV disease. Even without these additional HIV-related costs, the 1993 figure would be nearly 3 percent of total projected Medicaid spending for that year.

Whatever the impact of HIV on Medicaid costs, it will be felt disproportionately in a few States. While the case load is beginning to grow in other areas, over the short term the HIV population will continue to be concentrated in the original centers of infection. Five States--New York, California, Florida, Texas, and New Jersey--accounted for 61 percent of all AIDS cases reported through June 1992.[19] Because of different Medicaid eligibility policies and different characteristics of the AIDS population in different areas, coverage rates in these States are likely to vary considerably. For example, Florida does not expect AIDS to account for more than 4 percent of total Medicaid spending in the near future, about the national average.[20] Spending in New York or New Jersey, on the other hand, could be much higher than average. A potential result could be increasing pressure to curtail services to other kinds of Medicaid beneficiaries.

IV. RECENT LEGISLATIVE INITIATIVES

The OBRA 90 added a new option that may assist persons with HIV disease in some States. States may now pay premiums for continuation of private insurance coverage for persons entitled to such benefits under COBRA. OBRA 90 also authorized a two-State demonstration of Medicaid coverage for early intervention services for HIV-infected persons; however, no State applied to participate.

---

[18]U.S. Congress. House. Committee on Energy and Commerce. Subcommittee on Health and the Environment. *AIDS Issues (Part 3)*. Hearings, Serial No. 101-162, 101st Cong., 2d Sess., Feb. 27, 1990. Testimony of Kenneth E. Thorpe. Washington, GPO, 1990. p. 99.

[19]The next five States, Illinois, Georgia, Pennsylvania, Massachusetts, and Maryland, along with Puerto Rico, accounted for another 16 percent of total cases.

[20]Clarke, Gary J. In his AIDS and the Medicaid Program: A View from the States. *Proceedings: AIDS Prevention and Services Workshop, February 15-16, 1990*. Princeton, Robert Wood Johnson Foundation, 1990. p. 167-70.

A. Continuation of Employer Group Coverage

The COBRA provided that an employer with 20 or more employees that offered a group health plan must offer employees the opportunity to continue coverage under that plan after certain "qualifying events," such as termination of employment or divorce from a covered employee, that would ordinarily end the coverage. For most qualifying events, coverage can continue for 18 months, with the employee responsible for the premium (up to 102 percent of the premium otherwise applicable). OBRA 89 (P.L. 101-239) allowed an extension of coverage up to 29 months for persons with a disability at the time they terminated employment. For months after the 18th month, the employee's maximum premium is 150 percent of the premium otherwise applicable. The 29-month extension of benefits is designed to carry beneficiaries through the sequential waiting periods for Social Security disability benefits (5 months after the onset of disability) and the waiting period for Medicare for the disabled (24 months after qualifying for Social Security).

The COBRA continuation coverage is thus designed to bridge the gap for a disabled person between the end of employment and eligibility for Medicare. However, not everyone eligible for the coverage can afford to pay the premiums, because income may drop sharply after the end of employment. As a result, some disabled persons might let the coverage lapse and qualify for Medicaid after incurring large medical bills. Some States concluded that it might be cost-effective to assist with COBRA premium payments and thus delay Medicaid eligibility. By the end of 1990, eight States had developed programs to pay for continuation coverage for persons with HIV disease: California, Colorado, Connecticut, Maryland, Michigan, Minnesota, Texas, and Wisconsin.[21] However, Federal Medicaid funds were not available for these programs, because they paid premiums on behalf of persons who did not necessarily meet the financial and other standards for Medicaid eligibility.[22]

The OBRA 90 allows a State Medicaid program the option of paying COBRA continuation premiums for individuals who are eligible for COBRA coverage, whose family income is no more than 100 percent of the Federal poverty level, and whose resources are no more than twice the limit applicable for SSI in the State. (Individuals need not meet the categorical tests for Medicaid eligibility, such as family status or disability.) The State must determine that payment of COBRA premiums would be cost-effective; that is, that resulting savings in direct Medicaid service costs are likely to exceed the cost of the premiums. In addition, premiums may be paid only on behalf of persons whose former employers have 75 or more employees. Note that the option is not restricted, as the State-funded programs were, to persons with HIV disease. Possibly for this reason, none of the States with existing programs for

---

[21]Unpublished data, AIDS Policy Center, Intergovernmental Health Policy Project, George Washington University.

[22]State Medicaid programs have always been permitted to pay health insurance premiums on behalf of beneficiaries who meet Medicaid eligibility standards.

persons with HIV disease appears to have adopted the OBRA 90 option. According to HCFA, only two States, Montana and Washington, were making use of the option as of March 1992.

B. Early Intervention Demonstrations

As noted earlier, restrictive disability criteria may mean that some HIV-infected persons are ineligible for assistance with early treatment for HIV disease but qualify for Medicaid as their illness progresses to clinical AIDS. Some people have suggested that it might be more appropriate for Medicaid to pay for early treatment and thus perhaps prevent or delay more serious problems later. OBRA 90 required the Secretary to provide for two State demonstration projects to test this concept.

Each demonstration was to provide Medicaid coverage to HIV-positive persons who met the State's financial standards for eligibility for the disabled but who did not necessarily meet the disability criteria. Enrollment in each project would have been limited to 200 persons, and each project would have been required to establish a control group of uninsured HIV-infected persons who would not be given early coverage (but who might become Medicaid-eligible later in the course of their illness). The aim of the demonstrations was to evaluate whether early intervention for the program participants was less costly than providing treatment at later stages of the disease.

Although HCFA in 1991 issued a request for proposals from States wishing to participate in the demonstration, no State applied. HCFA is now attempting to assess why no States were interested. (One possibility advanced by HCFA officials is that States were concerned about the control group requirement, which would have meant giving some people access to early intervention and denying it to others.)

V. MEDICAID COVERAGE AND REIMBURSEMENT OF SERVICES FOR HIV DISEASE

Persons infected with the HIV virus have widely varying service needs, depending on how far the disease has progressed and how it has manifested itself. Those with asymptomatic HIV infection require monitoring and counseling and may benefit from early interventions that can slow deterioration of the immune system or prevent opportunistic infections. Those whose disease has progressed further may still benefit from the many treatments for specific opportunistic infections that have been developed in recent years. The most severely ill may be only intermittently in need of the level of treatment provided by inpatient hospitals; the rest of the time they could remain at home if they had access to adequate home health care and support services. Those in the final stages of the disease could benefit from hospice care. Finally, some patients, particularly those with central nervous system problems and resulting dementia, may require care at the nursing home level. The effects of Medicaid coverage and reimbursement policies on the care of individual HIV patients may vary, depending on those patients' particular needs.

Patients requiring acute care services, such as those of hospitals and physicians, may encounter limitations on access comparable to those faced by other beneficiaries. In some States, Medicaid coverage of inpatient services is limited to a fixed number of days per patient. In others, payment is made at fixed rates, regardless of costs. Many hospitals have reported that Medicaid reimbursement is inadequate to meet the high costs they incur in treating AIDS patients. Some facilities may respond by referring persons with AIDS to public or teaching hospitals which are prepared to accept Medicaid reimbursement. Low payment levels may also affect access to other kinds of services, such as nursing home and hospice care.

In addition, there are some services that State Medicaid programs may not cover at all. While all States must offer some form of home health care, coverage may be limited and may not include the highly intensive nursing care required by some AIDS patients or the personal care services required by others. While States might consider adding additional services to meet the needs of persons with AIDS, they may be prevented from doing so by a general Medicaid rule against discrimination by diagnosis. Services provided to beneficiaries must be uniform; new services usually cannot be added just for persons with a particular condition (two exceptions, the "2176" waiver program and the targeted case management option, are discussed below).

Nevertheless, some States have begun to explore ways to improve access to existing services for persons with AIDS or to develop new services, and Congress has taken some steps to assist them. The following is a discussion of some of the more important issues relating to specific services.

A. Home and Community Care

Although there has been some change in recent years, much of the treatment for persons with AIDS occurs in inpatient hospital settings. This is not only costly, but could eventually strain the physical capacity of hospitals in the localities most heavily affected. The alternative to expanding hospital capacity is to find ways of treating more persons with AIDS in other settings. Many localities have sought to develop comprehensive care systems, combining acute AIDS treatment units with community support services. San Francisco's system, coordinating a specialized inpatient treatment center with a network of outpatient and community services, has served as a model for many of these programs and is reported to have reduced average per patient costs while at the same time providing more humane care.[23] Both the Public Health Service and private sources have supported efforts to develop similar systems elsewhere, and further support is provided in the Ryan White AIDS care act.

Medicaid programs ordinarily may not reimburse for the nonmedical social and support services that are an integral part of these systems. In addition, although home health care is a mandatory Medicaid benefit, many States offer

---

[23]Scitovsky, Anne A., Mary Cline, and Philip R. Lee. Medical Care Costs of Patients with AIDS in San Francisco. *Journal of the American Medical Association*, v. 256, no. 22, Dec. 12, 1986. p. 3103-3106.

only limited home health services. They may not cover the intensive services some persons with AIDS may need if they are to remain in the community, such as parenteral (intravenous) nutrition. Again, these coverage policies usually cannot be modified in order to help persons with a particular diagnosis.

A State may obtain an exception to these rules, with the approval of HCFA, through a waiver for the provision of home and community-based services. Under a waiver, the State may offer a special package of services to a defined population as an alternative to institutional care. The package may include expanded home health care, case management, and other services needed to help chronically ill beneficiaries remain in community settings. These waivers, known as section 2176 waivers after the provision of the Omnibus Budget Reconciliation Act of 1981 (OBRA 81, Public Law 97-35) that created them, are discussed more fully in *Chapter VI, Alternate Delivery Options and Waiver Programs*.

The COBRA made technical changes in the waiver authority to make it easier for States to develop programs for persons with AIDS. The changes clarified that a State could establish a waiver program for persons at risk for hospital care; prior to the changes, a program could serve only persons at risk of needing nursing home services. As of January 1991, 13 States had developed section 2176 waiver programs targeted specifically at persons with HIV disease: California, Colorado, Florida, Hawaii, Illinois, Iowa, Missouri, New Jersey, New Mexico, Ohio, Pennsylvania, South Carolina, and Washington. (Some other States may be serving persons with AIDS under waiver programs targeted at more general populations of the physically disabled.) In addition, four States, Delaware, Illinois, North Carolina, and Virginia, have made use of the "model waiver" option, an expedited waiver process for limited groups of disabled children.

A 1989 study of the HIV waiver programs then in operation found that, while services offered varied widely, the most common were case management, personal and homemaker care, adult day care, private duty nursing, and home-delivered meals. Four programs also had special support services targeted to children in foster care. The study also found that States generally saw the 2176 waiver option as a way of broadening the array of available services, and not necessarily a way of saving money. The authors question whether savings can in fact be achieved through home and community-based services for HIV patients. While the San Francisco program apparently saved money, it relied heavily on volunteer services; similar savings might not be achieved if the same services have to be paid for.[24]

Under another option added by COBRA, States may offer case management services to special populations without a waiver. This "targeted" case management option allows a State to improve the coordination of available medical and social services for members of the target group. Unlike the 2176

[24]Jacobson, Peter D., Phoebe A. Lindsey, and Anthony H. Pascal. *AIDS-Specific Home and Community-Based Waivers for the Medicaid Population*. The RAND Corporation, Dec. 1989. [R-3844-HCFA]

waiver option, however, the case management option does not allow the State to cover more services for the target group than for other Medicaid beneficiaries. At least five States (Alabama, Maine, Maryland, Pennsylvania, and Washington) have established case management services specifically targeted at persons with HIV disease.[25] As in the case of section 2176 waivers, some States may be covering persons with AIDS under more general case management programs for the disabled.

B. Hospice and Nursing Home Care

1. Hospice

The COBRA authorized States to cover hospice services as an optional Medicaid benefit. As *Chapter IV, Services* indicates, 32 States had elected to cover hospice services as of October 1990.

Hospices are programs that provide "palliative treatment," care intended to comfort rather than cure, to terminally ill patients. Although some hospices maintain their own facilities, most hospices provide care to patients in their own homes. Under Medicare and Medicaid rules, a hospice is not a facility but a coordinated system for providing intensive home health care, counseling, and related services. Patients are expected to spend most of their time at home, usually with a family member or friend as a routine care-giver. Reimbursement for hospice services furnished on an inpatient basis is strictly limited, and the hospice may be financially penalized if patients are treated on an inpatient basis more than 20 percent of the time. The effect of this rule has been to limit the usefulness of the hospice option as an alternative to hospital care for persons who have AIDS and who are without a stable living situation. The Omnibus Budget Reconciliation Act of 1987 (OBRA 87, Public Law 100-203), permits waivers of the inpatient care limitations for Medicaid hospice patients with AIDS. OBRA 90 further expands Medicaid hospice coverage by eliminating an overall 210-day limit on hospice care to any individual. Care may now continue beyond this limit if the patient is still determined to be terminally ill.

One other possible problem in access to hospice care may be low reimbursement rates. The Omnibus Budget Reconciliation Act of 1989 (P.L. 101-239) included enhanced daily reimbursement rates for hospices under Medicare and Medicaid and provided for regular updates in the future. However, most States require hospices to cover the cost of prescription drugs as part of the all-inclusive daily rate. Because drugs for AIDS can be especially costly, some hospices are reporting that a daily rate which is adequate for other kinds of patients is too low for patients with AIDS.

2. Nursing Home

Persons with AIDS requiring the level of services provided by nursing homes have faced continuing problems in obtaining access to care. Some facilities are afraid of potential infection, or may even be forbidden by State law

---

[25]National Governors' Association. Unpublished survey data, Dec. 1990.

to accept patients with infectious diseases. Others may argue that they are simply not equipped to deal with the special needs of some persons with AIDS, particularly those suffering from mental illness or those addicted to drugs. One State, Minnesota, has taken legal action to compel nursing homes to accept persons with AIDS. On a national basis, however, the number of nursing homes accepting AIDS patients remains very small.

The access barriers faced by persons with AIDS may be compounded if they have no financial resources of their own. As *Appendix H, Medicaid as Health Insurance: Measures of Performance* indicates, facilities in areas with high nursing home occupancy rates may have incentives to adopt preferential admission policies. They may accept private pay patients before Medicaid patients and, when they accept Medicaid patients, select those requiring the least intensive services. One solution to this problem, adopted by 12 States as of 1989, is to vary Medicaid payment according to the "case mix" at a particular facility. Facilities receive higher reimbursement if they treat patients requiring more intensive care. At least seven States have attempted to improve nursing home access by offering higher Medicaid reimbursement specifically for AIDS patients.[26]

C. Prescription Drugs

While there is still no prospect of a "cure" for HIV disease in the near future, there has been considerable progress in developing therapeutics that can slow the effects of the virus on the immune system, can prevent the occurrence of certain opportunistic infections, or can be used to treat those infections when they appear. The most widely publicized treatment directed at the virus itself, AZT (azidothymidine or Retrovir), was approved for therapeutic use by the FDA in early 1987. Alternatives now in use include DDI (dideoxyinosine) and DDC (dideoxycytidine). Widely used treatments or preventives for specific opportunistic diseases include aerosolized pentamadine for pneumocystis pneumonia (PCP) and ganciclovir for cytomegalovirus infection.

Many of these treatments are useful for patients who have not yet progressed to AIDS. As was noted earlier, however, access to these treatments may be limited by problems in establishing Medicaid eligibility for these patients. One response has been the authorization of the Medicaid early intervention demonstrations cited earlier. In addition, since shortly after the approval of AZT, Congress has provided limited grants to States to provide HIV drugs to non-Medicaid low-income patients. The Ryan White AIDS care act authorizes further such grants, and FY 1991 Department of Health and Human Services (DHHS) appropriations include $45 million in non-Medicaid funding for drugs and other early interventions in HIV-related illness.

---

[26]Unpublished data, Intergovernmental Health Policy Project, George Washington University, June 1990. Simply to pay higher rates for persons with AIDS would potentially conflict with the general Medicaid prohibition against discrimination by diagnosis. Instead, the States have defined new provider types or new types of specialized services for persons with AIDS and have established separate payment rates for those providers or services.

Even patients who have qualified for Medicaid benefits may face additional barriers because of varying State policies on coverage of experimental therapies or new drugs. Medicaid programs, like Medicare and other health insurers, will generally cover only therapies which are already proven effective and which have been approved by FDA. In the past there was a relatively clear distinction between these approved drugs and drugs still under investigation, which were usually available only to participants in clinical trials and were paid for by the researchers. Partly in response to pressures from persons with HIV disease, FDA has recently developed procedures under which patients who are not participating in clinical trials can obtain promising new drugs before the drugs have received full FDA approval. Investigational new drugs (INDs) may be made available to patients with a serious or life-threatening disease for which no satisfactory alternative treatment exists. Unlike participants in clinical trials, who ordinarily do not pay, patients receiving drugs under a "treatment IND" may be charged the costs of the drugs.[27] Because the drugs are not approved, however, most Medicaid programs (like most other insurers) will not assist with these costs. As a result, Medicaid beneficiaries may not have early access to these treatments or may have to pay for them on their own.

Many States have restricted coverage even of drugs that have received FDA approval. As of July 1990, 19 States had restrictive "formularies," limited lists of drugs they will cover, which may not include every drug approved for clinical use by FDA. Some of these States require applications and lengthy approval processes before adding new drugs to their formularies. In addition, State Medicaid programs may approve the use of a drug only for certain classes of patients. For example, AZT was originally tested on patients who had already had an episode of PCP pneumonia and was formally approved by FDA for treatment of such patients. Although physicians commonly prescribed the drug for other HIV-infected patients, some States would not cover this "off-label" use. (Off-label use is prescription of a drug for a medical indication other than those specifically approved by FDA and hence appearing on the drug's packaging information.)

As is discussed in *Chapter V, Reimbursement*, OBRA 90 requires States to include in their formularies nearly all the approved drugs manufactured by a pharmaceutical company that has entered into a Medicaid rebate agreement with DHHS (there are exceptions for certain types of drugs, such as those for weight loss or infertility and abusable drugs). States may require preauthorization before a drug is dispensed, but may not exclude it entirely; preauthorization requirements may not apply to new drugs for the first 6 months after FDA approval. In addition, off-label use of an approved drug must be covered if the use is supported by peer-reviewed medical literature or is accepted by one or more of specified standard drug references. These changes are likely to provide more rapid access to new treatments once they win FDA approval, but will not affect access to drugs in the investigational stage.

---

[27] For further information, see U.S. Library of Congress. Congressional Research Service. *Drug Approval: Expediting Access to Drugs for Severely Ill Patients*. Issue Brief No. IB90016, by Blanchard Randall IV, Jan. 24, 1991 (Archived). Washington, 1991.

D. Special Problems of Children

As of October 1992, 4,051 cases of AIDS in children under 13 had been reported to the CDC. In 86 percent of the cases, the child apparently contracted the disease from an infected mother; CDC estimates that 30 percent of children born to infected mothers will also be HIV-infected. The course of the disease is different in children than in adults. They suffer from different types of opportunistic infections, and fewer treatments have been developed.[28] The 1987 U.S. hospital AIDS survey found that children with AIDS are more likely to be hospitalized than adults over the course of a year and are likely to stay in the hospital longer.[29] Little is known about the health care costs incurred by children with HIV disease. As was suggested earlier, however, children may be more likely to qualify for Medicaid early in the course of the disease. A study of pediatric AIDS-related discharges in 1986-1987 found that 57.1 of pediatric cases were covered for by Medicaid, compared to 27.2 percent of adult AIDS-related cases in the same hospitals.[30]

Hospitals and social services agencies have consistently reported problems with children who have AIDS or are HIV-infected and who are abandoned by their mothers, or whose mothers are themselves too sick to care for their children. The children sometimes must remain in the hospital, even though they do not require acute care, because no alternative placement can be found. Potential foster parents may be reluctant to accept these children, and there may be concerns about placing possibly infected infants with other children in group homes or shelters. As a result there have been cases in which children have spent their entire lives in hospitals, often at enormous cost. These so-called "boarder babies" include, not only children born with HIV infection, but also children who are addicted to drugs at birth because their mothers used drugs during pregnancy.

The Medicare Catastrophic Coverage Act of 1988 (Public Law 100-360) established a new home and community-based services waiver program under Medicaid, similar to the section 2176 waivers described earlier but specifically targeted at boarder babies. States could develop special support programs for children up to age 5 who are HIV-infected or addicted to drugs at birth, or who

[28]U.S. General Accounting Office. *Pediatric AIDS: Health and Social Service Needs of Infants and Children.* Report to the Chairman, Committee on Finance, U.S. Senate. GAO/HRD-89-96, May 1989. Washington, 1989.

[29]U.S. Congress. House. Committee on the Budget. Task Force on Human Resources. *Pediatric AIDS.* Hearings, Serial No. 5-7, 101st Cong., 2d Sess., Mar. 13, 1990. Testimony of Christine Sarrico, on behalf of National Association of Children's Hospital and Related Institutions. Washington, GPO, 1990.

[30]Ball, Judy K., and Susan Thaul. *Pediatric AIDS-Related Discharges in a Sample of U.S. Hospitals: Demographics, Diagnoses, and Resource Use.* Agency for Health Care Policy and Research Provider Studies Research Note 16, Feb. 1992.

have developed AIDS after birth. However, no State has ever applied for a waiver under this option. As was noted earlier, some States have used the existing section 2176 option (including model waivers) to provide special services for HIV-infected children. Several of these programs include support services targeted specifically at children in foster care.

ADDENDUM I

INDEX TO THE MEDICAID STATUTE

Many have remarked on the complexity of the Medicaid statute, which is found in Title XIX of the Social Security Act. In Schweiker v. Gray Panthers, 453 U.S. 34, 43 (1981), the U.S. Supreme Court, per Mr. Justice Powell, observed that "The Social Security Act is among the most intricate drafted by Congress. Its Byzantine construction, as Judge Friendly has observed, makes the Act almost unintelligible to the uninitiated."

The statutory changes that have occurred in the eleven years since Mr. Justice Powell's observation have made Title XIX even more complex, so that even the initiated have difficulty locating provisions. The purpose of this index is to make the statute more accessible to the initiated and the uninitiated alike.

This index was prepared in November, 1992. At that time, a number of technical corrections to Title XIX were pending. These amendments were designed to correct errors resulting from the enactment of the Omnibus Budget Reconciliation Act (OBRA) of 1990, P.L. 101-508. The index was compiled on the basis of the uncorrected version of Title XIX. If the pending technical corrections are adopted, a number of the references in this index may change.

The citations in this index are to the Social Security Act itself. For those using the United States Code, there is a conversion table at the conclusion of the index.

This Addendum was assembled by the majority staff of the Subcommittee on Health and the Environment and does not represent the work product of the Congressional Research Service. The Subcommittee gratefully acknowledges the assistance of Edward G. Grossman and Noah L. Wofsy of the House Office of Legislative Counsel; the staff of the Health Care Financing Division of the Office of General Counsel; and Sara Rosenbaum, Senior Staff Scientist, George Washington University Center for Health Policy Research.

INDEX TO MEDICAID STATUTE AND RELATED LAWS

Term	Social Security Act Section
Advance Directive.................	1902(a)(57),(58); 1902(w); 1919(c)(2)(E)
AFDC Maintenance of Effort.........	1902(c); 1903(i)(9)
Agreements........................	See Buy-in; Prescription Drugs
AIDS (Acquired Immune Deficiency Syndrome):	
Boarder Babies...................	1915(e)
COBRA Continuation Coverage......	1906
Demonstration Project for HIV-Positive Individuals........	Section 4747 of OBRA 90 (P.L. 101-508)
Home and Community-Based Care.....	1915(c)
Hospice..........................	1905(o)(1)(B)
Targeted Case Management.........	1905(a)(19); 1915(g)(2)
Alcoholism and Drug Dependency Treatment.......................	last sentence of 1905(a)
Aliens............................	1137(d); see Illegal Aliens

(1115)

Social Security Act Section	U.S.Code Section
1901	42 U.S.C. 1396
1902	42 U.S.C. 1396a
1903	42 U.S.C. 1396b
1904	42 U.S.C. 1396c
1905	42 U.S.C. 1396d
1906	42 U.S.C. 1396e
1907	42 U.S.C. 1396f
1910	42 U.S.C. 1396i
1911	42 U.S.C. 1396j
1912	42 U.S.C. 1396k
1913	42 U.S.C. 1396l
1914	42 U.S.C. 1396m
1915	42 U.S.C. 1396n
1916	42 U.S.C. 1396o
1917	42 U.S.C. 1396p
1918	42 U.S.C. 1396q
1919	42 U.S.C. 1396r
1920	42 U.S.C. 1396r-1
1921	42 U.S.C. 1396r-2
1922	42 U.S.C. 1396r-3
1923	42 U.S.C. 1396r-4
1924	42 U.S.C. 1396r-5
1925	42 U.S.C. 1396r-6
1926	42 U.S.C. 1396r-7
1927	42 U.S.C. 1396r-8
1928	42 U.S.C. 1396s
1929	42 U.S.C. 1396t
1930	42 U.S.C. 1396u

○